Medical Microbiology

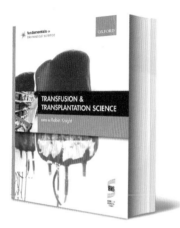

TRANSFUSION &
TRANSPLANTATION SCIENCE

edited by Robin Knight

BIOMEDICAL SCIENCE
PRACTICE

EXPERIMENTAL & PROFESSIONAL SKILLS

*edited by Hedley Glencross, Nessar Ahmed,
Chris Smith & Qiuyu Wang*

CYTOPATHOLOGY

edited by Behdad Shambayati

CLINICAL BIOCHEMISTRY

edited by Nessar Ahmed

IMMUNOLOGY

edited by Angela Hall & Christine Yates

HAEMATOLOGY

*Andrew Blann, Gavin Knight,
& Gary Moore*

MEDICAL
MICROBIOLOGY

edited by Michael Ford

CELL STRUCTURE
& FUNCTION

edited by Guy Orchard & Brian Nation

HISTOPATHOLOGY

edited by Guy Orchard & Brian Nation

fundamentals OF
biomedical science

Medical Microbiology

Second edition

Edited by

Michael Ford
Microbiology Department, Freeman Hospital,
Newcastle Upon Tyne

OXFORD
UNIVERSITY PRESS

Great Clarendon Street, Oxford, OX2 6DP,
United Kingdom

Oxford University Press is a department of the University of Oxford.
It furthers the University's objective of excellence in research, scholarship,
and education by publishing worldwide. Oxford is a registered trade mark of
Oxford University Press in the UK and in certain other countries

First Edition published 2010

Impression: 2

Published in the United States of America by Oxford University Press
198 Madison Avenue, New York, NY 10016, United States of America

British Library Cataloguing in Publication Data
Data available

Library of Congress Control Number: 2013945733

ISBN 978-0-19-965513-7

Printed in Great Britain by
Bell & Bain Ltd, Glasgow

Contents

An introduction to the Fundamentals of Biomedical Science series

Biomedical scientists form the foundation of modern healthcare, from cancer screening to diagnosing HIV, from blood transfusion for surgery to infection control. Without biomedical scientists, the diagnosis of disease, the evaluation of the effectiveness of treatment, and research into the causes and cures of disease would not be possible. However, the path to becoming a biomedical scientist is a challenging one: trainees must not only assimilate knowledge from a range of disciplines, but must understand—and demonstrate—how to apply this knowledge in a practical, hands-on environment.

The *Fundamentals of Biomedical Science* series is written to reflect the challenges of biomedical science education and training today. It blends essential basic science with insights into laboratory practice to show how an understanding of the biology of disease is coupled to the analytical approaches that lead to diagnosis. Produced in collaboration with the Institute of Biomedical Science, the series provides coverage of the full range of disciplines to which a biomedical scientist may be exposed.

Learning from this series

The *Fundamentals of Biomedical Science* series draws on a range of learning features to help readers master both biomedical science theory, and biomedical science practice.

Case Studies illustrate how the biomedical science theory and practice presented throughout the series relate to situations that are likely to be encountered routinely in the biomedical science laboratory.

CASE STUDY 4.1 Multidrug-resistant or

A 70-year-old male admitted via the Emergency Department with symptoms of septicaemia has a blood culture and urine sample collected. After overnight incubation the positive blood culture showed Gram-negative bacilli. The positive bottle was subcultured to purity plates

1. What would you sus of the organism?
2. How would you conf you perform and wh

The organism was ident

Method boxes walk through the key protocols that the reader is likely to come across in the laboratory.

METHOD Catalase test

- Using a plastic loop, sample a single colony and rub this inoculum onto a glass sli The inoculum should be sufficiently large to be visible to the naked eye.
- Place a drop of 30% hydrogen peroxide onto a glass coverslip and place the cov slip onto the slide, exposing the bacterial inoculum to the hydrogen peroxide.

Health and Safety boxes raise awareness of key health and safety issues related to topics being discussed with which the reader should be familiar.

HEALTH & SAFETY

General requirements of Containment Level 3 are as follows.

Facilities:

1. Spacious, self-contained room.
2. Dedicated equipment.
3. Easily cleanable surfaces.
4. Negative air pressure.
5. Microbiological safety cabinet.

CLINICAL CORRELATION

Serious fungal infections

Most serious fungal infections occur in patients with some other underlying illness which redu immunity to infection. Common underlying conditions include AIDS, cytotoxic therapy malignancy, the use of steroid therapy, immunosuppression for transplantation, diabetes and lowing abdominal surgery.

Clinical Correlation boxes emphasize at a glance how the material sits in a clinical context.

Further features are used to help consolidate and extend students' understanding of the subject

Key Point

Most fungi exist in one of two forms – a yeast for Certain fungi are dimorphic, i.e. they can exist in form depending on environmental conditions.

Key points reinforce the key concepts that the reader should master as they work through each chapter, while **Summary** points act as an end-of-chapter checklist for readers to verify that they have remembered the principal themes and ideas presented within the chapter.

prozone

Prozone is the phenomenon exhibited by some sera, in which agglutination or precipitation occurs at higher dilution ranges, but is not visible at lower dilutions or when undiluted.

adding the enzyme conjugate by washing (see antibodies in the serum. The method is simple, not **prozone** in the presence of high titre antibo detecting low-affinity antibodies. If antibodies they block binding sites and prevent the hydrol This lack of colour change indicates a positive

Key terms in the margins provide instant definitions of terms with which the reader may not be familiar; in addition, each title in the series features a **glossary**, in which the key terms featured in that title are collated.

The role of cell culture in the diagnosis of viral infections is being increasingly challenged rapid diagnostic methods. Therefore, the role of cell culture is expected to decline and is lik to be restricted to large central reference laboratories.

SELF-CHECK 13.7

Why is cell culture still used when there are so many more rapid diagnostic meth available?

Self-check questions throughout each chapter provide the reader with a ready means of checking that they have understood the material they have just encountered; answers to self-check questions are presented at the end of each volume.

 Discussion questions

13.1   Discuss the provision of a diagnostic virology service to a district general hospital.

13.2   'There is no longer a need for diagnostic laboratories to attempt isolation of viruses tissue culture.' Comment on this statement.

13.3   What factors would you consider before selecting a commercially available diagnos assay?

Discussion questions are provided at the end of each chapter, to encourage the reader to analyse and reflect on the material they have just read. Hints and tips for answering the discussion questions are provided at the end of each book.

Cross reference

Antimicrobial susceptibility testing methods are discussed in Chapter 4.

• The patient's age.
• Pregnancy.
• Drug allergies, e.g. penicillin.
• Local factors, e.g. known circulation of resista

As with other infections, patients with an LRTI wi biotic, based on likely pathogens. Once the resu prescribed if appropriate.

Cross references help the reader to see biomedical science as a unified discipline, making connections between topics presented within each volume, and across all volumes in the series.

Online learning materials

Each title in the *Fundamentals of Biomedical Science* series is supported by an Online Resource Centre, which features additional materials for students, trainees, and lecturers.

www.oxfordtextbooks.co.uk/orc/fbs

online resource centre

Guides to key experimental skills and methods

Video walk-throughs of key experimental skills are provided to help you master the essential skills that are the foundation of biomedical science practice.

Biomedical science in practice

Interviews with practicing biomedical scientists working in a range of disciplines give a valuable insight into the reality of work in a biomedical science laboratory.

Virtual microscope

Visit the library of microscopic images and investigate them with the powerful online microscope, to help gain a deeper appreciation of cell and tissue morphology.

Lecturer support materials

The Online Resource Centre for each title in the series also features figures from the book in electronic format, for registered adopters to download for use in lecture presentations, and other educational resources.

To register as an adopter visit **www.oxfordtextbooks.co.uk/orc/fbs** and follow the on-screen instructions.

Any comments?

We welcome comments and feedback about any aspect of this series. Just visit www.oxfordtextbooks.co.uk/orc/fbs and share your views.

Contributors

Jenny Andrews
Clinical Scientist, City Hospital NHS Trust, Birmingham

Steve Davies
Microbiology Department, Northern General Hospital, Sheffield Teaching Hospitals Foundation Trust

Dr Lynn G. Dover
Head of Biomedical Sciences, School of Life Sciences, Northumbria University, Newcastle upon Tyne

Dr Michael Ford
Microbiology Department, Freeman Hospital, Newcastle Upon Tyne

Dr Clive Graham
Consultant Microbiologist, Microbiology Department, West Cumberland Hospital, Whitehaven, Cumbria

Jayne Harwood
Chief Biomedical Scientist, Serology Department, Freeman Hospital, The Newcastle Upon Tyne Hospitals NHS Foundation Trust

Louise Hill-King
Team Leader, Microbiology Department, Frimley Park Hospital, Camberley

Dr Malcolm Holliday
Laboratory Manager, Microbiology Department, Freeman Hospital, The Newcastle Upon Tyne Hospitals NHS Foundation Trust

Dr Derek Law
Head of Microbiology, Microbiology Department, F2G Ltd, Eccles, Manchester

Sheila Morgan
Nurse Consultant, Microbiology Department, Freeman Hospital, The Newcastle Upon Tyne Hospitals NHS Foundation Trust

Kathy Nye
Consultant Microbiologist, Health Protection Agency, West Midlands Regional HPA, Birmingham Heartlands Hospital, Birmingham

Dr John Perry
Clinical Scientist, Microbiology Department, Freeman Hospital, The Newcastle Upon Tyne Hospitals NHS Foundation Trust

Mark Tovey
Microbiology Department, Northern General Hospital, Sheffield Teaching Hospitals Foundation Trust

Dr Tony Worthington
Senior Lecturer in Clinical Microbiology, School of Life and Health Sciences, Aston University, Birmingham

Online materials developed by:

Dr Sarah Atchia
Senior Lecturer in Biomedical Sciences, Faculty of Life Sciences, London Metropolitan University

Dr Ian Hancock
Lecturer in Biomedical Sciences, Faculty of Human Sciences, London Metropolitan University

Sheelagh Heugh
Principal Lecturer Biomedical Sciences, Faculty of Human Sciences, London Metropolitan University

Dr Ken Hudson
Lecturer in Biomedical Sciences, Faculty of Human Sciences, London Metropolitan University

Dr Pamela McAthey
Academic Leader for Undergraduate Programmes, Faculty of Life Sciences, London Metropolitan University

Abbreviations

4-MeU	4-methylumbelliferone		CF	cystic fibrosis
7-AMC	7-amido-4-methylcoumarin		CFT	complement fixation test
AAFB	acid–alcohol-fast bacilli		CFTR	cystic fibrosis transmembrane conductance regulator
ABHG	alcohol-based hand gels		CFU	colony forming units
ABPA	allergic bronchopulmonary aspergillosis		cGMP	cyclic guanosine monophosphate
ACDP	Advisory Committee on Dangerous Pathogens		CLED	cysteine lactose electrolyte deficient
ACV	acyclovir		CLSI	Clinical Laboratory Standards Institute
ADH	arginine dihydrolyase		CMV	cytomegalovirus
ADPR	adenosine diphosphate		CNS	coagulase-negative *Staphylococcus*
ADPR	ADP-ribose		COSHH	Control of Substances Hazardous to Health
A/E	attaching and effacing		CPE	cytopathic effect
AFB	acid-fast bacilli		CRP	C-reactive protein
AIDS	acquired immune deficiency syndrome		CSF	cerebrospinal fluid
API	analytical profile index		CSU	catheter stream urine
ASO	antistreptolysin O		CT	computed tomography
ATCC	American Type Culture Collection		CV	coefficient of variation
ATP	adenosine triphosphate		CVA	cerebrovascular accident
AUC	area under curve		DAEC	diffusely adherent *E. coli*
AZT	azidothymidine		DAG	diacylglycerol
β-HS	β-haemolytic streptococci		dATP	deoxyadenosine triphosphate
BAL	bronchoalveolar lavage		DCA	deoxycholate citrate agar
Bcc	*Burkholderia cepacia* complex		DFA	direct fluorescent antibody
BCG	Bacille Calmette–Guérin		DGI	disseminated gonococcal infection
BCR	B-cell receptor		dGTP	deoxyguanosine triphosphate
BCYE	buffered charcoal yeast extract		DNA	deoxyribonucleic acid
bDNA	branched DNA		DNase	deoxyribonuclease
BEAV	bile esculin azide vancomycin		dNTP	deoxyribonucleotide triphosphate
BEB	bile esculin broth		DTT	dithiothreitol
BHI	brain heart infusion		dTTP	deoxythymidine triphosphate
BSAC	British Society for Antimicrobial Chemotherapy		EAEC	enteroaggregative *E. coli*
BV	bacterial vaginosis		EBV	Epstein–Barr virus
C390	9-chloro-9-(4-diethylaminophenyl)-10-phenylacridan		ECM	extracellular matrix
cAMP	cyclic adenosine monophosphate		EDTA	ethylenediaminetetraacetic acid
CAPD	continuous ambulatory peritoneal dialysis		EF-2	elongation factor 2
CAT	chloramphenicol acetyltransferase		EHEC	enterohaemorrhagic *E. coli*
cCTP	deoxycytidine triphosphate		EHO	Environmental Health Officer
CDC	Centers for Disease Control		EIA	enzyme immunoassay
CDC	cholesterol-dependent cytolysin		EIEC	enteroinvasive *E. coli*

ELISA	enzyme-linked immunosorbent assay
EM	electron microscopy
EPEC	enteropathogenic *E. coli*
EPS	exopolysaccharide
EPU	eyepiece units
ESBL	extended spectrum β-lactamase
ETEC	enterotoxigenic *E. coli*
E-Test	epsilometer test
EUCAST	European Committee on Antimicrobial Susceptibility Testing
FEC	formalin–ether concentration
FIC	fractional inhibitory concentration
FPIA	fluorescence polarization immunoassay
GAP	GTPase activating protein
GC	guanylate cyclase
GDI	guanine nucleotide dissociation inhibitor
GDP	guanosine diphosphate
GEF	guanine nucleotide exchange factor
GI	gastrointestinal
G6PD	glucose-6-phosphate dehydrogenase
GP	General Practitioner
GTP	guanosine triphosphate
GU	genitourinary
GUM	genitourinary medicine
HA	haemagglutination
HACEK	group of CO_2-dependent organisms – *Haemophilus* spp., *Aggregatibacter actinomycetemcomitans* (previously named *Actinobacillus*), *Cardiobacterium hominis*, *Eikenella corrodens*, and *Kingella* spp.
HAI	health-care-acquired infection
HAV	hepatitis A virus
HBV	hepatitis B virus
HCAI	health-care-acquired infection
HCV	hepatitis C virus
HEPA	high efficiency particulate absorption
Hib	*Haemophilus influenzae* type b
HIV	human immunodeficiency virus
HPLC	high-performance liquid chromatography
HPU	Health Protection Unit
HSV	herpes simplex virus
HVS	high vaginal swab
IA	invasive aspergillosis
IATA	International Air Transport Authority
ICU	Intensive Care Unit

IE	infective endocarditis
IFAT	indirect fluorescent antibody test
IgA	immunoglobulin A
IgG	immunoglobulin G
IgM	immunoglobulin M
I3P	inositol trisphosphate
INF	interferon
IL	interleukin
ISTB	Iso-Sensitest broth
IUCD	intrauterine contraceptive device
KES	*Klebsiella–Enterobacter–Serratia*
KOH	potassium hydroxide
LAP	leucyl aminopeptidase
LCR	ligase chain reaction
LD50	median lethal dose
LD50	median time to death
LEE	locus of enterocyte effacement
LJ	Löwenstein–Jensen
LOS	lipooligosaccharide
LRTI	lower respiratory tract infection
LV-PVA	low viscosity polyvinyl alcohol
MAC	*Mycobacterium avium* complex
MAC	membrane attack complex
MAMP	microbial associated molecular pattern
MAPK	mitogen-activated protein kinase
MBC	minimum bactericidal concentration
MDR	multidrug resistant
MHB	Mueller–Hinton broth
MHC	major histocompatibility complex
MIC	minimum inhibitory concentration
MICE	minimum inhibitory concentration evaluation
MIRU-VNTR	mycobacterial interspersed repetitive units variable number tandem repeats
MRSA	methicillin-resistant *Staphylococcus aureus*
MSA	mannitol salt agar
MSCRAMM	microbial surface components recognizing adhesive matrix molecules
MSU	midstream urine
MSM	men who have sex with men
MTB	*Mycobacterium tuberculosis*
NAAT	nucleic acid amplification test
NAC	N-acetyl-L-cysteine
NAD	nicotinamide adenine dinucleotide
NCTC	National Collection of Type Cultures

NEQAS	National External Quality Assurance Schemes		SDA	strand displacement amplification
NHS	National Health Service		SIC	streptococcal inhibitor of complement
NNT	number needed to treat		SM-ID	*Salmonella* identification
NOD	nucleotide oligomerization domain		SPA	suprapubic aspirate
NPA	nasopharyngeal aspirate		SPS	sodium polyethanol sulphonate
NSU	non-specific urethritis		STI	sexually transmitted infection
O129	2,4-diamino-6,7-diisopropylpteridine phosphate		SU	stage unit
			TAA	trimeric autotransporter adhesin
ONPG	*o*-nitrophenyl-β-d-galactopyranoside		TB	tuberculosis
PABA	*para*–aminobenzoic acid		TCBS	thiosulphate citrate bile salt sucrose agar
PBP	penicillin-binding protein		TCR	T-cell receptor
PCP	*Pneumocystis jirovecii* pneumonia		TLR	Toll-like receptor
PCR	polymerase chain reaction		TPHA	*Treponema pallidum* haemagglutination
PID	pelvic inflammatory disease		TPPA	*Treponema pallidum* particle agglutination
PIP2	phosphatidylinositol-4,5-biphosphate		T3SS	type III secretion system
PK	protein kinase		TSS	toxic shock syndrome
PMC	pseudomembranous colitis		TSST	toxic shock syndrome toxin
p-NA	*para*-nitroaniline		TST	tuberculin skin test
POC	products of conception		TV	*Trichomonas vaginalis*
PPE	personal protective equipment		UBA	urine bacterial analysis
PRR	pattern recognition receptor		UCP	urine collection pad
PUO	pyrexia of unknown origin		UPEC	uropathogenic *E. coli*
PVC	polyvinyl chloride		UTI	urinary tract infection
PVE	prosthetic valve endocarditis		UV	ultraviolet
PVL	Panton–Valentine leukocidin		VDRL	Venereal Disease Reference Laboratory
RAPD	random amplified polymorphic DNA		VHF	viral haemorrhagic fever
RBC	red blood cell		VP	Voges–Proskauer
RCA	regulators of complement activation		VRE	vancomycin-resistant *Enterococcus*
RFLP	amplified fragment length polymorphism		VTEC	verocytotoxin-producing *E. coli*
RNA	ribonucleic acid		VZV	varicella zoster virus
RPR	rapid plasma reagin		WBC	white blood cell
RSV	respiratory syncytial virus		WHO	World Health Organization
RT-PCR	real-time PCR		WD	washer disinfector
SAF	sodium acetate–acetic acid–formalin		XLD	xylose lysine deoxycholate
SAH	subarachnoid haemorrhage		ZN	Ziehl–Neelsen
SCBU	Special Care Baby Unit			

Introduction to microbiology

Michael Ford

There can't be many subjects that students study where on a frequent basis an article on the subject attracts high profile media attention. Almost all members of the general public will have heard of numerous species of bacteria and viruses contained within these chapters, as so many of them can impact dramatically upon people's lives. Most students will have already heard of many organisms described in this book from history lessons, including plague, anthrax, and cholera to name a few. Even those who have not studied biology will almost certainly be familiar with some viral pathogens such as HIV and will have some knowledge of the severity and consequences of *Clostridium difficile* and MRSA. This makes microbiology one of the most fascinating subjects to study, as microorganisms and their effects on all of us is clear and well documented.

Even though technology for the diagnosis of infectious disease has improved dramatically, and continues to improve, many of the techniques used every day in the diagnosis of infectious disease were used over 100 years ago. Microbiologists still use microscopes and read culture plates every day, and still use the basic colonial appearance of an organism to help identify it.

The principles and techniques used by some of the pioneers of microbiology, such as Louis Pasteur and Robert Koch, are still very evident today.

In this introduction, you will discover the basic properties of microorganisms such as growth characteristics, colonial and microscopic appearance, as well as principles of sterilization and disinfection. This will aid you when studying the other chapters in this book.

Learning objectives

After reading this chapter you should:

- Have a basic understanding of classification.
- Understand bacterial cell anatomy and key features.
- Understand principles of bacterial growth in liquid and on solid media.

■ Perform basic colony recognition.

■ Understand how and where microscopy is used and be able to identify certain cellular types.

■ Understand the basic principles of sterilization and disinfection.

1.1 Classification

All living things, including microorganisms are placed into a system of classification. This system highlights characteristics that are common among certain groups while giving order to the huge variety of microorganisms that exist on our planet. This science of classifying living things is known as taxonomy. For all organisms, a species is defined as a population of individuals that breed among themselves. For microorganisms, a species is defined as a group of organisms that have a similarity of greater than 70%.

In bacterial classification the numerous species which exist are grouped together to form a genus. For example, the Gram-negative species *Klebsiella pneumonia* and *Klebsiella oxytoca* are both contained within the genus *Klebsiella* as both organisms are highly similar. Whilst the colonies of both organisms are identical in culture they possess different traits, which warrant different species names. Various genera are then grouped as a family, and various families grouped further to form an order. Orders are then grouped together as a class, and several classes are then categorized as a single phylum or division. The various phyla or divisions are placed in the broadest classification – the kingdom.

By establishing a species, and then placing them together in broader classification categories, numerous characteristics are considered. These include cell morphology, cell structure, biochemical properties, and genetic characteristics.

1.1.1 Prokaryotes and eukaryotes

Microorganisms join all other living organisms in two major groups: prokaryotes and eukaryotes. Bacteria are prokaryotes (simple organisms having no nucleus or organelles) because of their cellular properties. Other microorganisms such as fungi, protozoa, and unicellular algae are eukaryotes (more complex organisms whose cells have a nucleus and organelles). Viruses are neither prokaryotes nor eukaryotes because of their simplicity and unique characteristics.

Cross reference
See Chapter 13.

1.2 The bacterial cell

Every living creature is made up of cells, and one of the simplest cellular forms is bacterial cells. Individual bacterial cells can only be seen down a microscope, in contrast to when they are growing as colonies on culture plates, where collectively they can be seen by the naked eye. Colonies on culture plates can only be seen following incubation (generally overnight) so each tiny bacterial cell has multiplied sufficiently into a huge number, all concentrated in the same place to be visible as a bacterial colony.

Bacterial cells have a **prokaryotic** type of cellular organization and exist as a single cell, that is until they start to divide, with a typical size of between 0.4 and 1.5 μm. Figure 1.1 shows the typical structure of a bacterial cell together with the main components. These are a rigid cell wall, flagella, fimbriae/pili, **ribosomes**, cytoplasmic membrane, nucleoid (circular DNA), and cytoplasm.

prokaryotic
An organism (bacteria and cyanobacteria) characterized by the lack of a distinct, membrane-bound nucleus or membrane-bound organelles. Also characterized by the fact that the DNA is not organized into chromosomes.

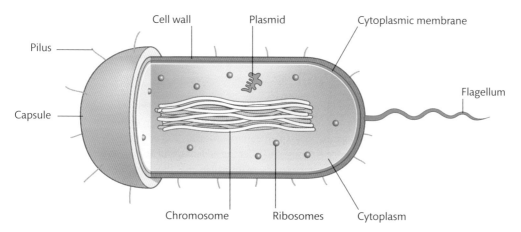

FIGURE 1.1
Diagram of a bacterial cell showing the cell wall and intracellular components.
Source: Courtesy of H. Ford

The rigid cell wall is there to hold the contents of the cell together, strengthened with a layer of **peptidoglycan**. This peptidoglycan layer is composed of N-acetylglucosamine and N-acetylmuramic acid linked together to form a strong chemical chain, which is cross linked for extra strength. It is important to note that the chemical structure of the bacterial cell wall differs considerably between Gram-positive and Gram-negative organisms. The cell wall is quite porous and is a physical barrier to the outside environment much like human skin, and is essential for the organism to survive and multiply. As you will see from later chapters, this part of the cell, especially the peptidoglycan component, is often a target for β-**lactam** antibiotics.

Underneath the cell wall is the cytoplasmic membrane which is an osmotic barrier and is responsible for maintaining the concentration differences between the inside and outside of the cell. It is supported in place and protected by the cell wall of the organism. The membrane is impermeable to both large and small solutes to help maintain this osmotic barrier. Nutrients are taken into the cell with the help of enzymes which facilitate the rapid transport of such nutrients. Water molecules can diffuse into the cell and waste products can diffuse out. Enzymes present in the cytoplasmic membrane facilitate a variety of key functions including chemical conversion into nutrients which are essential for both the cell wall and cell membrane.

The cytoplasm contains numerous **ribosomes** (around 72,000 in *Escherichia coli*) and itself is comprised of a watery jelly solution in which is dissolved a variety of organic and inorganic compounds. The cytoplasm is >80% water and, as well as containing structures such as ribosomes, it can contain energy stores. These include the metachromatic granules found in *Corynebacterium diphtheriae*.

On the outer parts of the cell are a variety of finger-like projections – these are flagella, fimbriae, and pili, and we will consider each one of these in turn.

1.2.1 Flagella

Not all bacteria possess flagella, only the ones which are motile and there may be several on a single bacterial cell. Their main roles are considered to be the ability to allow the cell to move quickly to new environments which have better or higher levels of nutrients. They also allow

peptidoglycan
A porous rigid layer composed of polysaccharide and protein. It is attached to lipoproteins in the outer membrane of the cell.

Cross reference
See Chapter 4.

ribosomes
Are found in both eukaryotic and prokaryotic cells. They are spherical-shaped structures contained within the cytoplasm of a cell. Each is composed of RNA and protein and is the site of protein synthesis.

the organism to move rapidly away from those areas depleted of nutrients or those where toxic substances exist. Migrating towards nutrients is known as **chemotaxis**.

1.2.2 Fimbriae/pili

Cross reference
See Chapter 15.

Cross reference
See Chapter 12.

These are generally more numerous across the cell than flagella and far shorter. These fimbriae are seen in both motile and non-motile cells and their main role is **adhesion**. On contact with a solid surface, including other cells (plant, animal, fungal), they will facilitate the cell to 'stick' or adhere to it. This adherence is thought to offer the advantage of holding the bacterium close to nutrient sources. The disadvantage to any mammalian cells they attach to is that the adhesion can be a major virulence factor in the disease process. This is because once the bacteria adhere to the surface of host cells they can subsequently initiate invasion, in addition some pathogenic bacteria secrete toxins, production of which can severely damage the host. Examples of this include the toxins of *Clostridium difficile* strains which cause pseudomembranous colitis.

1.2.3 Sex pili

These are involved in the attachment of bacteria to each other. Their main function is in the transfer of DNA from one bacterial species to another. This is one way in which genes coding for antibiotic resistance are transferred between bacterial species.

SELF-CHECK 1.1

What are the main differences between flagella, fimbriae, and pili?

Other important cellular components include spores and capsules that are not associated with all bacteria. Bacterial spores are most commonly found in *Clostridium* and *Bacillus* species and are a resting stage of the organism. When environmental conditions worsen, spore-forming organisms can survive in a dormant state for long periods of time and will germinate when conditions improve. They are often more resistant to killing by disinfectants than the vegetative cells they derive from. They are also very resistant to killing by heat. Using spores and demonstrating they are dead is one way of testing the efficiencies of heat sterilization devices such as autoclaves.

Capsules are found often in some of the most pathogenic organisms to humans including *Bacillus anthracis* (anthrax), *Streptococcus pneumoniae*, and *Neisseria meningitidis*. The bacterial cells are surrounded by a sticky gel which is mainly composed of water plus some carbohydrates/proteins. Their role is most likely to be protection of the cell from enzymes and **bacteriophages** which can quite easily kill the cell. However, when these organisms enter the host bloodstream they also protect against attack from the host immune response including phagocytes. This makes capsulate organisms often highly virulent to the host as they can survive an onslaught from host cells and continue to multiply.

a bacteriophage
A bacteriophage is a virus which is capable of penetrating a bacterial cell and causing its destruction by lysis.

1.3 **Bacterial growth**

This is a complex process but it is extremely important that these complexities are understood as the diagnosis of disease often depends upon growing the organisms in either solid or liquid media. This growth allows the organisms to reach a critical mass so that the laboratory scientist can examine them and use the information to determine the cause of an infection. Most bacteria will grow under a variety of conditions, but some have a very narrow growth spectrum and require either specific nutrients or atmospheric conditions in order to grow at all.

Bacterial growth in liquid media (Figure 1.2) is one of the most well-documented areas of microbiology. When bacteria are placed into an optimal nutritional and atmospheric environment they will begin to grow and divide. When inoculated into a liquid medium (broth), at first there is no cellular division, this is known as the **lag phase** whereby the cell is preparing to initiate growth and cell division. On the assumption that these optimal conditions remain constant, the next phase is exponential growth where the cells are dividing in the shortest timescale possible. During the **exponential phase**, the growth can be visible in a liquid medium as the number of cells rises dramatically. As the growth of the organism is so rapid, the nutrient levels in the medium start to deplete. In the exponential phase some Gram-negative organisms such as *E. coli* can divide in a few minutes. If these conditions are mimicked in the human body you can see how some organisms can produce a severe infection in a relatively short time. Eventually this exponential growth slows and the bacterial numbers reach their maximum as nutrients disappear. At this point the bacterial growth enters a **stationary phase**, if organisms were sampled during this phase they would all form colonies, known as colony forming units (CFU), on an agar plate as they are still alive. However, towards the end of this stationary phase, the organisms will begin to die and this will be shown if a sample of organisms is taken, as the number of CFU will be lower as the cells perish. This is known as the decline (or death) phase and eventually all of the organisms in the growth medium will die off.

In order to measure the number of bacteria in a particular population a variety of simple methods are available. The first of these is the plate count method whereby a known volume of the sample of bacteria is diluted, generally in saline or buffer. Known volumes of the sample dilutions are inoculated onto nutrient agar plates and incubated overnight. Following incubation, the numbers of colonies are counted per plate and the number multiplied by the dilution factor to give the number of CFU/mL. The reason for the dilutions is that it is impossible to count colonies by eye accurately if there are more than 200 CFU present. If the dilutions are optimal then one of them will reveal a plate where the number of colonies can be easily counted. Other methods include a direct microscopic count in a counting chamber. A known volume of bacterial suspension is added to the counting chamber and the number of organisms is counted. Multiplying by a reference figure will give an acute measure of the number of organisms present. The disadvantage of this method is that both live and dead bacteria are counted so it does not give the number of CFU.

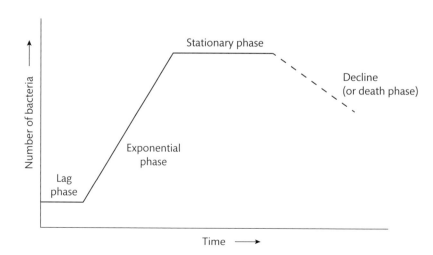

FIGURE 1.2

Growth curve of a bacterium growing in a nutrient-rich liquid medium. Note the various stages of growth over time.

Source: **Courtesy of D. Ford**

SELF-CHECK 1.2

What are the phases of growth in a liquid medium and what are the main differences?

Key Point

Bacterial cells will multiply at very different rates generally depending upon the composition of the media used and length of incubation. When examining bacterial colonies the biomedical scientist needs to consider all of the above in determining a provisional identification.

1.4 Sterilization and disinfection

It is important to understand the difference between these two terms as it is often confusing. Essentially **sterilization** is the complete killing of all living organisms; this includes bacteria, fungi, viruses, and spores. The latter are notoriously difficult to kill, even with extremes of heat. Disinfection is more about removing any pathogenic organisms, so with disinfection there may still be some organisms present but they are either considered harmless or in such low numbers that they are unlikely to cause any harm.

1.4.1 Sterilization

There are several methods to ensure the complete killing of microorganisms. These are:

Heat

This is the most commonly used method of sterilization and is used in a number of settings. In order to achieve sterilization, temperatures above 120°C need to be used. Whilst most microorganisms are killed well below this temperature (around 70°C) the killing of bacterial and fungal spores requires very high temperatures. The most common method is to use moist heat in an **autoclave**, which can be looked on as just a very large pressure cooker you would use at home. It works as steam is piped into the autoclave and when under atmospheric pressure, the temperature of the steam rises above boiling point. As the pressure rises then so does the temperature. Using moist heat, it is generally considered that a temperature of 121°C for a time of 15 minutes will achieve sterilization. Using moist heat is advantageous as it disperses through all of the contents of the autoclave and thus penetrates all areas and achieves complete kill. There are some caveats to this, however, as it can depend on the organic content, the microbial load, and the type of organisms (spore vs non-spore forming) but generally moist heat at this temperature will achieve the desired result. The commonest uses of autoclaves in microbiology are for disposing of laboratory waste (blood samples, culture plates, etc.) and to sterilize culture media before it is poured into plates to be used in the laboratory.

Dry heat is used in some circumstances, most commonly for disposal of particular types of pathological waste (anatomical parts), in hospitals these are normally sent for incineration. More generally it is used to sterilize surgical instruments as there is no reason to use moist heat because it is the surface of the instrument which needs to be sterilized. In the laboratory, dry heat is used to sterilize the loops the scientists use between working with different organisms, although this practice is being replaced with pre-sterilized plastic disposable loops.

Filtration

As you can imagine there are certain things which cannot be sterilized using heat as they would be destroyed or broken down so they would be of no use. The best example of this is in the production of culture media, particularly selective media, as, in order to make the medium selective for a certain pathogen(s), antibiotics need to be added. Antibiotics are particularly heat sensitive and need to be added to culture media after the medium has cooled to around 50°C. Antibiotics therefore need to be filter-sterilized before adding to cooled culture media, and the best way of achieving this is by filter sterilization. This is performed using a membrane filter with a pore size of 0.22 μm. These membrane filters are made of cellulose or other polymers and the antibiotic solution is placed into a syringe and gently pushed through the filter. Strictly speaking it should not be termed filter sterilization as viruses and certain bacteria, such as mycoplasmas, will pass through the filter.

Cross reference
See Chapter 3.

SELF-CHECK 1.3

Why would there be little consequence if some viral particles were able to pass through the filter and into a sterile selective agar plate?

Irradiation

All types of ionizing radiation are lethal to all cellular types including mammalian cells. Due to the nature of the ionizing source and the dosage required to kill bacterial cells these are generally used in niche areas, such as industrial environments to sterilize plastic which are used across the healthcare spectrum. This would range from plastics used for patient care such as syringes and IV catheters to laboratory consumables such as the plastic petri dishes and containers used for sample collection.

Other types of sterilization include the use of gases, most commonly used for medical devices as the gas (**ethylene oxide**) is highly penetrative. The main problem is the toxicity of the gas and the fact that it is flammable. Special precautions therefore need to be taken and the process is mainly confined to specialized facilities. Formaldehyde is another gas that can be used for sterilization purposes and it has an advantage in that it kills spores. However, like ethylene oxide toxicity issues make its use confined to specialized areas. Finally, microwave ovens can in theory be used for sterilization of laboratory media and waste but they have not yet been widely adopted.

1.4.2 Disinfection

Most people will use a type of disinfection on an almost daily basis when they use chemicals to clean the bathroom or kitchen or even when washing the dishes. The process begins with removing any waste or dried-on debris so the maximum surface contact with the disinfectant can be obtained. One of the problems with disinfection is that bacteria can be trapped inside bits of debris and thus never come into contact with the disinfectant used. As a result they can multiply and cause infection. There are several types of disinfection and the main ones will be considered next.

The most common type of disinfection is chemical disinfection, which is anything from the soap used for hand washing to use of a variety of well-known brands used for environmental/surface disinfection. It is vitally important to first get the concentration of the disinfectant correct as if it is too weak it will have limited or no effect. Also of great importance is the pH as some disinfectants such as gluteraldehyde are generally more active at an alkaline pH

(7.8–8.5). The choice of the disinfectant is also significant as some will work only in certain areas and they can also have a limited range of bactericidal activity. The most commonly used disinfectants are:

Alcohols

Cross reference
See Chapter 12.

Generally they are used in high concentrations (around 80%) and in the form of alcohol wipes are used throughout health care institutions. A major drawback is that they are not active against spores (e.g. *C. difficile*) and poorly penetrate organic material. As a result they are often used on already 'clean' surfaces so their effect is maximized.

Halogen disinfectants

These are chlorine-releasing disinfectants and will kill a wide range of bacteria and viruses. Like alcohols they are not optimal in areas where organic material is present, other disadvantages include corrosion of metals and damage to the person using them, especially if they come into contact with mucosal areas. They also corrode metals so constant use will see the item needing to be replaced. A major advantage of using halogen disinfectants is that they are sporicidal and low cost. Iodine in an aqueous form is often used in conjunction with alcohols and is widely used for disinfection of the skin before surgical procedures. The side effects are the obvious staining of the skin as well as some irritant effects and hypersensitivity.

Aldehydes

The commonest of these is glutaraldehyde which is used widely in hospitals in particular. Glutaraldehyde, whilst highly active against a wide range of organisms including fungi and viruses, has a limited action against bacterial spores. The main drawback of glutaraldehyde is that it is an irritant to mucous membranes in particular and the person using it must wear personal protective equipment.

SELF-CHECK 1.4

What is the spectrum of action associated with each type of disinfectant? Why can health care environments not just use one type?

> ### Key Point
>
> It is important that all healthcare staff know the limitations of disinfectants as using the wrong disinfectant can have serious clinical consequences as transmission of infection can occur.

1.5 **Bacterial colony recognition**

Cross reference
See Chapters 2 and 3.

One of the most important stages in the identification process is determining if an organism is a pathogen and this is initially based on the colonial appearance of the organism in a routine diagnostic microbiology laboratory. On initial examination of the culture plates following incubation, laboratory scientists can often tell the genus of the organism growing simply by looking at the size, shape and colour of the colony. Whilst this not an exact science, because colonial appearance is dependent on the length of incubation, the sample isolated from, which may contain inhibitory substances, the media it is growing on, and the atmosphere it was incubated in, laboratory scientists are highly skilled in colonial recognition.

There are several types of colonial appearance and some examples of these are shown in Figure 1.3. The most common colonial types, seen from colonies growing from patient samples, are either entire or **undulate**. In addition it is important to determine the height of the colony and its colour, as some are translucent (clear/transparent) or opaque. The pigment of the colony can be useful in identification but can vary considerably even amongst the same species. Using growth on blood agar as an example, most staphylococcal colonies will be white with streptococci and enterococci often grey. Most enterobacteriaciae (*E. coli/ Klebsiella/Salmonella* etc.) will also appear as grey colonies on blood agar; however, they are much larger than streptococci. This is one of the reasons that other media, especially chromogenic media, are used which can help speciate the organism further, simply on colonial appearance.

Cross reference
See Chapter 3.

The laboratory scientist also needs to record any distinguishing features such as the ability of the colonies to cause haemolysis of the medium (β-haemolytic streptococci), or produce any colonial pigments (*Pseudomonas* spp.) as these can often narrow the identification process down considerably. It must also be noted that the lack of growth on some media but not others can give a clue as to the identity of the isolated organism. For example, the bile salts in media such as CLED (cysteine lactose electrolyte deficient) are inhibitory to most species of *Streptococcus* so a typical colonial appearance on blood agar is reinforced by its lack of growth on CLED.

Throughout the various chapters in this book you will see examples of how different the colonial types of various bacteria are and how little has changed over the years in isolation and identification of them. It is still a manual process and despite many attempts at automating these processes the real love of a biomedical scientist is still examining culture plates and

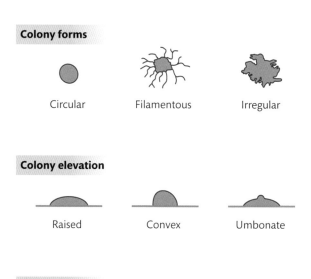

Colony forms

Circular   Filamentous   Irregular

Colony elevation

Raised   Convex   Umbonate

Colony margin

Entire   Undulate   Filamentous

FIGURE 1.3
Diagram of the commonest colony types seen in diagnostic microbiology departments.
Source: Courtesy of H. Ford

identifying pathogens on a daily basis. Whether this is detecting *Salmonella* in a faeces sample or MRSA in a patient's bloodstream it is through your skills as a scientist that you make a real contribution to the diagnosis and management of infections in clinical patients.

SELF-CHECK 1.5

What are the most common bacterial colony types and what other colonial features do laboratory scientists use to identify bacteria?

Key Point

In examining bacterial colonies you need to examine all culture media the sample has been inoculated onto as growth/no growth on a particular medium can be very important in determining the organism's identity. Always look for clues such as haemolysis, pigment production, and even smell to narrow down the identity of the organism.

 Chapter summary

After reading this chapter you should know and understand:

■ The importance of microbiology and its place in the detection and prevention of infection.

■ Key components of the bacterial cell.

■ Principles and methods of disinfection. Common disinfectants used in health care environments.

■ Growth of bacteria in liquid media and the limiting factors to bacterial growth.

■ Sterilization of bacterial cultures and methods used.

■ Simple colonial appearance and the key features used in the first stage of the identification process.

 Further reading

● **Collins CH, Lyne PM, Grange JM, eds. *Collins and Lyne's Microbiological Methods*, 8th edition. CRC Press, 2004.**

This is a useful text which provides further detail on many aspects of this chapter. An essential laboratory handbook.

- **Mackie TJ, McCartney JE, *Medical Microbiology*, Volume 1, 13th edition. Churchill Livingstone, 1985.**

  Useful text which covers many basic principles of microbiology.

- **Hawkey P, Lewis D, eds. *Medical Bacteriology*, 2nd edition. Oxford University Press, 2004.**

  General text covering many aspects of sample processing and other areas of microbiology.

 # Discussion questions

1.1   What are the basic colonial characteristics which help identify bacterial colonies? Provide some examples with your answer.

1.2   Why would organisms inoculated into a simple liquid medium from a patient sample grow poorly or not at all? What measures could you take to help the organisms to grow?

1.3   What disinfectants would you chose for the following situation and give your reasons to justify your choice(s):

   a.   General cleaning of laboratory surfaces.

   b.   Waste from an analyser which is used for HIV testing.

   c.   Cleaning an isolation bay where a patient has a severe *C. difficile* infection.

1.4   Why is the cell wall important both to the bacterial cell and also in the fight against infection?

2

Identification tests

John Perry

This chapter will concentrate principally on the biochemical reactions that allow for differentiation of clinically important bacteria. The application of other identification tests, including immunological tests, will be discussed.

Bacterial identification is traditionally based on a presumptive assignment to a genus or species based on morphological and cultural characteristics, followed by confirmation using biochemical tests. Bacteria are usually first isolated on agar-based culture media and this allows morphological and cultural features to be gathered first. These include: colony size, shape, and colour; degree and type of haemolysis on blood-based media; size, shape, and Gram reaction of cells on microscopy; atmospheric requirements for growth (e.g. failure to grow anaerobically). The assessment of these features will, in many cases, enable a presumptive assignment of the bacterial isolate to its family or genus.

For example, a Gram stain of colonies that only form under anaerobic conditions revealing spore-forming Gram-positive bacilli, would suggest that the isolate belongs to the genus *Clostridium*. Similarly, small α-haemolytic colonies confirmed as Gram-positive cocci and showing both aerobic and anaerobic growth would be presumptively regarded as *Streptococcus* spp. If there is any doubt about the likely family or genus to which an isolate belongs, two very simple biochemical tests for catalase and oxidase may be useful and results can be achieved within minutes.

Learning objectives

After studying this chapter you should be able to:

- Explain how bacterial hydrolases (e.g. glycosidases, peptidases, esterases) can be detected and give examples of specific hydrolases produced by pathogens.
- Give examples of how carbohydrate metabolism by bacteria can be exploited in bacterial identification.
- Give examples of how amino acid metabolism by bacteria can be exploited in bacterial identification.
- Give examples of how susceptibility tests can assist microbial identification.
- Explain the basis of simple immunological tests for the rapid identification of bacteria.

2.1 **Biochemical tests**

2.1.1 Catalase test

Detection of catalase is a highly useful test in bacterial diagnostics and this enzyme is commonly found in a wide range of bacterial species. Catalase results in the decomposition of potentially toxic hydrogen peroxide into water and oxygen. Detection of catalase is most useful for discrimination between genera, for example, allowing differentiation between staphylococci (+) and streptococci (–) or listeria (+) and lactobacilli (–).

2.1.2 Oxidase test

The oxidase test is able to distinguish bacteria that possess cytochrome *c* as a respiratory enzyme (Figure 2.1). The test is simple and requires only a single reagent. Most commonly, the choice of reagent is *N,N,N,N*-tetramethyl-*p*-phenylenediamine dihydrochloride. This reagent is water soluble and colourless in solution. On exposure to oxidase-positive bacteria the reagent is rapidly oxidized to produce a purple–blue dye (Wurster's blue). As with catalase, detection of oxidase activity is useful for differentiation of bacterial families and genera. For example, all genera among the Enterobacteriaceae such as *Escherichia* or *Enterobacter* are oxidase negative (*Plesiomonas* is an exception) and this differentiates them from genera such as *Pseudomonas* and *Aeromonas* (oxidase positive). Among Gram-negative cocci, *Acinetobacter* (oxidase negative) may be differentiated from *Moraxella* and *Neisseria* (oxidase positive).

Although the oxidase test has its greatest use for differentiation of Gram-negative bacteria, a few Gram-positive species demonstrate oxidase activity and this can be useful, for example in the differentiation of *Staphylococcus sciuri* from many other species of staphylococci, e.g. *Staphylococcus aureus*.

FIGURE 2.1
Oxidase reagent applied to a
***P. aeruginosa* susceptibility**
test plate. The blue–violet
coloration shows the
organism is oxidase positive.
Source: Courtesy of M. Ford.

METHOD Catalase test

- Using a plastic loop, sample a single colony and rub this inoculum onto a glass slide. The inoculum should be sufficiently large to be visible to the naked eye.
- Place a drop of 30% hydrogen peroxide onto a glass coverslip and place the coverslip onto the slide, exposing the bacterial inoculum to the hydrogen peroxide.
- Observe for immediate generation of oxygen bubbles (catalase positive).
- Discard the slide and coverslip into disinfectant.
- Precautions:
  - Avoid the use of metal loops or inoculating wires as these may cause false-positive results.
  - False-positive results are commonly obtained when colonies have been selected from blood agar as blood cells contain catalase.
  - Hydrogen peroxide is quite unstable and controls must be used to ensure optimal performance of the test.

SELF-CHECK 2.1

What problems are associated with the catalase test and how can these be overcome?

2.1.3 Detection of bacterial hydrolases: glycosidases

Glycosides are sugar derivatives that occur naturally and are found commonly, for example, in plants. It has long been recognized that most clinically important bacteria produce glycosidase enzymes. These are enzymes that hydrolyse (or 'break down') glycosides to release the sugar part of the molecule, which is then used for generation of energy. Any non-sugar part of the molecule is referred to as an '**aglycone**' and detection of this free aglycone can be used to demonstrate the presence of a **glycosidase.** The nomenclature of the glycosidase enzyme is governed by the type of derivative it hydrolyses. So, for example, a galactosidase will hydrolyse derivatives of galactose (i.e. galactosides) and a glucosidase will hydrolyse glucosides, etc. It is important to remember that these enzymes do not hydrolyse the sugars themselves, but rather, sugar derivatives. So, for example, a glucosidase will not act on glucose and a glucuronidase will not act on glucuronic acid, etc.

The linkage between the sugar and the aglycone is also very important. This glycosidic linkage may have alpha or beta orientation and this will determine whether the enzyme is able to act. So, for example, a β-galactosidase will only hydrolyse substrates containing galactose that is linked to another molecule or group via a beta linkage.

In microbiology, one of the best known glycosides is esculin, a naturally occurring glucoside that can be extracted from the bark of the horse chestnut tree (*Aesculus hippocastanum*). Esculin is hydrolysed by a glycosidase known as β-glucosidase. Hydrolysis of esculin leads to the release of glucose and an aglycone known as esculetin. In the presence of iron salts (for example ferric ammonium citrate) esculetin forms a brown/black complex or 'chelate', which

aglycone
A molecule that is not a sugar but is linked to a natural sugar (e.g. galactose) via a glycosidic bond (example: nitrophenol in *ortho*-nitrophenyl galactopyranoside).

glycosidase
A **glycosidase** is an enzyme that hydrolyses compounds consisting of a sugar molecule linked to another molecule in a glycosidic linkage. The other molecule may or may not be another sugar. Natural substrates include esculin or disaccharides such as lactose.

(a)

(b)

FIGURE 2.2

(a) The structure of esculin and the complex formed upon hydrolysis. (b) Colonies of E. faecalis showing hydrolysis of esculin on agar-based medium.
Source: Courtesy of J. Perry.

indicates that esculin has been hydrolysed and β-glucosidase is present. The structure of esculin and the complex formed after hydrolysis are shown in Figure 2.2a. Since 1926, the hydrolysis of esculin in the presence of bile has been recognized as a useful identification test to differentiate enterococci and group D streptococci from other streptococci (Figure 2.2b). The esculin hydrolysis test is also useful for differentiation of species within the Enterobacteriaceae.

As a convenient assay for glycosidases, sugars may be linked to coloured dyes (via alpha or beta linkages) to form **synthetic enzyme substrates**. A key feature of such substrates is that when the dye is linked to the sugar, its colour is quenched. Hydrolysis of the substrate then leads to the release of the dye and the restoration of colour. This is, therefore, a very convenient and simple means of demonstrating bacterial enzyme activity. Such substrates that release coloured dyes when hydrolysed are known as 'chromogenic substrates' because a visible colour is produced and this can be interpreted by the biomedical scientist.

The best-known synthetic chromogenic substrate in clinical microbiology is o-nitrophenyl-β-D-galactopyranoside (ONPG), which comprises galactose in beta linkage with a yellow compound, o-nitrophenol. When in solution ONPG is virtually colourless, but the presence of bacteria that produce β-galactosidase causes hydrolysis, leading to the generation of a bright yellow colour. The ONPG test is a very useful test for differentiating *Salmonella* (–) from many other genera within the Enterobacteriaceae, for example *E. coli* (+) and *Citrobacter* spp. (+). The reaction is illustrated in Figure 2.3.

As well as linking sugars to coloured dyes, they may also be linked to fluorescent molecules to form non-fluorescent compounds that are highly sensitive **'fluorogenic' enzyme substrates**. Hydrolysis leads to restoration of fluorescence, which may be measured by using a fluorimeter or simply observed under a suitable ultra violet light source. The most commonly used fluorescent molecule or 'fluorophore' is 4-methylumbelliferone (4-MeU), which emits a powerful sky-blue fluorescence under UV light. A commonly used **fluorogenic substrate** is 4-methylumbelliferyl-β-D-glucuronide, which is useful for the detection of β-glucuronidase produced by *E. coli*.

Other glycosidase enzymes useful in microbial identification include N-acetyl-β-D-glucosaminidase produced by *Candida albicans*, which distinguishes it from most other yeasts.

synthetic substrate
Synthetic enzyme substrates are not obtained from natural sources but are chemically synthesized in order to demonstrate enzyme activity. A synthetic substrate that releases a coloured dye when it is hydrolysed is referred to as a chromogenic substrate.

fluorogenic substrate
A fluorogenic substrate may be natural or synthetic but is metabolized (usually by a hydrolase) to release a fluorescent compound.

o-Nitrophenyl β-D-galactopyranoside
(colourless)

β-Galactosidase + H₂O

Galactose

o-Nitrophenol
(yellow)

FIGURE 2.3
Hydrolysis of ONPG to release yellow o-nitrophenol.
Source: Courtesy of J. Perry.

> ### Key Point
>
> It is important to remember that the compounds released by bacterial enzyme action will readily diffuse through agar and it will be impossible to pick out the target organism in a mixture. Hence most of these tests are performed in tubes or other enclosed containers.

2.1.4 Peptidases

Many bacteria produce a wealth of peptidases involved in the breakdown of the peptide linkages that exist between amino acids. Synthetic substrates have been devised that link an amino acid to a coloured dye to form a colourless enzyme substrate. Hydrolysis then releases the amino acid, which is used for metabolism, and the coloured dye. One such dye that is widely used is *p*-nitroaniline. This compound diffuses readily through agar and can also be quite toxic to bacterial cells.

The amino group of this molecule can be linked to the carboxyl group of various amino acids to generate aminopeptidase substrates. Whether or not the substrate is hydrolysed depends to a large extent on the nature of the amino acid. L-alanine-*p*-nitroanilide is a colourless substrate comprising L-alanine linked to *p*-nitroaniline. All Gram-negative bacteria demonstrate a strong L-alanyl aminopeptidase activity, resulting in hydrolysis of this substrate and release of a yellow dye. The enzyme is referred to as an 'aminopeptidase' because the amino group (NH_2) of the amino acid is free. An alternative name for the enzyme is L-alanyl aryl amidase.

L-Pyroglutamic acid may also be linked to *p*-nitroaniline to form a chromogenic substrate for detection of pyroglutamyl aminopeptidase (also known as pyrrolidonyl peptidase). Detection of this enzyme is highly useful for differentiation of enterococci (+) and group A streptococci (+) from other streptococci (–); and differentiation of *Salmonella* and *Shigella* (–) from many other genera of Enterobacteriaceae, for example *Citrobacter* (+) and *Hafnia* (+).

A number of other aminopeptidases are useful for biochemical identification including γ-glutamyl aminopeptidase that can discriminate *Neisseria meningitidis* (+) from other *Neisseria* (–). Detection of prolyl aminopeptidase differentiates *Neisseria gonorrhoeae* (+) from other *Neisseria* (–) and is a useful identification marker for *Clostridium difficile*. β-alanyl aminopeptidase is a useful identification marker for *Pseudomonas aeruginosa*. Finally, leucyl aminopeptidase (LAP) is useful for the discrimination of *Leuconoctoc* spp. and *Aerococcus viridans* from the streptococci.

As well as chromogenic methods for the demonstration of aminopeptidase activity, fluorogenic substrates based on amino acids linked to 7-amino-4-methylcoumarin are commercially available and widely used. Like many other released compounds, the fluorogen will readily diffuse through agar and the whole plate will fluoresce and the target pathogen will be impossible to pick out.

We have shown that various aminopeptidase enzymes are useful for identification but other types of peptidase may also be valuable taxonomic markers. Hippuric acid (or in its salt form, sodium hippurate) comprises the amino acid glycine linked to benzoic acid in a peptide linkage. This substrate is found naturally as a product of excretion in the urine of horses and other herbivores. Many species of bacteria hydrolyse hippurate to form benzoic acid and glycine and the latter is usually detected by addition of ninhydrin reagent. This enzymatic activity is referred to as hippurate hydrolase (Figure 2.4) and is essentially a 'carboxypeptidase' activity as the carboxyl group of the glycine is free. Detection of this enzyme activity is useful for discrimination of group B streptococci (+) from most other streptococci (–); discrimination of *Campylobacter jejuni* (+) from *Campylobacter coli* (–) is also a useful marker for *Legionella* spp.

SELF-CHECK 2.3

Why do you think there are both chromogenic and fluorogenic substrates available?

2.1.5 Esterases

Coloured dyes such as *p*-nitrophenol and fluorophores such as 4-methylumbelliferone may be derivatized with carboxylic acids ('fatty acids') to form esters such as acetate, butyrate, propionate, etc. Removal of the carboxylic acid by hydrolysis of the ester link is accomplished by bacterial esterases and results in generation of colour or fluorescence

Cross reference
See Section 2.1.3, this chapter.

FIGURE 2.4
Hydrolysis of hippuric acid to glycine and benzoic acid.
Source: Courtesy of J. Perry.

respectively. Short chain esters are easily hydrolysed and the vast majority of bacteria (if not all) hydrolyse acetate esters. Hydrolysis of butyrate esters is less common and is useful for discrimination of *Moraxella catarrhalis* from *Neisseria* spp. *Salmonella* spp. hydrolyse longer chain esters such as octanoate (C8) and nonanoate (C9) derivatives and this activity is an excellent diagnostic marker for the discrimination of *Salmonella* (+) from most other Enterobacteriaceae (–).

2.1.6 Phosphatase

Phosphatases are produced by a wide range of clinically important bacteria. They are most conveniently detected using phosphate esters of coloured or fluorescent dyes such as *p*-nitro-phenol and 4-methylumbelliferone, respectively. Enzymatic hydrolysis liberates inorganic phosphate and restoration of colour or fluorescence. Phosphatase activity can be used as an identification marker for *S. aureus* but, depending on the choice of substrate and the length of incubation, the enzyme can be readily demonstrated in species of coagulase-negative staphylococci. Phosphatase is also a useful identification marker for *Clostridium perfringens* if an appropriate substrate with high specificity is used such as phenolphthalein diphosphate.

2.1.7 Deoxyribonuclease (DNase)

Deoxyribonuclease or DNase is an extracellular enzyme capable of hydrolysing DNA to release oligonucleotides. A heat-resistant DNase or thermonuclease is produced by *S. aureus* and detection of this enzyme is a useful diagnostic marker as other staphylococci produce lower amounts of the enzyme or none at all. Traditionally, the enzyme has been detected by incorporating DNA into an agar-based medium and inoculating the test organism. After incubation, the medium is flooded with hydrochloric acid. The addition of acid results in precipitation of the DNA, which is visible in the agar; however, if the DNA is hydrolysed a clear zone will be apparent around bacterial colonies. Alternative assay formats have been developed to avoid the inconvenience of flooding agar plates with acid. One such adaptation of the method involves the inclusion of a metachromatic dye such as toluidine blue O. This dye complexes with intact DNA to produce a blue colour; however, when DNA is hydrolysed, this dye forms a pink colour with oligonucleotides. As well as being a useful identification marker for *S. aureus*, DNase is also produced by some streptococci (e.g. *S. pyogenes*), *Serratia marcescens*, and *Corynebacterium diphtheriae*.

2.1.8 Hydrolysis of gelatine

Some bacteria demonstrate a proteolytic activity that results in digestion or liquefaction of gelatine, resulting in the generation of polypeptides and/or amino acids. There are various assay formats involving both solid and liquid media. In one of the most effective assays, finely powdered charcoal particles are bound to a small amount of solid gelatine. Digestion of the gelatine by bacterial enzymes results in the release of the charcoal particles into suspension, this forming a clearly visible black precipitate. Hydrolysis of gelatine is a useful diagnostic marker for several species of Enterobacteriaceae including *Proteus* spp. and *Serratia* spp. Gelatinase is also produced by members of the Vibrionaceae, for example *Vibrio cholerae* and *Aeromonas hydrophila*, as well as being useful for the differentiation of non-fermentative Gram-negative rods and for differentiation between *Clostridia* spp.

2.1.9 Amino acid metabolism

Amino acids may be metabolized by bacteria in a variety of ways depending on their ability to produce certain enzymes. Lysine and ornithine are atypical amino acids in that they each contain two amino groups and a single carboxyl group. Some Gram-negative bacteria decarboxylate either lysine or ornithine, or both, to generate diamines (cadaverine and putrescine respectively), which are very alkaline. This activity can be conveniently detected using an appropriate pH indicator such as bromocresol purple or phenol red. Pyridoxyl phosphate may be included as a coenzyme to enhance activity. Detection of lysine or ornithine decarboxylase activity provides excellent discrimination between species of Enterobacteriaceae (see Table 2.1).

Some bacteria are able to split the amino acid arginine via a complex dihydrolase reaction, also generating ammonia as an end-product, which may be detected using a pH indicator. The demonstration of arginine dihydrolase (ADH) is a useful marker for some species of Enterobacteriaceae including *Enterobactercloacae* and *Salmonella* spp. and also related bacteria such as *Aeromonas hydrophila*. It is also useful for differentiation within the staphylococci, enterococci, and streptococci.

When testing for either decarboxylase or dihydrolase activity it is preferable to perform the tests in tubes in which the test medium is overlaid with mineral oil to create anaerobic conditions for growth. In the presence of air, bacteria readily oxidize peptone to form alkaline end-products which may lead to false positive results.

As well as the removal of the carboxyl group of amino acids, an amino group may be removed by deaminase enzymes. Deamination of aromatic amino acids such as tryptophan and phenylalanine leads to the release of ammonia and the generation of organic acids (indole pyruvic acid and phenylpyruvic acid respectively) which may be detected by their formation of coloured complexes in the presence of ferric ions. Deaminase activity is largely restricted to the three related genera *Proteus*, *Providencia*, and *Morganella*, and it is therefore an excellent diagnostic marker for this group.

In addition to being a target for deaminases, certain species are able to split tryptophan to form pyruvate, ammonia, and indole. The latter is detected by specific reagents such as Kovac's or James' reagent to generate a red colouration. Generation of indole is a very useful identification test for differentiation of Enterobacteriaceae and as a marker for many other species of Gram-negative bacteria such as *Aeromonas hydrophila*, *Pasteurella multocida*, and *Fusobacterium necrophorum*. The ability to generate indole from tryptophan is rare amongst Gram-positive bacteria but it is useful for identification of certain species, for example *Clostridium tetani*.

TABLE 2.1 A simple biochemical test scheme for identification of Enterobacteriaceae from urine samples.

		Biochemical profile				
Lysine	Ornithine	Glucose	Indole	Cellobiose	Urea	Identification
–	+	+	+	+	–	*Citrobacter koseri*
–	–	+	–	–	–	*Citrobacter freundii*
+	+	+	–	+	–	*Enterobacter aerogenes*
–	+	+	–	+	–	*Enterobacter cloacae*
+	+ or –	+	+	–	–	*Escherichia coli*
+ or –	+	+	+	–	–	*Escherichia coli*
+	–	+	+	+	+ or –	*Klebsiella oxytoca*
+	–	+	–	+	+ or –	*Klebsiella pneumoniae*
–	+	+	+	–	+	*Morganella morganii*
–	+	+	–	–	+	*Proteus mirabilis*
–	–	+	–	–	+	*Proteus penneri*
–	–	+	+	–	+	*Proteus vulgaris*
–	–	+	+	–	–	*Providencia* species
+	+	+	–	–	–	*Serratia* species

2.1.10 Carbohydrate oxidation/fermentation

Most species of clinical importance utilize sugars via either oxidation or fermentation to generate organic acids. This activity is generally detected by use of a suitable pH indicator such as phenol red or bromothymol blue. The ability to acidify glucose under anaerobic conditions (fermentation) is a fundamental test that can differentiate major groups of bacteria, for example distinction of all members of the family Enterobacteriaceae (+) from non-fermentative genera such as *Pseudomonas* (–), *Acinetobacter* (–) and *Stenotrophomonas* (–), or the differentiation of staphylococci (+) from micrococci (–).

Not only is the ability to ferment glucose of fundamental importance to bacterial identification, so is the way in which it is fermented. Fermentation of glucose may lead to the formation of different end-products and this varies between species. For example, when *Klebsiella* spp. and *Enterobacter* spp. ferment glucose, 2,3-butanediol is a major end product of metabolism whereas the closely related *E. coli* does not generate this compound. These differences in metabolism are exploited by the Voges–Proskauer (VP) test. In the VP test bacteria are allowed to ferment glucose and, after incubation, 40% potassium hydroxide and 5% α-naphthol (dissolved in ethanol) are added. These reagents react with acetoin (the precursor of 2,3 butanediol) to form a pink coloration indicating a positive VP reaction. The VP test is highly useful for differentiation of species within the Enterobacteriaceae and also within staphylococci and streptococci.

For differentiation of very closely related species within a genus (e.g. *Staphylococcus* or *Enterococcus*) it is often necessary to test a range of appropriate sugars to obtain a biochemical profile. A wide range of compounds are acidified by bacteria and these include pentoses (e.g. L-arabinose, D-xylose), hexoses (e.g. D-glucose, L-sorbose), deoxysugars (e.g. L-rhamnose), disaccharides (e.g. sucrose, lactose), trisaccharides (e.g. melezitose, raffinose), polysaccharides (e.g. inulin, starch), glycosides (e.g. esculin, salicin), and sugar alcohols (e.g. adonitol, D-mannitol).

For most bacteria, such tests are generally straightforward and consist of peptone, 1% sugar, and a suitable pH indicator, for example phenol red. When testing fastidious bacteria, such as *Neisseria* spp., it may be necessary to include 2% serum to allow growth. Serum should be heat-treated to ensure that potentially interfering enzymes (e.g. maltase) are inactivated.

SELF-CHECK 2.4

Having read the above, what tests would you use to differentiate between the following?

(a) *Pseudomonas* and Enterobacteriaceae
(b) *Proteus mirabilis* and *E. coli*
(c) *Salmonella* spp. and *E. coli*
(d) *Staphylococcus* spp. and *Streptococcus* spp.

2.2 Miscellaneous biochemical tests

2.2.1 Urease

This enzyme is found in a range of diverse species and causes the hydrolysis of urea into carbon dioxide and ammonia. Ammonia is a strong base and consequently there is a notable rise in pH caused by hydrolysis of urea. This is usually detected with a suitable indicator such as phenol red (Figure 2.5). Detection of urease is useful for the differentiation of genera within the Enterobacteriaceae. A strong urease reaction is generated by *Proteus* spp. and weaker reactions are common in *Klebsiella* spp. and occasionally in *Serratia* spp. On media for the isolation of enteric pathogens, *Proteus* often resembles *Salmonella* and *Shigella* and a rapid test for urease can be useful to identify *Proteus* and thus exclude these two pathogens.

Helicobacter pylori produces a urease with exceptional activity that may be detected in minutes and detection of this enzyme is highly useful in the diagnosis of gastritis.

2.2.2 Hydrogen sulphide production

Some bacteria are able to generate hydrogen sulphide from compounds containing sulphur, including sodium thiosulphate and sulphur-containing amino acids such as cysteine or methionine. The release of hydrogen sulphide is detected using a suitable metal ion that forms an insoluble black precipitate with hydrogen sulphide. Commonly, this involves incorporation of an iron salt into the growth medium (e.g. ferric ammonium citrate) or the use of filter paper

FIGURE 2.5

Urease test showing positive (*P. mirabilis*: pink) and negative (*S. enteritidis*: no colour change) results.

Source: **Image reproduced by permission of Thermo Fisher Scientific.**

soaked with lead acetate to detect hydrogen sulphide liberated into the atmosphere above the growth medium. The test is mainly applied to the differentiation of Enterobacteriaceae and few species are positive including *Salmonella* spp., *Proteus* spp., and *Citrobacter freundii*.

2.2.3 Reduction of nitrate

Nitrate may be reduced by a wide range of bacteria to produce either nitrite or nitrogen gas. To test for nitrate reductase, bacteria are incubated in a nutrient broth supplemented with 0.1% potassium nitrate. After incubation, two reagents are added, N,N-dimethyl-α-naphthylamine and sulphanilic acid, and these will cause the development of a red diazonium compound if nitrite is present. A red coloration therefore indicates a positive result, that is, nitrate has been reduced. Lack of colour upon addition of reagents does not necessarily indicate a negative result as denitrification may have led to decomposition of nitrite and generation of nitrogen gas. This can be resolved by addition of powdered zinc to the test medium, which will cause reduction of intact nitrate to nitrite, resulting in a red coloration in the presence of the reagents. If the test medium remains colourless after addition of zinc, it can therefore be concluded that nitrate has been completely reduced resulting in formation of nitrogen gas, that is, the test is positive.

Most bacteria encountered in the clinical laboratory reduce nitrate and the test is therefore a useful marker for species that do not. These include a number of Gram-negative non-fermenters such as *Acinetobacter* spp., *Alcaligenes faecalis*, and *Sphingobacterium* spp. The nitrate reduction test is also highly useful for division of the mycobacteria where only a minority of species, including *Mycobacterium tuberculosis*, are able to reduce nitrate.

2.2.4 Coagulase

Outside of the urinary tract, *Staphylococcus aureus* is the most predominant pathogen encountered in clinical microbiology. Detection of staphylocoagulase or 'free' coagulase using the tube coagulase test is a highly reliable means of confirming the identification of *S. aureus*. Among other staphylococci, coagulase is only produced by rarely encountered species such as *S. schleiferi* and *S. intermedius*. *S. aureus* strains lacking staphylocoagulase are uncommon.

The biochemical mechanism of the coagulase enzyme is complex and the subject of much debate. The enzyme reacts with a thermostable thrombin-like substance present in plasma, resulting in the formation of a fibrin clot. Human or rabbit plasma are recommended for the test and suitable preparations (containing anticoagulant, e.g. citrate) are available from a number of commercial sources. To perform the test, the plasma is mixed with an equal volume of an overnight broth culture of the test strain in a test tube; alternatively a loopful of growth from solid media may be directly suspended in the plasma to produce an equivalent turbidity. The tube is incubated at 37°C and examined after 1, 4, and 18 h of incubation. If staphylocoagulase is present, a visible clot is normally apparent within 4 h of incubation.

As well as producing free staphylocoagulase most strains of *S. aureus* possess a bound coagulase or 'clumping factor' that may be detected in slide tests (the tube method detects both types). A loopful of growth from solid medium is mixed in physiological saline to produce a heavy suspension. The suspension must be homogeneous and show no evidence of autoagglutination after thorough mixing. Autoagglutination is common if strains are selected from media containing a hypertonic salt concentration, for example mannitol salt agar, and this will invalidate the test. If the saline suspension is suitable, a loopful of plasma may then be added and mixed into the suspension. The presence of *S. aureus* will result in immediate, coarse clumping of the plasma (Figure 2.6). Any delayed reactions (i.e. >20 seconds) should be confirmed by the

FIGURE 2.6

Slide coagulase test showing negative control (*S. epidermidis*: left) and positive result (*S. aureus*: right).

Source: Courtesy of M. Ford.

tube coagulase test (see start of this section). For both tests, positive and negative controls are essential and must give expected reactions before interpretation is made.

Chromogenic and fluorogenic substrates have been developed for detection of staphyloco-agulase. Examples include those based on the chemical formula N-t-boc-Val-Pro-Arg-X where X is a fluorescent or coloured label such as 7-amino-4-methylcoumarin (7-AMC) or p-nitroan-iline (p-NA), respectively. Prothrombin also needs to be incorporated in the assay. The presence of staphylocoagulase results in release of the label, which may be detected visually as colour or fluorescence or by a suitable optical device. A number of commercially available assays are available that employ chromogenic or fluorogenic methods. An example is the Staphychrom II, which is able to detect staphylocoagulase with high specificity in a 2-h test.

SELF-CHECK 2.5

Why are two types of coagulase test available to identify *S. aureus*? What are the differences and when would you use them?

2.2.5 Lecithinase (phospholipase C)

A major component of lecithin is phosphatidylcholine, which may be hydrolysed by bacteria to generate phosphorylcholine and insoluble digylceride. Egg yolk is a rich source of lecithin and this may be incorporated into agar media in order to demonstrate lecithinase activity. Colonies that produce lecithinase produce a halo of opalescence due to the precipitation of diglyceride which is released from lecithin by enzyme activity.

Demonstration of lecithinase is characteristic of a number of species of *Clostridium* including *C. perfringens*, *C. sordellii*, *C. novyi*, and *C. bifermentans.* It is also produced by a number of *Bacillus* spp. including the pathogenic species *B. cereus* and *B. anthracis*. Most commonly, the lecithinase reaction is used for the identification of *C. perfringens*. The α toxin of *C. perfringens* is responsible for lecithinase activity and its reaction on egg yolk media can be neutralized using a specific antitoxin. This is known as the Nagler reaction (Figure 2.7). To test for the Nagler reaction, an agar plate medium containing egg yolk is prepared and specific antitoxin is spread on the surface of half of the plate. A suspect strain of *C. perfringens* is then streaked across the medium so that both halves of the plate are inoculated. After incubation *C. perfringens* shows a clearly visible opalescence, which is inhibited on one side of the plate due to neutralization by a specific antitoxin.

FIGURE 2.7

Clostridium perfringens growing on Nagler egg yolk medium. Note the diffuse opacity due to production of lecithinase C. This opalescence is neutralized with a specific antitoxin.

Source: Courtesy of M. Ford.

2.3 **Carbon source utilization tests**

These are used widely for bacterial identification and are particularly useful for relatively 'unreactive' bacteria, for example those that do not acidify sugars. The best known carbon source utilization test is the citrate test. Bacteria are incubated with various salts including ammonium phosphate (as a sole nitrogen source) and citrate (as a sole carbon source). Bacteria that are able to utilize citrate are able to grow and visible growth is used as an endpoint to indicate a positive test. Alternatively, bromothymol blue may be included and an alkaline (blue) reaction indicates growth due to the release of ammonia from ammonium phosphate. Classically, the citrate test is used in the differentiation of the Enterobacteriaceae and can help differentiate *E. coli* and *Shigella* spp., which in contrast to most other genera are unable to utilize citrate as a sole carbon source.

A range of other organic acids may also be used in carbon source utilization tests to help differentiate species. These include sodium salts of acetate, benzoate, lactate, oxalate, propionate, pyruvate, succinate, tartrate, malate, gluconate, and malonate. When performing such tests care must be taken to ensure that nutrient media (containing additional sources of carbon) are not accidently included with the bacterial inoculum and the inoculum itself should generally be low.

SELF-CHECK 2.6

Why are carbon source utilization tests used and not carbohydrate fermentation tests for some organisms?

2.4 **Susceptibility to antibiotics and chemical inhibitors**

The susceptibility of bacteria to antimicrobial agents can provide useful information to assist the identification process. *Staphylococcus saprophyticus* is a urinary tract pathogen that possesses an intrinsic resistance to novobiocin, thus differentiating it from most other commonly encountered species of staphylococci, although some other species (e.g. *S. xylosus*) are also resistant. Among Gram-negative bacteria, resistance to colistin can be a useful identification marker, for example for distinction of *Burkholderia cepacia* complex (always resistant) from *Pseudomonas* species (usually susceptible). Susceptibility to bacitracin has been used for many years for the differentiation of *Streptococcus pyogenes* from other β-haemolytic streptococci. Finally, susceptibility to metronidazole can help to differentiate anaerobes from non-anaerobes. The use of antibiotic resistance markers as tools in identification should be used with care as acquired resistance can emerge during antimicrobial chemotherapy. Nalidixic acid was widely recommended as an identification marker in the 1980s to differentiate *Campylobacter laridis* (resistant) from other thermophilic campylobacters. However, widespread use of quinolones in subsequent years led to a large proportion of *Campylobacter jejuni* expressing resistance to nalidixic acid. Despite these limitations, an experienced biomedical scientist will always review the biochemical identification of a pathogen in the light of all other available information, including its antibiogram.

Susceptibility to non-antibiotic substances may also be of diagnostic use. Optochin (ethyl hydrocupreine hydrochloride) is a highly useful test to differentiate *Streptococcus pneumoniae* from other α-haemolytic streptococci. 2,4-diamino-6,7-isopropylpteridine phosphate (O/129) is an agent that inhibits the growth of *Vibrio* spp. providing differentiation from closely related genera (e.g. *Aeromonas* spp.). Resistance to 9-chloro-9-(4-diethylaminophenyl)- 10-phenylacridan (C390) is a highly useful marker for *Pseudomonas aeruginosa* among non-fermentative Gram-negative bacteria, although around 4% of strains are susceptible. Tolerance to various salts has also been used as an identification marker. For example, the ability to grow in the presence of 6.5% sodium chloride is a characteristic of enterococci but not streptococci and growth in the presence of potassium cyanide (0.0075%) has been shown to be useful for differentiation of species of Enterobacteriaceae. Finally, the ability to grow in the presence of various dyes (e.g. thionin, basic fuchsin, and safranin O) has been used to distinguish between the three main pathogenic species of *Brucella*.

SELF-CHECK 2.7

Which do you consider to be the better tests to differentiate between organisms — biochemical or substance susceptibility testing? What are your reasons?

2.5 Tolerance to environmental conditions

Clinically important bacteria grow at pH 7 at 37°C, although that may not be their optimum growth temperature or pH. The ability to withstand deviations in temperature and pH varies between different groups of bacteria and tests for tolerance to such deviations can be useful for identification. For example, it has been recognized for many years that enterococci are particularly robust and will typically grow at temperatures between 10 and 45°C and at a pH as high as 9.6. They are also able to maintain viability after being heated at 60°C for 30 min and these features may contribute to their differentiation from closely related genera. *Pseudomonas aeruginosa* is able to grow at 42°C unlike the closely related *Pseudomonas fluorescens* and *Pseudomonas putida*. *Listeria* spp. are able to grow at 4°C thus distinguishing them from *Erysipelothrix* and *Lactobacillus* spp.

As well as the ability to grow or survive at extremes of temperature, the behaviour of bacteria may vary according to the temperature of incubation. This is not surprising, as 37°C is higher than the optimal temperature for a number of pathogenic bacteria. For example, *Listeria* spp. show characteristic tumbling motility at 22°C but are sluggishly motile or non-motile at 37°C. *Yersinia pseudotuberculosis* is also motile at 22°C but not at 37°C. Biochemical characteristics of bacteria may also vary and this is classically seen with *Yersinia* spp. For example, *Yersinia enterocolitica* is much more likely to demonstrate motility, ornithine decarboxylase, β-galactosidase and a positive VP reaction at 22°C rather than 37°C. The ability to grow in different atmospheric conditions may also be highly useful in bacterial identification.

2.6 Requirement for growth factors

The growth requirements of bacteria can be exploited for the identification of species as best illustrated by the requirements of *Haemophilus*. On primary isolation, all species of *Haemophilus* require either X factor (haemin or haematin) or V factor (nicotinamide adenine dinucleotide), or both, for growth. These requirements can be demonstrated by inoculating a suspect strain of *Haemophilus* onto a basic medium (without blood) and placing paper discs impregnated with X, V, and X + V onto the surface of the medium. Nutrient agar has traditionally been used for X and V tests but brain heart infusion agar, trypticase soy agar, and Mueller Hinton agar have also been recommended. Following incubation, growth should only be visible around the discs that provide the factors necessary for growth. For example, *H. influenzae* is the most frequent *Haemophilus* spp. isolated in clinical laboratories and requires both X and V factors to grow. Growth will therefore only occur around the disc containing both growth factors. Identification of the requirement for X and V assists with discrimination between species. The requirement for growth factors (particularly the requirement for X) can be lost during serial subculture and this has been well documented with certain species, for example *H. aphrophilus*. As with any test for growth factor dependence, great care should be taken to use a modest inoculum and to avoid the transfer of nutrients that may contaminate the bacterial inoculum.

2.7 **Identification schemes**

We have discussed the principles of a range of biochemical tests. To assign a bacterial strain to a particular species, it is often necessary to perform a battery of tests to obtain a 'biochemical profile'. The choice of which biochemical tests to perform will be based on the results of preliminary observations such as colonial appearance, interpretation of Gram stain, etc. Table 2.1 shows a simple test scheme for identification of a suspect strain of Enterobacteriaceae from a urine sample using six biochemical tests for fermentation of glucose and cellobiose, hydrolysis of urea, production of indole, and decarboxylation of lysine and ornithine. For most commonly encountered species, a reliable identification is provided. Problems arise when uncommon urinary pathogens such as *Salmonella* spp. or *Kluyvera* spp. are encountered and these are likely to be misidentified.

To ensure accurate identification of a wider range of species, including those that are rarely encountered, a wider range of biochemical tests must be employed and, in general, the more tests that are used, the more accurate the identification. This is facilitated by the availability of commercial identification kits and automated identification systems.

Cross reference

See Chapter 3.

Biochemical tests may be useful for the rapid exclusion of pathogens such as *Salmonella* species. For example, xylose lysine deoxycholate (XLD) medium is used to screen for the presence of *Salmonella* which typically forms black colonies on this medium. The black colour results from production of hydrogen sulphide and indicates that the colonies are likely to be produced by one of three genera (*Proteus*, *Citrobacter*, or *Salmonella*). These three genera can be distinguished by two simple biochemical tests as follows:

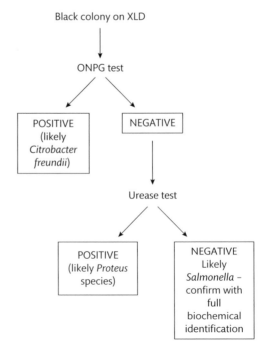

Alternatively, the use of a greater number of biochemical tests can be used to confirm a species identification. In this example four tests can be used to confirm the likely species of a lactose-fermenting 'coliform' recovered from a urine sample on CLED or MacConkey medium. Six species can be differentiated in this way.

Lactose-fermenting Gram-negative rod

2.8 **Commercial kits**

A wide range of commercial kits are available from a number of manufacturers for the identification of bacteria. Typically, these consist of a plastic strip with compartments or wells containing dehydrated growth media and metabolic substrates. Manual inoculation of a bacterial suspension of known density is then required to re-hydrate the contents of the wells. Following incubation, the wells of the strip are observed for growth and/or colour changes. Manual addition of reagents is often required for some of the tests to be interpreted. In 1971, the first evaluation of the API 20 E was reported. This strip comprised a gallery of 20 biochemical tests including nine distinct sugar fermentation tests. Following addition of reagents to three of the tests, and interpretation of colour changes in all 20 wells, a seven-digit profile is generated. This profile number is then computed using dedicated software to give the most likely identification of the strain. These strips allow for the discrimination and identification of over 100 species and are widely used today.

FIGURE 2.8

Identification of *Stenotrophomonas maltophilia* using the API 20 NE. The strain shows reduction of nitrate, hydrolysis of esculin, liquefaction of gelatin, and production of β-galactosidase. In addition, the strain is able to utilize any of several substrates as a sole source of carbon, including glucose, mannose, *N*-acetyl glucosamine, maltose, malic acid, and citrate.

Source: Courtesy of J. Perry.

The last 30 years have seen the development of API galleries designed for the identification of most other clinically important species. Some groups of bacteria do not readily acidify sugars and the most useful way to identify these is with the use of 'assimilation tests'. In such tests, a minimal growth medium in which the bacteria do not grow is supplemented with a single substrate, which offers the bacteria its only significant source of carbon. The ability of the bacteria to metabolize this substrate will result in growth and therefore a positive test. Carbon source assimilation tests are a major feature of the API 20 NE (Figure 2.8) (for non-enteric Gram-negative bacteria, e.g. *Pseudomonas* spp.) and the API Campy strip (for *Campylobacter* spp.).

In addition to the API strip, a wide range of identification systems based on similar principles are available from a number of manufacturers. Examples of kits for the identification of Enterobacteriaceae include the GN2 MicroPlate (Biolog Inc.), the Crystal E/NF (Becton Dickinson), the Microbact (Oxoid), and the Micro-ID (Remel). There are ample comparisons of the performance of these kits published in microbiology journals to allow potential users to assess their relative attributes and limitations.

SELF-CHECK 2.8

What are the advantages of using commercial kit systems such as API for the identification of microorganisms?

2.9 Automated systems

Biochemical tests that do not require addition of reagents after incubation lend themselves to automation. Cards containing panels of miniaturized biochemical tests (Figure 2.9) may be inoculated with a standardized bacterial suspension and then monitored during incubation by sophisticated optical readers for changes in turbidity or development of colour or fluorescence due to hydrolysis of enzyme substrates. Since the early 1980s, automated instruments have been available for both bacterial identification and antimicrobial susceptibility testing. A number of systems are available for automated identification including the Microscan WalkAway (Siemens), Vitek 2 (bioMérieux), BD Phoenix (Becton Dickenson), Trek Sensititre (Sensititre), and the GN2 MicroPlate (Biolog). For some rapidly growing bacteria (e.g. strains of Enterobacteriaceae) some automated systems may generate an identification result in as little as 2–3 h.

A somewhat different approach is employed in the GN2 MicroPlate system (Biolog). The system utilizes a 96-well microtitre plate and each test well contains a different carbon source. The test strain is inoculated into all wells, which also contain a tetrazolium dye. If the strain is able to utilize the carbon source, microbial growth causes reduction of the dye and generation of a purple colour. This results in the generation of a carbon source metabolic 'fingerprint'. The trays can be used manually with visual recording of the results or as part of a fully automated system. Identification of at least 526 species or taxa is possible including Enterobacteriaceae, non-fermenters, and fastidious organisms. For some species, identification can be achieved in 4 h.

Scientific evaluations of commercially available products may show a wide range of accuracy, most often due to differences in study design, and it is prudent to review a number of published evaluations. There are a number of systems with essentially equivalent performances and other factors such as cost, patient population, throughput, and workflow play an important part in selection. A detailed description of some of these systems has recently been reviewed (see Further reading).

FIGURE 2.9

Identification cards used in the Vitek 2 automated system for the identification of bacteria. The 64-well card includes 47 biochemical reactions which are all colorimetric and are monitored by the optical readers of the instrument. Chromogenic substrates for detection of hydrolases include those based on *p*-nitrophenol and indoxyl (for detection of glycosidases and esterases) and *p*-nitroaniline and dichloroaminopenol (for detection of peptidases). The identification profile that is generated for Gram-negative organisms allows differentiation of 55 genera and 130 species of Enterobacteriaceae and non-fermentative Gram-negative bacilli.

Source: Courtesy of M. Ford.

Matrix-assisted laser desorption ionization time-of-flight (MALDI-TOF) mass spectrometry is increasingly used for microbial identification by many large diagnostic laboratories. The technique is used to generate a spectrum or profile of the most highly abundant proteins that are present in bacteria and other microbes (e.g. fungi) to generate a 'molecular fingerprint'. The generated spectrum (Figure 2.10) is then matched to an extensive library of spectra from known species in order to assign identification to species level.

In its simplest format, a smear of the test microbe is inoculated onto a steel plate or 'target'. A small amount (1 µL) of matrix solution is then added and allowed to dry. The target is then introduced to the fully automated mass spectrometer and species-level identification can be available in less than 10 minutes. The target can accommodate up to 96 different isolates thereby allowing batch testing.

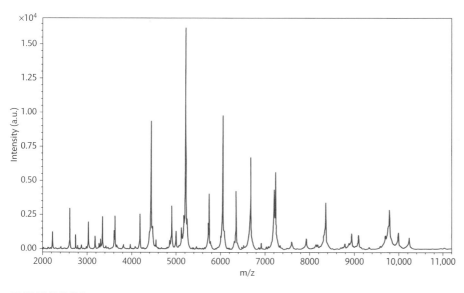

FIGURE 2.10

MALDI-TOF generated spectrum of *P. aeruginosa* showing the protein peaks which identify the organism.

Source: Courtesy of Craig Parker: Bruker.

The method is extremely simple and requires no previous knowledge or expertise with mass spectrometry. Although the instrumentation is relatively expensive (> £100,000) the consumable costs are very inexpensive when compared with conventional biochemical identification systems. This makes MALDI-TOF an attractive option for laboratories with a high throughput of isolates for identification. The main advantages are its speed and simplicity and also the fact that (for most organisms) only a single colony is required for testing. There are limitations of MALDI-TOF in its ability to differentiate between certain closely related species. Some of these are significant such as its inability to reliably differentiate *E. coli* from species of *Shigella*, and its inability to differentiate *Streptococcus pneumoniae* from some commensal streptococci. An extraction protocol is available to obtain identification results directly from positive blood cultures with a success rate of around 80%.

2.10 Immunological tests

The surface of a bacterial cell contains a variety of antigens that may be targeted by antibodies so that a signal is generated when a specific antigen–antibody reaction occurs. In the simplest immunological tests, a bacterial suspension is mixed on a glass slide with a suspension of unlabelled antibody and the mixture is gently agitated and observed for visual agglutination. This results from an antibody, which has two identical variable regions that can interact with antigen, interacting with more than one bacterial cell and causing clumps of organisms bound to antibody. Such agglutination tests are widely used for the detection of somatic polysaccharide ('O' antigens) present in the Gram-negative outer membrane. Agglutination tests are widely used for differentiation of species of *Shigella*, for typing within the genus *Salmonella* and for differentiation of *E. coli* that cause diarrhoea (e.g. *E. coli* O157). Typing of *Salmonella* flagella (H) is also routinely sought using agglutination tests. Cross reactions between *Salmonella* antibodies and other species of Enterobacteriaceae are common and it is necessary to confirm the identity of *Salmonella* and *Shigella* spp. using biochemical tests as well as agglutination tests.

The interaction of antibody and antigen resulting in agglutination can be magnified by using a latex agglutination test. In such a test, latex particles of approximately 1 µm in diameter are coated with antibody and then mixed with a bacterial suspension. If specific antigens are present on the cell surface agglutination is readily visible as the latex particles leave the milky suspension and form clumps due to the antigen–antibody reaction. Commercially available latex reagents have become widely used for the detection of Gram-positive pathogens such as *S. aureus* and *S. pneumoniae*. Latex particles for detection of *S. aureus* may be coated with a number of distinct monoclonal antibodies targeting cell surface antigens and may also be coated with fibrinogen to detect 'clumping factor'. Some other species of staphylococci can generate specific agglutination reactions such as *S. intermedius* and *S. lugdunensis* although these are relatively uncommon.

The latex agglutination test is also widely used for identification of haemolytic streptococci of groups A, B, C, F, and G. The letters designate carbohydrate antigens present in the cell wall and these may be readily extracted using simple enzymatic methods or chemicals such as nitrous acid. Some bacteria are capable of causing apparent clumping of latex particles that is unrelated to specific antigen–antibody reactions. For this reason it is essential to perform a negative control, usually consisting of latex reagent without specific antibody, to exclude non-specific latex agglutination.

2.11 Pitfalls and quality issues with biochemical identification tests

The most fundamental point for any identification test or kit is the necessity for pure cultures. Ideally, the inoculum for identification tests should originate from a single well-isolated colony but this is not possible for some commercial kits as they require a high inoculum. Some selective culture media will inhibit bacterial growth but do not kill bacteria and it is possible that viable bacteria that are not visible may be inadvertently included in the inoculum for identification tests.

When bacteria are inoculated into identification media and incubated overnight, a suitable non-selective culture plate should always be inoculated and incubated concomitantly. Before the results of any biochemical tests are interpreted, the purity of the inoculum must be confirmed by examination of the subculture (often termed a 'purity plate'). This safeguard is compromised when rapid identification tests are performed and results are reported in 4–6 h, before purity can be verified. Some automated systems may be able to detect the likelihood of a mixed inoculum but this cannot be guaranteed and if there is any question about the purity of the inoculum, this should be resolved before any conclusions are drawn.

Biochemical identification is also compromised by bacteria that behave atypically. For example, auxotrophic mutants may arise that are dependent on growth factors, for example thymidine-dependent S. aureus or E. coli, and such strains may not produce expected reactions in identification tests. With highly atypical or rarely encountered strains the identification process can seem more like an art form than a scientific process and the microbiologist must assimilate all of the available information about the strain and use all of his or her experience. In addition to the results of biochemical tests, all of the following may prove useful to point the microbiologist in the right direction: colony morphology, Gram stain, atmospheric growth requirements (e.g. requirement for carbon dioxide), antimicrobial susceptibility pattern, ability to grow on a range of media (e.g. requirement for blood), and seemingly extraneous information such as the site of isolation (blood, urine, etc.), clinical details of the patient, antibiotic therapy, etc.

Reagents for performing identification tests such as catalase and oxidase reagents or latex agglutination reagents should be tested with control organisms that give positive and negative results to ensure adequate performance, and results should be documented. This should be performed either daily or whenever a test is carried out. Identification media should also be inoculated with controls. Strains obtained from recognized culture collections with well-defined characteristics should be used as control organisms.

Chapter summary

After reading this chapter you should know and understand:

- The importance of biochemical tests in the identification process.

- The most important biochemical tests used in microbiology and how these tests work and are performed.

- How susceptibility patterns can aid in the identification of specific organisms or groups of organisms.

- How tests are performed routinely by use of commercial kit systems, e.g. API kits.

- The role and methodology of immunological tests for bacterial identification.

- The advantages and disadvantages associated with automated identification of microorganisms, including MALDI-TOF.

- Problems associated with identification of bacteria.

 Further reading

- **Barrow GI, Feltham RKA, eds.** *Cowan and Steel's Manual for the Identification of Medical Bacteria*, **3rd edition. Cambridge University Press, 2008.**

  A recommended, comprehensive overview of biochemical tests for identification of medically important bacteria.

- **MacFaddin J.** *Biochemical Tests for Identification of Medical Bacteria*. **Williams & Wilkins, 1999.**

  Another recommended, comprehensive overview of biochemical tests for identification of medically important bacteria.

- **O'Hara CM. Manual and automated instrumentation for identification of Enterobacteriaceae and other aerobic Gram-negative bacilli.** *Clinical Microbiology Reviews* **2005; 18: 147–162.**

  A useful review for further information on automated systems for microbial identification and susceptibility testing.

- **Orenga S, James AL, Manafi M, Perry JD, Pincus DH. Enzymatic substrates in microbiology (review).** *Journal of Microbiological Methods* **2009; 79: 139–155.**

  A detailed overview of enzyme substrates used in microbiology including automated instruments.

 Discussion questions

2.1   Do you believe it is necessary to identify all organisms isolated from culture? If not, which organisms do you need to identify? Provide reasons for your answer.

2.2   Do you believe automated identification systems will replace biochemical and immunological identification tests? If not, why not?

3

Culture media

John Perry

In 1890, Robert Koch published four criteria designed to establish a causal relationship between a microbe and a disease. One of these stipulated that the microorganisms must be isolated from the diseased individual and grown in pure culture. Despite over 120 years of advances in diagnostic microbiology, the use of culture media remains central to the diagnosis of most bacterial and fungal infections in any clinical microbiology laboratory.

Pathological specimens are referred to the laboratory for diagnosis and are typically inoculated onto one or more culture media. Following incubation, microbial colonies are identified to detect pathogenic bacteria thus assisting the diagnosis of infection. A wide range of media are available for assisting the isolation and identification of numerous pathogenic species and this chapter will review the types of media available, how they work, and how they are prepared.

Learning objectives

After studying this chapter you should be able to:

- Identify the basic growth requirements of bacteria including some fastidious bacteria.
- Identify the basic ingredients of culture media and the contribution of specific supplements.
- Give examples of selective, differential, and enrichment media and what they are used for.
- Explain the principles of chromogenic media and provide examples of their use.
- Understand the principles and pitfalls of media preparation.
- Explain how media are assessed for quality and performance.

3.1 Microbial requirements for growth

A bacterial culture medium must provide all of the nutritional requirements for the bacterial species it is expected to recover. All bacteria require a range of elements in order to grow; these include carbon, oxygen, hydrogen, and nitrogen which are constituents of amino acids; sulphur for the synthesis of amino acids such as cysteine and methionine; phosphorus for nucleic acids. Potassium, magnesium, and calcium are major cellular cations and iron is an important component of cytochromes. Trace elements such as manganese, cobalt and zinc are also important as co-factors for enzymes.

Bacteria encountered in the clinical laboratory are heterotrophic and therefore need to be supplied with organic compounds in order to grow. Their requirements may vary widely, for example some species such as *Pseudomonas aeruginosa* are able to grow on a culture medium containing only a single source of carbon, such as acetate. This is remarkable when one considers the vast diversity of carbon-containing compounds that *Pseudomonas* spp. will need to synthesize in order to grow. Other bacteria may be more demanding and require other **growth factors** such as vitamins, purines, and pyrimidines, or specific amino acids. Bacteria that require a range of growth factors are termed **fastidious**. Occasionally, strains of bacteria lose their innate ability to synthesize a compound essential for growth. Such strains are termed auxotrophic and therefore rely upon the addition of this compound as a growth factor.

growth factor

A growth factor is a specific compound that is required for growth of a particular organism. As it cannot be synthesized it must be added to culture media in order to allow growth.

fastidious

Fastidious organisms require a number of growth factors.

SELF-CHECK 3.1

Why do microorganisms require so many different types of nutrients for growth?

3.2 Ingredients of culture media

Media may be 'chemically defined', which means that the composition has been formulated using known amounts of pure chemical compounds. Such media are invaluable for studying the growth requirements of bacteria and for studies of bacterial metabolism. In practice, culture media used by diagnostic laboratories are not defined as they contain extracts of complex biological materials of which the exact composition is unknown. The reasons for this are convenience and the fact that bacteria generally grow better on complex undefined media. Some common constituents of complex culture media are listed in the next subsections.

3.2.1 Water

A culture medium typically comprises >90% water. Water makes up 80–90% of the bacterial cell and is the solvent in which all metabolic processes take place. Deionized water is usually recommended for media preparation as tap water may have a variable mineral content and some constituents can be harmful to microorganisms.

3.2.2 Protein derivatives

Digests or extracts of protein are major constituents of most culture media. 'Peptones' are very commonly used and these consist of the water-soluble products generated when a suitable protein source is digested with proteolytic enzymes, for example, trypsin. Suitable protein sources include meat, soya flour, and casein. The products of digestion include a variety of compounds to support bacterial growth including peptides, amino acids, phosphate, various metal ions in trace amounts, and potential growth factors such as nicotinic acid and riboflavin. A good peptone can be dissolved in water, and without other additives can provide a good medium for growth of many commonly encountered bacteria, for example *E. coli* and *S. aureus*.

Another common source of nutrients is provided by extracting the water-soluble components of protein. For example, using methods originally devised by Liebig, lean finely divided beef may be infused with boiling water to extract its water-soluble components. Following removal of fats, these components may be concentrated to produce a powdered 'meat extract' or 'meat infusion'. This is a rich source of nutrients and includes nitrogenous compounds such as amino acids, purines, and glutathione as well as salt and other minerals and a range of potential growth factors. The combination of peptone and meat extracts is frequently used in the formulation of commercially produced culture media.

Key Point

Media used in clinical microbiology are not strictly defined in terms of their chemical composition and are mostly based on extracts or digests of animal or plant tissues that are chemically complex.

3.2.3 Yeast extract

Cells of brewer's or baker's yeast may be lysed by gentle heat or chemical methods and the insoluble cellular material (e.g. cell walls) removed by filtration. The resulting product is a rich mix of a wide range of amino acids, carbohydrate (e.g. glycogen), minerals, and growth factors (especially of the vitamin B group).

3.2.4 Gelling agents

In order to separate different bacterial species from a polymicrobial inoculum it is necessary to obtain isolated colonies on a solid medium. Agar is by far the most widely used and convenient gelling agent for solidifying culture media. Agar is a product of various seaweeds and is extracted as an aqueous solution at temperatures above 100°C. Its attributes include the fact that it is relatively inert, it has convenient solidifying and melting temperatures (38°C and 84°C respectively), and has high gel strength at a relatively low concentration (1%). Agar may contain unwanted, or even toxic, substances including inorganic salts and long chain fatty acids. These are normally removed during processing to produce a final product with low toxicity and high clarity. Typically, microbial culture media are poured into sterile Petri dishes, normally 90 mm in diameter. Media can also be poured as slopes so organisms can be stored for long periods or onto plastic carriers which are used as dipslides.

Other solid media that do not contain agar have been used for the isolation of pathogenic bacteria. Gelatine was used as a solidifying agent to create some of the earliest solid culture media and serum or egg can be coagulated by inspissation to create solid media. Löwenstein–Jensen medium is the most widely used egg-based medium and is an effective and economical option for the culture of mycobacteria, including *Mycobacterium tuberculosis*. Whole egg is aseptically removed from its shell and added to a sterile solution of minerals and malachite green. This suspension is then dispensed into sterile bottles and heated at 80–85°C for 45 min using an inspissator. This procedure is used to solidify the medium rather than sterilize it.

3.2.5 Buffers

All bacteria have an optimal pH for growth and a pH range within which they are able to grow but this can vary widely for different bacteria. During growth bacteria may generate acid from carbohydrate or alkali from oxidation of peptone resulting in deviation from optimal pH. For some species this may adversely affect growth or even cause loss of viability.

Phosphate buffers are most commonly used but a wide range is available and the choice of buffer is determined chiefly by the starting pH of the medium. Typically, general-purpose agars are formulated to give a pH of between 7 and 7.5, but use of a different pH may be advantageous. For example, *Vibrio cholerae* is susceptible to acid but grows readily under alkaline conditions. Hence, media for *V. cholerae* are often formulated to give a pH of around 8.5 and this limits the growth of competitors. In contrast, media for the isolation of pathogenic yeasts, such as Sabouraud agar, have a pH of around 5.6.

SELF-CHECK 3.2

Why do you think most culture media have a pH of 7 to 7.5 and why is it important to maintain this pH during bacterial growth?

3.2.6 Blood and serum

Blood from various mammals (including man) may be collected aseptically and used to supplement or enrich sterilized media to improve the growth of fastidious bacteria. Horse blood (mainly) or sheep blood are most commonly used. Blood is normally defibrinated to prevent it from clotting and this is preferable to the addition of anticoagulants that may interfere with bacterial growth. It is also important, as with any culture ingredient derived from biological material, to ensure that the blood is free from infective agents and antibiotics. Addition of blood or serum improves the growth of a range of fastidious bacteria and allows the demonstration of haemolysis, which may be useful for identification.

SELF-CHECK 3.3

What are the advantages of using horse blood as the main blood supplement in culture media? Why is human blood not routinely used?

3.2.7 Charcoal

Activated charcoal is porous and has a very large surface area. It has a tendency to adsorb a range of molecules to its surface by both physical and chemical means and it is used in culture media to bind compounds that may be toxic to growth. Some bacteria have a tendency to generate toxic products such as peroxide free radicals that can inhibit growth. Activated charcoal has been shown to be beneficial when used in culture media for pathogenic Gram-negative rods such as *Bordetella pertussis*, *Campylobacter* spp., *Haemophilus ducreyi*, and *Helicobacter pylori* and it is indispensable for growth of *Legionella* spp. Because of the non-toxic nature of pure activated charcoal, it can be used in general-purpose broth media for the culture of blood and can assist in the adsorption of antimicrobial compounds. Other substances included in media, such as starch and blood, may also reduce the effect of potentially toxic products of metabolism.

3.2.8 Other additives for fastidious bacteria and anaerobes

Glucose may be added to culture media as a ready source of energy and promotes the growth of a number of species. For example, it is included in agar media for *Brucella* spp. and in brain heart infusion broth, which is used for the cultivation of fastidious organisms. For fastidious bacteria, growth factors may need to be added. If the exact growth requirements are known, specific compounds can be added, for example, nicotinic acid is added to culture media for the isolation of *Bordetella pertussis*. Alternatively, commercial companies supply nutritional supplements that consist of a concentrate of vitamins and other potential growth factors. Examples include Vitox and IsoVitaleX and these are particularly useful for inclusion in media for the isolation of *Neisseria gonorrhoeae*.

Cultivation of anaerobic bacteria can be particularly challenging as some Gram-negative species are fastidious in their growth requirements and oxygen may be toxic to some anaerobes, although tolerance varies between species. To address these needs specialized media have been developed that are supplemented with growth factors and reducing agents to maintain a low redox potential in the culture medium. Growth factors include haemin, menadione, and succinate for fastidious Gram-negative rods such as *Porphyromonas* spp., *Prevotella* spp., and *Bacteroides* spp. Reducing agents may include L-cysteine, dithiothreitol, and sodium thioglycolate.

Isolation of spore-bearing anaerobes may also be difficult, but for different reasons. *Clostridium difficile*, as implied by its name, is a case in point. Spores may take some 'persuasion' to germinate on synthetic media and compounds that initiate spore germination can substantially increase the yield of *C. difficile* from stool samples. Examples of such compounds include lysozyme and certain bile salts such as sodium taurocholate.

3.3 **Selective media**

Antibiotics or other chemical inhibitors of growth can be added to general-purpose media to inhibit the growth of commensal bacteria and thus increase the likelihood of isolating target pathogens. *Staphylococcus aureus* is the most commonly encountered pathogen associated with infections of skin and wounds. Some wounds, particularly from the lower body, may be dirty and contain faecal flora including strains of Enterobacteriaceae such as *Escherichia coli* and *Proteus* spp. The large colonies formed by Enterobacteriaceae and the swarming growth of *Proteus* sp. may mask the presence of *S. aureus* colonies on general-purpose culture media such as blood agar. It can therefore by advantageous to include a **selective agent** to inhibit the growth of Gram-negative bacteria and increase the likelihood of recovering *S. aureus*. A useful selective agent for this purpose is aztreonam, which inhibits Gram-negative bacteria including most strains of Enterobacteriaceae and *Pseudomonas aeruginosa* (Figure 3.1). Studies have shown that the use of blood agar containing up to 32 mg/L of aztreonam can increase the isolation rate of *S. aureus* from wound swabs compared with blood agar alone.

The growth of Enterobacteriaceae may also mask the presence of anaerobic bacteria such as *Bacteroides fragilis* and anaerobic streptococci. The inclusion of 30 mg/L nalidixic acid inhibits

selective agent
A selective agent is an antimicrobial substance that is incorporated into culture media to inhibit the growth of unwanted commensal bacteria thus assisting the isolation of target pathogens.

FIGURE 3.1
Culture of a leg ulcer swab on blood agar with an apparent pure growth of coliform (left). Culture of the same swab on blood agar plus aztreonam (right) reveals the presence of *Staphylococcus aureus*.
Source: Courtesy of M. Ford/J. Perry.

the growth of most Enterobacteriaceae and allows the growth of these anaerobes. Nalidixic acid is generally inhibitory to strains of clostridia, and if *Clostridium* infection is suspected on clinical grounds, a more appropriate selective agar would be blood agar supplemented with neomycin. The commonest pathogen from upper respiratory tract infection is *Haemophilus influenzae* and this is typically diagnosed by culture of sputum. If *H. influenzae* is present, it is typically there in large numbers and isolation on chocolate agar is normally straightforward. In some cases, sputa may be heavily contaminated by oral streptococci and these may complicate the isolation of small numbers of *H. influenzae*. Many laboratories therefore employ chocolate agar supplemented with an anti-Gram-positive antimicrobial, bacitracin, to increase the isolation rate of *H. influenzae*.

In some cases, a cocktail of antibiotics may be employed to drastically reduce the amount of normal flora and therefore optimize the chances of recovering target pathogens. Stool samples typically contain a wide variety of Gram-negative and Gram-positive flora and consequently the isolation of *Campylobacter* spp. would be almost impossible without the use of selective agents. Traditionally, a cocktail of agents has been used, for example, Skirrow's formulation includes vancomycin, polymyxin, and trimethoprim for inhibition of commensal faecal flora. A similar cocktail of agents is applied in the isolation of *Neisseria gonorrhoeae* from urethral and endocervical swabs. For example, modified New York City medium contains vancomycin, colistin, trimethoprim, and amphotericin B. Vancomycin may be inhibitory to a small proportion of *Neisseria gonorrhoeae* strains and the inclusion of lincomycin, in place of vancomycin, is preferred by some laboratories. The activity of trimethoprim is reduced or abolished in the presence of thymidine, which may be present in small amounts in nutrient media. It is therefore customary to include either lysed or laked blood in selective media that contain trimethoprim. Erythrocytes from horses contain an enzyme, thymidine phosphorylase, which can inactivate thymidine thus allowing trimethoprim to exert its activity.

SELF-CHECK 3.4

What would be useful antimicrobial agents for the selective isolation of (a) Gram-negative bacteria and (b) Gram-positive bacteria?

3.4 Differential media

Ideally, for dedicated media that target a specific pathogen, the growth of all other bacteria and fungi would be suppressed using selective agents. In such a scenario only growth of the pathogen would occur and biochemical identification would be unnecessary. In practice, it is extremely difficult to inhibit all unwanted bacteria using selective agents and particularly those that are closely related to the target pathogen. In such cases it may be useful to incorporate a 'detection system' into the culture medium that will highlight a particular metabolic activity thus providing differentiation of the target pathogen from other species that are able to grow on the medium. Such media are described as **differential media**.

By far the commonest means of highlighting a metabolic feature is the use of carbohydrates, which may be used by bacteria to generate acid and this can be highlighted using a suitable pH indicator. A suitable example is cystine lactose electrolyte deficient (CLED) medium, which is a non-selective medium used principally for the cultivation of urinary tract pathogens. The inclusion of lactose, and bromothymol blue as a pH indicator, allows the differentiation of species and provides clues to their likely identity. So, for example, *Proteus* spp. produce medium-sized, blue colonies due to an inability to acidify lactose whereas enterococci form much smaller yellow colonies due to acidification of lactose. The swarming of *Proteus* spp. is inhibited by the absence of electrolytes (e.g. sodium chloride) in the medium. Some brands of CLED medium include Andrade indicator in addition to bromothymol blue to provide a greater range of colours produced by lactose fermenters (red–yellow) and thus provide enhanced differentiation of colony types.

Key Point

Differential media allow the distinction of different species based on their biochemical reactions. This results in different species forming different coloured colonies, usually as a result of their ability to produce acid from a sugar in the presence of a pH indicator.

In practice, most differential media incorporate selective agents and may therefore be described as selective and differential. A suitable example is mannitol salt agar, which highlights *S. aureus* as large yellow colonies due to mannitol fermentation in the presence of phenol red indicator. This provides differentiation from some other species of staphylococci and most notably the commonest commensal of the skin, *Staphylococcus epidermidis*, which fails to ferment mannitol (Figure 3.2). However, mannitol salt agar is also selective due to the inclusion of a high concentration of sodium chloride (up to 7.5%) resulting in the inhibition of most Gram-negative bacteria and some Gram-positive species.

The use of media that are both selective and differential is employed for the detection of enteric pathogens such as *Salmonella* and *Shigella*. Traditional media for isolation of *Salmonella* have relied on the fact that *Salmonella* (a) does not usually ferment lactose and (b) typically generates hydrogen sulphide from sulphur-containing compounds such as thiosulphate. One of several media that exploits these attributes of *Salmonella* is desoxycholate citrate agar (DCA). This medium employs sodium desoxycholate and sodium citrate as selective agents and also contains a pH indicator (neutral red) plus lactose as well as chemicals for the demonstration of hydrogen sulphide production (sodium thiosulphate/ferric citrate). Most species of Enterobacteriaceae ferment lactose and therefore grow as pink/red colonies; *Shigella* are unreactive on the medium and are therefore colourless or very pale pink due to late fermentation of lactose. Salmonella are colourless due to the absence of lactose fermentation but colonies usually show a black centre due to generation of hydrogen sulphide, which subsequently reacts with iron to form the black precipitate (Figure 3.3). This classical methodology has been widely used for detection of *Salmonella* and *Shigella* but is relatively non-specific. For example, *Proteus* spp. are common in stool samples, are always non-fermenters of lactose and frequently generate hydrogen sulphide. They are therefore frequently confused with *Salmonella*

FIGURE 3.2
Differentiation of *Staphylococcus aureus* (left) from *Staphylococcus epidermidis* (right) using mannitol salt agar.
Source: Courtesy of J. Perry.

FIGURE 3.3

Growth of *Salmonella enteritidis* showing typical black colonies on XLD.

Source: Courtesy of Emma Marrs.

or *Shigella* and require other tests such as biochemical screening to differentiate them from *Salmonella* in particular.

A much more ingenious approach is utilized in xylose lysine deoxycholate medium (XLD), which can detect up to five distinct metabolic activities and can therefore detect *Salmonella* and *Shigella* with higher specificity. This medium contains three carbohydrates, xylose, lactose, and sucrose, any of which may be fermented to generate acid and thus cause bacterial colonies to appear yellow in the presence of phenol red. The vast majority of Enterobacteriaceae, except *Shigella* spp., ferment at least one or more of these three sugars and therefore appear as yellow colonies. *Salmonella* spp. typically ferment the small amount of xylose present to generate acid but then proceed to decarboxylate lysine to cause a rise in pH to at least 7.0. At this pH, the generation of hydrogen sulphide is possible and *Salmonella* therefore generate black colonies. Other common producers of hydrogen sulphide (e.g. *Proteus* spp. and *Citrobacter freundii*) do not possess the enzyme to decarboxylate lysine and are not able to demonstrate hydrogen sulphide production at low pH. Some species of Enterobacteriaceae (e.g. *Providencia* spp.) may not undergo any of these reactions and consequently may resemble *Shigella* spp.

> **Key Point**
>
> In practice, most differential media contain selective agents and may also be classed as selective media.

3.5 Enrichment media

Enrichment media are broth media that are useful for recovery of small numbers of target pathogens that may be present in clinical samples alongside larger numbers of non-target commensal bacteria. Some broth media are completely non-selective and their function is simply to amplify the numbers of any bacteria that are able to grow. Brain heart infusion broth (BHI) is one such medium and is useful for supporting the growth of fastidious bacteria. Robertson's cooked meat broth is another example and is helpful for the isolation of anaerobes. Non-selective broth media that can support fastidious bacteria (e.g. BHI and trypticase soy broth) are used for the culture of blood to detect bacteraemia and these are discussed in more detail in Chapter 5.

Enrichment media are broth media that are designed to favour the growth of target pathogens and discourage the growth of commensals. By achieving this, small numbers of pathogenic bacteria are able to multiply more rapidly than competitors and may then be readily isolated following subculture of the broth onto solid media. A good example is alkaline peptone water, which is used for the isolation of *V. cholerae* from stool samples. Alkaline peptone water has a high pH (8.4) and includes sodium chloride (0.5–2%) to encourage rapid growth of *Vibrio* spp. and suppress the growth of other flora (e.g. most Enterobacteriaceae). The alkaline peptone water can then be subcultured after 6–8 h of incubation onto agar media such as thiosulphate–citrate–bile–sucrose (TCBS) to isolate colonies and confirm identification. Selenite F broth is an enrichment medium that is very useful for the isolation of *Salmonella* spp. from stool samples and various modifications are available to optimize the growth of *Salmonella* spp.

3.6 **Chromogenic media**

In Chapter 2, the principles of chromogenic enzyme substrates were described. Chromogenic substrates may be incorporated into agar-based culture media to form **chromogenic media**. Such media often contain selective agents and are therefore both selective and differential. A limited range of chromogenic substrates may be used in an agar-based medium because it is critical that the coloured dye released by hydrolysis does not diffuse in agar. By ensuring that the colour generated remains highly localized on bacterial colonies, this allows differentiation of bacterial colonies producing a particular enzyme from those that do not. For agar media the most widely used substrates are those based on indoxyl (or its halogenated derivatives). Indoxyl may be derivatized to form a phosphate, a glycoside (sugar-derivative) or an ester with a fatty acid (e.g. indoxyl octanoate). Removal of these groups by hydrolysis by a specific enzyme yields free indoxyl, which, in the presence of oxygen, forms an insoluble blue-grey dye. Compounds closely related to indoxyl produce different coloured dyes, for example, 6-chloro-indoxyl forms a pink coloured dye, 5-bromo-6-chloro-indoxyl forms a magenta dye and 5-bromo-4-chloro-indoxyl forms a green dye. Figure 3.4 shows the structure of indoxyl and some halogenated derivatives and all of these may be derivatized to form substrates that are suitable for use in agar media.

> **chromogenic media**
> Chromogenic media are sophisticated differential media. Target pathogens are distinguished on the basis of colour, and the colour originates from hydrolysis of a chromogenic enzyme substrate.

3.6.1 Detection of *Salmonella* and *E. coli* O157 using chromogenic media

One of the first chromogenic media applicable to clinical microbiology was Rambach agar and its performance was first reported in 1990. Rambach agar relies on the fact that the vast majority of *Salmonella* strains encountered in clinical specimens do not produce β-galactosidase. The medium therefore employed a chromogenic substrate for β-galactosidase to enable most common strains of Enterobacteriaceae (e.g. *E. coli*, *Klebsiella* spp., *Enterobacter* spp., *Citrobacter* spp.) to form blue colonies. In order to differentiate *Salmonella* from the remaining flora (e.g. *Proteus* spp., *Pseudomonas* spp.), the medium also contained neutral red indicator and propylene glycol. The latter was fermented by *Salmonella* to generate pink–red colonies. SM-ID agar was designed at around the same time and worked on identical principles except that glucuronic acid was used in place of propylene glycol.

Indoxyl

5-Bromo-4-chloro-indoxyl ('X')

6-Chloro-indoxyl ('Rose')

5-Bromo-6-chloro-indoxyl ('Magenta')

FIGURE 3.4

Structure of commonly used indoxylic dyes.

Source: Courtesy of J. Perry.

Over the last 18 years, chromogenic media for detection of *Salmonella* have evolved and a variety are now available from different manufacturers. Most of these media rely on the fact that *Salmonella* can hydrolyse long chain esters, for example octanoate or nonanoate derivatives of chromogenic dyes. Only a few other species of Enterobacteriaceae produce such esterases and these can be made to produce a different coloration by incorporation of a second chromogenic substrate (e.g. for β-glucosidase). Esterases are also produced by non-fermentative Gram-negative rods and yeasts but their growth can be limited by incorporation of selective agents, for example cefsulodin and amphotericin, respectively.

The main advantage of chromogenic media for isolation of *Salmonella* is their high specificity. Coloured colonies are usually confirmed as *Salmonella* and, when compared with the use of conventional (i.e. non-chromogenic) media, there are far fewer species that resemble *Salmonella*. A disadvantage of chromogenic media for *Salmonella* is that, unlike deoxycholate agar and XLD medium, they do not accommodate the isolation of *Shigella* spp. and therefore two different media need to be used if both pathogens are sought.

E. coli O157 is a cause of haemorrhagic colitis and its presence is sought in diarrhoeal stool samples. Traditional methods rely on the fact that, unlike most *E. coli* strains, this serotype fails to ferment sorbitol. *E. coli* O157 also fails to produce β-glucuronidase and a chromogenic substrate for this enzyme may be used for differentiation. Several media have been developed and marketed using this approach.

SELF-CHECK 3.5

What are the advantages of using chromogenic media for the isolation of *Salmonella* spp. from stool samples?

3.6.2 Detection of *Staphylococcus aureus* (including MRSA) with chromogenic media

The presence of *S. aureus* is routinely sought in swabs from skin and soft tissue infection and there is widespread demand in many hospitals for screening patients and staff for colonization with methicillin-resistant strains (MRSA). Such demand has led to the development of chromogenic media both for the specific detection of *S. aureus* and the specific detection of MRSA. Such media exploit selective agents for the inhibition of Gram-negative bacteria and enterococci. If only methicillin resistant strains are sought, the medium is further supplemented with a β-lactam antibiotic (e.g. oxacillin or cefoxitin) to inhibit methicillin-sensitive strains of staphylococci. There is now good evidence to show that cefoxitin is the preferred of these two options. A chromogenic substrate is then used for the differentiation of *S. aureus* from other staphylococci. Substrates for phosphatase activity or α-glucosidase activity have been shown to be suitable for this purpose.

Cross reference
See Chapter 12, Section 12.2.

3.6.3 Chromogenic media for urinary tract pathogens

E. coli is the predominant species associated with urinary tract infections and other species of Enterobacteriaceae and enterococci are also commonly isolated. Non-selective chromogenic media have been designed to isolate and differentiate all common pathogens associated with urinary tract infection. A number of media are available and most rely on the same principles.

They include chromogenic substrates for the detection of two enzymes, β-galactosidase and β-glucosidase, as well as tryptophan with iron salts in order to detect deaminase activity in the *Proteus–Providencia–Morganella* (PPM) group of species. Production of β-galactosidase generates colonies with a red–pink coloration due to hydrolysis of the chromogenic substrate, whereas production of β-glucosidase generates blue or green colonies. Deamination of tryptophan in the presence of iron results in a diffuse brown coloration.

Approximately 99% of *E. coli* strains produce β-galactosidase, but not β-glucosidase, and they therefore grow as pink or red colonies. The *Klebsiella–Enterobacter–Serratia* (KES) group of species typically produce both of these enzymes and colonies appear predominantly blue. Enterococci also have a strong β-glucosidase activity and also appear blue but are smaller in size. Colonies of the PPM group produce a brown coloration. The reactions shown by representatives of these species are shown in Figure 3.5. Several brands of chromogenic media are available that target the same enzyme activities including UriSelect 4, Chromogenic UTI medium, and CHROMagar Orientation. Additional biochemical tests may be used to confirm the identification of colonies on these chromogenic media including a spot indole test to confirm the identity of *E. coli*. *Citrobacter freundii* is infrequently found in urine samples but, when present, it often grows as pink colonies due to its strong β-galactosidase activity and weak or absent β-glucosidase activity. A rapid indole test can be used on pink colonies to exclude *C. freundii* and thereby provide reliable confirmation of *E. coli* (indole positive).

The CPS ID brand of media (CPS ID2, CPS ID3) operate on slightly different principles in that a chromogenic substrate for β-glucuronidase is used in place of a substrate for β-galactosidase. This strategy has advantages and disadvantages. Firstly, β-glucuronidase is largely restricted to *E. coli* among urinary tract pathogens – the enzyme may be found in *Salmonella*, *Shigella*, and *Yersinia* but these are only rarely encountered in urine. This means that only *E. coli* produce pink colonies and there is arguably no requirement for further confirmation of identity. The disadvantage is that only 94% of *E. coli* strains from urine produce β-glucuronidase and appear as pink colonies and the remaining strains form colourless colonies requiring identification. Members of the KES and PPM groups, as well as enterococci, are distinguished as on the media described previously.

FIGURE 3.5

Differentiation of common urinary tract pathogens using a chromogenic medium. (a) *E. coli* **(producing β-galactosidase), (b)** *Proteus mirabilis* **(producing tryptophan deaminase), (c)** *Klebsiella pneumoniae* **(producing β-galactosidase and β-glucosidase), and (d)** *Enterococcus faecalis* **(producing β-glucosidase).**

Source: Courtesy of J. Perry.

FIGURE 3.6

A contaminated urine specimen cultured on UriSelect 4. On CLED medium (right), a mixture of large and small lactose-fermenting colonies are visible. On the chromogenic medium (left) differentiation of *E. coli* (pink), *Klebsiella pneumoniae* (large blue), and *Enterococcus faecalis* (small turquoise) is significantly easier.

Source: Courtesy of J. Perry.

The most useful aspect of all of these media is their ability to differentiate mixed cultures, which are commonly encountered in urine samples and are often an indication of contamination rather than true polymicrobial infection. Figure 3.6 shows a urine sample that has been cultured simultaneously on cystine–lactose–electrolyte-deficient (CLED) medium and on a chromogenic medium, UriSelect 4. The sample contains *E. coli*, *K. pneumoniae*, and *Enterococcus faecalis*. All of these grow as lactose-fermenting (pink) colonies on CLED medium and their respective numbers are difficult to estimate due to their similar appearance. On UriSelect 4 medium, colony differentiation is much easier due to the different colours generated. Several large studies comparing chromogenic media with conventional media (e.g. MacConkey agar or CLED) have demonstrated that mixed cultures may be detected with significantly higher frequency when using chromogenic media, thus allowing a more accurate diagnosis to be performed. Despite this, many laboratories still use traditional urine media such as MacConkey or CLED, mainly due to cost considerations. Growth of *E. coli* and *P. mirabilis* on MacConkey agar is shown in Figure 3.7.

Key Point

Chromogenic media for urines allows for the specific identification of *E. coli* and the differentiation of other species, thus assisting the recognition of mixed cultures.

FIGURE 3.7

Growth of *E. coli* (left) showing typical pink/red colonies of lactose fermentation. For contrast *P. mirabilis* (right) is shown which fails to ferment lactose.

Source: Courtesy of J. Perry.

3.6.4 Chromogenic media for detection and differentiation of yeasts

A range of chromogenic media is available for detection of yeasts. Such media enable micro-biologists to differentiate between different species unlike conventional media such as Sabouraud agar. There are sound clinical reasons for this, as some *Candida* spp. are intrinsically resistant to some antifungal agents. On conventional media it is virtually impossible to deter-mine if more than one species of *Candida* is present.

A principal feature of these media is the inclusion of a chromogenic substrate for N-acetyl-β-D-glucosaminidase, thus allowing the differentiation and identification of the most frequent and clinically important species, *Candida albicans*. Use of such a substrate (e.g. 5-bromo-4-chloro-3-indolyl-β-D-N-acetyl-glucosaminide) results in *C. albicans* forming characteristic green–blue colonies, although *Candida dubliniensis* cannot be differentiated.

Some chromogenic media for yeasts include a second chromogenic substrate (e.g. for phos-phatase activity) and enable the recognition of species other than *Candida albicans*. CAN2 agar (Figure 3.8) employs two substrates and enables the differentiation of *C. albicans* as green colonies and also the identification of *Candida tropicalis* (blue colonies). Other species form either pink or white colonies. *Candida krusei* may be recognized by the formation of charac-teristic pink, flat colonies.

FIGURE 3.8

The use of chromogenic *Candida* agar to detect mixed yeast cultures. The plate on the left is Sabouraud's dextrose agar and on the right CAN2 agar (bioMérieux) which shows pink colonies of C. *tropicalis* and blue colonies of C. *albicans*. This mixture is very difficult to detect on non-chromogenic media. *Source*: Courtesy of M. Ford.

SELF-CHECK 3.6

Why would it be clinically important to be able to determine that a culture contains more than one species of *Candida*?

3.7 Media for antimicrobial susceptibility testing

As discussed earlier in the chapter, media used in clinical microbiology are not strictly defined in terms of their chemical composition and are mostly based on extracts or digests of animal or plant tissues that are chemically complex. In spite of the great deal of knowl-edge that has been accumulated by microbiologists regarding the growth requirements of bacteria, it has not proved possible to produce chemically defined media that match the performance of complex undefined media. This is not a problem media provided that the performance of different batches of media is consistent. However, complex media are prob-lematic for antimicrobial susceptibility testing. The action of various antibiotics may be adversely affected by media components. For example, thymidine is antagonistic to the action of trimethoprim and the various cations may impact upon the activity of aminoglycosides such as gentamicin.

One solution has been to design culture media that are 'semi-defined' so that complex components are kept to the minimum required for good growth, the presence of antagonists is minimized, and batches of agar may be produced with reproducible performance. Iso-Sensitest agar (or broth), which is widely used in UK laboratories, is specifically designed for susceptibility testing and comprises only around 1.4% (w/v) of undefined content. Over 25 other chemically defined ingredients are included in the medium including glucose, buffer, minerals, and vitamins to ensure satisfactory growth of most commonly encountered bacteria. Fastidious organisms such as streptococci may require the addition of 5% defibrinated horse blood in order to grow well and *Haemophilus* spp. require the further addition of 20 mg/L NAD.

Cross reference
See Chapter 4, Section 4.3.

Mueller–Hinton agar is less defined than Iso-Sensitest agar and contains some 30% (w/v) solids derived from infusion of beef. Historically, the medium has shown problems with batch-to-batch variation in its content of divalent cations and thymidine leading to problems with its consistency of performance. However, Mueller–Hinton agar remains the standard medium for antimicrobial susceptibility testing recommended by the Clinical Laboratory Standards Institute (CLSI) and is used widely in many countries including the United States. Problems have been overcome by ensuring that batches conform with strict performance criteria published by the CLSI, before distribution from manufacturer to laboratory. Wilkins–Chalgren agar has been recommended for the susceptibility testing of anaerobic bacteria. It contains a range of growth factors to support the growth of anaerobes without requiring the addition of blood.

Cross reference
See Section 3.2, this chapter.

3.8 Preparation and sterilization of culture media

Although an increasing number of diagnostic laboratories rely on the purchase of ready-made culture plates from commercial suppliers, many laboratories continue to prepare their own culture media. Invariably, culture media are prepared from fully formulated, dehydrated powders supplied by commercial manufacturers. Therefore, for simple media, laboratory personnel simply have to add water to the powder, sterilize, and dispense the medium into Petri dishes. More complex media may require a number of additives. Some general principles of media preparation are outlined next.

Commercially supplied, dehydrated media should be stored and prepared in strict accordance with manufacturers' instructions. An expiry date will be supplied for each batch of media and this should be strictly adhered to. Dehydrated media are adversely affected by heat and should be stored away from sunlight and other sources of heat such as autoclaves and hot air ovens. They are hygroscopic and therefore highly susceptible to moisture. They must therefore be kept in tightly closed containers and not exposed to the atmosphere unnecessarily. If the medium is no longer 'free-flowing' (i.e. shows evidence of clumping due to absorption of moisture) or becomes discoloured, it should be discarded.

Dehydrated media commonly contain hazardous materials, often incorporated as selective agents, and examples include bile salts, lithium chloride and various dyes. Any hazardous ingredients will be detailed in the Material Safety Data Sheet accompanying the product. Weighing out fine powders is hazardous and requires the use of a weighing station, in which the powder is removed from the air by filters. Personal protective equipment such as a mask and gloves should also be used and laboratory personnel should be familiar with relevant COSHH assessments. To reduce the potential problem of inhalation of toxic substances, some media suppliers offer granulated media containing a lower proportion of fine powder.

Media should be rehydrated with either distilled or deionized water in glassware that has been meticulously cleaned. Thorough mixing is essential to ensure that none of the powder remains adherent to the glassware or floating on the surface of the water. Bottles of media should be clearly labelled using heat sensitive tape that will change colour if the medium has passed through the autoclave, although this is not an indication of sterilization.

3.8.1 Sterilization

This is normally achieved by autoclaving using a standard sterilization cycle, for example 116°C for 20 min or 121°C for 15 min. Bottles of media should be autoclaved with the lids loosened and personal protective equipment should be employed when sterilized media are removed. The autoclave should be dedicated to media preparation and should not be used, for example, for sterilization of bacterial cultures or clinical samples. The temperature of the autoclave should be monitored during the sterilization cycle and records of performance should be kept. After removal from the autoclave, agar media should be cooled to 50°C in a water-bath and dispensed as soon as possible. Prolonged exposure to heat is very damaging to culture media resulting in autooxidation and the formation of **superoxides**.

The use of semiautomated media preparators is advisable for sterilization of large batches of agar-based media (>1 litre). Such instruments perform continuous stirring of the media and therefore allow excellent heat dispersal and minimal overheating. Care must be taken, however, to ensure meticulous rinsing of the drum which holds the medium and the tubing used for dispensing, particularly if different types of media are being prepared using the same instrument. Cross contamination of antimicrobials between batches occurs very readily and is a common source of error. It is therefore advisable to have dedicated instruments (or at least dedicated tubing) for selective media.

Although all culture media will suffer from prolonged heating, some ingredients are more sensitive than others and sugars are particularly susceptible to breakdown. When preparing some selective agars, such as XLD and TCBS, it is sufficient to boil the medium briefly to dissolve all of the constituents and then dispense the medium into Petri dishes. This does not constitute sterilization but the exposure to 100°C combined with the selectivity of the medium obviates any problems of contamination.

For non-selective broth media that do not withstand sterilization via autoclaving, a process known as tyndallization has been traditionally used. This process involves heating the medium at 100°C for 30 min and then incubating overnight at 37°C. This process is then repeated twice. The heating process kills all vegetative bacteria but may not kill all spores. The incubation period is designed to allow the vegetation of any spores, which will subsequently be killed by a further round of heating, and so on. This process is not ideal as it allows for the germination of spores and subsequent bacterial growth that may alter the constituents of the medium. For this reason, and for its general lack of convenience, the method is now infrequently used.

SELF-CHECK 3.7

What types of media supplements are heat sensitive and how is this problem overcome?

3.8.2 Dispensing media

Once the culture medium has been sterilized by an appropriate method, heat sensitive additives such as blood, serum, egg yolk, or antimicrobials may be added as sterile supplements to cold broth media or molten agar at 45–50°C. When adding to agar, supplements should be warmed up to at least room temperature. If supplements are added, these may alter the pH of the medium and checking and/or adjustment of the pH may be necessary. After addition of heat-sensitive supplements, media should be dispensed without delay.

Media should be dispensed into sterile containers (e.g. Petri dishes) in a dedicated, thoroughly clean preparation area using all aseptic precautions. Individual culture plates must be labelled or coded with a unique batch number so that a user can easily tell the exact type of media and its expiry date. Generally, culture plates may be stored for a week at 4°C without loss of performance, or longer if they are sealed to avoid loss of moisture. Some ingredients, such as antibiotics, are relatively labile and it is important for laboratories to establish the 'shelf life' of any culture media. For every batch of media, a record should be available to access the lot numbers of its ingredients as well as details of the sterilization cycle and, if applicable, the automated preparator used for dispensing the media (Figure 3.9).

FIGURE 3.9

An automated media preparator for production of culture plates. The autoclave (left) sterilizes a batch of agar, which is then automatically dispensed at 42°C into sterile Petri dishes.
Source: Courtesy of J. Perry.

3.9 Quality control

Laboratories have an obligation to assess the performance of culture media and they should not be used for diagnostic procedures until performance criteria have been met. The physical attributes of the media may be assessed by simple visual examination and measurement of pH. If these are acceptable, sterility testing and assessment of microbiological performance are then required.

3.9.1 Sterility testing

A random sample of each batch of culture plates and broth media should be incubated at 30°C for at least 24 h and closely examined for microbial colonies. This does not guarantee sterility as some microbes may take days to appear, but most contamination events will be detected by these measures. Any indication of contamination on the surface of the medium or within the medium should prompt disposal of the batch.

3.9.2 Choice of bacterial strains

Microbiological assessment involves the inoculation of culture media with microbial strains of known characteristics to examine their growth and colony appearance. Strains should be derived from a recognized culture collection that is accessible to others such as the National Collection of Type Cultures (NCTC) or the American Type Culture Collection (ATCC). If problems are encountered, testing can then be reproduced by other laboratories or commercial suppliers using the same strains. Such strains are often referred to as 'control strains' and they are generally susceptible to antimicrobial agents. When strains are first obtained from a culture collection, they should be stored to provide a 'seed lot' that can be accessed for subculture at least once a month. The use of control strains that have undergone serial subculture for many weeks should be avoided as strains may lose their characteristics or become contaminated.

Microbiological assessment should be designed to test the major characteristics of the medium and to ensure that media are 'fit for purpose'. So, for example, if a medium is differential, microbiology tests should be performed to demonstrate its ability to differentiate between relevant species and if a medium is selective then the ability of the medium to inhibit relevant species should be demonstrated and so on. So, for example, a general purpose non-selective medium such as blood agar could be inoculated with control strains of *Staphylococcus aureus*, *Escherichia coli*, and *Streptococcus pyogenes*. This will demonstrate the growth of commonly encountered pathogens (both Gram-positive and Gram-negative) as well as the ability of *S. pyogenes* to demonstrate typical β-haemolysis. CLED medium could be inoculated with *E. coli*, *Proteus mirabilis*, and *Enterococcus faecalis* thus assessing the growth of three commonly encountered urinary tract pathogens (both Gram-positive and Gram-negative) and showing the ability of the medium to differentiate between *E. coli* and *P. mirabilis* (based on lactose fermentation) and prevent the swarming growth of *Proteus*. As well as inoculation of test media, it is important to inoculate a medium of proven performance (i.e. from an in-use batch) in order to demonstrate the viability and inoculum level of the test bacteria.

3.9.3 Inoculum

The most common pitfall associated with the assessment of culture media is the use of high inocula. When attempting the isolation of a bacterial pathogen from a pathological sample (e.g. a cerebrospinal fluid) success may depend upon the isolation of only a handful of bacterial colonies. It is therefore of little relevance to assess the performance of a culture medium by inoculating a loopful of growth containing $>10^8$ colony forming units (CFU); however, such practice is commonplace. An ideal inoculum for control strains should deliver no more than 100 CFU onto the culture medium. This will allow a colony count to be performed and this count can be monitored to allow batch to batch comparison of media in order to detect deterioration of performance. Various methods may be used to achieve such inocula and most commonly this involves the preparation of a standardized suspension by measurement of turbidity followed by serial dilution. This is cumbersome and prone to errors and some products are now commercially available to deliver a controlled inoculum onto culture media. Examples include lenticule discs and vitroids, which consist of a small inoculum of microorganisms preserved in a water soluble solid matrix.

There are occasions when it may be appropriate to use a higher inoculum (e.g. at least 1000 CFU) of a control strain. For example, this may be useful for demonstrating the ability of a selective agent to inhibit growth of unwanted bacteria. Similarly, an enrichment broth is most usefully assessed using a low inoculum of target pathogen (100 CFU) along with a higher concentration (1000 CFU) of an unwanted commensal. For example, selenite broth could be inoculated with 100 CFU of *Salmonella enteritidis* and 1000 CFU of *E. coli*. After incubation, subculture onto a medium that demonstrates lactose fermentation (e.g. CLED or MacConkey agar) should demonstrate a predominance of *Salmonella* colonies (non-lactose fermenting). This illustrates that the selenite broth has performed effectively as an enrichment medium for *Salmonella*.

3.9.4 Batch failure

There are a number of potential sources of error that can lead to unacceptable quality or performance of culture media. Assuming that the sterilization cycle has been monitored effectively, most contamination events are due to the inadvertent addition of non-sterile additives. For example, batches of sterile blood may become contaminated during storage and this is usually detected after overnight incubation of culture media. The inclusion of an excessive amount of a selective agent, due to a dilution error, is also a potential source of error. In the event of a failure, all media from the batch should be discarded and an audit conducted to examine all of the steps and ingredients involved in production of the batch.

Once a batch has passed quality assessment it can be released for use in the laboratory. Batch rotation is essential to ensure that media are used in chronological order.

SELF-CHECK 3.8

Why is quality control of media so important?

Chapter summary

After reading this chapter you should know and understand:

- Why culture media are essential in the diagnosis of infection.

- How culture media are produced and the ingredients essential for optimal bacterial growth.

- How the various types of media such as selective media are used in routine microbiology and the types of selective agents used.

- How and why enrichment media are used in the routine laboratory.

- How and why susceptibility test media are used and why they are so different to other culture media.

- The importance of chromogenic media over other more conventional media, and also the advantages and disadvantages of using such media.

- How media are sterilized and the processes involved.

- The importance of quality control of media and how batches of media can fail quality control and what action should be taken.

Further reading

- ***The Oxoid Manual*. Available from Oxoid Ltd, Basingstoke, UK.**

  A comprehensive source of references for conventional culture media and an excellent resource in itself. Contains detailed descriptions of a wide range of media for clinical and food microbiology.

● **Perry JD, Freydiere AM. The application of chromogenic media in clinical microbiology.** *Journal of Applied Microbiology* 2007; **103**: 2046–2055.

Provides a review of the chromogenic media available for detection of clinical pathogens and how they work.

 Discussion questions

3.1 Chromogenic media are gradually replacing more conventional media for the isolation of specific pathogens from clinical samples. Why is this change happening and what are the advantages of this change?

3.2 Do you think the future of microbiology will be to move away from traditional methods of culture and towards more rapid detection methods such as PCR? If not, why not?

3.3 Many laboratories now purchase all media used in their laboratory – do you think this is a good or bad practice? Explain your reasoning.

4

Susceptibility testing and antibiotic assay

Jenny Andrews

antibiotic
An antibiotic is classed as a chemical compound that has the ability to kill or inhibit the growth of microorganisms. They are sufficiently non-toxic to be administered to the host.

Antibiotics have played a major role in the treatment of infectious disease since the discovery of penicillin in the 1920s. Since then hundreds of antibiotics have been made or discovered with a wide range of different properties and activities. Although some antibiotics have been rendered useless by the development of bacterial resistance, there are still a large number available for clinicians to use for the treatment of infection. However, whilst numerous antibiotics are available, laboratory support is required to determine if this is the correct antibiotic for the treatment of a particular infection. Throughout this chapter you will be shown the importance of the laboratory in determining the susceptibility of an organism to an antibiotic, and in the monitoring of the patient's serum for the correct concentration of antibiotic.

The primary purpose of an antimicrobial susceptibility test performed in the laboratory (*in vitro*) is to assist clinicians in the choice of appropriate agents they can use for therapy. As such, it is an essential component of the management of patients that antimicrobial susceptibility is performed and reported in the timeliest manner. Antibiotics are one of the most widely prescribed drugs in the world and almost everyone will undergo at least one course of antibiotics in their lifetime. The importance of antimicrobial therapy is enormous, from both a clinical and laboratory perspective.

Learning objectives

After studying this chapter you should confidently be able to:

- Understand why antimicrobial susceptibility tests are performed.
- Discuss current national/international guidelines and methods available.
- Describe what is meant by intrinsic resistance and in which pathogens it occurs.
- The types and importance of β-lactamases.
- Have a thorough knowledge of commonly used susceptibility test media.
- Assess the significance of MIC and MBC.

- Understand the difference between bacteriostatic and bactericidal agents.
- Understand why combination therapy is used and common synergistic combinations.
- Give clinical reasons for combination therapy and examples.
- Understand procedures for testing for antibiotic synergy between two different agents.
- Understand how resistance markers may prove useful in detecting more widespread resistance to that class of antibiotic (e.g. ESBLs).
- Know the types of antibiotics that require patient's serum level monitoring.
- Understand procedures for monitoring serum antibiotic levels and the principles of the methodology.
- Understand acceptable ranges of peak and trough serum levels for the commonly monitored antibiotics.
- Understand the role of reference laboratories.

4.1 Rationale for antimicrobial susceptibility testing

It is essential that for the management of patients with an infection that the organism isolated is tested for susceptibility against a relevant set of antimicrobial agents. Without susceptibility test results, the clinician would be uncertain as to whether an infection was being treated with the correct therapy. However, it is not quite as clear-cut as this because if a patient is admitted to hospital then the clinician has no choice but to prescribe the most appropriate antimicrobial in the hope that the patient will respond (**empiric antibiotic therapy**). The results of susceptibility tests will follow and hopefully confirm that the correct therapy was administered.

Routine laboratory susceptibility testing, in addition to providing a result to the clinician, also provides essential current and relevant accumulated data that are used in the formulation of hospital prescribing policies, the selection of the most suitable agents for empirical use, surveillance of resistance studies, and the future development of new agents.

empiric antibiotic therapy
Empiric antibiotic therapy is antibiotic therapy commenced before the identification of the causative microorganism is available. Typically, full identification and susceptibility testing of bacteria from clinical specimens is not available for 48–72 h after collection of the specimen from the patient.

Key Point

A prescribing policy is where clinicians are guided in the use of antimicrobials rather than prescribing any drug.

In a clinical setting, agents are commonly used empirically and the laboratory test is used to confirm susceptibility, explain treatment failures, and to provide suitable alternative agents. Just consider GP surgeries for a moment; a patient showing signs of infection would have an antimicrobial agent prescribed. The patient wouldn't be happy if they had to return to the practice several days later for treatment, while their symptoms continued, waiting for the laboratory to isolate the organism and test it against the antibiotic prescribed.

4.2 Commonly used antibiotics

A wide variety of antibiotics are used for patient therapy and a number of different classes of antibiotics exist. Some antibiotics are active only against Gram-positive organisms and some only against Gram-negative strains or anaerobes. Whilst it would be impossible to list them all, the commonest antibiotics used are as follows:

- β-lactams – active against bacterial cell walls and include penicillins and cephalosporins.
- Macrolides – often used as alternatives to β-lactam agents if the patient is allergic, particularly for respiratory and soft tissue infections. Examples include erythromycin and clindamycin.
- Glycopeptides – active virtually exclusively against Gram-positive organisms and resistance is uncommon. Examples are vancomycin and teicoplanin.
- Aminoglycosides – these are **broad-spectrum antibiotics** which are normally administered IV. Common examples include gentamicin and tobramycin.
- Quinolones/fluoroquinolones – these are broad-spectrum antibiotics with Gram-negative organisms showing good susceptibility. A common example is ciprofloxacin.

broad-spectrum antibiotic

Broad-spectrum antibiotics are those that show activity against a wide range of organisms, typically both Gram-negative and Gram-positive species.

4.3 Antimicrobial susceptibility testing

It is essential that tests are performed in such a way that accurate and reproducible results are obtained because of the clinical implications to individual patients. The need for standardization of *in vitro* testing was recognized by the World Health Organization (WHO) in the 1950s when a first expert committee was convened in Geneva. Since that time, several national committees have developed standardized methods, taking into consideration all the components of the test. This includes media constituents, concentration of antimicrobial used in discs, rate of organism growth, supplements required, atmospheric conditions, and length of incubation.

It is important that laboratories are aware that standardized methods of susceptibility testing have to be followed precisely and that the procedure cannot be modified. Alterations in the procedure may result in inaccurate interpretation of susceptibility.

Cross reference

See Chapter 3, Section 3.7.

4.3.1 Disc susceptibility testing

The most widely used method of determining antimicrobial susceptibility is by the use of disc diffusion tests. The method involves inoculation of an organism onto a specific medium and application of paper discs containing antimicrobials of known strength. All of the above must be standardized. The discs used for susceptibility testing may contain either the antibiotic that is to be used for therapy or **indicator antibiotics**.

indicator antibiotic

Indicator antibiotics are agents that are generally the least microbiologically active members of a family of antibiotics and are therefore more likely to detect low-level resistance. Examples of agents that have been used for this purpose include oxacillin for the detection of penicillin resistance in *Streptococcus pneumoniae* and methicillin-resistant *S. aureus*.

4.3.2 Disc susceptibility testing – inoculum required

The method involves the application of paper discs containing different antibiotics to the surface of an agar plate containing a known inoculum of the organism to be tested. Several methods are available for this process including those recommended by the Clinical Laboratory Standards Institute (CLSI) or the British Society for Antimicrobial Chemotherapy (BSAC), both of which require standardization of inoculum, media, disc content, and incubation time, the results of which determine if the organism is termed sensitive, intermediate, or resistant to the antibiotic(s) tested. It is appropriate to test more than one antibiotic – routinely up to

FIGURE 4.1

Examples of a range of inoculum densities for disc susceptibility testing with the ideal being semi-confluent growth (middle plate: BSAC methodology).

Source: Courtesy of M. Ford.

six antibiotics are tested against any organism. This saves the need for further testing if the organism is resistant to one particular antibiotic and results can be reported after overnight incubation.

Essentially, the target pathogen is inoculated into an appropriate medium (e.g. Iso-Sensitest broth) with a standardized inoculum, made by reference to McFarland standards. Suspensions are accurately prepared using a spectrophotometer, or more commonly a bench-top nephelometer, to ensure the inoculum is correct. According to the methodology used, a dilution of the suspension may be required before the plate is inoculated. The plate is then inoculated and spread to achieve the required 'lawn'; this can be confluent or semiconfluent depending on the standardized method. For the disc diffusion test, the inoculum density has been shown to be one of the most important factors in ensuring the correct result is obtained. Studies have shown that intra- and inter-laboratory reproducibility is affected most by an inoculum which was considered 'too heavy', whereas a lighter inoculum gave less variation. Figure 4.1 shows the types of lawn, from too light to confluent.

4.3.3 Depth of agar

In the case of disc susceptibility testing, the depth of agar affects performance; very thin medium results in pronounced increase in zone sizes and vice versa with very thick media. The medium should have a depth of 4 mm (± 0.5 mm). It is therefore essential that proper quality control is carried out on all media, especially susceptibility test media.

SELF-CHECK 4.1

What would happen to the zone sizes if the plate was (a) too thin and (b) too thick? What consequences could this have for the patient?

4.3.4 Application and storage of discs

Discs are applied using sterile forceps to the plate or more conveniently by use of disc dispensers. The dispensers generally hold six different antibiotics and are 'stamped' onto the agar plate by the operator. The plates are then incubated under the required conditions and examined for the zones around the various antibiotic discs. The following points are important:

- Discs must be firmly applied to the surface of the agar.
- Discs should be stored correctly as potency of the antibiotic is lost following exposure to heat, light, and moisture.

- Discs must be stored in sealed containers with a desiccant and protected from light – this is important for light-susceptible agents such as metronidazole, chloramphenicol, and the quinolones.
- Stock discs should be stored at −20 °C unless otherwise advised by the manufacturer.
- To prevent condensation, allow discs to warm to room temperature before use.
- Discs must be discarded on, or ideally before, the expiry date shown on the side of the container.

4.3.5 Incubation and atmospheric conditions

Generally, incubation of disc susceptibility tests is in air at 35-37 °C for 18-20 h. However, there are exceptions to these recommendations. There is much debate about the effect of atmospheric conditions on the *in vitro* activity of antibiotics. In the case of the respiratory pathogens *Haemophilus influenzae* and *Streptococcus pneumoniae* there are two diametrically opposed opinions, one stating that for optimum growth of newly isolated clinical strains, an atmosphere enriched with 4-6% CO_2 is needed. Other opinions advise against the addition of CO_2 because of its effect on the macrolide antibiotics such as erythromycin – agents that are used to treat respiratory infections. The argument for incubating in 4-6% CO_2 is based on observations that 20% of *H. influenzae* and 40% of *S. pneumoniae* isolates from clinical samples required an atmosphere enriched with CO_2 to give semiconfluent growth. Also, it has been suggested that *in vivo* the acid within the respiratory tree may reduce the efficacy of the macrolide/azalide antibiotics.

The detection of glycopeptide resistance in enterococci has proved unreliable by disc testing methods. However, detection is improved if the plates are incubated for at least 24 h before examination, which allows time for the resistant microcolonies to be visibly detectable.

When using cefoxitin as an indicator antibiotic for the detection of methicillin resistance in *S. aureus* the temperature should not exceed 36 °C because this will result in the unacceptable merging of the susceptible and resistant populations. When methicillin or oxacillin is used to detect resistance, plates must be incubated at 30 °C to ensure the detection of the minority resistant population. Incubation conditions for all disc susceptibility testing are available on the BSAC web site (http://www.bsac.org.uk) or in CLSI publications.

Key Point

It is essential that all parameters are standardized in order that the zone size result can be interpreted correctly.

SELF-CHECK 4.2

Why are temperature and atmospheric conditions so important in disc susceptibility testing?

4.3.6 What do zones of inhibition mean – what do they relate to?

Just because an organism shows a zone around an antibiotic disc doesn't mean the organism is susceptible to it. Is a zone of 15 mm sensitive, or is a zone of 30 mm? If so, does this mean you can reliably treat the patient? Because of this, it is important that you understand how zone

FIGURE 4.2

Example of a regression line correlating the zone diameters to agar dilution MICs.

Source: Courtesy of J. Andrews.

sizes relate to the concentration of antibiotic that is required in the body to inhibit growth or kill the infecting organism. There have been several approaches to obtain a relationship between **minimum inhibitory concentration (MIC)** and zone of inhibition, so that critical zone diameters can be obtained that separate the susceptible, intermediate and resistant populations. One approach uses regression analysis where zone diameters (arithmetic scale plotted on the x axis) and corresponding MICs (logarithm to base 2 plotted on the y axis) for 100–150 representative clinical isolates with an MIC evenly distributed over the range studied are tested simultaneously by MIC and disc diffusion (Figure 4.2).

By applying the MIC **breakpoint** the critical zone diameters can be calculated, keeping the number of major discrepancies (organism resistant by MIC, yet susceptible by disc testing) as low as possible. A disadvantage of this method is that it relies on an even distribution of MIC over the range tested. This is not always possible, particularly when new agents are introduced.

In view of the inconsistencies of regression analysis, Metzler and DeHaan devised a bivariate 'error minimization' or 'error rate bounded' classification scheme for relating MIC values to zone diameters which is not concerned with regression analysis. Figure 4.3 illustrates a scattergram where the zone diameter breakpoint is calculated by taking into consideration the

minimum inhibitory concentration (MIC)

Minimum inhibitory concentration is the lowest concentration of an antibiotic needed to inhibit bacterial growth.

breakpoint

The breakpoint refers to when only certain antibiotic concentrations are tested, normally two. These concentrations would be appropriate for differentiating between susceptible, intermediate, and resistant microorganisms.

FIGURE 4.3

Example of error rate bounded analysis.

Source: Courtesy of J. Andrews.

MIC breakpoint and applying a false susceptible and false resistant limit of ≤1 and 5%, respectively. This method of analysis has been used by the BSAC.

To convert zones of inhibition into susceptible, intermediate, or resistant categories, thus inferring whether it is possible to treat an infection with a given antibiotic, reference is made to these data in conjunction with pharmacokinetic (time course of antibiotics in serum, tissues, and body fluids), pharmacodynamic (the relationship between drug concentration and antimicrobial effect), and clinical response data. All of the data together are analysed and a zone size calculated, which can be termed sensitive, intermediate, or resistant. It is important to define what these terms mean and how they relate to the clinical management of the patient:

- Clinically resistant: level of antimicrobial susceptibility that results in a high likelihood of therapeutic failure.
- Clinically susceptible: level of antimicrobial susceptibility associated with a high likelihood of therapeutic success.
- Clinically intermediate: a level of antimicrobial susceptibility associated with uncertain therapeutic effect. It implies that an infection due to the isolate may be appropriately treated in body sites where the drugs are physically concentrated or when a high dosage of drug can be used; it also indicates a buffer zone that should prevent small, uncontrolled, technical factors from causing major discrepancies in interpretation.

It must be noted that national MIC breakpoints are based on the standard dosing used in that particular country and that dosage may vary between Europe, the USA and the rest of the world.

SELF-CHECK 4.3

How does the zone size relate to the effectiveness of the antibiotic being tested? What methods have been used to determine this?

4.3.7 Interpretation of disc susceptibility tests

In the laboratory setting, the zones of inhibition must be read for each antimicrobial susceptibility test set up (Figure 4.4). These zones are measured from the back of the plate where clear media are used or from the front if supplemented media are used. The zone diameter is measured (to the nearest millimetre) with a ruler, callipers, or an automated zone reader, taking the zone edge, as judged by the naked eye, as the point of inhibition. Tiny colonies at the edge of the zone, films of growth due to the swarming of *Proteus* spp. and slight growth within sulphonamide or trimethoprim zones should be ignored. Colonies growing within the zone of inhibition should be subcultured and identified, and the test repeated if necessary. The biomedical scientist must confirm that the zone of inhibition for the control strain falls within acceptable ranges before interpreting the test.

A template (Figure 4.5) can also be used for interpreting susceptibility and a program for preparing templates is available from the BSAC web site (www.bsac.org.uk). The susceptibility test plate is placed over the template and the zones of inhibition are examined in relation to the template zones. If the zone of inhibition of the test strain is within the area marked with an 'R' the organism is resistant. Antimicrobial susceptibility using discs is reported qualitatively, as sensitive, intermediate, or resistant. For example, if the zone of inhibition is equal to or larger than the marked area the organism is susceptible. The results would then be reported according to laboratory policy with reference to the hospital prescribing policy. It is important to remember that it is essential to have more than one antibiotic to which an organism is deemed susceptible. This is because the patient may have developed an allergic response or the drug

FIGURE 4.4

Showing growth of *E. coli* on Iso-Sensitest agar and zones of inhibition around antibiotic containing discs.

Source: Courtesy of J. Collins.

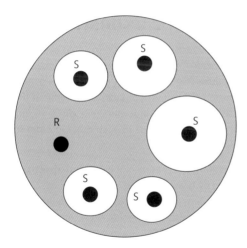

FIGURE 4.5

Template for interpreting disc susceptibility tests. R indicates the zone size which will be interpreted as resistant, and S is susceptible.

Source: Courtesy of J. Andrews.

may not be well tolerated. If the organism shows multi-drug resistance then further antibiotics may need to be tested.

SELF-CHECK 4.4

What would be the consequences of mis-reporting the result of an antibiotic susceptibility test?

In an attempt to overcome some of the problems associated with reading antibiotic zone sizes, commercial companies have produced automated instruments. Such instruments allow zone sizes to be read rapidly and input into the host computer, and as a result transcription errors are removed. There are, however, problems with this instrumentation, in that colonies growing inside a susceptible zone may be missed and problems can be encountered with diffuse zone edges. It is believed the performance of these instruments will improve in the future with more powerful processing power and image recognition.

4.3.8 Direct susceptibility testing

As you have read earlier, disc susceptibility tests require a standardized inoculum in order to interpret the result correctly. However, there are some situations where it can be important to have a susceptibility test result at the same time as the culture is available. This, however, bypasses the standardized approach to susceptibility testing in order to achieve a potentially clinically useful result. Direct susceptibility tests are performed exactly as previously described but the sample is applied directly to the agar and antibiotic discs applied. This is often performed on positive blood cultures where a susceptibility result is often very important. Direct susceptibility tests are also performed on urine samples, which may have been highlighted as positive using an automated analyser or organisms have been seen using inverted microscopy. Some studies have shown only small variations between direct and conventional standardized tests. For urine samples, this will result in improved turnaround times and less labour as a suspension need not be made. However, it is essential that if the correct inoculum has not been achieved, then the test must be repeated – this is especially important for direct susceptibility results obtained from positive blood cultures.

SELF-CHECK 4.5

What are the potential problems in performing and reading direct susceptibility tests? Are there clinical benefits in performing them?

4.3.9 Double disc/combination disc techniques

Double disc tests have been used to detect inducible resistance in organisms that classically have inducible **Amp C** β**-lactamase** (e.g. *Enterobacter* spp. and *Serratia* spp.) or for detecting dissociated resistance in Gram-positive organisms (Figure 4.6). This is seen when testing erythromycin and clindamycin and occurs because erythromycin induces an enzyme in the test organism and as a result the organism is resistant to similar antibiotics (e.g. clindamycin). It must be remembered that the two antibiotic discs must be close to each other in order to demonstrate this particular type of resistance.

One of the main uses of combination discs is to confirm the presence of **extended-spectrum** β**-lactamase** (ESBLs). These are enzymes produced by Gram-negative organisms which break down a range of β-lactam antibiotics, including penicillins and cephalosporins. Since these are such widely used antibiotics, it is imperative that organisms producing these enzymes are detected and their presence reported. Delayed recognition of ESBL strains has been associated with increased patient mortality.

Essentially, a plate is inoculated in the same manner as any other susceptibility test but a comparison is made between discs containing a cephalosporin, such as cefpodoxime, and the same disc containing clavulanic acid. The zone diameters are compared, and if the zone size is increased by >5 mm (or equal to) in the presence of clavulanic acid then this implies ESBL production. The advantage of combination discs is their low cost when compared to other methods such as the use of ESBL E-test strips.

Methods for detecting dissociated resistance and confirmation tests for ESBLs are available on the BSAC web site (www.bsac.org.uk).

4.3.10 Gradient method of susceptibility testing

This is a method of susceptibility testing where an actual MIC as a numerical value is achieved rather than a zone size. The gradient method of testing is available commercially (E-test, bioMérieux, and MICE Thermo Fisher, Basingstoke, UK). For this method, antibiotic is applied as a gradient to an inert strip. When the strip is applied to the surface of an agar plate, previously inoculated with a lawn of the organism, there is instantaneous diffusion of the antibiotic into the medium and the gradient is maintained. After overnight incubation the ellipse is examined to determine the amount of antibiotic that has inhibited the growth of the organism (Figure 4.7). Gradient methods have mainly been used to confirm resistance rather than for primary susceptibility testing. This is because generally a whole plate is required for the test and it is very expensive when compared to conventional disc susceptibility tests.

Gradient methods are not considered a 'gold standard' for evaluating the performance of other methods of testing. They should not be used to elucidate equivocal results when detecting methicillin resistance in staphylococci because they are subject to variation in the conditions of testing like any other microbiological method. A molecular method for **mecA** should be used to determine resistance, or for *S. aureus* a latex method for detecting PBP2 or PBP2a is available commercially (Mast, Merseyside, UK).

4.4 Broth methods

Broth MIC determinations are considered the 'gold standard' by the CLSI and this method of testing is preferred for determining organism susceptibility by the pharmaceutical industry as part of drug development programmes.

Amp C

Amp C is an inducible enzyme occurring in clinically isolated Gram-negative strains such as *Enterobacter* spp. They hydrolyse broad- and extended-spectrum cephalosporins.

extended-spectrum β-lactamase

Extended-spectrum β-lactamases are enzymes that can be produced by bacteria, making them resistant to penicillins and cephalosporins such as cefuroxime, cefotaxime, and ceftazidime. These antibiotics are some of the most important antibiotics available for the treatment of infectious disease.

FIGURE 4.6

Dissociated resistance in *Staphylococcus aureus* detected using a double disc technique shown with erythromycin (left) and clindamycin (right) discs.

Source: Courtesy of M. Ford.

mecA

mecA is a gene that codes for an altered penicillin binding protein (PBP2 or PBP2a). These proteins have a lower affinity for β-lactam antibiotics and confer resistance to the organism.

Broth MICs are undertaken infrequently in the UK and are generally only required when the **minimum bactericidal concentration (MBC)** of an organism is needed, for example as a possible aid in the treatment of endocarditis or for determining the susceptibility of slow-growing organisms. Mueller–Hinton broth (MHB) and Iso-Sensitest broth (ISTB) are available for undertaking broth susceptibility tests. For MHB the formula is the same as for the agar method (without the addition of agar) and with a Ca^{2+} and Mg^{2+} concentration of 20–25 mg/L and 12–25 mg/L, respectively. Broth methods have been adapted for use in automated systems that are available commercially. Some products use microtitre trays that require reconstitution of freeze-dried antibiotic with MHB. It must be remembered that if MHB is used, the CLSI MIC breakpoints must be applied to interpret susceptibility; those of BSAC cannot be used.

For broth MIC testing the inoculum should be 5×10^5 CFU/mL, except when testing organisms with extracellular β-lactamase where an inoculum of 10^6 CFU/spot is required. Methods for preparing inocula for MIC testing are freely available on the BSAC web site (www.bsac.org.uk) or in a variety of other publications.

Briefly, the organism for broth MIC testing is placed into broth and this is incubated overnight. This is then diluted to the required concentration of the organism. A rack of tubes containing sterile broth is prepared containing doubling dilutions of the test antibiotic. A known suspension of organism is placed into each tube, with an antibiotic-free tube as a control. A culture plate is inoculated with the organism suspension as a purity check. The tubes are then incubated overnight under the required conditions and examined for turbidity. After incubation it is essential to ensure that the test and control organism have grown on the antibiotic-free control plate, in the broth control tube and no contaminants are present. The MIC is determined as the lowest concentration that completely inhibits growth. This produces a numerical value which can be compared to published data to determine if the organism is sensitive, intermediate or resistant.

For broth MICs a problem may be seen where one tube or well with no growth is observed but obvious growth is seen at higher and lower concentrations. The 'skipped' tube or well should be ignored and the concentration that finally inhibits growth should be recorded as the MIC. If more than one 'skipped' tube or well occurs the MIC should be repeated. Trailing endpoints may be seen with **bacteriostatic** agents such as sulphonamide and trimethoprim. Trailing endpoints are generally not observed with **bactericidal** agents such as gentamicin. In these cases, a 90% decrease in growth as compared with the growth control should be recorded as the MIC. Partial inhibition may also be seen with growth of resistant variants or if there is contamination. Subculture of all tubes or wells is advised.

It must be remembered that the stability of the antibiotic must be assessed if prolonged incubation is undertaken. ISTB is the medium used most frequently.

FIGURE 4.7
E-test strip showing susceptibility of *S. pneumoniae* to erythromycin.
Source: Courtesy of M. Ford.

> **minimum bactericidal concentration (MBC)**
> Minimum bactericidal concentration is the lowest concentration of an antibiotic which is cidal to ≥99.9% of the test inoculum.

> **bacteristatic/ bactericidal**
> Bacteristatic refers to an antibiotic which inhibits the growth of an organism but doesn't necessarily kill it. Bactericidal antibiotics are those which are likely to kill the organism.

SELF-CHECK 4.6

What are the main differences between broth and agar susceptibility tests and the results obtained?

4.5 **Automated susceptibility testing**

Over the last few years, many routine laboratories have switched a large part of the susceptibility test workload onto automated platforms. This is in a bid to further improve standardization, as operator error in recording zone sizes is eliminated. In addition, these instruments

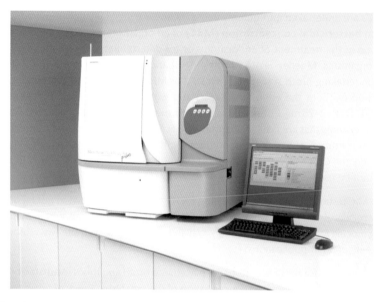

FIGURE 4.8
Siemens Walkaway automated susceptibility test instrumentation.
Source: Courtesy of Siemens.

can provide an identification which is very beneficial; as we have learned, some organisms can give large zone sizes but have mechanisms of resistance whereby the antibiotic may not work *in vivo*.

There are several instruments available, the most common being the bioMérieux VITEK and the Siemens Walkaway (Figure 4.8). For both of these instruments, interpretation of results is based on CLSI MIC breakpoints; however, in the future, it is likely that some standardization will occur and the instruments will be programmed with EUCAST breakpoints. With these instruments, operator time is minimal and the main inoculation process can be easily deskilled.

The Siemens Walkaway instrument uses a broth dilution susceptibility test method where the components are dehydrated. The various antibiotics used are diluted in broth (Mueller–Hinton) with all of the required supplements necessary for optimal test performance. After the panels are inoculated with a standardized suspension, they are placed onto the instrument and incubated at 35 °C for a minimum of 16 h before reading. The panels are read automatically by the instrument in comparison with growth controls contained within the panel. Growth in the panels results in turbidity and this is recorded by the instrument. The results are reported as susceptible, intermediate or resistant. The actual MIC is also recorded. Depending upon the panel type used, either an MIC or a breakpoint concentration is achieved. Numerous panel types are available for both Gram-negative and Gram-positive organisms. Figure 4.9 shows a typical antibiotic/identification panel used in the instrument.

Whilst the instruments provide excellent results and overcome the problems associated with reading disc susceptibility tests, there are some drawbacks. They cannot be used for performing direct susceptibility tests, for example on positive blood cultures. In addition, there are a number of organisms where these tests give poor results, for example on mucoid *Pseudomonas* strains. As a result, it is unlikely these instruments will totally replace conventional disc susceptibility tests.

FIGURE 4.9

Microtitre panels containing dehydrated antibiotics used in the Siemens Walkaway system.

Source: Courtesy of Siemens.

4.6 Enzymatic methods of resistance (β-lactamases)

β-lactamases are enzymes, produced by a wide range of bacteria which provide the organism with resistance to β-lactam antibiotics. These antibiotics include penicillins (penicillin/amoxicillin), cephalosporins, and carbapenems (ertapenem) and they are probably the most important and widely used of all types of antibiotics. These enzymes breakdown the characteristic β-lactam ring, which is a common structure of all β-lactam antibiotics (Figure 4.10). The enzyme breaks down this ring through hydrolysis and as a result the antibiotic has no effect on the organism. This allows the organism to gain an advantage in environments where β-lactams are widely used.

How β-lactamases are characterized depends upon the nucleotide and amino acid sequences of the enzyme itself. There are four classes (A–D); classes A, C, and D act by a serine mechanism; class B requires zinc for its action and as a result, these β-lactamases are known as metallo-β-lactamases.

β-lactam ring ——— Penicillin → β-lactamase hydrolysis → Penicilloic acid

FIGURE 4.10

Core structures of penicillin showing the β-lactam ring (highlighted). The β-lactamase breaks a bond in the β-lactam ring, inactivating the effect of the antibiotic

Source: Courtesy of D. Ford.

4.6.1 Class A β-lactamases

Enzymes in this Ambler class are the most commonly encountered enzymes associated with resistance to β-lactam antibiotics. Most of the resistance to amoxicillin in *E. coli* is due to the production of the class A enzyme known as TEM-1 (named after the patient it was first isolated in). In some countries *E. coli* resistance to amoxicillin is greater than 80%. Although common in *E. coli* they are also found in a wide range of other Gram-negative organisms such as *Klebsiella* spp., *H. influenza*, and *N. gonnorhoeae*. These TEM enzymes are also known as extended-spectrum β-lactamases (ESBLs) as production confers resistance to many β-lactam antibiotics including aztreonam. Amino acid substitutions at various positions result in slightly different TEM types. TEM-10 and -26 are the most common types seen in the USA. Other types of class A enzymes include SHV types (sulphydryl variable) and CTX-M enzymes which are particularly active against the cephalosporin cefotaxime (hence CTX-M). Over 80 types of CTX-M enzymes are known and are widespread throughout the world in Gram-negative organisms such as *E. coli* and *Salmonella* spp. These enzymes are usually susceptible to β-lactam inhibitors such as clavulanic acid and sulbactam.

4.6.2 Class B β-lactamases

Also known as metallo-β-lactamases (or carbapenemases) they are again found in a range of commonly encountered Gram-negative organisms including *Pseudomonas aeruginosa* and *Acinetobacter* spp., and are picked up from other species via plasmids. This is the case with the IMP type enzymes. A second type, known as the VIM enzymes, again have a worldwide distribution, and occur most commonly in *P. aeruginosa* and occasionally in some species of Enterobacteriaceae. These VIM enzymes confer the ability of the organism to hydrolyse all β-lactam antibiotics, the action of which is not inhibited by clavulanic acid. The ability of these enzymes to break down many commonly used antibiotics including carbapenems is of huge importance to future public health as the number of antibiotics patients can be treated with successfully is diminishing.

4.6.3 Class C β-lactamases

These are *AmpC* type β-lactamases and are commonly found in *Citrobacter*, *Enterobacter*, and *Serratia* spp. These enzymes are inducible (produced when exposed to the antibiotic) and can be produced in very high quantities (hyper production) and typically hydrolyse cephalosporin antibiotics. These antibiotics are widely used to treat UTIs and they are generally considered broad-spectrum antibiotics, as they are active against a wide range of organisms. As a result they are often used in hospitals as prophylactic agents, e.g. for patients undergoing abdominal surgery, where a mixture of aerobic and anaerobic organisms will be encountered.

4.6.4 Class D β-lactamases

These are the OXA group of enzymes (short for oxacillinase) which hydrolyse carbapenems and are widely distributed in some of the more antibiotic-resistant Gram-negative bacteria, including *Acinetobacter baumannii* and *P. aeruginosa*. The expression of OXA enzymes can confer either a narrow or wide spectrum of hydrolysis (including carbapenems: MIC >128 mg/L – resistant) depending which one of the 150 enzyme variants is expressed.

> ### Key Point
>
> Organisms are continually becoming resistant to more and more antibiotics through changes to existing enzyme structures. Efforts need to be strengthened so new antibiotics are developed to counteract bacterial resistance.

4.7 Detection of mechanisms of resistance and the application of expert rules

Results of susceptibility testing are normally reported as sensitive, intermediate, or resistant based on the results for individual antibiotics. Often only limited agents are tested and organisms are not identified to species level, which precludes the detection of some underlying mechanisms of resistance (e.g. *AmpC* β-lactamases).

In France and in some commercial systems (VITEK 2) a comprehensive panel of 16–20 antibiotics are tested in conjunction with an accurate identification of the test organism. This allows the full potential of interpretative reading to be exploited, including the application of expert rules which have implications for antibiotic therapy. A comprehensive publication on this subject is available on the BSAC website (www.bsac.org.uk).

It is also important for laboratories to recognize unusual or unexpected susceptibility patterns, for example Group A streptococci resistant to benzyl penicillin, vancomycin, teicoplanin, or linezolid. Table 4.1 shows examples of exceptional resistance phenotypes that are worthy of further investigation. In these cases, if resistance is confirmed, organisms should be sent to a reference laboratory for further analysis and confirmation.

TABLE 4.1 Examples of exceptional resistance phenotypes.

Organism	Exceptional resistance/susceptibility
Enterobacteriaceae except *Proteus* spp.	Resistance to meropenem/imipenem
E. coli	Resistance to ertapenem, tigecycline
Klebsiella spp.	Susceptibility to ampicillin/amoxicillin
P. aeruginosa	Resistance to colistin
Pseudomonas spp.	Susceptibility to ampicillin/amoxicillin, cephalosporins other than ceftazidime of the fourth-generation cephalosporins[1]
N. meningitidis	High-level resistance to penicillin or resistance to ciprofloxacin
N. gonorrhoeae	Resistance to any third-generation cephalosporin[2]
S. aureus	Resistance to vancomycin, teicoplanin, linezolid, quinupristin/ dalfopristin, daptomycin, tigecycline

continued

TABLE 4.1 Examples of exceptional resistance phenotypes. (*Continued*)

Organism	Exceptional resistance/susceptibility
S. pneumoniae	Resistance to meropenem, vancomycin, teicoplanin, linezolid, quinupristin/dalfopristin
β-Haemolytic streptococci	Resistance to penicillin, vancomycin, teicoplanin, linezolid, quinupristin/dalfopristin, daptomycin, tigecycline
Enterococcus spp.	Resistance to linezolid, daptomycin, tigecycline. Resistant to teicoplanin but not vancomycin
E. faecalis	Susceptible to quinupristin/dalfopristin
E. faecium	Resistant to quinupristin/dalfopristin

[1] Fourth-generation cephalosporins: cefepime, and cefpirome.
[2] Third-generation cephalosporins: cefotaxime, cefpodoxime, ceftazidime, and ceftriaxone.

4.7.1 Natural (inherent/intrinsic) resistance

Resistance to antibiotics can be divided into that which is intrinsic/inherent resistance (naturally occurring) and that which is acquired. Naturally occurring resistance is shared by most or all of the species and is therefore considered a characteristic of that species. This type of resistance is less of a problem because it is well recognized during the early development of a drug. Of greater importance is acquired resistance, which implies that an originally susceptible organism has developed resistance to an agent to which it was originally susceptible.

It is important that laboratories are aware of natural (inherent/intrinsic) resistance of common pathogens before antibiotic susceptibility testing is undertaken. Examples of natural resistance are shown in Table 4.2; a more comprehensive list of resistance phenotypes of common pathogens can be found on the BSAC website (www.bsac.org.uk).

TABLE 4.2 Examples of natural (inherent) resistance in common clinical isolates.

Organisms	Natural (inherent) resistance
All Enterobacteriaceae	Penicillin, glycopeptides, fusidic acid, macrolides, clindamycin, linezolid, daptomycin, quinupristin/dalfopristin, mupirocin
Klebsiella	Ampicillin (*Klebsiella* have chromosomal penicillinases)
Proteus mirabilis	Colistin, nitrofurantoin, tetracyclines
Salmonella spp.	Cefuroxime and aminoglycosides (active *in vitro*, not active *in vivo*)
All Gram-positive bacteria	Aztreonam, temocillin, colistin, nalidixic acid
Methicillin-resistant *Staphylococcus aureus*	All β-lactams
Moraxella catarrhalis	Trimethoprim
Listeria	Cefotaxime, cefpodoxime, ceftazidime and ceftriaxone, fluoroquinolones

Why is it considered important that the identity of the organism is known at the same time as the susceptibility results are determined?

4.8 Additional tests

4.8.1 Antibiotic combination and synergy testing

Combinations of antibiotics have been used clinically to prevent the emergence of resistance when treating *Mycobacterium tuberculosis*, for the treatment of bacterial endocarditis and also in the treatment of patients with cystic fibrosis. *In vitro* methods that have been used to observe the effect of combining one or more antibiotics are the chequerboard titration, time kill curves, and double disc techniques.

4.8.2 Chequerboard titrations

Chequerboard titrations have been used to calculate the fractional inhibitory concentration (FIC) using the following formula:

$$FIC = \frac{MIC_A \text{ (in combination)}}{MIC_A \text{ (alone)}} + \frac{MIC_B \text{ (in combination)}}{MIC_B \text{ (alone)}}$$

where A is one drug and B is the other.

Interpretation of the combination is as follows:

$$\text{Synergistic FIC} = \leq 0.5$$

(positive interaction where the combined effect is significantly greater than the expected result when drugs are tested alone);

$$\text{Additive FIC} = 1.0$$

(indifferent response);

$$\text{Antagonistic FIC} = \geq 2.0$$

(negative interaction where the combined effect is significantly less than their independent effect when tested separately).

The value of this test in the clinical setting has been debated. MacGowan *et al.* demonstrated synergy when erythromycin was tested in combination with itself and therefore doubted the value of the test. Others have recommended using synergy testing to aid in the treatment of patients with cystic fibrosis as *P. aeruginosa* isolates from these patients in particular are often resistant to numerous antibiotics.

Cross reference
See Chapter 9.

4.8.3 Time kill curves

These tests are mainly used as a research tool due to the labour intensity of performing the test. They have been used to compare the activity of drugs both alone and in combination, to measure the effect of increasing the concentration of drug on *in vitro* activity, and to detect the emergence of resistance.

The test to measure the effect of increasing the concentration of drug on *in vitro* activity has been used to determine if drugs have concentration or dose-independent activity (very little difference in the rate of bactericidal activity when the concentration exceeds four times the MIC, observed with the β-lactam antibiotics) or concentration or dose-dependent activity (number of organisms decrease more rapidly with each rising MIC concentration, seen with the quinolones and aminoglycosides). The *in vivo* pharmacodynamic parameters that correlate with clinical response in man and animals for agents that have concentration or dose-independent activity or concentration or dose-dependent activity respectively are as follows:

$$\frac{Time}{MIC}$$

where the concentration above the MIC should be 50–75% of the dose interval;

$$\frac{AUC \text{ or } C_{max}}{MIC}$$

where:

a ratio of 30–60 is needed

AUC = area under the curve

C_{max} = peak concentration following standard dosing

4.9 Control of antimicrobial susceptibility testing

4.9.1 Control strains

Susceptible control strains have been recommended for monitoring test performance (not for interpreting susceptibility) and resistant strains to ensure that particular mechanisms of resistance can be detected. Ideally, appropriate controls should be included with every batch of tests performed in the laboratory on a daily basis as some antibiotic discs show reduced activity if not stored correctly. Control strains are available from the American Type Culture Collection (ATCC) and the National Collection of Type Cultures (NCTC) and limited controls are available commercially (several suppliers). Table 4.3 provides examples of susceptible and resistant control stains that can be used.

4.9.2 Maintenance of control strains

The method used for the maintenance of control strains should minimize the risk of mutation. The following procedure is suggested (www.bsac.org.uk). Briefly, store control strains at −70 °C in glycerol broth or on beads in glycerol broth. Non-fastidious organisms may be stored at −20 °C. Ideally, two vials of each control strain should be stored, one for an 'in-use' supply, the other for archiving. Each week, a bead or glycerol broth from the 'in-use' vial should be subcultured onto appropriate non-selective media and checked for purity. From this pure culture,

TABLE 4.3 Control strains for antimicrobial susceptibility testing.

Organism	Strain		Characteristics
	Either	**Or**	
Escherichia coli	NCTC 12241 (ATCC 25922)	NCTC 10418	Susceptible
Escherichia coli	NCTC 11560		TEM-1 β-lactamase producer
Staphylococcus aureus	NCTC 12981 (ATCC 25923)	NCTC 6571	Susceptible
Staphylococcus aureus	NCTC 12493		*MecA*-positive, methicillin resistant
Pseudomonas aeruginosa	NCTC 12934 (ATCC 27853)	NCTC 10662	Susceptible
Enterococcus faecalis	NCTC 12697 (ATCC 29212)		Susceptible
Haemophilus influenzae	NCTC 11931		Susceptible
Haemophilus influenzae	NCTC 12699 (ATCC 49247)		Resistant to β-lactams (β-lactamase negative)
Streptococcus pneumoniae	NCTC 12977 (ATCC 49619)		Intermediate resistance to penicillin
Neisseria gonorrhoeae	NCTC 12700 (ATCC 49226)		Low-level resistance to penicillin
Pasteurella multocida	NCTC 8489		Susceptible
Bacteroides fragilis	NCTC 9343 (ATCC 25285)		Susceptible
Bacteroides thetaiotaomicron	ATCC 29741		Susceptible
Clostridium perfringens	NCTC 8359 (ATCC 12915)		Susceptible

prepare one subculture for each of the following 5 days. For fastidious organisms that will not survive on plates for 5 or 6 days, subculture the strain daily for no more than 6 days.

In the case of disc diffusion tests, acceptable ranges for control strains are published. For monitoring laboratory performance of disc diffusion a 20-point reading frame has been suggested (Figure 4.11) (www.bsac.org.uk). The problems that can occur with disc susceptibility testing are listed in Table 4.4.

FIGURE 4.11

Use of a 20-point reading frame to monitor the performance of disc susceptibility testing where one observation outside the range is acceptable.

Source: Courtesy of J. Andrews.

TABLE 4.4   Potential sources of error for disc susceptibility testing.

Source	Error
Test conditions	Incorrect inoculum Uneven inoculum Excessive pre-incubation before discs applied Excessive pre-diffusion before plates incubated Incorrect incubation temperature Incorrect incubation atmosphere Incorrect incubation time Inadequate illumination of plates when measuring zones Incorrect reading of zone edges Incorrect zone criteria used to interpret susceptibility
Medium	Required susceptibility testing agar not used Not prepared as required by the manufacturer's instructions Batch-to-batch variation Antagonists present (e.g. with sulphonamides and trimethoprim) Incorrect pH Incorrect divalent cation concentration Incorrect depth of agar plates Agar plates not level Expiry date exceeded
Antimicrobial discs	Wrong agent or content used Labile agent possibly deteriorated Light sensitive agent left in light Incorrect storage leading to deterioration Disc containers opened before reaching room temperature Incorrect labelling of disc dispensers Expiry date exceeded
Control strains	Contamination Mutation Incorrect inoculum density Uneven inoculation Old culture used

4.10 **Antibiotic assays**

Antibiotic assays are performed for many reasons. New agents are assayed as part of drug development to establish their pharmacokinetic properties, initially in animals and later in man. Concentrations of a drug may also be measured as part of clinical trials to ascertain levels at various sites of infection. There has been a trend away from performing these assays in microbiology departments over the last few years and into biochemistry, where they are performed on modern fully automated analysers. However, many microbiology laboratories still perform these tests and the results are often interpreted by senior biomedical scientists or medical staff. Which department performs these tests is of little consequence as the tests need to be performed for a variety of reasons.

In a clinical setting, therapeutic drug monitoring is performed for the following reasons:

- To ensure that serum concentrations are high enough for clinical efficacy.
- To ensure that toxicity is minimized for those agents with a narrow **therapeutic index**, e.g. the aminoglycosides.
- To monitor patient compliance, e.g. in the treatment of tuberculosis.

Antibiotics that require monitoring primarily to minimize adverse effects are gentamicin, tobramycin, netilmicin, amikacin, and vancomycin. In Tables 4.5 and 4.6 the normal levels for these agents are shown. For agents not commonly assayed, a service is generally provided by antimicrobial reference laboratories.

therapeutic index

Therapeutic index is the ratio between the toxic dose and the therapeutic dose of a drug, used as a measure of the relative safety of the drug for a particular treatment. A drug with little difference between toxic and therapeutic doses is referred to as having a narrow therapeutic index.

TABLE 4.5 Normal ranges for gentamicin, tobramycin, netilmicin, and amikacin in patients following once or twice daily dosing.

Antibiotic	Once daily dosing predose level (mg/L)	Twice (BD) or three times (TDS) daily dosing		
		Site of infection	Predose level (mg/L)	Postdose level (mg/L)
Gentamicin Tobramycin Netilmicin	<1	Gram-negative pneumonia	<2	<7
		Infective endocarditis	<1	2–3
		Most other infections	<2	>5
Amikacin	<5		<10	>20

TABLE 4.6 Normal ranges for patients receiving vancomycin therapy.

Antibiotic	Concentration (mg/L)		
	Predose only	1 h postdose	2 h postdose
Vancomycin	10–20	20–40	18–26

4.10.1 Assay methods – microbiological assays

Methods that have been used to measure concentrations of antibiotics are divided into micro-biological and non-microbiological techniques.

Many of the original assay methods were developed by the pharmaceutical industry to monitor commercial products. However, microbiological assays have been used in clinical laboratories particularly with the introduction of potentially toxic agents such as the aminoglycosides. Although microbiological assays are relatively easy and cheap to perform, they are now used infrequently in clinical laboratories because patients are often prescribed more than one antibiotic, which affects the specificity of the assay and they have long 'turnaround' times with results only being available after 18–24 h. Table 4.7 shows the antibiotic profile for a resistant *Klebsiella* sp. (NCTC 10896) that has been used to measure concentrations of gentamicin. A more detailed account of methods can be found in *Clinical Antimicrobial Assays* (see Further reading at the end of the chapter).

Advantages of microbiological assays:

* Relatively cheap.
* Relatively quick to develop.
* Can be more sensitive than chemical methods.
* Measure antimicrobial activity.

TABLE 4.7   Antibiotic profile for resistant *Klebsiella* sp. NCTC 10896 that has been used to measure concentrations of gentamicin in clinical samples.

Antibiotic	Susceptibility	Antibiotic	Susceptibility
Penicillin	R	Gentamicin	S
Ampicillin	R	Neomycin	R
Cloxacillin	R	Trimethoprim	R
Carbenicillin	R	Chloramphenicol	R
Methicillin	R	Tetracycline	R
Fusidic acid	R	Streptomycin	R
Lincomycin	R	Co-trimoxazole	R
Erythromycin	R	Mecillinam	R
Rifampicin	R	Cefazolin	MIC 16 mg/L
Sulphadimadine	R	Cephradine	MIC 8 mg/L
Colistin	S	Cefoxitin	S
Tobramycin	S	Cefuroxime	S
Kanamycin	S	Carbapenems	S

Disadvantages of microbiological assays:

- Mixtures of antibiotics are difficult to measure.
- Active metabolites may interfere with the assay.
- Concomitant antibiotics may affect the result.
- Often clinical details do not indicate if the patient is on more than one antibiotic.
- Results are obtained after overnight incubation and therefore these assays are not suitable for urgent tests.
- If the organism fails to grow there is a delay of 24 h before a result is available.

SELF-CHECK 4.8

Why are antibiotic assays performed only for a limited number of antibiotics?

4.10.2 Non-microbiological methods – enzyme-based assays

There are three broad classes of non-microbiological assay methods used to measure concentrations of antibiotics in clinical samples: enzyme-based assays, immunoassays, and physicochemical assays, which includes chromatography.

Specific enzymes, which inactivate an antibiotic, have been used to assay specific antimicrobials. Examples of enzymes that have been used are chloramphenicol acetyltransferase (CAT) and aminoglycoside modifying enzymes; this method of testing involves the use of a radiolabelled cofactor. Enzyme-based assays were introduced to overcome the effect of concomitant antibiotics and to improve turnaround time, both disadvantages of microbiological assays. Although this method of testing gives results in approximately 1 h, the safety precautions associated with radioactive material (including the disposal of radioactive material) and the need for expensive scintillation counters have made this a costly procedure. In comparative studies it has been found that enzyme-based assays compared favourably with other methods of testing.

Advantages of non-microbiological methods:

- Assay not affected by concomitant antibiotics.
- Results available in approximately 2 h.
- Suitable for on-call purposes.

Disadvantages of non-microbiological methods:

- Reagents not available as a kit, therefore preparation of enzymes and other reagents is undertaken by the laboratory.
- Radiolabelled cofactor is expensive.
- Involves the use of radioactive material, requiring special handling and disposal.
- Expensive scintillation counter is needed.

4.10.3 Immunoassays

For immunoassays the antibiotic being assayed acts like an antigen and binds with a specific anti-drug antibody. Most antibiotic assays are of the competitive binding type where a fixed concentration of tracer-labelled drug (the drug to be assayed labelled with a radioactive atom, fluorophore, or an enzyme) competes with the drug to be assayed in the sample for a limited amount of anti-drug antibody. The greater the amount of drug in the sample, the smaller the amount of tracer-labelled drug that can bind to the anti-drug antibody. Examples of commercial assays are the fluorescence polarization immunoassay (FPIA, Abbott) and the kinetic interaction of microparticles in solution immunoassay (KIMS, Roche Diagnostics, Indianapolis, USA). The antibiotics that are generally assayed by immunoassay are the aminoglycosides and vancomycin.

Advantages of immunoassays:

- Rapid and easy.
- Fast turnaround time.
- Small samples can be processed and therefore they are applicable to paediatric samples.
- Kits supplied commercially.
- Continual upgrade of technology.
- Can be assayed using clinical chemistry platforms and therefore results can be available 24 hours a day, 7 days a week.
- Perform well in National External Quality Assurance Schemes (NEQAS).

Disadvantages of immunoassays:

- Equipment may be expensive.
- If the machine is purchased a laboratory could be committed to a system that is superseded.

4.10.4 High-performance liquid chromatography

High-performance liquid chromatography (HPLC) is used when immunoassays are not available and microbiological assays are inappropriate. For HPLC, a form of liquid chromatography, the drug to be assayed is separated from other components in the sample and then quantified using a non-specific property such as ultra violet (UV) absorption.

In HPLC a mobile phase (liquid) is pumped through a column packed with a stationary phase on which separation takes place. The sample is introduced into the mobile phase by means of an injector and passes through the column where separation occurs by differential retention on the solid phase. After elution from the stationary phase, the mobile phase containing the separated solutes passes through a detector where the separated substances cause a response. The output from a detector is called a chromatogram. By comparing either the peak height or the area under the curve of a calibrator with those of the test, the concentration in the test sample can be calculated. Concentrations can be calculated using a calibration curve or a single-point calibration. For a single-point calibration the following formula is used:

$$C = C\,(R_{sample}/R_{calibrator})$$

where:

C = concentration of the calibrator

R_{sample} = peak height or peak area of the sample

$R_{calibrator}$ = peak height or peak area of the calibrator

HPLC is normally only undertaken by reference laboratories or research departments.

Advantages of HPLC:

- Very versatile and mixtures can be measured.
- Large numbers of samples can be processed using autosamplers.
- High precision coefficient of variation (CV) 5% or less.
- Result within 2–3 h.

Disadvantages of HPLC:

- Costly.
- Operator dependent.
- New assay development is lengthy.

SELF-CHECK 4.9

Which method of antibiotic assay would be the best for routine monitoring of antibiotics in patients' serum? Give reasons for your answer.

CASE STUDY 4.1 Multidrug-resistant organisms

A 70-year-old male admitted via the Emergency Department with symptoms of septicaemia has a blood culture and urine sample collected. After overnight incubation the positive blood culture showed Gram-negative bacilli. The positive bottle was subcultured to purity plates and direct disc susceptibility tests performed. The urine sample was 'flagged' as positive on automated microscopy and the organism cultured onto CLED agar and a direct susceptibility test performed.

The next day the culture results yielded a 'coliform', which showed resistance to cefuroxime, ceftazidime, cefpodoxime, gentamicin, and ciprofloxacin. The organism was susceptible to amikacin.

1. What would you suspect from the susceptibility pattern of the organism?

2. How would you confirm this and what other tests would you perform and why?

The organism was identified as *E. coli* and the ESBL combination discs gave the following results:

Cefpodoxime 10 µg No zone

Cefpodoxime 10 µg + clavulanic acid 20 mm zone

The organism also showed susceptibility to both ertapenem and meropenem.

3. What would be your conclusions and what antibiotics would you report as therapeutic options?

CASE STUDY 4.2 MRSA sepsis

A 60-year-old man with an abscess in his sternum has blood cultures taken from which an MRSA is isolated. The patient is prescribed vancomycin and antibiotic assays confirm adequate dosing. However, repeated blood cultures grow an MRSA.

1. What would you suspect from these results?

2. What susceptibility tests would you undertake to confirm this?

A gradient method of susceptibility testing on Mueller Hinton agar gave a vancomycin MIC of 3 mg/L.

3. What would be your conclusions?

4. Would you send the isolate to a Specialist Laboratory for further testing and what test would you request?

5. How would you report the susceptibility of the organism?

CASE STUDY 4.3 *Problem susceptibility testing*

A 50-year-old man with ventilator-associated pneumonia has a Gram-negative, oxidase-negative rod isolated from a respiratory sample. The organism is resistant to the carbapenems on primary testing.

1. What would you suspect from these results?

2. What susceptibility test/tests would you undertake?

The organism is confirmed as *Stenotrophomonas maltophilia*.

3. Which antibiotics can be reported as resistant without further testing?

4. How would you report the susceptibility of the organism?

CASE STUDY 4.4 *Difficult to grow organisms*

The sputum sample from a 12-year-old child with cystic fibrosis grows a mucoid oxidase-positive Gram-negative rod that grows very poorly on culture media.

1. What would you suspect from these results?

2. How would you undertake susceptibility testing?

The organism is confirmed as *Pseudomonas aeruginosa*, but has failed to grow confluently on susceptibility testing media.

3. What further testing would you undertake?

4. How would you report the susceptibility of the organism?

5. Would you send the isolate to a Reference Laboratory for further testing?

Chapter summary

After reading this chapter you should know and understand:

- Why antimicrobial susceptibility tests are performed and why some are required more urgently than others.

- Why national guidelines are in place and the importance of them.

- The methods involved in performing disc susceptibility tests and the pitfalls involved.

- How the zone size relates to the MIC of the organism.

- The types and importance of β-lactamases.

- Why and when automated methods can be used.

- Which organisms are naturally resistant to some antibiotics.

- The controls required for antibiotic susceptibility testing.

■ The difference between bacteriostatic and bactericidal agents.

■ Why and when combination therapy is used, common synergistic combinations, and the relevance of the test.

■ Which antibiotics are required to be monitored in a patient's serum and the methods involved in determining the concentration.

■ The importance of reference laboratories.

 # Further reading

● Finch R, Davey P, Wilcox M, Irving W. *Antimicrobial Chemotherapy*, **6th edition.** Oxford University Press, 2012.

● Andrews JM. BSAC standardized disc susceptibility testing method (version 6). *Journal of Antimicrobial Chemotherapy* 2007; **60**: 20–41.

● Bush K. Proliferation and significance of clinically relevant β-lactamases. *Annals of the New York Academy of Science* 2013; **1277**: 84–90.

● The European Committee on Antimicrobial Susceptibility Testing (EUCAST). www.eucast.org.

● Livermore DM, Winstanley TG, Shannon KP. Interpretative reading: recognizing the unusual and inferring resistance mechanisms from resistance phenotypes. *Journal of Antimicrobial Chemotherapy* 2001; **48** (Suppl. 1): 87–102.

● Louie L, Matsumura O, Choi E, Louie M, Simor AE. Evaluation of three rapid methods for detection of methicillin resistance in *Staphylococcus aureus. Journal of Clinical Microbiology* 2000; **38**: 2170–2173.

● Reeves DS, Wise R, Andrews J, White LO, eds. *Clinical Antimicrobial Assays.* Oxford University Press, 1999.

● CLSI. *Performance Standards for Antimicrobial Susceptibility Testing,* **Twenty Third** Informational Supplement. Clinical and Laboratory Standards Institute, 2013.

 # Discussion questions

4.1 Discuss the advantages and disadvantages of both automated and non-automated susceptibility tests. In conclusion, state which method you feel is best for routine laboratory testing.

4.2 Direct susceptibility tests are used widely despite the possibility of incorrect results being obtained. What reasons can you give to justify their continuation?

4.3 Do you think the antibiotic level in serum should be monitored for all antibiotics? Provide detailed reasons for your answer.

4.4 Do you think we will ever win the battle against microbial resistance or do you think microorganisms will always find ways of combating antimicrobial agents?

5

Blood cultures

Derek Law

This chapter will describe what a blood culture sample is, and when and why they are taken. It will cover in detail the procedures for taking and processing blood culture samples in the clinical laboratory, the organisms commonly found in blood cultures, and the methods used to identify them.

Learning objectives

After studying this chapter you should confidently be able to:

- Understand how blood cultures are taken and processed.
- Understand the principles of common blood culture systems.
- Work safely with blood cultures.
- Know which organisms are commonly isolated from blood cultures, their likely significance, and their source.
- Be aware of the usefulness of a blood culture Gram stain in providing a rapid diagnosis of septicaemia.
- Understand culture methods for commonly encountered organisms and tests available for rapid identification.
- Be aware of the problems of blood culture contamination.
- Recognize samples requiring specialized testing, e.g. endocarditis, samples from children or immunocompromised patients.

5.1 Laboratory investigation of blood culture samples

bacteraemia
Bacteraemia is the term given to the presence of bacteria in the bloodstream; bacteraemia may be transient, intermittent, or continuous.

Blood cultures are extremely important clinical samples, and are requested by clinicians when the signs and symptoms suggest the possibility of **bacteraemia** or **septicaemia**, a systemic (widespread) infection where organisms have disseminated from a localized site of infection.

When there is a strong suspicion of septicaemia the patient is usually started on empirical antimicrobial therapy aimed at several target organisms. If the patient's symptoms are not clear-cut and evidence of an infection is inconclusive, the clinician must decide whether to start broad-spectrum antimicrobial therapy or wait until further information is available. The use of antibiotic therapy increases costs, may cause side effects, and may complicate the achievement of an accurate diagnosis, although an appropriate antibiotic may improve the outcome of an infection. A positive blood culture may help the clinician to confirm an existing presumptive diagnosis and to adjust therapy to a more appropriate or narrow-spectrum anti-microbial. Blood cultures are important tools in the management of patients and prompt processing of positive bottles can help in this process. Early recognition of a positive blood culture is crucial in guiding antimicrobial therapy and influencing patient management. Following recognition of a positive sample, appropriate laboratory techniques must be used to allow prompt and accurate identification and susceptibility testing of the infecting organism.

septicaemia
Septicaemia is the presence of bacteraemia with symptoms of systemic infection. Typical symptoms include pyrexia, chills, rigors, hypotension, shock, and, in more severe cases, multiple organ failure.

Key Point

It is essential that the Gram stain result of a positive blood culture is telephoned as a matter of urgency to the clinician.

Because of the importance of obtaining rapid results with blood cultures we will see that this is one area of microbiology where automation is commonplace. In addition, considerable research has been done over the years to improve culture media and detection methods.

SELF-CHECK 5.1

Why would the patient be started on antibiotics before the sample in the bottle is even positive if septicaemia is suspected?

5.1.1 Blood culture methods

As blood cultures are important samples, which can provide vital information to clinicians on the condition of their patients, it is important that they are taken and processed correctly and promptly. The following section will deal with these aspects.

5.1.2 Procedures for sample taking, transport, and processing

A blood culture involves taking a sample of blood from a patient and inoculating the blood into a blood culture bottle; the bottle is then transported to the laboratory for incubation. The procedure has three main stages: sample taking, transport, and processing.

When taking blood cultures, blood is usually collected from a patient's vein via a syringe. This is known as venepuncture. The venepuncture site must first be disinfected, usually with alcohol (70% isopropyl alcohol is preferred) followed by iodine to remove normal skin organisms. Blood is withdrawn into the syringe and then used to inoculate the blood culture bottles. Occasionally, blood may be taken through a catheter in the skin. Depending on the blood culture system used, there may be a cap that has to be removed to expose a septum; in some systems the septum is not sterile and must be first swabbed with alcohol.

Cross reference
See Chapter 1, Section 1.3.

Cross reference
Chapter 4, Section 4.1.

There are several factors to consider when taking blood cultures:

- They should be taken by experienced personnel, familiar with the blood culture system, and familiar with taking blood cultures.

- The person taking the blood culture should wash their hands with an antimicrobial agent and water (e.g. chlorhexidine gluconate) and wear gloves when the samples are being taken.

- Attention to **aseptic technique** is vital to avoid contamination. Contamination of blood cultures is discussed later in this chapter.

- If other samples of blood are required, e.g. serological (antibody) testing or biochemical or haematological analysis, the blood culture bottles should always be inoculated first. Many types of blood tube are non-sterile and inoculation of these tubes before the blood culture bottles may introduce contamination.

- Bottles should be inoculated with the recommended blood volume.

Many blood culture systems comprise pairs of bottles – an aerobic bottle and an anaerobic bottle; it is usual to inoculate a single pair of bottles on each sampling. In some systems pairs of aerobic bottles are used and anaerobic bottles are added if infection with anaerobic organisms is suspected. Further pairs of bottles should be taken at intervals of several hours, as this both increases the yield of positive results and may allow better recognition of contamination. Two sets of bottles are usually adequate in most cases, although in cases of **endocarditis** (discussed in more detail later in this chapter) more blood culture sets should be taken. For very young children special paediatric blood culture bottles are available, as often only a small amount of blood sample will be available.

Figure 5.1 shows a typical set of commercially available blood culture bottles. In this system, one of the bottles is aerobic and the other is anaerobic. Note the caps on the top of the bottles which cover the septum where the sample is inoculated. The barcode labels are used to identify the bottle. It is important that the barcode is not covered by any patient identification labels as the barcode must be accessible by the incubating instrument.

It is common practice to take blood cultures at the time of, or shortly after, a **pyrexial spike** as this is the time when bacteria are more likely to be found in the bloodstream. It is usual to inoculate 5–10 mL of blood into each of a pair of bottles at each sampling point, depending on the blood culture system used. The manufacturer's recommended blood volume should be used at all times. Lower volumes should be avoided as there is a relationship between the

aseptic technique

Aseptic technique is the use of sterile equipment and procedures to avoid possible contamination.

endocarditis

Endocarditis is an infection of the heart valves.

pyrexial spike

A pyrexial spike is a transient increase in the patient's body temperature.

FIGURE 5.1

A pair of commercially available blood culture bottles. One bottle is an aerobic bottle (left) and the other is an anaerobic bottle (right). Note also the barcodes which help identify the bottle.
Source: Figure kindly provided by R. Dopierala, bioMérieux.

volume of blood cultured and positivity rate. However, larger volumes should also be avoided as it may interfere or overwhelm the neutralization capacity of the bottle. Instead, further sets of bottles should be inoculated.

Once blood culture bottles have been inoculated they should be clearly labelled with full patient details; accompanying report forms should also include patient's symptoms and current and/or recent antibiotic therapy and be sent to the laboratory as soon as possible. It is important that full clinical details are provided as this gives information to laboratory staff on organisms likely to be encountered, further tests that may need to be carried out on positive bottles, and whether bottles require additional procedures such as extended incubation or **terminal subculture**.

terminal subculture
Terminal subculture is where the blood culture bottle is inoculated onto culture media at the end of the incubation period regardless of whether it is positive or not.

Once samples are taken and labelled:

- They must be transported to the laboratory as quickly as possible.
- They should be placed in a clearly labelled incubator, provided and maintained by the microbiology laboratory.
- On no account should blood culture bottles be refrigerated – it may adversely affect some organisms, delay organism growth, and lengthen time for the bottle to become positive.
- If no incubator is available then they should be kept at ambient temperature.
- Once received in the laboratory, samples should be loaded onto any automated system as soon as possible to allow positive samples to be identified quickly.

Key Point

Blood cultures should be transported to the laboratory without delay and should be incubated as soon as possible.

HEALTH & SAFETY

Safety aspects of handling blood cultures

Blood cultures should be treated with great care: breakages can occur and many systems use glass bottles which can cause cuts. Blood may harbour many dangerous pathogens including HIV, various types of hepatitis, and potentially haemorrhagic fever viruses, particularly in patients presenting with pyrexia of unknown origin (**PUO**). Any breakages should be handled with care using locally approved disinfectant and disposal methods, and the disinfectant used must have virucidal activity. Any blood stains on the outside of bottles should be wiped with an appropriate disinfectant, with the operator wearing suitable gloves.

5.1.3 Principles of common blood culture systems

The principle of all blood culture systems is to encourage rapid growth of any bacteria present in the blood sample inoculated into the blood culture bottle. Rapid growth is obtained by using highly nutritious media and incubation at an optimal temperature. Eventually, the number of organisms in the blood culture will reach a threshold where they can be detected either by some biochemical signal or by changes in turbidity.

5.1.4 Types of media used in blood culture systems

In all blood culture systems highly nutritious culture media are an absolute necessity. Many systems employ brain heart infusion broth or tryptic soya broths, which are able to support the rapid growth of a wide range of pathogenic bacteria including fastidious organisms. Equally importantly, the media must be capable of supporting growth from very small inocula. The amount of fermentable carbohydrate (usually glucose) is important, although high concentrations promote rapid growth and acidic conditions produced from glucose may cause autolysis of some organisms unless the medium is highly buffered. In anaerobic bottles the medium will often contain a reducing agent to promote anaerobiosis. The bottle will also be filled with an anaerobic gas mixture to further reduce oxygen tension and stimulate growth of anaerobic bacteria. Although fungi may grow in blood culture broths designed for bacteria, specialized fungal blood culture bottles are available with media optimized for fungal growth and detection, and these should be used if fungal infection is suspected. Similarly, for mycobacteria specialized blood culture bottles are available. In both cases prolonged incubation is the norm – up to 6 weeks for mycobacteria.

Key Point

Blood culture bottles contain highly nutritious culture media to promote rapid growth of pathogens.

SELF-CHECK 5.2

Why is it so important to use highly nutritious media in blood culture systems?

5.1.5 Traditional non-automated blood culture systems

Traditional blood culture systems use bottles filled with culture medium inoculated with a sample of the patient's blood (usually 5–10 mL in adults, 1–3 mL in children). Growth of organisms is identified by an increase in turbidity of the medium and/or haemolysis (breakdown of red blood cells (RBCs)). There are several drawbacks with this approach. Firstly, it takes several hours for RBCs to settle to the bottom of the bottle before turbidity associated with bacterial growth can be observed. Secondly, the degree of turbidity varies from organism to organism: coliforms and staphylococci grow rapidly and produce obvious changes in turbidity, whereas some organisms, such as streptococci and many fastidious organisms, produce less obvious turbidity and may be missed. Frequent checking of bottles in the first 48 h after receipt and **blind subculture** at 24–48 h and at the end of incubation is required. This frequent checking is a highly labour intensive process and every time the bottle is opened to sample it, there is a risk of contamination being introduced and also a potential infection risk to staff.

Because of the drawbacks of traditional systems, various improvements in methods have been made. The biggest improvements in speed and sensitivity came in the 1980s with the development of automated continuous monitoring systems.

5.1.6 Automated blood culture systems

Traditional blood culture systems rely on bacterial growth and turbidity to indicate positivity. As we saw in the previous section, this can be problematic. Newer blood culture methods are able to detect bacterial growth earlier and this can reduce the time to positivity. Because **time to positivity** is critical in diagnosing septicaemia, most laboratories now use blood

blind subculture

Blind subculture is subculture of the bottle regardless of the presence or absence of turbidity or indications of growth.

time to positivity

Time to positivity is the time taken from when a blood culture bottle is inoculated to when it is identified as being positive. Methods that reduce time to positivity are preferred.

culture methods that can reduce this. Next is a description of some of the commonly used methods.

5.1.7 Radiometric methods

The first automated systems used radiometric methods. These involved using culture media containing C^{14} **radiolabelled** glucose; metabolic activity by bacteria or fungi converted the labelled glucose to radiolabelled CO_2 which could be detected in the **headspace** of the bottle. This is achieved by sampling a small volume of the headspace gas and detecting radiolabelled CO_2 in a beta particle counter. Bottles are typically tested two to three times per day in the first 2–3 days and then once or twice daily for the remaining incubation period. Because bottles were not examined for turbidity they could be agitated during incubation, stimulating bacterial growth and shortening detection times. Although such methods were popular and widely used, issues with safety and disposal of radioisotopes led to the development of non-radioactive detection methods.

radiolabelled
Radiometric methods involve the use of radiolabelled substrates to detect bacterial growth.

headspace
Headspace is the gas in a blood culture bottle above the liquid.

5.1.8 Non-radioactive detection methods

Several commercial systems are now available that work by detection of CO_2 produced as a consequence of glucose metabolism during microbial growth. The production of CO_2 from glucose causes a change in fluorescence or reflectance in a sensor located in the bottom of the bottle. In both cases bottles are placed in a dedicated incubator/detector where they are agitated and the sensor is continually monitored to assess the CO_2 content in the bottle. Agitation increases the growth rate of bacteria and reduces the time to positivity, especially in aerobic bottles. In traditional manual systems the lack of agitation may delay detection of a positive bottle. This is one of the main advantages of automated systems.

The bottles are routinely incubated in the incubator/detector for up to 7 days and are then discarded. Bottles can become positive at any time during the incubation period as monitoring is continuous and a signal alerts the user that a bottle is positive. Bottles can then be removed and processed as soon as they become positive. Many laboratories have blood cultures checked outside of normal working hours, allowing early detection and processing of positive bottles. The majority of blood cultures received in the laboratory are negative and reducing the amount of work required on these bottles is beneficial. Because automated methods do not require all bottles to be manually subcultured they produce savings in the time spent processing negative bottles and reduce the amount of culture media used.

Key Point

Although radiometric blood culture methods were commonly used these have largely been replaced by non-radiometric methods which detect CO_2 production by bacteria using sensors that respond to the concentration of CO_2 in the bottle. These methods avoid issues associated with use and disposal of radioisotopes.

Lysis centrifugation methods

Other systems have been developed such as the lysis centrifugation system. In this blood culture system, agents are added to the blood sample, to lyse both red and white cells. The blood

Cross reference
See Chapter 9.

is centrifuged and the deposit containing organisms is harvested and used to inoculate various solid media. This allows a quantitative assessment of the number of bacteria per millilitre of blood. Such techniques are labour intensive but have found value where quantitative cultures are required and in mycobacterial and fungal blood cultures where they can speed up the time to detection for these organisms.

Neutralization of antimicrobial agents and other inhibitory factors

Blood contains many antibacterial components including antibodies and complement. It may also contain a wide variety of antibiotics that the patient has received. These can reduce or inhibit the ability of bacteria to grow and to produce a positive signal either by turbidity or an automated signalling method. Most blood culture systems employ at least one method of inactivating some of these antibacterial systems; simple dilution by the addition of 5 mL of blood to 50–100 mL of medium can reduce the activity of many of these inhibitors. In other systems, special resins or charcoal are added to the medium. These bind many antibacterial agents and reduce their effect. Sodium polyethanol sulphonate (SPS) is added to media and is an effective neutralizer of innate bacterial inhibitory agents in blood. Some systems also contain para aminobenzoic acid (PABA) and thymidine to neutralize the effects of sulphonamides and trimethoprim respectively. In some cases commercially available β-**lactamase** can be added to bottles to neutralize β-lactam drugs.

β-lactamases

β-lactamases are enzymes that breakdown penicillin and related antibiotics (β-lactams) such as ampicillin and destroy their antibacterial activity.

Key Point

Traditional blood culture systems are labour intensive, requiring frequent examination of bottles and blind subcultures. Automated systems often rely on CO_2 production by bacteria as they grow – such systems offer increased positivity rates, shorter time to positivity, and reduced labour costs.

5.2 Procedure for dealing with negative bottles

The majority of blood culture bottles received in the laboratory show no growth and should be discarded after 5–7 days' incubation. If a continuous monitoring system is used a terminal subculture need not be carried out. However, if a traditional manual blood culture system is used it is common for a blind subculture to be carried out. There are some exceptions where bottles may sometimes require longer incubation before being discarded, for example endocarditis (discussed later in this chapter) or in specific patients where there is a possibility of an infection with a fastidious or slow-growing organism. For negative bottles a written report is typically issued to the ward at 48 h and at the end of incubation stating that the culture shows no growth.

5.3 Procedure for dealing with positive bottles

It is important for patient management that positive blood cultures are processed rapidly – in this section we will cover the procedures used to deal with positive blood cultures. There are three stages in this process, namely microscopy, culture and sensitivity tests, and finally iden-tification of the pathogen.

The first stage in processing is to carry out a Gram stain on the blood culture:

- The aim of a Gram stain of a positive blood culture bottle is to provide the clinician with a guide to the identity of a possible pathogen, allowing initiation of appropriate antibiotics. Up to 24 h may elapse before susceptibility test results and the organism's identity are known; initial therapy is therefore frequently guided by the Gram stain result.

- A presumptive identification of the bacteria in a positive blood culture is invaluable to clini-cians in assessing the requirement for and type of antimicrobial therapy appropriate for a patient.

HEALTH & SAFETY

Safety aspects of processing positive blood cultures

In most cases positive blood cultures can be handled on the bench; it is good practice to wear gloves to protect against infection from spillages. Disinfectants with virucidal properties should be used to clean up blood culture spillages. If there is a suspicion that a Category 3 organism may be present (e.g. *Salmonella typhi*, *Brucella abortus*, or *Neisseria meningitidis*) all work must be performed in a Class I safety cabinet. *In some institutions it is standard practice to process all posi-tive blood cultures in a safety cabinet because of the potential risk of such organisms being present.* Removing fluid from blood culture bottles and preparing Gram stains can result in the generation of potentially infectious aerosols, and therefore use of a safety cabinet is mandatory. In such cases all materials for working with blood cultures (e.g. microscope slides, loops, hotplates) must be contained in the safety cabinet.

A venting needle is used to aspirate liquid from a blood culture bottle. Used needles must not be resheathed but should be placed into suitable containers for incineration. Where organisms such as *Brucella* spp., *Francisella tularensis*, *Yersinia pestis*, or *Bacillus anthracis* are suspected on the basis of clinical details and occupational information, it is both appropriate and prudent to send bottles direct to a laboratory better equipped for working with these pathogens.

Brucella spp. are pathogens of farm animals and are most frequently isolated from vets or farm-ers. The other organisms are potentially organisms associated with bioterrorism threats.

5.3.1 Microscopy of positive blood cultures

When a bottle becomes positive, either because of turbidity in a manual bottle or from a positive signal from an automated system, it is removed from the incubator and a sample of the fluid is taken for a Gram stain. Special venting needles can be used to aspirate a sample or in some systems the top can be removed and some fluid aspirated. Experience is required to ensure that the smears are neither too thick nor too thin. The slide should be fixed on a hotplate and flaming in a Bunsen burner should be carried out to completely kill all bacteria.

Key Point

Gram staining is the first stage in processing positive blood culture bottles. The result of the Gram stain plays an important role in patient management and antibiotic therapy is often started on the basis of the Gram stain result.

5.3.2 Differentiation of bacterial types based on microscopy results

Gram staining of the slide is carried out as normal using neutral red as a counter stain, although some laboratories prefer to use dilute carbol fuchsin as the counter stain to aid visualization of small Gram-negative rods. In the majority of cases abundant bacteria are clearly visible and the type, arrangement and staining reaction should be recorded. This can provide important information on the identity of the organism; for example pairs of lanceolate Gram-positive diplococci may be *Streptococcus pneumoniae*, clusters of large Gram-positive cocci may be staphylococci.

In some cases the morphology and arrangement of bacteria may not be characteristic and it may not be possible to presumptively identify an organism in a positive bottle. This typically occurs with Gram-positive cocci occurring singly, in pairs and in small groups, which may be staphylococci or streptococci. Although a certain bacterial type may be immediately evident on a smear, for example Gram-positive cocci in clusters, further examination of the smear should be carried out to identify smaller numbers of other bacterial types. Mixed infections, although uncommon, do occur.

Microbiology medical staff should be informed of the Gram stain results and provisional identity so that advice on therapy can be provided to the ward clinicians. A written report should also be issued to the ward with the Gram stain result.

SELF-CHECK 5.3

Why is it important that the result of the Gram stain is reported to clinicians as quickly as possible?

5.3.3 Procedures in the event of negative microscopy

Occasionally, we come across situations where a blood culture bottle is positive but the Gram stain does not show any organisms even after careful examination. There may be several reasons for this:

- Bacteria may be present but too small or too poorly stained to see.
- In manual systems turbidity in bottles may be due to blood lipids or red blood cells that have not settled out.

In automated detection systems false positives do occur – most often due to metabolic activity of white blood cells in the bottle. Large numbers of white cells will often be seen on the Gram stain. Examine the signal from the bottle; Figure 5.2 shows typical traces from a negative blood culture bottle, a true positive bottle and a bottle that has become positive because of white blood cell metabolism. The traces of the true positive bottle and false positive bottle are clearly distinct and it is relatively easy to identify cases where a positive signal occurs because of white blood cell metabolism.

In all cases the procedures listed in the Method Box for organisms not showing on Gram stain of positive blood culture should be carried out.

FIGURE 5.2

Typical growth indices obtained from a commercial blood culture system, highlighting the differences in profile between a true positive bottle and a false positive caused by a high white cell count.

Source: Courtesy of D. Law.

 METHOD *Organisms not showing on Gram stain of positive blood culture*

- Repeat Gram stain – consider alternative counter stain, e.g. dilute carbol fuchsin.
- If still negative, consider alternative stains, e.g. acridine orange, or Giemsa.
- If no bacteria are seen on further smears, subculture the bottle onto blood agar, incubated aerobically and anaerobically, plus a chocolate agar plate incubated in CO_2 for 4 days. Plates should be examined daily to detect any slow-growing organisms.
- The blood culture bottle should always be reincubated.

Key Point

Positive bottles with negative microscopy must be investigated further. A repeat Gram stain is the first step in this process. Positive bottles with negative microscopy should be cultured and the bottle reincubated. False-positive blood cultures do occur.

5.3.4 Culture regimes following microscopy

When a blood culture becomes positive, microscopy is the first stage of the process to identify and characterize the infecting organism. Following microscopy, the blood culture is cultured to isolate and identify the infecting organism. At the same time sensitivity tests to antibiotics should be carried out and identification tests set up if appropriate. The aim for the laboratory is to have a culture result, a presumptive identification of the pathogen, and a sensitivity test result to appropriate antibiotics within 24 h of the bottle becoming positive. The efforts of the laboratory must be focused on achieving these aims; with the most common blood culture pathogens this is certainly possible.

5.3.5　Culture of positive bottles

When a blood culture bottle becomes positive, microscopy is carried out, and once the result of microscopy is known the bottle should be cultured. The results of microscopy dictate the type of culture plates set up for each positive blood culture bottle.

In all cases, a minimum of blood agar plates incubated aerobically and anaerobically and a chocolate agar plate incubated in CO_2 should be inoculated for each positive sample. The most common bacterial pathogens will grow on at least one of these media in 24 h with some requiring 48 h. In some cases, prolonged incubation may be required, particularly for anaerobic or fastidious organisms. If there is no growth on the plates at 24 h, the Gram stain should be repeated on the bottle to ensure that no errors have been made.

Cultures should be set up on positive bottles depending on Gram stain results and clinical details. Some suggested culture regimes for commonly encountered organisms are listed in Table 5.1. These can be modified based on local experience and local prevalence rates of pathogens.

If mixtures of organisms are seen on Gram stain then appropriate susceptibility tests should be carried out against all organisms expected to be isolated. Selective media should be set up to assist isolation of slow-growing organisms or those likely to be overgrown, for example in a mixture of streptococci and possible coliforms, neomycin or naladixic acid containing media can help isolate the *Streptococcus*. Or in the case of swarming *Proteus* and staphylococci the use of mannitol salt agar or MacConkey's/CLED agar with appropriate antibiotic discs (gentamicin, naladixic acid or aztreonam) may help isolate the *Staphylococcus*.

5.3.6　Direct susceptibility tests

It is important that direct susceptibility tests are carried out on all positive blood cultures, so that a provisional sensitivity result is available as soon as possible. **Direct susceptibility tests** should be carried out on media and under incubation conditions (CO_2/anaerobic) appropriate for the target organism. The antibiotics used in susceptibility tests should reflect those of the local antibiotic policies and local resistance patterns and must be continually re-evaluated.

direct susceptibility test

A direct susceptibility test is a sensitivity test carried out directly on a sample rather than on an isolated bacterial culture. It is more difficult to standardize inocula on direct sensitivities and mixtures of organisms can be problematic.

Cross reference

See Chapter 4.

It is important when carrying out a direct susceptibility test that the inoculum is acceptable. Whilst getting the correct inoculum is a matter of trial and error there are some guidelines. For Gram-negative organisms likely to be coliforms, a drop of blood culture fluid should be mixed with 5 mL of water and used to inoculate plates. For potential staphylococci three drops of blood culture should be mixed with 5 mL of water. For other organisms a single drop of fluid from the blood culture is used to inoculate the plate.

Disc susceptibility tests can be carried out on different media and incubated under different conditions depending on the Gram stain results and the likely identity of the organism. Disc tests also allow the identification of mixed cultures. Although direct susceptibility tests on blood cultures are important, susceptibility tests should always be repeated with a pure culture using the laboratory's standard methodology where inoculum and incubation time can be more carefully controlled.

TABLE 5.1 Culture media and identification tests required for organisms seen in positive blood culture bottles.

Gram stain result	Target organism	Media	Identification aids	Confirmatory tests
Gram-positive cocci in clusters	S. aureus Coagulase-negative Staph.	Blood agar in air Chocolate agar in CO_2 Blood agar anaerobically Susceptibility test in air + methicillin/cefoxitin at 30°C Chromogenic MRSA medium	DNase medium MRSA agar Slide coagulase	Slide and tube coagulase test Or latex agglutination test for S. aureus Commercial kits
Gram-positive cocci in pairs or chains	Streptococci S. pneumoniae Enterococcus spp.	Blood agar in air Chocolate agar in CO_2 Blood agar anaerobically Susceptibility test in CO_2	Granada plate if child or expectant mother Optochin discs on CO_2 or anaerobic plate High level gentamicin susceptibility	Catalase test Lancefield group Commercial identification kits
Gram-positive bacilli Coryneform	Listeria spp. Corynebacterium spp. Propionobacterium spp.	Blood agar in CO_2 Chocolate agar in CO_2 Blood agar anaerobically + metronidazole disc Susceptibility test in CO_2	Aerobic growth Anaerobic growth Selective Listeria medium Broth for tumbling motility	Commercial identification kits
Large, Gram-positive bacilli +/- spores	Clostridium spp. Bacillus spp.	Blood agar in air Chocolate agar in CO_2 FAA anaerobically + metronidazole disc Susceptibility test in O_2 and anaerobically	Anaerobic growth Aerobic growth	Commercial identification kits
Gram-negative cocci	N. meningitidis N. gonorrhoeae	Blood agar in air Chocolate agar in CO_2 Blood agar anaerobically Susceptibility tests in CO_2	Latex agglutination on blood culture broth	Initial confirmation with oxidase reaction and serological tests Confirm with serological tests
Gram-negative rod Coliform type morphology	Coliforms Pseudomonas spp. Non-fermenters, e.g. Acinetobacter spp.	Blood agar in air Chocolate agar in CO_2 Blood agar anaerobically + metronidazole disc CLED/MacConkey Chromogenic coliform media Susceptibility test in air	Oxidase test Reaction on chromogenic medium Serology on possible Salmonella spp.	Confirm with biochemical tests, and serology where appropriate (Salmonella)
Gram-negative rod Small, poorly staining OR Growth in anaerobic bottle or appearance suggestive of anaerobes	Anaerobes Haemophilus spp. Cardiobacterium Eikenella Kingella	Blood agar in CO_2 Chocolate agar in CO_2 Blood agar anaerobically + metronidazole disc CLED/MacConkey FAA anaerobically Susceptibility test in CO_2 Susceptibility test anaerobically	Growth in CO_2 Growth anaerobically	Susceptibility to metronidazole X and V factor dependence Commercial identification kits

If both bottles in a pair of blood cultures show the same types of organism on Gram stain then both bottles should be cultured, although a direct sensitivity test is often only carried out on one of the pair, unless the morphology in each bottle is distinct.

SELF-CHECK 5.4

Why is it important to perform direct susceptibility tests on positive blood cultures?

5.3.7 Additional tests

As well as carrying out direct susceptibility tests other media can be set up to aid in the identification and characterization of the organisms in the blood culture. Chromogenic media can be used which may help in identifying many common pathogens, for example MRSA, coliforms, and yeasts, depending on the result of the Gram stain.

There are some specific tests that can be carried out directly on the blood culture bottle to assist in identification of the organism.

Gram-positive cocci in clusters are often staphylococci but it is important to differentiate between *S. aureus* and coagulase-negative staphylococci, the latter frequently occurring as contaminants (this is discussed later in this chapter). Methods are available to differentiate *S. aureus* from coagulase negative staphylococci in blood cultures such as the heat-stable nuclease test, although this is not widely used. More commonly, DNase plates are set up with confirmation of identity by slide coagulase test on isolated colonies.

Cross reference
See Chapter 3, Section 3.6.

Key Point

The DNase test is commonly used to differentiate *S. aureus* from other staphylococci. This is typically carried out using DNase agar. *S. aureus* is DNase positive whereas most coagulase-negative staphylococci are DNase negative.

S. pneumoniae can be identified by carrying out a pneumococcal antigen test on a sample of the blood culture. This uses a commercially available latex reagent. Similar methods may also be available for identification of *N. meningitidis* in blood culture containing Gram-negative cocci.

Commercially available identification tests such as API strips and VITEK cards may be inoculated directly from blood culture bottles. However, blood and blood culture media components may interfere with the interpretation of certain tests and so results obtained in this way may produce incorrect identifications and often have to be repeated. For rapidly growing organisms such as *E. coli* and other coliforms, if plates are inoculated early in the day, there may be sufficient material growing on an aerobic blood agar plate 6–8 h later to allow an identification test to be set up and read the following day with the culture plates and susceptibility test. In all identification tests a non-selective culture plate must be set up to ensure that the culture is pure. However, most laboratories wait until the culture has grown sufficiently to provide single colonies to carry out identification tests or serological identification. Identification methods will vary from laboratory to laboratory but when commercial kits are used the manufacturer's instructions must be followed.

PCR
PCR (polymerase chain reaction) is a technique involving amplification of specific DNA sequences which can be used to rapidly identify pathogens.

Although not widely available yet, it is likely that in the future commercially available **PCR** (polymerase chain reaction) tests will be used to provide rapid identification of pathogens found in blood cultures.

> ### Key Point
> It is imperative to set up sufficient cultures to allow a preliminary identification of the organism seen in the Gram stain. Direct sensitivity tests must also be set up. The antibiotics tested should reflect both the possible identity of the organism and local guidelines and local susceptibility patterns.

5.4 Bacterial pathogens

It is important for anyone dealing with blood cultures that there is an understanding of the common organisms isolated, the conditions associated with these organisms, and possible sources of infection. We will now consider the organisms commonly found in blood cultures and discuss these aspects.

5.4.1 Pathogens likely to be a cause of septicaemia and bacteraemia

A search of the literature will show that a very wide range of bacteria can be isolated from blood cultures as a cause of septicaemia.

Although figures vary from one survey to another, most studies show that the majority of positive blood cultures yield one of the following pathogens: *S. aureus*, *E. coli* or other enterobacteria, *S. pneumoniae*, *Enterococcus* spp., *Pseudomonas aeruginosa*, or *Candida albicans*. As you can see from Figure 5.3 the number of bacteraemias caused by *E. coli* alone across the UK is rising year on year. Gram-negative organisms such as *E. coli* are a significant cause of morbidity and mortality.

> ### Key Point
> The incidence of various pathogens varies from hospital to hospital and reflects to some extent the medical/surgical specialities in a given institution.

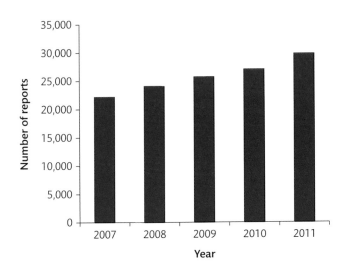

FIGURE 5.3

E. coli bacteraemia reports, England, Wales, and Northern Ireland: 2007 to 2011.

S. *aureus* is one of the most frequent pathogens isolated from blood cultures; this organism enters the bloodstream from an infected site in the body. Common sites of infection include abscesses in various tissues and organs, infected lesions in skin, for example cellulitis, and infected joints; occasionally pneumonia can be caused by S. *aureus* and septicaemia is often associated with this. The isolation of S. *aureus* from a blood culture is usually indicative of an infection at another body site and should prompt further clinical and microbiological investigation to identify the source.

E. *coli* is one of the other frequent causes of septicaemia. In most cases it is associated with an infection in the urinary tract, such as **pyelonephritis**, or in the elderly or immunocompromised a simple UTI may result in E. *coli* bacteraemia. Other sources of the organism include intestinal lesions and infections of the biliary tract. Similarly, other members of the Enterobacteriaceae also cause UTI and may be found in the blood as a result. *Salmonella enterica* may be found in cases of severe food poisoning or occasionally as a result of biliary sepsis. S. *typhi* and S. *paratyphi* cause enteric fever and rapid diagnosis and treatment of such infections is essential; any non-lactose fermenting, oxidase-negative colonies isolated from blood cultures should therefore be checked using antisera to see if they are *Salmonella*.

pyelonephritis

Pyelonephritis is an infection of the kidney, which is a complication of urine infection.

Key Point

Check all non-lactose fermenting, oxidase-negative, Gram-negative bacilli isolated from blood culture with antisera to exclude *Salmonella* spp.

Coagulase-negative staphylococci are frequently encountered in blood cultures but as we will see later in the chapter they are often contaminants, being derived from the skin during the taking of blood. They can be occasionally pathogenic, and cannot therefore be discarded without looking closely at the patient's symptoms; in particular they are often associated with infections of catheters and indwelling lines.

S. *pneumoniae* is often isolated from patients with chest infections (e.g. pneumonia) or occasionally meningitis. For some patients with pneumonia, blood culture may be the best means of microbiological diagnosis, as sputum production may be poor or the sample may be overgrown with normal flora.

Enterococci are frequently encountered as pathogens in blood cultures and have two principal sources: firstly, the urinary tract where they are a common cause of infection; and, secondly, the bowel is an important source. There is a strong association between *Streptococcus bovis* endocarditis and cancer of the bowel. Enterococcal septicaemia can be problematic to treat because of the limited range of active therapeutic agents.

β-haemolytic streptococci, principally those of Lancefield groups A, C, and G, are encountered in blood, usually as a result of a skin infection (e.g. cellulitis and infected leg ulcers). *Streptococcus agalactiae* (group B *Streptococcus*) is most commonly encountered in cases of neonatal sepsis.

Pasteurella multocida may occur in blood cultures, often associated with an abscess or skin infection following an animal bite. It may also be associated with chest infections.

α-haemolytic streptococci are encountered most frequently in patients with endocarditis where the organisms are derived from the oropharynx; however, they do occur as contaminants in blood cultures, often through oral contamination during venepuncture.

Anaerobic Gram-negative rods, such as *Bacteroides* spp. and *Prevotella* spp., occur in blood cultures of patients with abdominal sepsis or following surgical procedures on the bowel, female reproductive system or oropharynx. Although prophylaxis with metronidazole has markedly reduced the incidence of anaerobic infections including septicaemia they may still occur.

N. meningitidis although rare is an extremely important pathogen, indicating septicaemia with the possible presence of meningitis. Suspicion of this organism in a blood culture should immediately be brought to the attention of a clinician; the clinical course of meningococcal septicaemia can be very severe with many complications and rapid, aggressive antibiotic therapy is required. Biochemical tests are required to differentiate the organism from *N. gonorrhoeae* which may occasionally occur in blood cultures, often as a complication of a joint infection, and oral *Neisseria/Moraxella* which are often found as contaminants.

Candida albicans is recognized as the fourth or fifth most common blood culture isolate in some studies. *C. albicans* is most common in **immunocompromised** patients, patients with central venous catheters, and in premature infants. Use of broad-spectrum antibiotics may predispose to *Candida* infection by removing bacterial flora and increasing colonization by yeasts. Cytotoxic therapy for cancer patients may damage the gut mucosa allowing *Candida* to move from the bowel into the bloodstream. *Candida* infections carry a high mortality, partly due to the underlying status of the patients; therefore rapid diagnosis and speciation is important. Some species of *Candida* (e.g. *C. glabrata* and *C. krusei*) are often resistant to azole antifungals and their identification is required to ensure that correct therapy is given.

Key Point

When a fungal infection is suspected specialized fungal blood cultures should be taken.

SELF-CHECK 5.5

What are the commonest pathogens associated with septicaemia?

5.4.2 Polymicrobial bacteraemia

Although most cases of bacteraemia or septicaemia are caused by a single organism, occasional cases of **polymicrobial bacteraemia** occur. Many cases of polymicrobial bacteraemia are associated with serious underlying illness and frequently arise from the bowel. Organisms likely to be associated with such infections include enterobacteria, enterococci and anaerobes. The death rate from cases of polymicrobial bacteraemia is often higher than that from **monomicrobial bacteraemia**; this reflects both the nature of the underlying condition and the requirement for aggressive therapy against two different pathogens.

SELF-CHECK 5.6

Would it be easier to treat a polymicrobial or a monomicrobial bacteraemia? What are the reasons for your answer?

5.4.3 Mycobacteria

Mycobacterium tuberculosis may occur in blood during the primary phase of tuberculosis. However, other mycobacteria, such as *Mycobacterium avium-intracellulare*, may also occur in blood particularly in immunosuppressed patients, and especially those with AIDS.

immunocompromised

Immunocompromised, or immunodeficient, is a state where the patient's immune function is absent or impaired so the ability to fight infection is impaired. This can be as a result of drug action (e.g. immunosuppressive drugs used for organ transplantation) or disease (e.g. HIV infection).

Cross reference

See Chapter 11.

polymicrobial bacteraemia

Polymicrobial bacteraemia is bacteraemia where two or more significant organisms are isolated.

monomicrobial bacteraemia

Monomicrobial bacteraemia is bacteraemia where only one significant organism is isolated.

Mycobacteria are unlikely to be detected in conventional blood culture systems because the length of incubation of the blood culture bottle and solid media is too short.

Various techniques have been developed to help isolate mycobacteria from blood. The lysis centrifugation technique (described in Section 5.1.8) is useful; however, automated systems similar to those for conventional bacterial cultures have been developed. These incorporate a mycobacterial medium with a CO_2 sensor system; bottles are incubated for 3–4 weeks and checked for a positive signal on a daily basis. When such a bottle becomes positive, Gram stain and acid–alcohol-fast bacilli (AAFB) stains are carried out on the material, as well as further subculture onto mycobacterial-specific media. PCR may be useful for rapid identification of an AAFB present in a blood culture bottle.

Cross reference
See Chapter 9, Section 9.4.

All work with mycobacterial blood cultures must be carried out in a Class II safety cabinet; such work is often carried out in specialized centres with dedicated automated systems for mycobacteria. It may be appropriate to send blood culture bottles for mycobacterial investigation to such centres for processing.

5.4.4 Bacteraemia in children

Although most of the organisms described in the previous sections can cause infection in children and babies there are certain pathogens that are more frequently encountered in children. In newborn infants bacteraemia is commonly caused by either *E. coli*, *S. agalactiae*, or *Listeria monocytogenes* and often leads to the development of meningitis. Coagulase-negative staphylococci are also responsible for a significant proportion of cases of bacteraemia in children, often in association with intravenous catheters. Coagulase-negative staphylococci may also occur as contaminants and distinguishing true infection from contamination can be problematic (blood culture contamination is discussed later in this chapter). The problem is compounded by the small volumes of blood cultured from babies and the number of bottles taken. Infection with a species of yeast, *Candida parapsilosis* is relatively common and is probably related to the use of intravenous lines, which are colonized with relative ease by this organism.

Key Point

It is essential to rapidly differentiate *S. agalactiae* from *Listeria monocytogenes* as soon as possible. This is because the patient is likely to have been started on a cephalosporin antibiotic and *Listeria* is resistant. In cases where *Listeria* has not been recognized early, neonatal deaths have occurred.

Until recently, *Haemophilus influenzae* type b (Hib) was a common cause of septicaemia in children, often associated with meningitis or epiglottitis. However, vaccination with the Hib vaccine has resulted in a marked decline in the incidence of Hib infections.

leucopenia
Leucopenia is a reduction in the total number of white blood cells.

5.4.5 Bacteraemia in immunocompromised patients

Many hospitalized patients are immunocompromised, most frequently because of concurrent therapy for transplants, cancer, disease such as AIDS, or congenital immunological defects. **Leucopenia** and **neutropenia** represent the greatest risk of infection and are related to the neutrophil count. Although pathogens found in immunocompetent patients also infect immunocompromised patients, many infections are caused by organisms of low virulence which are commonly members of the normal flora. Many of the patients have underlying illnesses, long hospital stays, indwelling venous catheters, and have received broad-spectrum antibiotics.

neutropenia
Neutropenia is a reduction in the number of phagocytic white blood cells.

Infections caused by coagulase-negative staphylococci, *Listeria* spp., non-fermentative Gram-negative rods such as *Flavobacterium* spp., and fungi such as *Candida* spp. and *Aspergillus* spp. are common. Infections may also involve two or more organisms. It is sometimes difficult to determine whether an organism isolated from a blood culture is a pathogen or a contaminant (methods to differentiate significant isolates from contaminants are described later in this chapter). Treatment of such infections is also problematic as the lack of defence mechanisms reduces the efficacy of many antimicrobial agents, and cidal agents or combinations should be employed wherever possible rather than static agents.

Key Point

Although many types of bacteria are isolated from blood cultures, the most common organisms are staphylococci, enterobacteria, streptococci, and *Pseudomonas*. Polymicrobial infections account for over 10% of cases of septicaemia.

5.5 False-positive results

We have seen the importance that a blood culture has in patient management and how antibiotic therapy may be started or changed on the basis of a Gram stain of a positive bottle. However, not every organism detected in a blood culture is a pathogen and in many cases the organism is considered not significant – its occurrence in the blood culture may be due to contamination of the bottle. We will discuss the implications of contamination, ways to differentiate significant isolates from contaminants, and ways to reduce contamination.

5.5.1 Blood culture contamination

Contaminated cultures are a source of frustration for clinicians and laboratory personnel alike. For the former it is not known whether treatment is warranted or not. In many cases, patients will be started on antibiotic therapy, which may then be stopped when the identity of the organism is determined. This results in increased drug costs, longer hospital stays, the possibility of side effects, and problems of achieving a diagnosis due to concurrent antibiotic therapy. For laboratory personnel processing of contaminated blood cultures takes up valuable time and resources.

Blood culture contamination rates vary widely from institution to institution with an average rate of around 2–3% of bottles. There is some suggestion that rates are increasing, possibly related to improved blood culture methods, greater use of indwelling catheters, and changes in phlebotomy practices to minimize the risk of **needlestick injuries**.

SELF-CHECK 5.7

What are the possible consequences for a patient whose blood culture becomes positive, but the isolated organism is later found to be a contaminant?

---

needlestick injury

A needlestick injury occurs when a needle used to take a blood sample from a patient accidentally pierces the skin of a health-care worker. There is an infection risk associated with needlestick injuries.

5.5.2 Determining the significance of a possible contaminated culture

How can contamination be recognized and differentiated from truly significant bacteraemia? The most useful clue for determining whether an organism is a possible contaminant is to determine its identity. Certain organisms, such as *E. coli* and other enterobacteria, *S. aureus*, *S. pneumoniae*, *P. aeruginosa*, and *C. albicans*, are almost always genuine pathogens. On the other hand, coagulase-negative staphylococci, *Corynebacterium* spp., *Bacillus* spp. (other than *B. anthracis*), and *Propionobacterium acnes* are contaminants in many but not all cases. Of these organisms coagulase-negative staphylococci are most frequently encountered as a cause of blood culture contamination, representing over 70% of contaminants. However, coagulase-negative staphylococci are also increasingly implicated as a cause of significant bacteraemia, especially in patients with prosthetic devices or central venous catheters. Some studies suggest that between 10 and 25% of coagulase-negative staphylococcal isolates may be significant.

Each case of possible contamination must be examined on its own merits with regard to the patient's clinical condition and other factors described next in Section 5.5.3. Where there is doubt as to the significance of an organism further blood cultures should be taken, and micro-biological samples from other body sites should be considered to identify the source or focus of infection.

5.5.3 Factors to consider when determining the significance of an isolate

When we isolate an organism from a blood culture and its significance is unclear we have to look at other data to help us interpret the result. A combination of factors is used to determine the significance of an isolate.

Three factors can be considered which may help determine the significance of the isolate; these are:

1. The number of positive bottles out of the number taken.
2. The time taken for the bottles to become positive.
3. Clinical information.

Number of positive bottles

The first factor that helps differentiate contamination from true infection is to examine the number of positive sets of blood cultures from the total number of sets taken. Growth of a possible contaminant organism from only one of two sets can usually be viewed as contamination. In cases of genuine bacteraemia the same organism is usually isolated from multiple sets of blood culture bottles taken at different times, highlighting the value of taking multiple sets of bottles. The number of positive bottles within a set of bottles is not as useful because of the use of mixed bottle sets. For example, the occurrence of growth in the aerobic bottle only may not necessarily indicate contamination, but may reflect poorer growth of the organism in the anaerobic bottle, which may take longer to become positive.

Time for the bottles to become positive

A further factor to consider is time to positivity: cultures that become positive in 3–5 days are more likely to represent contamination than cultures that become positive in the first 48 h. This may reflect the organism load injected into the bottle. In cases of bacteraemia or septi-caemia the number of organisms in each millilitre of blood may be in excess of 100. Organisms may be multiplying rapidly, and consequently growth is rapid and time to positivity is short and may be measured in hours. In contrast, contamination in many cases is likely to be caused by injection of small numbers of organism into the bottle, growth is slow and time to positivity may stretch to several days.

Clinical information

Perhaps the most useful clue to assessing the significance of a blood culture isolate is the use of clinical information including: the presence of sepsis, hypothermia or pyrexia, high white cell counts, and high or rising **C-reactive protein** levels.

The presence of such symptoms, along with the isolation of a potential contaminant organism, warrants an assessment of both the patient and organism. In such situations further blood cultures may be taken, and therapy with an appropriate antibiotic may be started. If a coagulase-negative staphylococci or other potential contaminant is isolated from a blood culture but the patient is generally well, with little or no fever at the time the culture becomes positive, the isolate is frequently regarded as a contaminant.

Many patients have vascular catheters inserted into veins and blood cultures are frequently drawn from such catheters. A positive culture taken via a catheter may represent true bacteraemia, true contamination or catheter colonization; up to a quarter of catheters are colonized by coagulase-negative staphylococci. It is sometimes advocated that samples are taken through the skin at the same time as catheter blood samples are taken to allow an assessment of contamination.

Frequent removal of vascual catheters is recommended to ensure that the risk of seeding the patient's blood through indwelling catheters is minimized. Biofilms can form in these devices and virtually any organism can then enter the bloodstream. In some cases pathogens such as MRSA can cause sepsis in this way. The end of the catheter can be sent in a sterile container to the laboratory for culture. The catheter is then rolled onto a blood agar plate and examined for growth after overnight incubation. Huge emphasis is placed on keeping catheter lines free from bacteria at ward level as the consequences to the patient (particularly on ITU) can be severe.

If there is doubt about the significance of an organism repeat blood cultures are frequently taken; if the same organism is isolated from further bottles the likelihood that it is a contaminant is lower.

> **C-reactive protein**
> C-reactive protein (CRP) is a protein found in blood; levels of CRP increase when there is inflammation or infection.

Key Point

Distinguishing whether an organism is a contaminant or pathogen is difficult. Factors to be considered include: the identity of the organism, the number of bottles positive, the time taken to become positive, and the patient's symptoms. Further bottles may need to be taken to confirm or refute contamination.

5.5.4 Non-cultural markers of septicaemia

Although cultures remain the gold standard for diagnosis of septicaemia there is a need to identify other (often biochemical) markers, which may give an early indication of sepsis. These surrogate markers may allow early presumptive therapy, and continual monitoring of the marker may yield information regarding the effectiveness of antimicrobial therapy. They may also help differentiate contamination from true cases of septicaemia.

A wide range of markers have been examined for their association with sepsis. Temperature measurements, white cell counts, and C-reactive protein are all frequently used as indicators of sepsis. However, they are relatively non-specific and may be raised in other conditions. Other markers have been investigated; these include procalcitonin, macrophage migration inhibitory factor, soluble urokinase-type plasminogen activator receptor, and soluble triggering factor expressed on myeloid cells. However, none has proven to be a specific marker of septicaemia in all patients. For some markers (e.g. procalcitonin) kits are available for the measurement of levels in blood.

5.5.5 Reducing the incidence of blood culture contamination

The most obvious way to reduce the problems caused by blood culture contamination for clinicians and laboratory staff is to reduce its incidence. The most common source of blood culture contamination is the skin of the patient at the site where the blood culture is taken. **Skin antisepsis** is therefore of crucial importance when taking blood cultures and inadequate skin preparation is the commonest cause of blood culture contamination.

There are various skin disinfectant regimes in use but whichever is used the length of time that the disinfectant is applied to the skin is important.

The septa of blood culture bottles through which blood is inoculated although covered before use are often not sterile and these must be wiped, usually with alcohol, prior to inoculation.

Staff specifically trained to take blood cultures have been found to have significantly lower contamination rates than non-specialized staff. The use of dedicated teams to take blood cultures should be encouraged wherever possible, as reducing blood culture contamination can have a major impact on laboratory workload, reduce antibiotic usage, and costs, and helps in clinical decision-making.

skin antisepsis
Skin antisepsis is preparing the skin with disinfectant to remove bacteria before the blood is taken.

Key Points

Contamination is a major problem but can be reduced by using trained, dedicated staff for taking blood cultures.

Differentiation of contamination from true bacteraemia can be difficult in some cases.

Various markers have been assessed to distinguish contamination from true septicaemia, but to date none is completely predictive.

SELF-CHECK 5.8

Would one contaminating organism cause a problem in a blood culture bottle?

5.6 Endocarditis

5.6.1 Principles of how bacteria cause endocarditis

Endocarditis is an infection of the endocardium, the inner lining of the heart and heart valves. It is a serious illness that is fatal if left untreated. Endocarditis arises when bacteria gain access to the bloodstream through brushing teeth, surgical procedures, or in drug addicts through the use of dirty needles. In most cases the immune system rapidly removes these organisms so that they pose no risk to health. However, bacteria may occasionally settle on a heart valve and cause disease. This is most likely to occur if there has been pre-existing damage to the heart valve, following surgery, or it may be caused by rheumatic fever or congenital heart defects. It can also occur on normal valves with certain pathogens such as *S. aureus*. Damaged valves are more prone to infection for several reasons. For example, they cause defects in blood flow, resulting in stagnation of blood around some areas of the valve. This allows bacteria to adhere more readily to valve tissue. Damaged valves may also have fibrin deposits to which bacteria adhere. Once bacteria have settled on a valve they grow and over time small clumps of material develop. These clumps are known as vegetations. The vegetations contain organisms, fibrin deposits, and blood clots. The vegetations cause valve dysfunction, resulting in abnormal blood flow, and can lead to heart failure.

Key Point

The aortic and mitral valves are the most commonly affected heart valves.

Figure 5.4 shows a heart that has been dissected to expose the mitral valve. In the normal heart this consists of smooth tissue but this heart, from a patient with endocarditis, shows numerous vegetations on the valve. These vegetations cause the valve to malfunction. Pieces of the vegetation can also break off and disseminate around the body.

5.6.2 Bacteria associated with endocarditis

The most common bacteria implicated in native valve endocarditis are oral streptococci, such as *Strep. mitis* and *Strep. oralis*; occasionally nutritionally dependent streptococci (*Abiotropha* spp.) are isolated from cases of endocarditis. *S. aureus* and *Enterococcus* spp. are also encountered with a reasonable frequency. Many other bacteria can cause endocarditis, for example the HACEK group of organisms (*Haemophilus* spp., *Aggregatibacter actinomycetemcomitans* (previously named *Actinobacillus*), *Cardiobacterium hominis*, *Eikenella corrodens*, and *Kingella* species). The primary source of these organisms is the oropharynx.

Vegetation

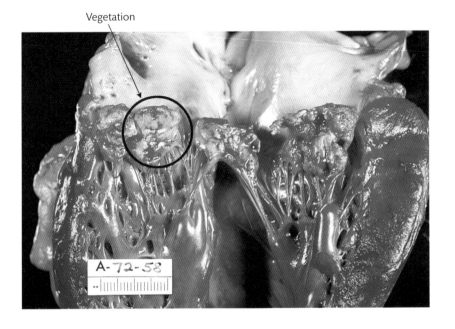

FIGURE 5.4

Dissection of the heart from a patient with endocarditis showing vegetations on the mitral valve.

Source: Figure kindly provided by CDC/Dr Edwin J. Ewing Jr.

Prosthetic valves as well as native heart valves may become infected to produce prosthetic valve endocarditis (PVE). The microbiology of this condition is different to that of native valve endocarditis. Two forms of PVE occur: early PVE and late PVE. Early PVE occurs within 2 months of surgery and is likely to be caused by contamination of the valve during replacement surgery. Infection is typically caused by coagulase-negative staphylococci, *S. aureus*, fungi such as *Candida* spp. and *Aspergillus* spp., and *Corynebacterium* spp. Late PVE occurs a year or more after surgery. The organisms isolated from such cases are similar to those causing native valve endocarditis and the source of these bacteria is the same as those causing native valve endocarditis.

Endocarditis is a particular risk for intravenous drug abusers; the organisms causing endocarditis in such patients may be quite different from those causing endocarditis in non-drug abusers; commonly *S. aureus* or enterobacteria are involved.

SELF-CHECK 5.9

What is the primary source of the commonest organisms that cause endocarditis?

5.6.3 Signs and symptoms of endocarditis

Symptoms of endocarditis develop slowly; it is often termed infective endocarditis (IE). Symptoms include feeling generally unwell, tiredness, and low-grade pyrexia. Note that these symptoms are non-specific and are found in many illnesses. Heart murmurs caused by faulty blood flow through damaged valves can be heard. Frequently, small parts of the vegetation break off and get carried through the bloodstream to other parts of the body causing nodules to develop in the eye or fingernails. Other symptoms include raised white cell count and enlarged spleen.

5.6.4 Diagnosis of endocarditis

The initial diagnosis of endocarditis is based on clinical signs. However, confirmation of the diagnosis is made in the laboratory by isolating and identifying the infecting organism. Prompt identification of the infecting organism and carrying out of antibiotic susceptibility tests are vital in order for the patient to receive the best possible therapy.

Numerous blood cultures are taken, often following a spike of temperature. Frequent sets are required to increase the likelihood of isolating the infecting organism as bacteraemia may be transient. Almost any organism can cause endocarditis; however, some of the causative organisms may be slow-growing and it has been common practice to increase the incubation time for all blood culture bottles from endocarditis patients to up to 28 days. During this incubation period an intermediate and terminal blind subculture of bottles are sometimes performed as some organisms may not always give a positive signal in automated systems. There is increasing evidence, however, that because of the high nutritional content of modern blood culture media extended incubation is not required as media support good growth of even slow growing organisms. Some cases of endocarditis are caused by an organism *Coxiella burnetti* which does not grow in blood culture media. Diagnosis of infection with this organism is based on clinical suspicion, (it is most common in farm workers and vets) and positive serology.

In some cases diagnosis of endocarditis may be made after culturing a heart valve that has been removed from a patient.

What symptoms would alert you to the possibility of endocarditis in a patient?

5.6.5 Identification and susceptibility testing

Once an organism has been isolated from a blood culture it should be identified to species level. Antibiotic susceptibility tests should be carried out; however, endocarditis is one of the few situations where disc or breakpoint susceptibility tests are often inadequate. To effectively eradicate bacteria from endocarditis vegetations requires that the antibiotics used are cidal rather than static. Minimum inhibitory concentration (MIC) tests should be carried out using either broth microdilution tests or E-test. The advantage of the former is that it allows bactericidal activity to be detected. In many cases of endocarditis a combination of drugs is often used to enhance cidal activity. Common regimes include the use of ampicillin and gentamicin for penicillin-sensitive streptococci or vancomycin and gentamicin in penicillin-allergic patients. Treatment is usually with intravenous antibiotics for the first 2 weeks of therapy and the patient may be switched to oral antibiotics if an improvement in condition is seen.

In some cases replacement of damaged valves is required once the valve has been sterilized by appropriate therapy. **Synergy testing** of various drug combinations may be warranted in some cases; however, such tests are difficult to carry out, standardize and interpret and are best left to specialized laboratories to carry out.

Patients who have had endocarditis have a risk of recurrence. Treated patients and those with damaged heart valves require antibiotic prophylaxis during various procedures such as surgery and dental extractions. The antibiotics used are dependent on the type of procedure and they remove bacteria entering the bloodstream during such procedures.

Cross reference
See Chapter 4.

synergy tests
Synergy tests are tests carried out on combinations of drugs to see if their effects are potentiated when combined. In some cases combinations may antagonize each other which reduces the effect of the combination.

Key Points

Blood cultures from endocarditis patients require extended incubation and blind subculture may be warranted.

Treatment of endocarditis requires prolonged doses of appropriate antibiotics often given in combination.

MIC tests are often used to guide antibiotic therapy rather than disc diffusion or breakpoint susceptibility methods.

CASE STUDY 5.1 Endocarditis

A 52-year-old man was admitted to the Emergency Department with a 2-week history of low-grade pyrexia, tiredness, and splinter haemorrhages. On examination he had an enlarged spleen, a CRP of 4.9 (normal range 0–1), an ESR of 49 mm/h (normal 1–15 mm/h), and a heart murmur. In the past he had surgery to correct a mitral valve defect. A diagnosis of subacute bacterial endocarditis was made and several sets of blood cultures were taken over a 24-h period.

The patient was started on a combination of ampicillin and gentamicin when all blood culture samples were taken, as streptococcal endocarditis was suspected. The aerobic bottle from the second set of blood cultures became positive 36 h after being taken. Gram stain revealed Gram-positive cocci in clusters. *S. epidermidis* was isolated from the bottle, and was regarded as a possible contaminant as no other bottles were positive at that time. After 72 h the first pair of bottles became positive. Initial Gram stain revealed no organisms; the Gram stain was repeated, and counter stained with carbol fuchsin. Numerous small Gram-negative coccobacilli were seen. The bottles were plated onto blood agar and chocolate agar incubated in CO_2 and blood agar and fastidious anaerobic agar incubated anaerobically. Disc sensitivities were carried out anaerobically on blood agar and in CO_2 on sensitivity agar enriched with lysed blood and NAD. Examination of the plates at 24 h revealed no growth. At 48 h, however, small grey colonies were evident on the chocolate plate incubated in CO_2. At this time a further three bottles became positive and Gram stain with carbol fuchsin revealed small Gram-negative coccobacilli in each of these.

Identification was carried out using X and V discs and commercial kits; the organism was not dependent on X or V factors but there was a requirement for CO_2. Identification by a kit confirmed identity as *Haemophilus aphrophilus*. Susceptibility tests revealed sensitivity to ampicillin and gentamicin and this was confirmed by E-test MICs on sensitivity test media in CO_2. The patient was treated with 2 g amoxicillin IV 6-hourly plus 1 mg/kg gentamicin daily for 2 weeks. Amoxicillin was continued for a further 2 weeks and the patient made a complete recovery. The damaged valve was replaced with a prosthetic valve several months later.

1. Why was the initial Gram stain on the positive bottle negative?

2. What precautions will the patient have to take when visiting the dentist?

CASE STUDY 5.2 *Unusual cause of sepsis*

A 65-year-old lady who worked on a farm was admitted to hospital with a 2-week history of fever, joint pains, and malaise with swollen glands. Blood cultures were taken and because the patient was a farm worker and the symptoms were possibly suggestive of brucellosis the bottles were sent to a specialized centre because of safety concerns to laboratory workers. Blood samples were also taken for *brucella* serological studies but tests were negative. After 7 days of incubation blood cultures were negative on an automated system and terminal subcultures on various standard media were also negative, further sets of blood culture were taken and were also negative. Specialized blood cultures for mycobacteria and fungi were also set up. Serological studies for Q fever, an infection frequently contracted from farm animals, were also negative. The patient's pyrexia continued and she remained unwell. Further questioning of the patient revealed that she kept many cats. Cat scratch fever caused by *Bartonella henselea* was suspected. Because this organism doesn't grow in conventional blood culture media alternative diagnostic tools are needed. Blood for serological studies demonstrated that the patient had high levels of antibody against *B. henselea*. A lymph node biopsy was taken and material sent to a specialist centre, *B. henselease* DNA was detected using PCR tests. A diagnosis of cat scratch fever was made and the patient was treated with a course of antibiotics. Her fever rapidly disappeared and her condition started to improve and she eventually made an uneventful recovery.

1. Why were the blood cultures sent to a specialized centre for handling?

2. Why was a terminal subculture of the bottles carried out?

3. Why were cultures for mycobacteria and fungi set up?

Chapter summary

After reading this chapter you should know and understand:

- Blood culture samples are one of the most important sample types processed in microbiology.

- Blood cultures must be taken using aseptic conditions to ensure no contaminating organisms are introduced into the sterile blood culture medium.

- One of the major symptoms of bloodstream infection is pyrexia. Blood cultures are taken around the time of a pyrexial spike to ensure maximum numbers of organism are present for detection.

- Blood cultures are routinely processed in the laboratory using an automated method.

- The Gram stain is the first stage in identifying the organism likely to be causing the bloodstream infection. This allows the patient to be managed optimally, based on the type of organism seen.

- Positive blood cultures are inoculated onto a wide variety of different media. In addition direct susceptibility testing is essential.

- It can be difficult to assess the significance of an organism in a positive blood culture bottle. The organism may be a skin contaminant. The role of medical staff in determining the significance of the isolate is extremely important.

- Endocarditis is a serious clinical condition where bacteria cause vegetations on heart valves. Multiple blood cultures and serology tests may be required to diagnose this type of infection.

Further reading

- Gould FK, Elliott TSJ, Foweraker J, *et al*. **Guidelines for the prevention of endocarditis: report of the Working Party of the British Society for Antimicrobial Chemotherapy.** *Journal of Antimicrobial Chemotherapy* 2006; **57**: 1035–1042.

  Text covering all aspects of endocarditis and guidance for laboratories.

- Elliott TSJ, Foweraker J, Gould FK, *et al*. **Guidelines for the antibiotic treatment of endocarditis in adults: report of the Working Party of the British Society for Antimicrobial Chemotherapy.** *Journal of Antimicrobial Chemotherapy* 2004; **54**: 971–981.

  Text detailing the complex regimes which can be used for the treatment of endocarditis.

- Hall KK, Lyman JA. **Updated review of blood culture contamination.** *Clinical Microbiology Reviews* 2006; **19**: 788–802.

- Yagupsky P, Nolte FS. **Quantitative aspects of septicemia.** *Clinical Microbiology Reviews* 1990; **3**: 269–279.

● **Standards Unit, Evaluations and Standards Laboratory, Centre for Infections.** *Investigation of Blood Cultures (for Organisms other than Mycobacterium Species).* **BSOP 37, 2005.**

National SOP for the processing of blood cultures used in many laboratories throughout the world. Essential background information on clinical conditions and investigations.

 ## Discussion questions

5.1 If a patient has suspected septicaemia the clinician will always treat before the blood culture becomes positive in the laboratory. How useful therefore are blood culture samples?

5.2 How useful is the Gram stain result on a positive blood culture?

5.3 What factors are involved in determining the significance of an isolate from a positive blood culture?

5.4 Is it important to have a full identification on every positive blood culture isolate?

5.5 Discuss the importance of ward procedures for taking blood cultures.

6

Investigation of urine samples

Clive Graham

Urinary tract infection (UTI) is considered to be the most common bacterial infection and urine the most common sample sent to the microbiology laboratory. In many laboratories hundreds of samples are received each day creating significant workload pressures, particularly when traditional labour-intensive methods are used.

The purpose of the laboratory is to provide a prompt result to the clinician but the laboratory needs to be mindful that therapy is often started empirically before the result is known. So perhaps rapid determination of the presence or absence of a significant infection followed by accurately assessing the significance and susceptibility of any growth should be regarded as its primary role.

Even then, these functions are confounded by the variability of samples received, both in quality and sample type, and the need for any laboratory method to cover all the eventualities. Often the methods used are designed simply to cover the majority of samples received.

Learning objectives

After studying this chapter you should confidently be able to:

- Describe the anatomy of the urinary tract.
- List the common specimen types used to diagnose urinary tract infection.
- List the common urinary tract pathogens.
- Describe the routine tests performed on urine.
- Describe which antibiotics are used to treat urinary tract infection.

6.1 **Overview of the urinary tract**

In order to appreciate the clinical setting of urinary tract infections we must have an understanding of the normal anatomy of the urinary tract (Figure 6.1) and those mechanisms in place that help prevent infection from occurring.

Urine is produced in the kidneys and passes through the ureter (a small tube) by a process known as peristalsis into the bladder. Urine collects in the bladder and is intermittently emptied via the urethra.

Ascending infection is the most common route of infection, that is to say microorganisms ascend the urethra into the bladder and may from there go on to infect the kidney. The organisms causing urinary tract infection are often from the gastrointestinal tract, for example, *Escherichia coli*. Less commonly, bacteriuria results from haematogenous spread (via the bloodstream). Haematogenous infection is uncommon and will not be considered in detail further in this chapter other than to say that infection is usually caused by a limited number of organisms that include *Staphylococcus aureus*, *Salmonella* spp., *Mycobacterium tuberculosis*, and *Candida* spp.

6.1.1 Normal flora of the urinary tract

Other than the distal urethra, the urinary tract is sterile.

6.1.2 Mechanisms designed to prevent infection

The bladder has a number of mechanisms designed to resist infection. The most basic of these is the physical washing out effect in the production of urine that dilutes any bacterial load and removes infecting organisms. This regular flushing helps prevent infection ascending either into the bladder or into the kidneys; furthermore a valve prevents reflux (backflow) of urine from the bladder into the ureter. One can imagine that the risk of infection would depend on

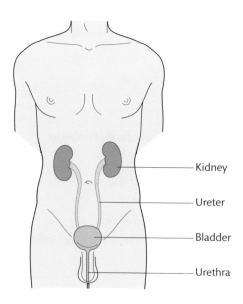

Kidney

Ureter

Bladder

Urethra

FIGURE 6.1
Anatomy of the urinary tract.

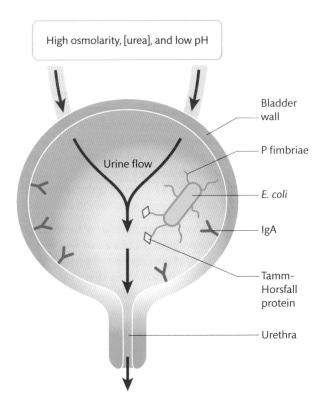

High osmolarity, [urea], and low pH

Bladder wall

P fimbriae

Urine flow

E. coli

IgA

Tamm-Horsfall protein

Urethra

FIGURE 6.2
Diagram to show some of the bladder mechanisms which promote resistance to urinary tract infection.
Source: Courtesy of M. Ford.

the initial inoculum and multiplication rate of the organism in addition to any residual urine within the bladder, urine flow, and frequency of voiding.

Obstruction to urine flow, for example through enlargement of the prostate gland in men, or if the bladder incompletely empties, for example through reflux of urine into the ureters (**vesi-coureteric reflux**) due to inadequate development of the one-way valve between ureter and bladder, increase the risk of urinary tract infection developing.

Other physical properties of urine, such as extremes of pH, high osmolality, immunoglobulin A (IgA), and high **urea** concentration, tend to be protective (Figure 6.2). Historically urine has been used as an antiseptic. Furthermore, the cells lining the urethra, bladder, and ureter resist colonization by bacteria. A type of antibody (IgA) secreted by immune cells within the bladder wall is also found in the urethra and stops bacteria binding. Finally, Tamm-Horsfall protein, a mucoprotein shed by the kidney, has also been shown to bind and trap *E. coli*.

SELF-CHECK 6.1

What is the commonest cause of a urinary tract infection and what are the common host defence mechanisms?

Key Point
Urinary tract infection is much more common in females than in males.

6.1.3 Mechanism of infection in the catheterized patient

A **catheter** is a tube that is passed into the urethra and then pushed into the bladder; a small balloon on the end of the catheter is then inflated to prevent it coming out. The tube can be made out of a number of different products, e.g. latex, silicone, PVC, or Teflon; some are coated with silver to reduce infection risk. Once inserted the catheter is connected to a collection bag. It is recommended that the system is kept closed, that is there are no breaks in the tubing to allow microorganisms to get into the inside (**intraluminal**) part of the tube. Catheters are required for a number of reasons; some are used for a short period of time, for example during an operation, whereas others are required for a prolonged period to deal with bladder or prostate problems. The insertion of the catheter is done aseptically to avoid introducing infection.

It is now considered that intraluminal colonization by reflux of bacteria from a contaminated bag or from a break in a closed drainage system is a rare event, and the most common route of infection is colonization of the exterior of the catheter by bacteria from the outermost part of the urethra, either at the time of catheterization or later as a film of mucus develops between the catheter and urethra. The rate of acquisition of high-level **bacteriuria** is estimated to be 5% per day; therefore the key way to reduce risk is to reduce catheter use and duration. When infection does arise it is often due to antibiotic-resistant bacteria.

> ### Key Point
> Urinary catheters are widely used in hospitalized patients and this bypasses many of the patient's defences designed to prevent UTI.

Although infection may be introduced through catheterization there is also a risk of infection being introduced with other surgical procedures such as operations to look into the bladder or remove the prostate gland.

SELF-CHECK 6.2

What are the advantages and disadvantages of catheterizing a patient?

6.2 Urinary tract pathogens

E. coli is by far the most common cause of urinary tract infection. Infection within hospital is more likely to be due to other organisms, many of which are resistant to the antibiotics commonly used to treat infection in the community (Table 6.1). This is because patients admitted to hospital are often given antibiotics either to treat a suspected infection or to prevent infection, for example, if they are having an operation. Such antibiotic use will select out skin and gut bacteria that are resistant to the antibiotic being used, and this may be a resistant strain of *E. coli* or another bacteria. These resistant strains in turn may cause infection in that patient or be passed on to another patient if infection control precautions are not followed.

The organisms causing community-acquired infection do vary, for example *Staphylococcus saprophyticus* is seen in sexually active young women but not in other groups. It also should be noted that antibiotic-resistant *E. coli* strains, in particular **extended-spectrum β-lactamase** (ESBL) producers, are increasingly being seen in patients who have had little or no contact with hospitals.

Cross reference
See Chapter 4, Section 4.3.

TABLE 6.1 Common bacterial causes of urinary tract infection in hospital and the community.

Organism	Community (%)	Hospital (%)
Escherichia coli	69.4	50.8
Proteus mirabilis	4.3	5.1
Klebsiella/Enterobacter spp.	4.7	7.3
Enterococcus spp.	5.5	11.9
Staphylococcus spp.	4.0	8.4
Pseudomonas aeruginosa	0	11.1
Others	12.1	5.4

Key Point

Commonly, the organisms causing UTI are from the patient's own gut flora.

Most community-acquired infections are in otherwise healthy individuals and are often termed 'uncomplicated' urinary tract infections. These infections respond well to antibiotics and recurrences are due to reinfections.

Complicated urinary tract infection describes infection in patients with a complicated urinary tract (e.g. abnormal because of structural or functional defects) or a patient generally more susceptible to infection, for example a patient on chemotherapy for cancer. These infections are due to a wider variety of bacteria, including other Gram-negative bacteria such as *Enterobacter* spp., *Pseudomonas* spp., *Providencia* spp., and *Morganella morganii*, and Gram-positive organisms such as enterococci, streptococci, staphylococci, and yeasts, especially *Candida* spp.; *E. coli* is less common. For infections in catheterized patients, the longer the catheter has been left *in situ* the greater the proportion of isolates other than *E. coli*, although interestingly *Candida* spp. are seen more frequently in those with short-term catheters.

Urinary tract infection is not a common feature in immunocompromised hosts unlike the higher rates of infection seen in those with structural and functional renal tract abnormalities. However, immune defects may mean that infections that do occur are not adequately controlled and that treatment of infection in such patients requires the use of antibiotics that achieve good tissue levels.

Complicated urinary tract infection is often equated to hospital-acquired infection but it should be noted that with increasingly complicated cases being managed in the community this distinction is less clear than it was in the past. With complicated infections, response to antibiotics is less and relapse with the same organism is more likely to occur.

SELF-CHECK 6.3

What is meant by a complicated urinary tract infection and in what type of patients do these occur?

6.2.1 Virulence factors of microbes causing urinary tract infection

There are many individuals who develop urine infection who do not have identifiable risk factors. Many of these infections are due to E. coli and indeed certain (uropathogenic) strains of E. coli are more strongly associated with urinary tract infection. They have certain characteristics that facilitate their ability to move from their normal residence in the gut and to colonize and infect the urinary tract. An example of such a mechanism is P fimbriae – these are hair-like projections on the surface of the bacteria which can bind to cells found in the kidney. These strains of E. coli commonly cause acute **pyelonephritis**.

pyelonephritis
A urinary tract infection which has ascended to reach the kidney. This is a serious infection.

6.2.2 Epidemiology

UTI is most common during the first year of life and is more common in young girls, except in neonates where UTIs in males predominate. Lowest rates are seen in 11–15-year-olds. The incidence of infection increases in young adult women where sexual activity is an important contributory factor; and increases again in old age. Indeed, around 20% of women develop a urinary tract infection during their lifetime; only after the age of 50 years is a similar incidence seen in males. Twenty-three per cent of all health-care-associated or **nosocomial infections** are urinary tract infections.

6.2.3 Infections of the lower urinary tract

Most cases (95%) of UTI are acute **cystitis**. It results from spread of organisms up the urethra and, like other sites of infection, E. coli is by far the most common cause. Symptoms of infection include pain when passing urine (**dysuria**), passing urine more frequently (often urgently) and pain in the lower abdomen (suprapubic pain).

The **urethral syndrome** is used to describe a patient who presents with the symptom of dysuria; this may (particularly in women) result from a urinary tract infection (due to E. coli or S. saprophyticus) sometimes with lower bacterial counts than anticipated with urinary tract infection. In both men and women, it may be part of an acute or chronic non-specific urethritis, classically due to Neisseria gonorrhoeae or Chlamydia trachomatis but Mycoplasma spp. may also be implicated.

There are other non-infective causes of the urethral syndrome. Prostatitis is inflammation of the prostate gland, a gland that in men surrounds the urethra just below the bladder. The causes of infection are usually sexually transmitted organisms such as Chlamydia trachomatis in young men, with more typical **uropathogens** causing infection in older men. It may follow instrumentation of the region by catheterization, etc. Inflammation may become chronic and in some of these cases there is no obvious earlier infection.

Acute epididymitis is inflammation of the epididymis, a tubing that connects the urethra to the testes. In older men this is usually due to typical UTI pathogens such as E. coli but in younger men it is more likely to be due to sexually transmitted bacteria.

6.2.4 Infections of the upper urinary tract

The hallmark symptoms of acute pyelonephritis are flank pain and fever; nausea, vomiting, and rigors may also occur. In most cases infection is from ascending lower urinary tract infection, resulting in bacteraemia in a third of cases. The most common organism responsible is E. coli.

Chronic pyelonephritis is chronic inflammation of the kidney, often associated with chronic obstruction of the urinary tract or, in young children, from backflow of urine from the bladder into the ureter (vesicoureteric reflux).

In general, which type of urinary infection is clinically the most important – upper or lower urinary tract infection?

6.2.5 Asymptomatic bacteriuria

This is commonly seen in elderly women and has no significant clinical consequence. Pregnant women should be screened for asymptomatic bacteriuria by culture as identification and treatment of asymptomatic infection reduces the risk of preterm birth. Treatment also reduces the risk of pyelonephritis developing (number needed to treat (NNT) = 7); recent evidence suggests it is thought that a single dose of antibiotic may be effective.

It is thought that the hormonal changes of pregnancy cause dilation of the ureters and increase the chance of ascending infection.

Key Point

Even though a urine sample may contain numerous pathogenic bacteria, there are occasions when they are not causing the patient harm. This is known as asymptomatic bacteriuria.

6.2.6 Asymptomatic pyuria

Asymptomatic pyuria is also found in patients with diabetes and the elderly (especially those with incontinence). In diabetics it is seen more frequently in those with **diabetic nephropathy**. In the elderly it can occur with or without bacteriuria and therefore in this patient group, pyuria should not be used to indicate whether a culture result is significant or not.

6.2.7 Common fungal pathogens

Fungal urinary tract infection is invariably due to *Candida* spp., usually *Candida albicans*. Most often infection is via the ascending route in a patient with a catheter *in situ* who is receiving antimicrobial chemotherapy. In asymptomatic patients, treatment may simply involve catheter removal (and stopping antibacterial therapy) with a repeat urine sample following catheter removal. For symptomatic patients or those with persistent infection, antifungal therapy is necessary. In women, vulvovaginal candidosis may give rise to positive cultures for *Candida* spp. in the urine; similarly, babies with 'nappy rash' may have urine contaminated with yeasts during collection especially if a bag or similar method is used for urine collection.

In neonates and immunocompromised patients, the presence of *Candida* spp. in the urine may indicate haematogenous spread of infection to the kidneys. Such infections have a significant morbidity and mortality associated with them and require prompt and aggressive antifungal treatment.

6.2.8 Atypical and fastidious organisms

Given that most urine cultures are done on a limited range of culture media, it should be noted that certain organisms that infrequently cause urinary tract infection may not be recovered on these media and additional culture methods may need to be considered in patients with persistent symptoms whose cultures are negative. For example *Haemophilus influenzae* (a cause of chest infections) is occasionally seen in children.

6.2.9 Mycobacteria

Cross reference

See Chapter 9, Section 9.4.

Mycobacterium tuberculosis infection of the renal tract may result in sterile pyuria and should always be considered in such patients. Infection of the kidney is due to blood-borne spread from a primary site elsewhere, invariably the lungs. The initial infection in the renal cortex, spreads to the papillae, casemates, and then discharges into the urine. Excretion of organisms is intermittent, hence the importance of collecting repeat samples on three consecutive days (early morning or first void). Such specimens need to be processed under Containment Level 3. As urine may contain *Mycobacterium smegmatis*, a normal commensal of the genital tract, staining of urine for mycobacteria is not recommended and the urine sample should be directly inoculated onto culture media.

6.2.10 Parasites

Parasitic infections of the urinary tract are rare in the UK but may be seen in those returning from abroad. *Schistosoma haematobium* (Figure 6.3) is the parasite that classically infects the urinary tract, causing haematuria and bladder irritation. A minimal volume of 10 mL should be examined as soon as possible after collection; if this is not possible the sample should be refrigerated. *S. haematobium* has a circadian rhythm; egg excretion peaks and is least variable from 10 a.m. to 2 p.m. Exercise before egg collection is unnecessary. Antigen detection methods have also been reported for urine (and serum) but are not widely available.

Other schistosomes and other parasites, such as *Entamoeba histolytica* and *Echinococcus granulosa*, can also rarely affect the urinary tract.

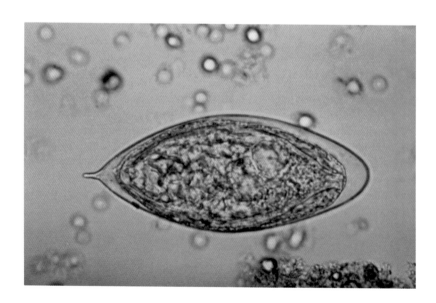

FIGURE 6.3

Image of a *Schistosoma haematobium* trematode parasite. Note the egg's posteriorly protruding, terminal spine, which is highly characteristic of the parasite.
Source: Courtesy of CDC.

Finally, the Amazonian Indians may be infected by a bloodsucking catfish known locally as *candirù* but with the Latin name *Vandellia cirrhosa*. This fish is said to be attracted to urine and capable of swimming up the urethra into the bladder.

Cross reference
See Chapter 17, Section 17.3.

SELF-CHECK 6.5

Why is it important for not just one sample to be sent to the laboratory to detect the presence of mycobacteria?

6.3 Urinary samples

6.3.1 Specimen collection

As is true for many aspects of microbiology, the quality of bacteriology results is only as good as the quality of the specimen. It is recognized that the distal urethra is colonized with bacteria, although it should be noted that this often involves skin commensal organisms such as anaerobes or *Lactobacillus* spp., which would rarely be considered significant in a urine culture. They may also have faecal organisms such as *E. coli* (which obviously could be deemed relevant) if the sample is not collected properly. There are a number of urine specimen types; these are listed next.

6.3.2 Midstream urine (MSU)

Patients should be given clear instructions on collection of urine. The first urine passed washes away organisms from the distal urethra and this should be discarded into a toilet or other receptacle. The midstream urine sample can then be collected into a suitable sterile container.

This process requires:

- Good control of micturition.
- Appropriate hand–eye co-ordination.
- Sufficient mobility to locate a sterile container in the urine stream.

It is obviously not suited to the very young, the elderly, or the infirm.

Some collection receptacles are associated with lower contamination rates.

6.3.3 Clean catch urine

This is the equivalent of midstream urine in young children where the volume passed can be relatively small and the sample is literally caught into a sterile container by the parent or staff member when the child happens to pass urine. It obviously takes patience and is not the method preferred by parents.

6.3.4 'Pad' urine

This is when an absorbent pad is located inside the nappy and checked every 10 minutes until wet. It is used in babies where obtaining a clean catch sample may be difficult. It is the preferred method of parents but does suffer the same problem with contamination that bag urines have; furthermore, if the pad becomes soiled it needs to be discarded. Pad urine samples may result in lower white cell counts on urine microscopy.

6.3.5 'Bag' urine

This is similar to pad urine but a sterile bag is placed in order to collect urine; such samples run a high risk of perineal contamination.

6.3.6 'In-out catheter urine'

This is the method of urine collection frequently used in children in North America. It has the advantage of being very rapid, not having to wait for urine to be passed spontaneously, but is relatively more traumatic and runs a risk of introducing infection into the bladder.

6.3.7 Catheter stream urine (CSU)

These are samples taken from patients with indwelling catheters, which may be either short term (for example used postoperatively) or long term where there is an underlying urological or other abnormality that requires the presence of a catheter. It should be noted that catheter-associated bacteriuria is common and in itself not significant; samples should only be taken if there is concern about a patient having an infection.

Samples need to be taken through a port or similar sampling point as breaking of a closed urinary catheter system runs the risk of introducing infection. An aseptic technique should be employed.

6.3.8 Suprapubic aspirate

These are samples taken from neonates and younger children only when it has been impossible to decide (based on pad or clean catch urine) if a child has a urine infection or not. The sample is taken by pushing a needle through the skin and aspirating urine directly from the bladder. Although there is a risk of contaminating the sample with skin organisms, the skin is cleaned thoroughly before the sample is taken and therefore any culture result must be viewed as significant.

Cross reference
See Chapter 1, Section 1.3.

Other samples from the urinary tract are sometimes received in the laboratory, in particular when that laboratory deals with samples from urology patients. Often these are from the upper renal tract, which should be sterile. Examples include those from nephrostomy – a tube that goes directly into the kidney.

SELF-CHECK 6.6

Why is it important not to collect the first few millilitres of a urine sample when collecting MSU?

6.4 Transport of specimens to the laboratory

Urine is a culture medium and delays in processing will allow bacteria to replicate, especially at higher temperatures, and this may result in either erroneous significant cultures being reported or mixed growths, where it is not possible to pick out the organism responsible for the patient's infection. When delay is anticipated, for example out of routine laboratory hours, the following methods should be considered to prevent deterioration in the sample:

- Refrigeration at 4°C: generally a maximum period of 24 h is recommended to preserve cellular elements. In terms of bacterial growth, surface viable counts of simulated specimens are said to remain constant for 72 h and Kass recommended 48 h (see Further reading, at the end of this chapter).

- Dip-slide technique: this involves commercially available agar-coated slides which are dipped into a freshly voided urine sample, placed back in their own containers, and then transported to the laboratory. Unfortunately, there is no record of the cellular or other components of the urine but conversion charts allow the quantification of culture results.

- Boric acid: boric acid is a preservative. It is designed to maintain bacterial and cellular components of urine where refrigeration is not practicable. The main disadvantage of this method is that bacterial counts may be reduced, and this is particularly important if counts are less than 10^5/mL to begin with (high inoculums are not affected) or if an inadequate volume of urine is dispersed into the container, as the concentration of boric acid would be higher than anticipated. Due to improvements in sample transport this preservative is now used very rarely.

6.5 Initial processing of samples

A clear, colourless urine sample is unlikely to grow significant numbers of bacteria but a cloudy sample can result from crystals, bacteria, red blood cells or white blood cells. Tests performed at the bedside or in the outpatient clinic can be used to help decide which samples should be sent for culture or if empirical therapy is appropriate. Catheters are foreign bodies and may elicit a raised white cell count or the patient may be infected with a nitrate-negative organism and therefore use of the dipstick tests described next should be avoided in this patient group. Reagent strip testing is often used; although a wide range of biochemical tests can be performed, two tests are particularly helpful in diagnosing infection.

6.5.1 Leucocyte esterase

Leucocyte esterase is an enzyme found in white blood cells called neutrophils; these are usually found in raised amounts in the urine of patients with infection. False-negative reactions occur with vitamin C, boric acid, glycosuria, high concentrations of protein, and certain antibiotics such as cefalexin, gentamicin, and nitrofurantoin; false-positive reactions occur with another antibiotic, clavulanic acid, contaminated samples, or in febrile children.

6.5.2 Nitrate reductase (Greiss test)

Nitrate reductase is an enzyme found in many, but not all, bacteria associated with urinary tract infection. Of particular note, *S. saprophyticus* does not produce this enzyme.

CASE STUDY 6.1 UTI in a child

A 6-month-old boy is taken by his mother to the Emergency Department with fever. Although the doctor suspects a viral infection a urine sample is collected by the nursing staff. The urine sample is tested by dipstick and found to be positive for leucocytes but negative for nitrates.

1. Should a urine sample have been tested by the GP?
2. What is the significance of a positive dipstick in a child?
3. What further tests should be carried out on the urine?
4. What are the implications if this child has a UTI?

METHOD The Rant–Shepherd method (Shepherd test)

- A urine specimen container is inverted and 80 μL of urine is transferred by pipette into a microtitre tray, and is allowed to settle for 10 min. This allows cells, casts, and crystals to sink to the well floor. The settled material is then observed using an inverted microscope.

- A cell count is performed but to determine the count per cubic millimetre of urine one has to know the field of view of the microscope and the fluid depth (which in turn depends on the radius of the microtitre well).

- Often such calculations have been done for the particular equipment in the laboratory to give a standard factor. The viewer then just needs to count the red and white cells seen on microscopy and multiply this by the standard factor to obtain the count per cubic millimetre.

6.5.3 Urine microscopy

Although a number of methods may be used for urine microscopy including Gram stain and phase contrast microscopy, one of the most widely accepted is the microtitre tray. This is known as the Rant–Shepherd method and is described in the Method Box. Interestingly, the first paper that described this method was refused publication as the editors thought that it would never gain wide acceptance.

Eucaryotic cell types in urine

Certain cell types are routinely reported when seen on microscopy.

- Leucocytes (white blood cells): in uncentrifuged urine, 10 leucocytes/μL is abnormal. Lower counts may be seen if there is a delay in microscopy as the hypotonicity of urine may cause cell disruption; furthermore if the peripheral cell count is low then the urine count may not be elevated. If no organisms are cultured the patient is said to have '**sterile pyuria**'; there are a number of potential reasons for this (Table 6.2).

- Erythrocytes (red blood cells): again any number of erythrocytes in urine is potentially abnormal although 'haematuria' may also be seen with menstruation. Haematuria may occur with infection but also occurs with renal calculi, malignancy and **glomerulonephritis**. Some automated methods reveal that a few red cells are seen in 'normal' individuals; indeed a cut off is required when an automated microscopy method is used. In healthy volunteers, 95% had less than eight erythrocytes/μL. In such individuals all red cells seen are dysmorphic (squashed appearance) suggesting a glomerular origin. Dysmorphic red cells are best detected by a special type of microscopy known as phase contrast.

- Epithelial cells: presence of epithelial cells indicates the urine has come into contact with the skin and may be contaminated.

sterile pyuria
Sterile pyuria is where the urine contains numerous white cells but no evidence of infection can be found.

glomerulonephritis
Glomerulonephritis is inflammation of the glomeruli, or small blood vessels of the kidney.

Significance of casts in urine wet films

Casts are proteinaceous imprints of the fine tubular network present in the kidneys; they may occur in a number of different renal pathologies. Although a number of cast types can be in urine, the most commonly seen are:

- Hyaline casts: these are made by aggregation of the Tamm–Horsfall protein and are seen in 'stressed individuals'. Epithelial cells are sometimes attracted to their surface (epithelial casts). Epithelial casts are said to occur with damage to the tubular epithelium and their morphology varies over time.

- Granular casts: these can be split into different types depending on how they are formed; four types have been described but only the first two will be considered:

  - Type 1 is associated with white blood cells casts and with degeneration of these casts. It results from a process of active inflammation within the kidney, white cells entering the tubular lumen, becoming bound in to the cast matrix and degenerating. In most instances this occurs with active tubular or interstitial injury and inflammation.
  - Type 2 is the most common type of granular cast. It consists of hyaline casts with granules (thought to be lysosomes, from associated epithelial cells) scattered throughout the matrix.

Key Point

Casts are tubular structures containing aggregates of particulate matter that form in the distal nephron. These can break off and pass into the urine and are seen on microscopy of the sample.

SELF-CHECK 6.7

Why is it important to carry out microscopy on a urine sample and report the result back to a clinician?

TABLE 6.2 **Causes of sterile pyuria.**

Chlamydia trachomatis and other sexually transmitted infections

Prostatitis

Neoplasia of the renal tract

Renal calculi

Catheter or other foreign body

Renal tuberculosis

Fever in children (regardless of cause)

Antimicrobial chemotherapy (resulting in negative cultures)

Types of pathological crystals found in urine

Crystalluria is a common finding and most cases are due to the precipitation of crystals of calcium oxalate, uric acid, triple phosphate, calcium phosphate, and amorphous phosphates or urates. Only in a minority of cases is it associated with pathological conditions such as urine stone formation or acute uric acid nephropathy. Crystalluria may also be associated with various drugs. Formation of urine stones has been linked to certain bacterial infections, especially those caused by urea splitting bacteria such as *Proteus* spp. Identification of urine crystals is not usually done in the microbiology laboratory.

Parasitic infection and detection

A method for examining urine for parasites is given in the Method Box.

METHOD *Examination of urine specimens for parasites: centrifugation method (Schistosoma haematobium)*

- Ensure specimen is in a conical-bottom container.
- Centrifuge at 500 g for 2 min.
- Decant and discard the supernatant, then mix the sediment.

- Using the whole deposit, place 1 or 2 drops onto a clean microscope slide and apply coverslips. Examine the entire area of each slide under low-power magnification.
- A filter method (with filter paper, polycarbonate, or polyamide) may also be used, and is often employed in epidemiological studies.
- It should be noted that egg excretion varies and although most patients with overt haematuria will have detectable eggs this may not be true for patients with more subtle urinary tract symptoms. See Figure 6.3.

6.5.4 Automated techniques available for processing urine samples in the laboratory and point of care testing (POCT)

It should be noted that routine microscopy and culture is still recommended for diagnosing infection in children less than 3 years of age and pregnant women.

A high proportion of urine samples generally grow insignificant amounts of bacteria or are culture negative. A procedure that would eliminate the need to culture those specimens that are unlikely to grow significant bacteria would be advantageous both in the laboratory, saving time and resources, and at the point of care where, potentially, antibiotic use could be reduced. Another advantage is that many of these methods are objective rather than subjective and therefore may be less prone to error or bias. Automated methods are suited to high-volume work but obviously the method employed will vary depending on cost and anticipated throughput.

Automated dipstick method

This has the advantage over manual reading of dipsticks because the result is not subject to interpretation but is read in a standard way, after the appropriate time interval, etc. Although mainly using leucocyte esterase and nitrite detection, other indices can also be measured. Automated systems include Clinitek (Siemens, Erlangen, Germany) and Urisys 1100 (Roche, Basel, Switzerland).

These methods continue to have the drawback of hand-held dipsticks, namely low specificity and positive predictive value. They are, however, cost effective if negative samples are not cultured.

Automated microscopy

Automated microscopy methods, such as Yellow Iris™ or R/S 2000, were designed to speed up standard urine microscopy methods. The latest marketed version, iQ200 (Iris Diagnostics, Chatsworth, California, USA) uses digital imaging and auto-particle recognition software to recognize 12 urine particles (erythrocytes, leucocytes, leucocyte clumps, hyaline casts, unclassified casts, squamous epithelial cells, non-squamous epithelial cells, bacteria, yeast, crystals, mucus, and sperm) and quantify results (Figure 6.4). The advantages over flow cytometry is that images that will be familiar to microbiologists can be viewed on demand rather than the scattergrams produced by flow cytometry.

FIGURE 6.4

Screen image from an iQ200 Sprint Urine Analyser showing the presence of epithelial cells in the sample.

Source: Courtesy of Instrumentation Laboratories.

Flow cytometry

Flow cytometry is widely used in non-microbiology laboratories, for example it is used in haematology laboratories for detection of the different cell types in blood. An early type, UF-50, was used to detect red blood cells, white blood cells, epithelial cells, casts, and bacteria in urine; detection of the latter was not optimal (false negatives were a problem) and various modifications have been made. The latest version, UF-1000i (Sysmex Europe GmbH, Hamburg, Germany), is said to be more sensitive.

To detect cells in urine, 200 µL of urine is diluted with a citrate buffer solution plus cationic surfactant. This mixture is supplemented with 40 µL of fluorescent dye that stains nuclei acid within the bacteria; the final mixture has a dye concentration of 1 ppm. This is then hydrodynamically focused and passed through a sheath flow illuminated with a laser beam. The forward scatter light intensity and lateral fluorescent intensity of each cellular component of the urine is converted into electrical signals by a photomultiplier and these are measured for each sample. Urine bacterial analysis (UBA) can distinguish bacteria from other cellular and non-cellular components of urine (e.g. erythrocytes, leucocytes, epithelial cells, fungi, and crystals).

This technology has been assessed for linearity (increasing bacterial suspensions give higher measurements); the carryover rate is estimated to be 0.029%. Variation (between and within runs) is less than with traditional culture methods especially with lower bacterial counts and correlation with culture results is excellent. The false-negative rate is low – 0.7% in one study.

Other automated methods for detecting bacteriuria

Other automated methods, such as bioluminescence and filtration, are available but are not widely used in the UK.

SELF-CHECK 6.8

What are the advantages of automated methods for the analysis of urine samples?

6.6 **Culture**

6.6.1 Significant culture results

A significant culture result is taken as greater than 100,000 (10^5) colony forming units (CFU)/mL of urine. Kass established a figure of equal to or greater than 10^5 organisms/mL of midstream urine as being able to distinguish women with acute pyelonephritis. Even in his original studies he noted that 6% of asymptomatic women had this degree of bacteriuria.

The significance of this value has been brought into question, with much lower counts (10^2 coliforms per mL) being deemed significant in symptomatic women. However, in the laboratory it is often difficult to be certain that a specimen has been collected properly and the use of such low counts could lead to the over-reporting of 'significant' results and, potentially, over-use of antibiotics, especially if one considers that most urine samples are subject to a delay before processing that may result in bacterial replication. For this reason, many laboratories use a cut off of a pure growth of 10^4 organisms per mL; indeed 90–95% of patients with acute pyelonephritis have bacteria at this concentration. For antibiotic studies, bacteriuria of $\geq 10^3$ CFU/mL of urine is used; this value has a specificity of 90% and sensitivity of 80% for the diagnosis of acute cystitis.

SELF-CHECK 6.9

Why is the number of bacteria isolated in urine samples considered very important?

6.6.2 Procedures for quantifying urine cultures

As indicated earlier, it is important to quantify the growth of bacteria. There are a number of methods one can use to do this; two are given in the Method Box. Other quantification methods are available, such as those used in dip-slides (previously) and the paper foot method (see Leigh and Williams, in the References list, end of this book).

METHOD *Quantification of urine cultures*

- *The calibrated loop technique* is based on the fact that using a calibrated loop a fixed volume (usually 1 μL or 10 μL) of urine is delivered to the agar plate.

- The urine is then streaked out so that individual colonies may be more easily counted. These can then be multiplied up to see if the colony count is significant: for example using a 1-μL loop, 1 colony would equate to 1000 CFU/mL of urine; using a 10-μL loop, 1 colony would equate to 100 CFU/mL and would be more appropriate, for example, when dealing with a suprapubic aspirate.

- *The multipoint inoculator method* uses a multipoint inoculator (0.3–2 μL depending on the pin size) to transfer urine from a tray onto agar for culture; the urine may require re-refrigeration until the inoculator is full.

- This method can be done manually or automated and is limited in its ability to detect growths of less than 10^5/mL. Modification of this method can be used to incorporate sensitivity testing and identification.

6.6.3 Common isolation media

Most bacteria and fungi associated with urinary tract infection can be isolated on standard agar. Often cysteine lactose electrolyte deficient (CLED) agar is used as a single plate, with more than one urine sample applied so that costs are contained. This agar gives a yellow

FIGURE 6.5
Growth of *E. coli* on CLED agar.
Source: Courtesy of bioMérieux.

colour with lactose fermenting colonies such as *E. coli* (Figure 6.5) and a blue colour with non-lactose fermenting colonies such as *Proteus* spp. It supports the growth of *Streptococcus pyogenes* and other fastidious organisms that do not require blood and it also inhibits the swarming of *Proteus* spp. Andrade indicator (fuchsin) may be incorporated into the medium to enhance colonial appearance. The colour changes seen depend on the pH of the media, ranging from bright red with a pH of 6.0 to deep blue with a pH of 7.4 (Table 6.3). CLED incorporating Andrade indicator should not be incubated for more than 24 h as lactose fermenters will cause pinkish coloration of the media, masking any non-fermenters present.

TABLE 6.3 Colony morphology on CLED agar with and without Andrade indicator.

Organism	CLED agar	CLED with Andrade indicator
Escherichia coli (lactose fermenting strains)	Yellow, opaque colonies with a slightly deeper coloured centre (1.25 mm diameter)	Bright pink, semi-translucent colonies with a surrounding pink halo
Proteus mirabilis	Translucent blue colonies around 1 mm	Blue-green translucent colonies
Klebsiella spp.	Mucoid, variable colour, yellow to whitish-blue	Grey-green mucoid colonies
Enterococcus faecalis	Yellow colonies, 0.5 mm in diameter	
Staphylococcus aureus	Deep yellow colonies about 0.75 mm diameter	Smooth, entire, opaque bright golden yellow colonies
Coagulase-negative staphylococci	Pale yellow or white colonies	Smooth, entire, opaque white colonies
Salmonella spp.	Flat, blue colonies	
Pseudomonas aeruginosa	Green colonies, matt surface and rough periphery	
Corynebacteria	Very small grey colonies	

Cross reference

See Chapter 3.

Differential agars are available for common urinary tract isolates; these give different colours depending on the organism present. Chromogenic agars contain substrates that when hydrolysed by bacterial (or in some cases fungal) enzymes produce coloured compounds. Several different media are available commercially; there are a number of studies comparing detection and identification rates and all are superior to CLED in detecting mixed culture results. As well as better detection of mixed cultures, they may also reduce inoculation and work-up time by laboratory personnel.

Fastidious bacteria such as *Streptococcus pneumoniae* may cause infection in children and these organisms would not be isolated if a selective agar is used alone. In highly specialized situations, depending on the clinical context, cultures for *Mycobacterium tuberculosis* or *Mycoplasma* spp. or *Ureaplasma* spp. may be performed.

SELF-CHECK 6.10

What culture medium would you consider to be the gold standard for isolation of urinary pathogens?

6.6.4 Confirmatory tests

Cross references

See Chapter 2 and Chapter 4, Section 4.3.

Experienced biomedical scientists can often identify organisms from primary culture plates. Organisms such as *Pseudomonas aeruginosa* have certain susceptibility profiles and may produce a pigment (pyocyanin) which produces a distinctive green discoloration to the agar.

Most presumptive identification needs to be confirmed; in most instances this is through biochemical tests. Historically, bacterial species used to be grouped together, for example '>10^5 coliform isolated'; however, it is now recognized that identification of the different bacteria responsible for urinary tract infection is essential for the accurate monitoring of susceptibility data and accurate determination of susceptibility using BSAC/CLSI or other methods.

6.6.5 Contaminated urine samples

Bacterial contamination of urine may be due to poor specimen collection, prolonged transport, or both. It is important as contaminated samples may need to be repeated, it may result in the wrong diagnosis (and inappropriate antibiotic use) or delay appropriate treatment of an infection, and it increases costs. Despite awareness of contamination as a problem, there has been little improvement in contamination rates over time, with recent studies having a median contamination rate of 15%.

Contamination is seen more commonly in women than in men and interestingly does not appear to be reduced where written collection instructions or collection kits are used; however, this may reflect the quality of instructions, the abilities of the instructor, the receptiveness of the patient, and where the instruction is given. Comparisons with other institutions can be used to assess the quality of specimen collection and processing.

Cross reference

See Chapter 4.

Mixed bacterial growth may indicate contamination of a specimen during collection although in certain clinical situations, for example in catheterized patients, such culture results may be significant; indeed mixed bacteraemia can occur in patients who have mixed urine cultures. Table 6.4 gives a guide to further processing of such mixed growths.

SELF-CHECK 6.11

How does the laboratory determine if the sample is contaminated?

TABLE 6.4 Significance and reporting of urine culture results.

No. of isolates		Specimen type	Microscopy result	Laboratory interpretation	Susceptibility testing
1	$\geq 10^4$/mL	All	Any	Probable UTI	Yes – consider comment if no WBC present
2	1 predominant at $\geq 10^5$/mL	All	> 10 WBC /µL present	Possible UTI	Yes
2	Both organisms ≥ 1	All	>10 WBC/µL present	Possible UTI	Yes
>2	No predominant organism	All except suprapublic aspirate	Any	Mixed growth	No
1 or 2	Any growth	Suprapubic aspirate	Any	Probable UTI	Yes
>2	Any growth	Suprapubic aspirate	Any	Possible UTI	Combined sensitivity

6.6.6 Antimicrobial susceptibility testing

As well as determining if any bacteria isolated from the urinary tract are significant, the laboratory also needs to report what antibiotics the organism appears susceptible to. Certain antibiotics are often used for urinary tract infection and these antibiotics would be tested in all cases but not necessarily reported to the requesting doctor.

Factors influencing the choice of antibiotics reported include:

- Susceptibility profile of the organism.
- Pregnancy.
- If the patient is in hospital or in the community.
- If the antibiotic is available in oral or IV form.
- Renal function.
- Broad or narrow spectrum.
- Antibiotic costs.

Microbiologists aim to promote the use of the most narrow spectrum, cost effective antibiotic therapy that has the least risk of adverse effects to the patient. Reporting of long lists of agents to which an organism is susceptible to may promote injudicious use of antibiotics.

Correct identification of organisms is necessary as certain antibiotics should not be used for certain coliforms that are naturally resistant to aminopenicillins, for example, see Table 6.5. These antibiotic–organism combinations should not be used; similar rules apply to Gram-positive organisms; for example enterococci should be regarded as having intermediate susceptibility to trimethoprim.

Antifungal susceptibility tests are not routinely performed; indeed most *Candida* other than *Candida albicans* do not need to be identified to species level.

6.6.7 Direct susceptibility testing

Susceptibility testing could be done at the time the urine is inoculated onto the culture plates or after culture results are complete, when only those urines harbouring significant growths

TABLE 6.5 Intrinsic resistance (R) in Enterobacteriaceae.

Organism	Amoxicillin	Co-amoxiclav	Piperacillin	Cefazolin	Cefoxitin	Cefuroxime	Aminoglycosides	Tetracycline/ tigecycine	Colistin	Nitrofurantoin
Citrobacter freundii	R	R		R	R					
Enterobacter cloacae	R	R		R	R					
Klebsiella spp.	R		R							
Morganella morganii	R	R		R		R		R	R	R
Proteus mirabilis				R		R		R	R	R
Proteus vulgaris	R			R		R		R	R	R
Serratia marcescens	R	R		R		R	*		R	

* All *Serratia marcescens* produce a chromosomal AAC(6')-Ic enzyme that may moderate the activity of all aminoglycosides except streptomycin and gentamicin.

would be inoculated. Most laboratories have systems in place where those urines likely to produce significant culture results (based on microscopy) are inoculated directly onto susceptibility test plates so that final culture results are available within 24 h of urine receipt; furthermore if further sensitivity work is required this is not delayed.

In terms of accuracy, direct susceptibility testing produces few errors with overall proportions of very major and major errors being low and comparable to the reproducibility of disc testing within the same laboratory.

CASE STUDY 6.2 *Antimicrobial prescribing policy*

An elderly lady is admitted to hospital with suspected urinary tract infection. A sample is sent to the laboratory and reports a significant growth of *E. coli* with a long list of different antibiotic susceptibilities.

The clinician caring for the patient reads the reports and decides to use IV cefuroxime to treat the patient. As a consequence the patient develops *Clostridium difficile* infection.

If a narrower range of antibiotics had been suggested then a more narrow-spectrum agent, such as trimethoprim, may have been used which would be less likely to result in this complication.

1. What are the disadvantages to using intravenous antibiotics?

2. Which antibiotics are associated with *Clostridium difficile* infection?

3. Is trimethoprim resistance common in urine isolates in your hospital? Why is this?

Key Point

It is important to use the most appropriate narrow-spectrum antibiotic to treat a urinary tract infection. Broad-spectrum antibiotics may promote resistance and wipe out the patient's normal flora.

Cross reference
Chapter 4, Section 4.3.

6.6.8 Automated identification and susceptibility

Many laboratories are using automated systems for identification and susceptibility testing. As resistance mechanisms are becoming more complex with one or more mechanism present in a particular bacteria, such systems may more accurately identify them. Such systems can either be rule based, for example, Microscan (Siemens, USA), Phoenix (Becton Dickenson, USA) and VITEK (bioMérieux, France), or pattern based, for example VITEK 2 (bioMérieux, France).

Cross reference
Chapter 3 and Chapter 4.

6.6.9 Hazardous organisms

Urine rarely contains hazardous bacteria but it should be noted that in cases of typhoid and paratyphoid *Salmonella* spp. may be excreted in the urine during the first week of the illness. When such infections are being considered urine samples should be processed under Containment Level 3.

6.7 **Urinary antibiotics**

Effective urinary concentrations are essential for the effective treatment of urinary tract infections. For certain infections such as pyelonephritis, adequate interstitial fluid concentrations are also required. Infection confined to the bladder in an individual with an anatomically and functionally normal system requires a shorter course of therapy than 'complicated cases' with known or suspected abnormalities.

Susceptibility data need to be interpreted with caution as many infections are treated in the community without resorting to bacterial culture; therefore samples received in the laboratory may be pre-selected and have higher resistance rates than those from patients in the community.

Key points relating to those antibiotics used to treat urinary tract infection are given in the next subsections.

6.7.1 Trimethoprim

It is recommended that trimethoprim is not used in the first trimester of pregnancy as its antifolate activity could potentially be linked to neural tube defects (spina bifida); it is automatically suppressed in antenatal clinics in some laboratories. The evidence for this approach is not conclusive and trimethoprim is unlikely to cause harm if the patient has adequate folate reserves. Some authorities suggest that trimethoprim should not be used for enterococcal urinary tract infections – this is based on the fact that there is some reversal of the antibacterial activity of trimethoprim by thiamine and 'folates' and documented treatment failures in the literature. The European Committee on Antimicrobial Susceptibility Testing (EUCAST) recommend that enterococci are reported as of intermediate susceptibility.

6.7.2 Cefalexin

Cefalexin is safe to use in all stages of pregnancy. Enterococci are intrinsically resistant.

6.7.3 Amoxicillin

Amoxicillin achieves high concentration in the urine but its use has decreased as many strains of E. coli are now resistant.

CASE STUDY 6.3 *Multidrug resistance*

Eleven days following a hip replacement, 75–year-old Mr Smith developed fever and loin pain. A catheter urine sample grew >10^5 E. coli, resistant to amoxicillin, cefalexin, trimethoprim, and ciprofloxacin but sensitive to nitrofurantoin.

1. Are there any other sensitivity tests you would like to perform?

2. How can such infections be avoided?

6.7.4 Co-amoxiclav

Co-amoxiclav is a combination of amoxicillin with the β-lactamase inhibitor clavulanic acid. It is too broad spectrum to be routinely used for urinary tract infection.

6.7.5 Nitrofurantoin

Nitrofurantoin is rapidly absorbed but produces low plasma levels and therefore despite a wide spectrum of activity is only used for treatment of urinary tract infections. It should be avoided in mild renal impairment because of inadequate urine concentrations. It is also contraindicated in children less than 3 months of age as it may cause neonatal haemolysis due to glucose-6-phosphate dehydrogenase (G6PD) deficiency, and is also contraindicated in pregnancy near to term and in the breast feeding mother.

6.7.6 Ciprofloxacin

Ciprofloxacin is a fluoroquinolone with high tissue concentration so, unlike many of the drugs listed above, it may be suitable for the treatment of complicated urinary tract infection. It should be avoided in pregnancy because of the risk of **arthropathy** and should be only used with caution in children.

arthropathy
Arthropathy is a disease or abnormality of a joint.

6.7.7 Gentamicin

Gentamicin is not absorbed in the gastrointestinal tract and must be given systemically, that is used intravenously or by intramuscular injection. It is nephrotoxic and is usually given in combination with a second agent.

Broader-spectrum agents – aztreonam, cefuroxime, carbapenems – may also be tested in resistant isolates and the laboratory needs to have a system in place for detection of extended spectrum β-lactamases. Less commonly used oral agents include fosfomycin and pivmecillinam.

Many antibiotics used to treat urinary tract infection are concentrated in the urine and because of this breakpoints that are used to determine whether an isolate is resistant or susceptible are higher for urinary isolates than for the same organism isolated from another body site.

SELF-CHECK 6.12

For a routine urinary tract infection would it be better to treat with oral or IV antibiotics? What are your reasons and which antibiotics would you suggest?

6.7.8 Treatment failure

Treatment failure is more likely to occur in the very young and the very old because they are more likely to have a functional or anatomical defect. This may warrant further investigation as only treatment of this defect may prevent further infections from occurring. It may also occur with empirical treatment if there is resistance to the initial agent used and therefore urine culture is mandatory in such patients.

> **Key Point**
>
> Most urinary tract infections are easily treated and result in few complications. However, the organisms can get into the bloodstream and cause life-threatening septicaemia.

6.7.9 Detection of antimicrobial substances

Some laboratories use methods to detect antimicrobial substances in urine; this usually consists of a susceptible organism to which you can simply look for inhibition of growth or as part of a microtitre plate assay based on a colorimetric substrate, p-nitrophenyl-β-D-glucopyranoside, in combination with a *Bacillus subtilis* strain. It may be useful in explaining cases of sterile pyuria, but as this should be recognizable by the clinician it is no longer performed in many laboratories. Interestingly, boric acid can interfere with this assay.

Chapter summary

After reading this chapter you should know and understand:

- The anatomy of the urinary tract is sterile and is difficult to infect in normal healthy individuals.

- Urinary tract infections are more common in females than in males.

- Uropathogenic strains have specific properties which allow them to colonize the urinary tract and cause infection.

- Which antibiotics accumulate in urine and are therefore commonly used to treat such infections.

- The common culture media used, e.g. CLED and chromogenic agars; chromogenic media enable a better presumptive identification of common infecting strains.

- The significance of isolating organisms from urinary catheters can be difficult as the catheter can be 'colonized' and there is difficulty in managing such patients.

- The reason for performing microscopy, either automated or manual, and how this can affect the significance of the organism isolated.

- The significance of the various cell types found in urine and the significance of these when detected on microscopy.

Further reading

- Bekeris LG, Jones BA, Walsh MK, Wagar EA. Urine culture contamination. A College of American Pathologists Q-probes study of 127 laboratories. *Archives of Pathology Laboratory Medicine* 2008; **132**: 913–917.

  Paper investigating why urine contamination is high in some institutions and how it can be reduced.

- Kass EH. Bacteriuria and the diagnosis of urinary tract infection. *Archives of Internal Medicine* 1957; **100**: 709–714.

  One of the original articles on which the quantitative examination of urine is based and the rationale for it.

- **NICE. Antenatal Care – Routine Care for the Healthy Pregnant Women. NICE Clinical Guideline March 2008. www.nice.org.uk/nicemedia/pdf/cg062niceguideline.pdf.**

  Report providing guidance for the clinical management of pregnant women, with reference to the problems associated with asymptomatic bacteruria.

- **Rubin RH, Shapiro ED, Andriole VT, Dais RJ, Stamm WE. Evaluation of new anti-infective drugs for the treatment of urinary tract infection.** *Clinical Infectious Diseases* 1992; **15**: S216–S227.

  Guidelines which discuss acute uncomplicated cystitis, acute uncomplicated pyelonephritis, and complicated infections of the urinary tract.

- **Brumbaugh AR, Mobley HL. Preventing urinary tract infection: progress toward an effective** *Escherichia coli* **vaccine.** *Expert Review of Vaccines* 2012; **11**(6): 663–676.

  Interesting article on recent advances on combating uropathogenic E. coli.

- **Hooton TM. Clinical practice. Uncomplicated urinary tract infection.** *New England Journal of Medicine* 2012; **366** (11): 1028–1037.

  Good review of UTI in general.

 # Discussion questions

6.1 What are the common causes of urinary tract infection? Why can the causes of UTI be different?

   a. In the community?

   b. In hospital?

6.2 What is meant by the term significant bacteriuria?

6.3 What methods can be used to screen patients for urinary tract infection?

6.4 Which antibiotics are commonly used to treat urinary tract infection?

6.5 A high proportion of urine cultures are negative – why is this?

6.6 What are the advantages and disadvantages of the different methods of urine culture?

7

Investigation of wound, tissue, and genital samples

Steve Davies and Mark Tovey

The skin and mucosa form an extremely effective physical barrier to the outside environment as part of the host's immune defence system. If this integrity is breached in any way, entry of bacteria can occur, which could potentially lead to infection. The majority of organisms associated with skin, mucosal and soft tissue infections are **commensals**; these may act as opportunistic pathogens once this defence has been overcome. This may occur in a number of ways: as a result of surgery or other medical intervention, trauma, burns, inflammation, or due to an underlying medical condition. Genital infections can also be a result of opportunism as well as sexual transmission.

The most common presentations of skin and tissue infections are:

- Cellulitis.
- Folliculitis.
- Boils and carbuncles.
- Abscess formation.
- Impetigo.
- Ulceration.
- Erysipelas.
- Discharging mucosal surfaces.

Wound, genital, eye, ear, nose, and throat swabs are some of the most commonly received samples in the clinical laboratory. This chapter describes the laboratory investigation of these and other specimens, and examines both commonly isolated and other significant pathogens.

Swab or tissue specimens can essentially be taken from any part of the body. This chapter therefore covers an extremely broad proportion of microbiology specimens; it is not conceivable to cover every possible infection of every possible site. We have deliberately separated skin and tissue infection from that of the genitalia. These infections are very much site-specific and can be found towards the end of the chapter. Before investigating types of infections it is important to briefly appreciate the anatomy of the skin.

Learning objectives

After studying this chapter you should be able to:

- Describe the ways in which the skin and mucosa act as a defence mechanism and how this barrier may be breached.
- Describe the different types of infection that occur in skin and soft tissue and on the genitals.
- List the most common pathogens and their virulence mechanisms, including toxins produced.
- Outline how these toxins are detected and the role of the relevant reference laboratory.
- Describe the media and incubation conditions used to isolate these organisms.

7.1 **The skin and mucosa**

7.1.1 **Overview of the skin**

The skin is the largest organ of the body. It consists of an external cellular layer, the epidermis, and a deep connective tissue layer called the dermis (Figure 7.1). The skin is critical in the body's defences against injury and dehydration, as well as against foreign bodies. It is equally important in sensation (e.g. pain) and the regulation of temperature.

Below the dermis is the **superficial fascia** (subcutis) consisting of looser connective tissue and fat. It is here you would find cutaneous nerves, blood and lymphatic vessels, and sweat glands. Finally, the deep fascia is a denser, more organized section of connective tissue that gives rise to structures such as muscle.

The skin acts as a primary defence system against unwanted bacteria or viruses. Physical trauma, such as burns, injury, or surgery, can breach the integrity of the skin and may create an infection opportunity. Mucosal membranes, including eyes, nostrils, and ears, are often easier to breach as they usually do not have skin as the primary defence mechanism.

Key Point

The skin is an excellent barrier to microorganisms and provided it remains intact it will act as a 'brick wall' to prevent infection.

7.1.2 **Normal flora of the skin**

Few areas of the body are sterile. The skin is exposed to the environment and so is colonized with **commensal organisms**. These are often transient – they may be temporarily removed, by washing for example, but will usually return by natural means. Common skin commensals include coagulase-negative staphylococci (CNS), viridans-type streptococci, *Corynebacterium* spp., and small numbers of *Staphylococcus aureus*, and *Candida* spp.

commensal organisms
Defined as those that live on a surface to the benefit of both host and organism. They constitute our 'normal flora'.

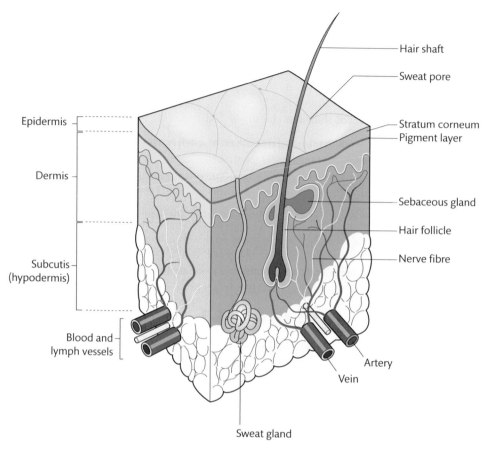

Epidermis

Dermis

Subcutis
(hypodermis)

Blood and
lymph vessels

Hair shaft

Sweat pore

Stratum corneum
Pigment layer

Sebaceous gland

Hair follicle

Nerve fibre

Artery

Vein

Sweat gland

FIGURE 7.1
Diagram of the skin.

pathogenic organisms

Although possibly part of our normal flora, their main role is to survive and multiply, often at the expense of the host. Such organisms possess more mechanisms by which to initiate infection.

Under normal circumstances we live in close harmony with these organisms, but as soon as the skin is damaged or our immune system is compromised in some way, the risk of infection increases. The normal flora may also be disrupted by hospitalization or by taking courses of antibiotics. Since most commensals and most **pathogenic organisms** are relatively sensitive to treatment, antimicrobials often select resistant bacteria by removing bacteria susceptible to the antibiotic. This is especially so in the hospital setting, which may lead to hospital-acquired infection, for example methicillin-resistant *S. aureus* (MRSA).

Cross reference

See Chapter 12.

7.2 **Skin infections and their causes**

Infections of the skin and/or subcutaneous tissue may be caused by a number of organisms. Traditionally, swabs are taken of suspected body sites, although tissue or biopsy specimens may often result in more efficient recovery of these bacteria. It is important that all organisms isolated from a particular swab (e.g. a wound swab) are assessed for clinical significance. Skin flora are often isolated along with pathogenic bacteria, and the qualified biomedical scientist is expected to know what should be investigated as a likely cause of infection and what should be regarded as insignificant.

7.2.1 Skin infections

The following are a few examples of different forms of skin infection.

Cellulitis

Cellulitis is a spreading skin infection often involving the superficial fascia, but may be caused by damage to venous or lymphatic systems, resulting in swelling (oedema), redness (erythema), tenderness, and pain. Common causes of infection include *S. aureus* and β-haemolytic streptococci (β-HS). These are shown side by side in Figure 7.2a and b.

Cellulitis due to wounds may also be infected by *Bacteroides* spp. and/or anaerobic cocci. Due primarily to the size of the wound, burns may result in severe skin infection involving one or more of the following: *S. aureus*, β-HS, *Pseudomonas aeruginosa*, Enterobacteriaceae, *Candida*, *Acinetobacter*, and *Bacillus* spp. (especially *Bacillus cereus*).

Bites are a common focus of infection; many bacteria have been implicated in human or animal bites, where organisms of an oral origin infect the wound (e.g. *S. aureus*, viridans streptococci and anaerobes). Similarly, the **HACEK** group of organisms is often implicated in human bites. Recognition of these organisms can be difficult due to their colonial similarity to other organisms often present in the sample. Their identification is also troublesome, mainly due to their fastidious nature and infrequent detection. *Pasteurella multocida*, *Capnocytophaga* spp. (dog), and *Streptobacillus* spp. (rat) have been specifically implicated in animal bites. Insect bites may also result in bacterial wound infection, but these are usually secondary infections with *S. aureus* and β-HS that may be residing on the skin surface.

Folliculitis

This occurs when a hair follicle becomes infected and inflamed. An erythematous pustule forms around the hair, often caused by *S. aureus*. Outbreaks of *P. aeruginosa* folliculitis have been traced back to swimming pools, while *Candida* species have been implicated in patients taking long-term antibiotics.

> **HACEK**
> A group of organisms, namely *Haemophilus* spp., *Aggregatibacter actinomycetemcomitans* (previously named *Actinobacillus*), *Cardiobacterium hominis*, *Eikenella corrodens* and *Kingella* spp., whose initial letters form the acronym. They are CO_2 dependent and initial infections can lead to complications such as endocarditis.

> **Cross reference**
> See Chapter 5.

(a)   (b)

FIGURE 7.2
(a) *Staphylococcus aureus* and (b) β-haemolytic *Streptococcus* on Columbia blood agar.
Source: Courtesy of M. Ford.

Boils and carbuncles

Boils are a localized area of inflammation caused by an infection under the skin, in a gland, or in a hair shaft, whereas carbuncles are deep subcutaneous abscesses, larger than a boil, usually with one or more openings draining pus onto the skin. *S. aureus* is the most common pathogen.

Abscesses

Abscesses are formed when pus starts to accumulate in the tissues. These may be superficial or of a deep-seated nature, associated with a particular organ. Essentially, any organism isolated may be of significance; however, common causes include *S. aureus* and anaerobes. For example:

- Brain abscesses may be caused by anaerobes, '*Streptococcus anginosus*' group, *S. aureus*, *Streptococcus pneumoniae*, β-HS, and, more rarely, *Haemophilus* and *Nocardia* species.
- Breast abscesses are most commonly caused by *S. aureus*, anaerobes, *Pseudomonas*, and *Proteus* species and often result in nipple discharge, oedema, and erythema.
- Dental abscesses are occasionally caused by the normal oral flora (e.g. viridans streptococci) but facultative or strict anaerobes are more common causes. '*S. anginosus*' group and occasionally *Actinomyces* species may also be responsible.
- Liver abscesses may be bacterial or amoebic in origin. They are often life threatening and require urgent drainage and/or antibiotic treatment. They are commonly caused by enteric organisms, e.g. Enterobacteriaceae, anaerobes, *P. aeruginosa*, and *Enterococcus* spp.

Impetigo

Impetigo is a superficial skin infection that results in swelling and pustules, often forming crusty sores. They are common around the mouth and are often associated with *S. aureus* or β-haemolytic streptococci.

Ulceration

Ulcers often form when circulation is compromised. This may be due to some form of vascular disease, neuropathic changes or as a result of too much pressure on already weakened skin (e.g. bedsores in hospitalized older patients). Chronic leg ulceration due to poor venous circulation is most commonly encountered. Ulcers are often longstanding and seldom sterile. It is thought that the presence of some organisms may be beneficial as they produce proteinases that may help break down necrotic tissue, but too many organisms may produce excessive proteinases and hinder the healing process, as any new tissue is also broken down. Organisms implicated in ulcer infections traditionally include *S. aureus*, β-HS, anaerobes, and *P. aeruginosa*. Water-related infections brought about by trauma during swimming or boating have given rise to rarer causes such as *Aeromonas* and non-cholera *Vibrio* species (e.g. *Vibrio parahaemolyticus* and *Vibrio vulnificus*).

Erysipelas

This is a superficial skin infection affecting mainly the dermis and the upper reaches of subcutaneous tissue. It largely involves the lymphatics within these regions, and results in marked swelling, often with small vesicles and a definite border. It is usually caused by β-HS Lancefield Group A, although Group G *Streptococcus* and *S. aureus* have also been implicated.

Some organisms have been mentioned a lot in the above list of common skin infections, e.g. *S. aureus*. Why do you think this is so?

Erysipeloid

Confusingly, the genus *Erysipelothrix* occasionally causes erysipeloid, and not erysipelas, in humans. The organism is a short, slim, Gram-positive non-sporing rod and *Erysipelothrix rhusiopathiae* is the only species known to cause erysipeloid. In 1886, however, Loffler had established this genus as the cause of 'swine erysipelas' and subsequently *Erysipelothrix* species have been proven to be of major economic importance, as they cause septicaemia and arthritis in swine, calves, lambs, turkeys, and other farm animals.

Necrotizing fasciitis

Necrotizing fasciitis is a rare condition affecting the lower reaches of epidermis and subcutaneous tissue. Toxin production results in extensive skin and muscle destruction and necrosis, often as a complication of trauma or surgery. It is often caused by Group A streptococci, *V. vulnificus*, and *Clostridium perfringens*, the so-called flesh-eating bacteria, but also heavy mixed populations, including several different anaerobes, can give similar effects.

Gangrene

Gangrene refers to the decay and death (necrosis) of tissue brought about by poor blood supply. It is commonly associated with trauma (e.g. gunshot wounds) and a common causative organism is *C. perfringens*. This bacterium and its spores are naturally found in the human and animal gut and in soil. After trauma, the oxygen potential at this site drops due to interruption to the circulation. If spores of *C. perfringens* contaminate this site they are able to become vegetative bacteria in the oxygen-free environment. *C. perfringens* then begins to produce toxin and initiates gangrene. The organism also produces gas as a by-product, causing the skin to 'bubble up', sometimes accompanied by a 'creaking' sound under the skin (**crepitus**). This collectively is known as **gas gangrene**. If treated early enough, the outcome is usually favourable. However, where treatment is delayed (e.g. in war situations) severely affected tissue and/or limbs may need to be amputated to prevent death as a result of sepsis.

C. perfringens is a strict anaerobe. Why would this organism be involved in gangrene?

Key Point

Remember how important clinical details are – you may look for different organisms if the patient has been bitten, or has been swimming abroad, etc. You may not receive such details and the biomedical scientist must consider every possibility when reading culture plates!

7.3 **Mucosal infections**

The mucosa or mucous membranes line various parts of the body that are either exposed to the environment or internal organs. They are primarily involved in either absorption or secretion, and include the eyes, ears, nostrils, and throat. Generally the sites are protected by the bacterial flora present at the site; the exception being the eyes, which are usually bacteria free due to the production of **lysosyme** and local IgA.

7.3.1 Eye infections

A wide range of microorganisms are capable of causing eye infections. Although it may be common to isolate contaminating skin flora from eye swabs, every organism should be assessed for significance before being ruled out as a causative agent.

Conjunctivitis – inflammation of the conjunctiva – is the most common ocular infection encountered and often results in red or 'sticky' eyes. Common causes include: S. aureus, S. pneumoniae, and Haemophilus influenzae. Examples are shown in Figure 7.3a and 7.3b. Other causes include β-HS, Moraxella catarrhalis, Neisseria gonorrhoeae, P. aeruginosa, and the Enterobacteriaceae.

Ophthalmia neonatorum – conjunctivitis of the newborn – is primarily caused by vertical transmission of N. gonorrhoeae or Chlamydia trachomatis from the mother at birth. If left untreated infection can result in blindness. In addition to the above causes, other pathogens include Group B streptococci. Adult conjunctivitis caused by N. gonorrhoeae is usually a result of concomitant genital infection, although it is also a risk to laboratory staff as it may be laboratory acquired.

Chlamydia and viral conjunctivitis – trachoma can be caused by serotypes A–C of C. trachomatis whilst inclusion conjunctivitis may be caused by serotypes D–K. The former serotypes are more associated with rural communities in under-developed areas, whilst the latter are more likely to be urban and associated with sexual transmission. Viral causes of conjunctivitis are predominantly adenoviruses.

FIGURE 7.3

Culture plates showing (a) S. pneumoniae, optochin sensitive, and (b) H. influenzae. Note how different the colonies are for two organisms that infect the same site.

Source: Courtesy of M. Ford.

(a)   (b)

Keratitis – inflammation of the cornea – may be caused by the protozoan *Acanthamoeba* species. They may be detected in corneal scrapings and are often associated with incorrect use and storage of contact lenses.

Orbital cellulitis – infection of orbital tissue usually as a consequence of trauma, either accidental or through surgical procedure and may lead to blindness or thrombosis. Tissue aspirates tend to be more appropriate specimens than eye swabs. Typically, *S. aureus*, β-HS, and anaerobes are implicated, whilst *H. influenzae* may still be isolated from children, although the use of the Hib vaccine has led to a fall in the prevalence of the type b strain.

7.3.2 Ear infections

Ear infections may be subdivided into otitis externa (external ear infection) and otitis media (middle ear infection).

Otitis externa may be caused by a similar range of organisms to those affecting the skin and soft tissues, with *P. aeruginosa* and *S. aureus* predominating. Group A streptococci, anaerobes, Enterobacteriaceae, and fungi (e.g. *Aspergillus* species) are also common.

Otitis media is diagnosed in symptomatic patients presenting with signs of acute illness along with the presence of fluid in the middle ear. Extreme untreated cases have led to deafness. It often occurs when organisms from the upper respiratory tract migrate along the Eustachian tube to reside in the middle ear. The main offenders are *S. pneumoniae*, *M. catarrhalis*, and *H. influenzae*. Other causes include *S. aureus*, β-HS, and Gram-negative bacilli.

7.3.3 Nasal swabs

Although between 15 and 40% of us carry *S. aureus* in our nostrils, nasal carriage markedly increases the risk of infection at other body sites, for example, post-surgery. It may also be associated with recurrent skin infections. Depending on the individual's circumstances, eradication of the organism from the nostrils may be required. Currently mupirocin nasal drops are extremely successful at eradicating carriage, but occasionally the use of systemic or other topical antibiotics is required.

Nasal swabs may also be employed to screen for certain 'target' organisms, especially MRSA screening on new hospital admissions and Group A streptococci on burns patients.

7.3.4 Throat infections

Sore throats are often of viral origin, are mild, and often get better without the need for specific treatment. This is one area where general practitioners were criticized by the government, as they were accused of helping cause the bacterial resistance problems by giving patients unnecessary antibiotics.

Severe sore throat or tonsillitis, however, will normally require appropriate antimicrobial therapy.

Pharyngitis – the most common cause of pharyngitis is the Group A *Streptococcus*. It can be spread by casual, close, or direct contact with infected individuals through respiratory droplets, and several outbreaks have been noted. The incubation period is between 2 and 5 days, and symptoms include sore throat, fever, headache, pyrexia, and occasionally nausea and vomiting. Group C and G streptococci can also cause pharyngitis.

Diphtheria – an acute upper respiratory tract disease caused by *Corynebacterium diphtheriae*. The organism is capable of producing a toxin (see later) which can damage the epithelium of the pharynx and form a pseudomembrane. Death can ultimately occur due to obstruction of the airways. This is one infection that is often diagnosed clinically and the laboratory is there for confirmation. Diphtheria is characterized by the patient having a characteristic 'bull neck' due to the effects of the toxin. Screening throat swabs for *C. diphtheriae* is recommended in patients with the following risk factors:

1.   Membranous pharyngitis/tonsillitis.

2.   Patients who have travelled abroad recently, particularly to Russia, former Soviet states, Eastern Europe, Africa, South America, and South East Asia.

3.   Contacts of the above.

Epiglottitis – an infection mostly associated with young children and the organism *H. influenzae*. The introduction of the Hib vaccine in 1992 has led to a fall in the number of cases; however, the organism should always be considered, especially in those who have not been vaccinated. In uncomplicated sore throats, the organism is not routinely investigated. However, this highlights the importance of clinical details and should epiglottitis be suggested, additional culture plates need to be inoculated.

Vincent's angina – an infection associated with poor oral hygiene or systemic disease and characterized by pharyngeal or gum ulceration. Also known as trench mouth as many WWI soldiers probably suffered from the disease due to very poor oral hygene (Figure 7.4). Laboratory detection is by direct microscopy and is confirmed by the presence of white cells, cigar-shaped fusiforms (*Fusobacterium* spp.) and spirochaetes (*Borrelia vincentii*).

Fusobacterium necrophorum – this anaerobic organism is now recognized as a cause of persistent sore throat, particularly in young adults, and may occasionally lead to **Lemierre's disease**, if undiagnosed. However, routine investigation is difficult as differentiation from anaerobic flora usually present in the mouth is troublesome and time-consuming.

•   Less common causes of pharyngitis include: *Arcanobacterium haemolyticum*, non- toxigenic *C. diphtheriae*, *N. gonorrhoeae*, *S. aureus*, and fungal infections.

•   Throat swabs may also be taken to check for carriage of *Neisseria meningitidis* from contacts of meningococcal meningitis.

> **Lemierre's disease**
>
> A disease mainly caused by *Fusobacterium necrophorum* but other fusobacteria can be involved. It mainly affects young adults. Lemierre's syndrome follows a streptococcal throat infection which has led to a peritonsillar abscess. *Fusobacterium necrophorum* can flourish in this abscess and can penetrate into the neighbouring jugular vein. Bacteria can then disseminate into the bloodstream. It is associated with a high mortality rate.

SELF-CHECK 7.3

Why do you think that GPs don't treat many throat infections with antibiotics? What would be the problem if they did?

FIGURE 7.4

Image of a patient with Vincent's angina. Note the pronounced gum disease which if untreated is likely to lead to ulceration.

Source: Courtesy of CDC/Minnesota Department of Health, R.N. Barr Library; Librarians Melissa Rethlefsen and Marie Jones.

Key Point

You should have noticed that a limited few pathogens are associated with the majority of the infections listed here. As a result the clinician can often have a good idea as to the infectious cause when the patient is first seen and thus prescribe accurately rather than waiting for culture results.

7.4 Organisms, virulence factors, and toxin production

In this section we will briefly look at some of the virulence factors and toxins produced by common pathogens discussed in this chapter. We will also consider the growing role reference laboratories play in the investigation of some organisms.

7.4.1 *Staphylococcus aureus*

As we have seen, *S. aureus* is capable of causing a wide range of infections. Its high level of invasiveness and pathogenicity is predominantly due to the ability to produce a wide range of extracellular enzymes and toxins:

- Coagulase – clots plasma, assists in spread throughout tissues, and can interrupt phagocytosis.
- Lipase – digests fat and allows faster spread of the organism.
- Haemolysin – destroys red blood cells and makes more nutrients available.
- Hyaluronidase – assists in spread of the organism in tissues by breaking down hyaluronic acid, a key component of connective tissue.
- Staphylokinase – helps induce fibrinolysis (affects clotting).
- Protein A – affects complement activation.
- Toxic shock syndrome toxin – causes rash, shock, and shedding of the skin.
- Enterotoxins – associated with food poisoning.
- Exfoliative toxin – causes skin loss.
- Leukocidin – destroys white blood cells.
- Panton–Valentine leukocidin (PVL) – a particularly aggressive toxin produced by *S. aureus* that is capable of forming pores in host cell membranes and has been associated with necrotizing pneumonia.

CASE STUDY 7.1 *An outbreak of S. aureus*

In 2007, an outbreak occurred in the UK of boils and skin infections in children. It initially centred around one school. It was noted that *S. aureus* with a distinctive antibiotic profile was isolated from several of the children. When the isolates were forwarded to the reference laboratory it was found that most were producing the Panton-Valentine

leukocidin toxin. Although this was not a particularly aggressive strain, this community-acquired outbreak of methicillin-sensitive *S. aureus* (CA-MSSA) spread rapidly throughout the school and affected a large number of children. The symptomatic children and their close family plus the majority of pupils in the school were screened for nasal carriage of *S. aureus*. Fortunately, the organism had a characteristic antibiotic profile (resistant to penicillin, gentamicin, tobramycin, and trimethoprim but sensitive to most other Gram-positive antibiotics, including methicillin and erythromycin). After receiving the initial results, it was possible to predict which families were carrying the toxigenic strain in their nostrils and hence needed to have mupirocin

treatment. Several months after the onset of this outbreak, sporadic cases still occurred, indicating the difficulty in eradicating community-based outbreaks.

1. What samples would have been taken?

2. What culture media would you have used?

3. What antibiotic therapy would have been initiated?

4. What agencies would need to have been informed?

Significant isolates, as well as organisms isolated from outbreaks, are often sent to reference laboratories to monitor local and national prevalence of particular strains.

7.4.2 Group A streptococci (*Streptococcus pyogenes*)

Infections caused by this pathogen range from sore throats to necrotizing fasciitis. The organism exists as Gram-positive cocci, typically in chains. As with *S. aureus*, a wide range of enzymes and toxins are produced. For example:

- Streptolysins – both types are responsible for digestion of blood and cause haemolysis of red blood cells, as seen on blood-containing agar plates. Streptolysin O is inactivated by oxygen, is antigenic, and induces production of antistreptolysin O (ASO) antibody in the host, whereas streptolysin S is oxygen stable and non-antigenic.

- Hyaluronidase – assists in spread of the organism in tissues by breaking down hyaluronic acid, a key component of connective tissue.

- Leukocidin – as previous.

- Streptokinase – helps induce fibrinolysis (affects clotting).

- M proteins – virulence factors associated with colonization and resistance to phagocytosis. More than 50 have been identified in different strains of Group A streptococci according to antigenic structure. R and T proteins are not involved in virulence, but play a key role in epidemiological typing.

adhesins

Adhesins appear to mediate bacterial adherence to host epithelial cells, thereby assisting in pathogenesis.

- Lipoteichoic acid – one of several **adhesins** that lends itself to colonization and ultimately infection at a given site, e.g. the pharynx.

- Streptococcal pyrogenic exotoxin (SPE) – formerly known as erythrogenic toxin, it is responsible for the rash seen with scarlet fever and occurs when the toxin disseminates in the blood. It is also associated with a streptococcal form of toxic shock syndrome, as well as necrotizing fasciitis.

SELF-CHECK 7.4

Just look how many toxins both *S. aureus* and Group A haemolytic streptococci produce! Think about the damage done to the host upon an infection with this organism. Why is it so significant epidemiologically?

Group A streptococci isolated from systemic infections (from positive blood cultures) are sent to reference laboratories due to the seriousness of the infection. In this way surveillance of infection and changes in trends are analysed both locally and nationally. From an epidemiological standpoint, this keeps the laboratory aware of circulating strains and may highlight a previously unrecognized outbreak.

Pseudomonas aeruginosa

P. aeruginosa is a Gram-negative rod, found in the human intestinal tract, water, soil and sewage and moist environments, such as sinks. It is an **opportunistic pathogen** of humans and infections are often hospital-acquired. It rarely affects healthy tissue, but can produce damage in tissue that is in poor condition or compromised in some way.

> **opportunistic pathogens**
> Opportunistic pathogens exploit weaknesses in host defences to create infections.

Virulence factors include:

- Fimbrae – are used to adhere to epithelial cells of the host, especially those of the upper respiratory tract of hospitalized patients.
- Alginate – production of this slimy substance, consisting of polysaccharide, also assists with respiratory tract adhesion. It enables the organism to form the basis (matrix) of the **biofilm** that *Pseudomonas* species create to survive within their environment.
- Elastase – is capable of cleaving collagen, immunoglobulin, and complement. It can interfere with the epithelial lining of the respiratory tract and affects ciliary operation.
- Cytotoxin – appears to be toxic to most eukaryotic cells.
- Phospholipase and lecithinase – act against lipid and lecithin within cells.
- Pyocyanin – the blue pigment produced by many *P. aeruginosa* which is a redox-active phenazine compound that kills both mammalian and bacterial cells alike by the generation of reactive oxygen intermediates. It has been linked to reduced bacterial clearance from the lungs of immunocompromised patients.

> **biofilms**
> Biofilms are complex masses of mono- or polymicrobial communities that are capable of secreting extracellular substances, producing a complex and sometimes highly organized glycocalyx structure within which they are embedded. This creates a protective layer that the organisms use to survive hostile environmental conditions or, in clinical situations, guard against host defence mechanisms, such as lymphocytes. They also prevent antibiotics from reaching their target sites, the most obvious example being the mucoid *P. aeruginosa* strains often found in the lungs of cystic fibrosis patients and the difficulty encountered in trying to eradicate the organism. In the microbiological diagnosis of infection, this biofilm may have to be disrupted in order to culture the responsible organisms.

Clostridium perfringens

Clostridium perfringens is an anaerobic Gram-positive rod that resides in the human gut and the environment. *Clostridium* spp. are capable of producing spores which allow the organism to survive in a dormant state until favourable conditions return. The organism is associated with gas gangrene.

Virulence factors include:

- α-Toxin (phospholipase C) is one of the toxins produced in cases of gas gangrene, resulting in rapid deterioration of tissue carbohydrate and gas production in necrotic tissue, especially muscles. Alpha toxin is the main cause of cellular breakdown and toxin spread, and is produced by *C. perfringens* type A1.
- Enterotoxin is produced by *C. perfringens* type A2 and causes self-limiting food-poisoning within 8–12 h of eating contaminated meat.
- β-Toxin causes a severe jejunitis known as **pigbel**. It is produced by *C. perfringens* type C, usually as a result of eating undercooked pig meat. Symptoms include abdominal pain, dysentery and vomiting. It is rare in the developed world, but has been recorded in China, Bangladesh, Papua New Guinea, and parts of East Africa.

Corynebacterium diphtheriae

The organism exists as a facultative Gram-positive rod, typically seen in palisades of 'Chinese letter' formation on Gram stain. Whilst uncommon in the UK, laboratories need to be aware that diphtheria is still present in several countries and consequently the need to maintain the capability of detecting *C. diphtheriae* remains, in terms of both experience and relevant media. There are four biotypes of *C. diphtheriae*, namely *C. diphtheriae* var. *gravis*, *intermedius*, *belfanti*, and *mitis*. As mentioned previously, both toxigenic and non-toxigenic strains can be found and the toxin is **bacteriophage induced**. Classical symptoms of diphtheria are presented only when toxin is produced and as a rule var. *gravis* is more pathogenic as it is known to produce the most exotoxin.

bacteriophage-induced toxin

A bacteriophage is a virus which infects bacterial cells and can transfer genetic material to it, which can code for production of toxins.

The pathogenesis of nasal, nasopharyngealm, and tonsillar diphtheria involves the production of this powerful and rapidly fatal toxin, which then disseminates into the bloodstream through the damaged mucous membranes of the upper respiratory tract. The patient requires urgent antitoxin to prevent potentially fatal cardiac and neural complications. In addition, an acute inflammatory response leads to the formation of the classical grey–yellow pseudomembrane at the site of infection. This can obstruct the larynx, block the passage of air, and may cause death by asphyxiation.

All isolates of *C. diphtheriae* should be sent to a reference laboratory for confirmation and toxin testing. This service is available 365 days a year in the UK and is traditionally performed using the ELEK plate (Figure 7.5) although molecular detection is currently being investigated.

Whilst many strains of *C. diphtheriae* prove to be non-toxigenic, increased travel to Eastern Europe and recent influxes of migrant workers from these regions increase the chances of isolating toxigenic forms. Some strains of *Corynebacterium ulcerans* and *Corynebacterium pseudotuberculosis* are also known to produce diphtheria toxin.

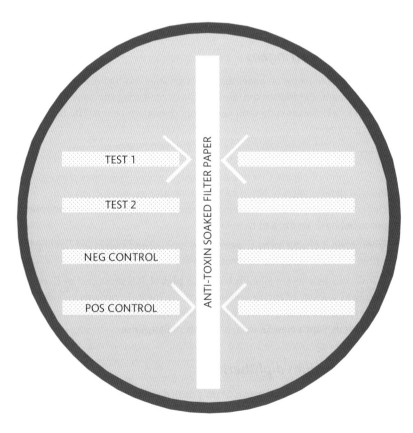

FIGURE 7.5
Image of an ELEK plate. Test strain 1 is toxigenic and is producing precipitation between the strain and the diphtheria antitoxin soaked filter paper (similar to the positive control). Test strain 2 is toxin negative (no precipitation).

7.4.3 Mycobacteria

Mycobacteria are unusual causes of skin infections but should be considered for certain case histories. For example, **fish tank granuloma** is particularly associated with keeping or handling tropical fish and may also be found in swimming pools. The condition is caused by *Mycobacterium marinum* giving rise to a red, scaly rash, often on the hands and arms.

Mycobacterium ulcerans should be investigated if the tropical '**Buruli ulcer**' is suspected. The organism is believed to enter the skin through cuts and abrasions. An ulcer develops, followed by necrosis and ultimately skin and bone destruction due to toxic events. Patients often undergo extensive surgery to remove the lesion.

7.5 Sample processing

Swab or tissue specimen may be collected from virtually any part of the body so it is virtually impossible to describe how each specimen is processed individually. However, it is important when processing these specimens that the scientist has some knowledge of the likely pathogens that may be encountered from these samples. This will help you decide which media should be selected.

7.5.1 Microscopy techniques

For most wound and mucosal swabs, the use of microscopy is unnecessary due to the large number of commensal organisms often present, resulting in the possibility of misleading information. Gram stains of pus samples or sterile fluids are less likely to be contaminated with skin flora and can give meaningful results.

Cross reference
See Chapter 9.

The presence of white blood cells along with organisms may be suggestive of an inflammatory response to the organism in question. Reporting this finding to a clinical microbiologist may give some immediate bearing on the treatment and management of the patient. Infections of this nature are rarely polymicrobial; hence you would expect to find only one type of organism present, for example Gram-positive cocci (Figure 7.6). Biomedical scientists should be wary of mixtures of different bacteria in normally sterile samples, as this is often the type of picture you may see from specimens such as drain fluids contaminated with gastrointestinal flora.

Gram stains from samples of connective tissue may also be of clinical benefit, but it is important to remember these specimens may be easily contaminated by normal skin flora and so results may be misleading. Tissues such as heart valves should be sterile and so should always have a Gram stain performed on them, due to the urgency of the request.

FIGURE 7.6
Photograph of Gram stain of staphylococci. Remember that whilst this could be suggestive of a pathogenic *S. aureus* infection, you can't tell from the Gram stain which staphylococcal species it is.
Source: Courtesy of D. Barclay.

SELF-CHECK 7.5

A Gram stain of a wound swab can give misleading information back to the clinicians. Why could this be?

Cross reference
See Chapter 9, Section 9.4.

Tissue samples from abscesses, particularly facial and dental abscesses, should be examined for 'sulphur granules' which may demonstrate the presence of *Actinomyces* species. The granules are clumps of organisms and should be crushed between two slides and Gram stained. *Actinomyces* species are branching Gram-positive bacilli.

As previously described, Vincent's stain is required to diagnose Vincent's angina and AFB staining techniques (either auramine or Ziehl–Neelsen) are required to demonstrate presence of *Mycobacterium* species.

> ### Key Point
>
> Sterile fluids, pus, and tissue specimens should have microscopy performed and the presence of bacteria should be reported to clinicians. Transport swab specimens are less appropriate for Gram staining, because both the swabbed site is more likely to contain normal flora and the transport media used (usually charcoal) may conceal the presence of organisms.

Cross reference
See Chapter 3.

7.5.2 Common isolation media

Most of the bacteria and fungi associated with skin and soft tissue infections can be isolated using routine cultural techniques. Whilst the precise selection of media used may vary between laboratories nationally, they will all tend to reflect the organisms that are likely to be encountered. Broadly speaking, selective and non-selective media are used in combination. Specific selective plates, however, may be employed for particular target organisms.

In general, the following types of media are routinely employed:

- Blood agar.
- Chocolate agar.
- MacConkey or CLED agar.
- Specific anaerobic agar with metronidazole disc added.
- Selective media relevant to isolation of specific pathogens, e.g. aztreonam agar for *S. aureus*.

Blood and chocolate plates should be incubated in an environment enriched with 5–10% CO_2. Selective media containing aztreonam or nalidixic acid are often used. These media suppress the growth of most colonizing Gram-negative organisms, allowing for the selection of Gram-positive organisms, such as staphylococci and streptococci.

Normally sterile fluid specimens that may yield fastidious organisms, such as *Haemophilus influenzae*, should be cultured to chocolate agar. These samples include ear and eye swabs, as well as knee aspirates and swabs from animal bites.

Specimens that may yield *Candida* spp. or other fungi, such as *Aspergillus* spp., should be cultured to Sabouraud dextrose agar. These samples include ear swabs, mouth swabs, where oral thrush is suspected, and swabs from moist or sweaty sites, for example feet.

Culturing for anaerobic bacteria requires an anaerobic environment. This is usually achieved by employing an anaerobic incubator or jars. Metronidazole discs ($5\,\mu g$) are usually added to the primary inoculum, and the presence of a zone of inhibition after incubation indicates the presence of anaerobes, although growth will often require prolonged incubation.

Key Point

By definition, anaerobic bacteria will not grow in the presence of oxygen. Fortunately, in the UK, the vast majority are still sensitive to metronidazole and hence metronidazole serves both a diagnostic and therapeutic role. NB Exceptions include *Actinomyces* and *Propionibacterium* species which are intrinsically resistant to metronidazole.

Throat swabs are routinely inoculated onto blood agar plates and are often incubated anaerobically to isolate any β-haemolytic streptococci that may be present. Not because these organisms are anaerobes but because haemolysis of the blood agar is enhanced anaerobically, making detection easier especially in mixed culture. If diphtheria is a possibility, the specimen should also be inoculated onto a Hoyle's plate (in CO_2) which contains potassium tellurite and is selective for *C. diphtheriae*.

SELF-CHECK 7.6

Why are the different media you use to isolate pathogens incubated under different atmospheric conditions?

7.6 Orthopaedic samples

Orthopaedic tissue samples are given a special mention due to the unique nature of the specimens. The costs to both the healthcare institution and the patient with the infected **prosthesis** are huge. Consequently, antibiotic cocktails are incorporated into the orthopaedic cement in an attempt to prevent infection. Hip replacements were pioneered by Sir John Charnley in the early 1960s and since then joint replacement (**arthroplasty**) has become commonplace. Arthroplasty is most commonly used for patients with osteoarthritis or inflammatory abnormality such as rheumatoid arthritis, with hip and knee replacements predominating. Modern surgical and anaesthetic techniques, appropriate patient selection, modified prosthesis design, prophylactic antibiotics, laminar airflow in operating theatres, and good post-operative care have reduced infection rates substantially, but there is still a finite risk associated with each procedure.

Infecting organisms may gain entry during primary implantation surgery or through the **haematogenous** (bloodstream) route and may establish either acute or chronic infection. The presence of a foreign body (the prosthetic device) in the joint creates a focus for invasion and means fewer organisms are required to establish infection.

The most common organism to cause acute infections is *S. aureus* and in chronic infections either *S. aureus* or coagulase-negative staphylococci (CNS) predominate. Many other organisms, including other skin flora, streptococci, coliforms, enterococci, and rarely anaerobes, mycobacteria or fungi, may also be implicated. This means that any organism cultured from a sample associated with a prosthetic joint or other orthopaedic device could be significant. Consequently, multiple samples should be taken including several tissue samples, bone, fluid samples, and swabs of the 'infected' site.

Once infection is established around a prosthetic joint, organisms may form a biofilm. Similarly, 'persisters' within the biofilm are very difficult to treat and removal of the prosthesis is often necessary.

SELF-CHECK 7.7

Why are organisms in a biofilm so difficult to eradicate?

7.6.1 Orthopaedic sample processing

The likely presence of antibiotics, either administered directly to the patient or in the cement used to support the replacement joint, indicates that both direct *and* broth enrichment culture is important. The obvious disadvantage of broth enrichment is the increased possibility of contamination. Additionally, as many chronic infections are due to skin flora, any organism cultured may be relevant, making differentiating infection from contamination difficult, especially when CNS are isolated. To aid this process, at least four to five tissue samples per site should be taken and processed individually. Under such circumstances the specificity of isolating CNS from two or more samples has been shown to be 97%.

Exclusion of contaminants during operative and laboratory processing is critical and strict aseptic technique and the use of a Class II cabinet is advocated. Subculture is normally onto standard media, although some workers recommend the use of chocolate agar, as this may help detect small-colony variants of staphylococci that may be isolated from deep samples as a consequence of antimicrobial therapy. Vancomycin, gentamicin, and tobramycin are the antibiotics that are generally incorporated into orthopaedic cement.

Key Point

Remember when a sample is placed into broth, a single organism can multiply to millions which makes detection easier. The laboratory scientist must ensure they process the sample to avoid any of their own skin organisms entering the broth. Think of how clinically misleading the result would be and the potential consequences to the patient if the broth was contaminated.

SELF-CHECK 7.8

Why would you need to use enrichment broth for culture orthopaedic samples when a direct culture is performed?

7.7 Genital tract and associated specimens

As with the skin, it is important to be able to distinguish between commensal and pathogenic organisms of the genital tract. Genital commensals can vary both by age and between the sexes, hence each patient's specimen needs to be considered individually and the microbiology assessed accordingly.

7.7.1 Normal flora of the genital tract

Due to the external nature of the penis, male genital commensals are similar to that of the skin. They consist of CNS, viridans-type streptococci, *Corynebacterium* species and possibly small numbers of *Staphylococcus aureus* and *Candida* species. Internally, however, the male genital tract is largely sterile; this is maintained by prostate secretions and the mechanical action of urination in flushing bacteria away.

Normal flora of the female genital tract is more variable and is strongly related to hormonal physiology and development. At birth, maternal hormones result in elevated levels of vaginal glycogen. Lactobacilli survive well in this environment, hence the initial flora of healthy neonates should reflect this, along with the presence of diphtheroids, staphylococci, streptococci, and *E. coli*.

The bacterial flora of babies soon changes and in female babies levels of glycogen soon fall and the normal flora in pre-pubescent girls may largely consist of coliforms and enterococci. The vaginal environment changes again during puberty; circulating oestrogens result in the elevation of glycogen levels and re-colonization by lactobacilli. Finally, hormonal changes at menopause lead to re-establishment of a flora consisting of an almost pre-pubescent state.

These are only general female changes that may occur with age. It is important to remember that the vaginal flora are constantly under other pressures, such as antibiotic therapy, pregnancy, and during menstruation. Organisms that may be harmlessly present in small numbers but can be implicated in disease if their numbers multiply include yeasts, anaerobes, *Gardnerella vaginalis*, and coliforms.

7.7.2 Specimen quality and type

Due to the nature of the sample, appropriate specimens are often difficult to obtain. Samples may be poorly collected, and incorrect samples are often received. Avoiding faecal contamination when collecting genital specimens can also improve the chances of recovering microbes causing infection. The types of specimen you may encounter include: high vaginal swab (HVS), vaginal discharge, endocervical swab, vulval swab, labial swab, penile swab, genital ulcer swab, urethral discharge/swab, semen, and screening swabs for gonorrhoea. Transport media play an important role in the support of delicate pathogens, such as *Neisseria gonorrhoeae* and *Trichomonas vaginalis*, although both survive for a very limited time in this media. Viral transport media contain antimicrobials to help prevent bacterial contamination of cell lines and hence are inappropriate for bacterial culture.

Aspirates may be collected from **Bartholin's gland**, **pouch of Douglas** fluid, or fallopian tubes. Intrauterine contraceptive devices (IUCDs) or products of conception (POC) may also be submitted to the laboratory for investigation.

SELF-CHECK 7.9

Why can it be so difficult to isolate an organism as important as *N. gonorrhoeae* from a genital sample?

7.7.3 Sexually transmitted infections (STIs)

There are a number of organisms that are capable of sexual transmission and result in a variety of clinical syndromes. It is advisable to screen for multiple infections once an initial STI is

Cross reference

See Chapter 13.

clinically suspected. Screening and contact tracing, performed by dedicated genitourinary medicine (GUM) departments, have a vital role in the control of gonorrhoea, syphilis, *Chlamydia*, and human immunodeficiency virus (HIV) infection.

Gonorrhoea is a form of urethritis involving the mucous membranes of the urethra and caused by the organism *N. gonorrhoeae*. It commonly results in a purulent urethral discharge, usually more apparent in the male than the female. Additionally, men may also experience pain in passing urine (dysuria). The most common complications are epididymitis (inflammation of the epididymis), prostatitis (invasion of the prostate) and orchitis (testicular infection) which can result in sterility. Rare complications include gonococcal cellulitis, urethral abscess and penile lymphangitis. Urethral discharge is the preferred specimen to collect from symptomatic males; urethral swabs are commonly collected from asymptomatic individuals.

Infection is confined to mucosal surfaces lined with columnar epithelia, that is the urethra, cervix, pharynx, rectum and conjunctiva. Vaginal squamous epithelial cells may not be infected by *N. gonorrhoeae*; hence endocervical or urethral swabs are preferred to HVS if gonorrhoea is suspected. Although endocervical infection is often associated with discharge, itching (pruritis) and dysuria, approximately 50% of infections in women are asymptomatic. Ascending spread from the cervix, through the uterus to the fallopian tubes can cause **salpingitis**, or to the ovaries, resulting in **ovaritis**. **Pelvic inflammatory disease** (PID) is the most important complication and can result in infertility.

Rectal infection (proctitis) can occur in women with endocervical infection. This is often caused by autoinoculation and is usually asymptomatic. Proctitis in men who have sex with men (MSM) is common through anal intercourse and can be symptomatic. Treatment of partners as well as the individual is essential to avoid reinfection.

Disseminated gonococcal infection (DGI) is a rare complication of gonorrhoea and results in spread to other body sites. Symptoms include joint and/or muscle pain (arthralgia/myalgia), polyarthritis, pustular rashes, septic arthritis, endocarditis, and meningitis (very rare). Blood culture and joint fluids are appropriate samples for diagnosing certain forms of DGI. Eye infections due to *N. gonorrhoeae* are discussed in Section 7.3.

Trichomoniasis, an infection caused by the protozoan *Trichomonas vaginalis* (TV), is predominantly spread by sexual contact. Patients may be asymptomatic for years, but for many patients infection causes symptoms including vaginal discharge, itching, and dysuria. Low birth weight and premature delivery can result from infection during pregnancy. There is also evidence that *Trichomonas* infection can predispose the person to an increased susceptibility to HIV infection after intercourse with an HIV-infected partner. The life cycle of the organism is shown in Figure 7.7.

Microscopy is generally the preferred method of diagnosis, although culture is still regarded as the 'gold standard', but this tends to be slower and more labour intensive. Consequently, wet preparation or acridine orange staining is employed by most UK laboratories, although the sensitivity of both methods is questionable. As conventional bacterial transport swabs do not offer optimal support for TV over longer periods of time, employing acridine orange may theoretically detect non-viable TV which may be overlooked in wet preparations. There are now molecular methods available for detection of *T. vaginalis* but with limited uptake generally due to high cost and very low prevalence in some areas.

Genital herpes is caused by the herpes simplex virus (HSV). Both types of the virus (1 and 2) are capable of causing genital disease, although type 2 is predominantly spread by sexual contact. Although a relatively common condition, infected pregnant women are at risk of serious systemic sequelae. Additionally, risks to the foetus include poor growth rates and death. Diagnosis

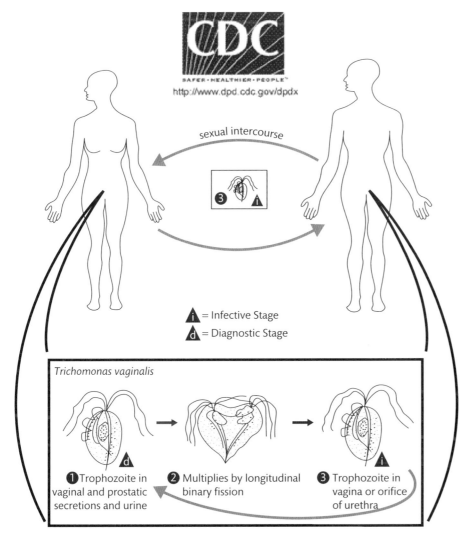

FIGURE 7.7
Life cycle of *Trichomonas vaginalis*.
Source: Courtesy of CDC/
Alexander J. da Silva, PhD/
Melanie Moser.

has traditionally consisted of viral culture, although PCR techniques have now superseded this. Site-specific viral swabs incorporating viral transport media to prevent bacterial overgrowth are the specimens of choice.

Chlamydia is the most common STI and may affect up to one in ten sexually active men and women, particularly those under the age of 25. There are over 100,000 cases per year in the UK. It is caused by the bacterium *Chlamydia trachomatis*. The organism is present in the semen and vaginal fluid of infected men and women. Infection can often be asymptomatic, but if left untreated can result in painful complications and infertility. In women, spread to other reproductive organs can cause PID, which may result in long-term pain, blocked fallopian tubes, infertility, and ectopic pregnancy. Men may experience urethritis, orchitis, and reduced fertility.

Traditionally, culture in McCoy cell lines and then detection of either inclusion or elementary bodies was deemed to be the gold standard. This was often supplemented with antigen detection using enzyme immunoassay (EIA) techniques. Both have now been completely superseded by nucleic acid amplification testing (NAAT), for example strand displacement

Cross reference
See Chapter 16.

FIGURE 7.8

Photomicrograph showing the characteristic spiral shape of the causative organism of syphillis (*T. pallidum*).
Source: Courtesy of CDC/W.F. Schwartz.

amplification (SDA) or ligase chain reaction (LCR). Although more expensive, it offers far greater sensitivity and specificity than antigen detection and is a lot less labour intensive than culture, and suitable for mass screening programmes. Furthermore, diagnosis does not heavily rely on invasive genital sampling, as routine urine samples, especially in males, or self-taken swabs can often suffice. Most manufacturers offer a combined *Chlamydia/N. gonorrhoeae* NAAT test which has now replaced culture in screening for the latter infection

Syphilis is caused by the spirochaete bacterium *Treponema pallidum* (Figure 7.8). Once regarded as an 'historical' infection, it has re-emerged as an STI and has been responsible for several recent outbreaks in many countries worldwide. The organism cannot be grown in routine culture.

Although sexual transmission predominates, IV drug use, blood transfusion, and congenital transmission from mother to unborn child are also possible. Primary syphilis begins with one or more painless sores called chancres. These are highly infectious and, as they are commonly situated on the genitals, are the main route of sexual transmission. The sores disappear after 3-6 weeks and, if untreated, the disease will usually progress further. Secondary symptoms occur 2-10 weeks after the appearance of the chancre, and include skin rash, sore throat, tiredness, and headaches. These symptoms typically disappear, even without treatment, although there may still be transient symptoms. A latent stage may follow where the patient suffers few symptoms and often feels 'cured'. Unfortunately, without treatment the infection may progress to tertiary syphilis. This can result in a variety of conditions including heart disease, dementia, and death.

Since all pregnant women are screened for syphilis, laboratories should be capable of testing large numbers of specimens, the majority of which will be negative. Confirmation of positive results may be conducted locally or by regional reference centres. Discrepancies should always be referred. The initial serology screen consists of an EIA to detect both IgM and IgG. This is highly sensitive, but not quite as specific as TPPA/TPHA (*Treponema pallidum* particle agglutination or *T. pallidum* haemagglutination) assays, which should be employed on patients' samples that are IgM/IgG positive or samples from contacts of positive patients. Final confirmation requires the VDRL/RPR test (Venereal Disease Reference Laboratory/rapid plasma reagin) to try to assess whether infection is likely to be recent or has been adequately treated.

SELF-CHECK 7.10

Why do you think sexually transmitted infections are on the increase, despite advertising campaigns, etc.?

Why are tests to detect antibodies to *T. pallidum* used rather than trying to grow the organism in culture?

Chancroid is a sexually transmitted infection caused by *Haemophilus ducreyi*. Painful genital ulceration is typical. The infection is traditionally regarded as a 'tropical disease', although distribution now appears to be spreading. Diagnosis is often made on clinical grounds; culture is often difficult. The organism is quite fastidious and requires specific media, not normally stocked by routine laboratories, lending the disease to molecular diagnosis.

7.7.4 Non-sexually transmitted genital tract infections

Candida albicans is responsible for about 85% of cases of vaginal candidiasis. Normally present in small numbers, candidiasis occurs when yeasts are able to proliferate and predominate over normal vaginal commensals. This may occur after antibacterial chemotherapy, during immunosuppression or pregnancy or whilst using oral contraception, all of which are known to disrupt the normal vaginal flora. Non-*albicans* species known to cause candidiasis include *C. krusei*, *C. tropicalis*, and *C. glabrata*.

Clinically, the patient may experience itching, dysuria and/or a creamy white discharge, although some women undergo soreness and swelling. Over-the-counter antifungal therapy creams are now widely available, but some only target *C. albicans*. Subsequently, less common yeast infections may often persist due to treatment failure. All genital swabs should be cultured to an appropriate medium for the isolation of yeasts (Sabouraud dextrose media). Use of the recently available chromogenic *Candida* media will help determine when a non-*albicans* species has proliferated.

Cross reference
See Chapter 14.

Vaginitis may be caused by *Candida* spp., *T. vaginalis*, β-HS, *S. aureus*, and coliforms amongst others. In young girls implicated organisms also include *H. influenzae*, although the cause may also be poor hygiene or simple irritation.

Ureaplasma urealyticum and *Mycoplasma hominis* are naturally stable bacteria that lack a cell wall. Whilst they may be present in small numbers within normal vaginal flora, they have been implicated in many infections of the genital tract of both males and females. Mycoplasmas have been associated with bacterial vaginosis (see later), postpartum endometritis, salpingitis, and PID. Both have been implicated in non-specific urethritis (NSU) in men, a condition that may be sexually transmitted in nature but cannot be attributable to a particular cause. Both organisms are rarely investigated as they are difficult to isolate and require specific media and technical expertise. For *M. hominis* it is essential that a serum-enriched clear medium is used so that the colonies can be visualized under a plate microscope after growth and they present with a 'fried-egg' appearance due to the lack of a cell wall. *U. urealyticum* colonies (previously known as T-strain mycoplasmas where 'T' equals tiny) are too small to be visualized using this methodology and often a chemical reaction within the media is relied on for their detection.

Bacterial vaginosis (BV) occurs when changes to the vaginal environment lead to a reduction in lactobacilli and an increase in other organisms, especially anaerobic bacteria (e.g. *Mobiluncus* species). BV is generally accepted as a polymicrobial condition and other organisms have also been implicated, including *G. vaginalis*. For this reason BV was previously described as *Gardnerella vaginalis* syndrome. The fact that this organism may be recovered from many asymptomatic women ensures that BV is now the more commonly used term. It is not fully understood what causes this imbalance, but changing soap, bath foam, and douching have all been implicated. A fishy smelling discharge is the most common symptom associated with BV and complications during pregnancy including **amnionitis,** premature labour, and PID have been noted.

Clinical diagnosis relies on the following criteria (three of four):

- Thin grey–white discharge.
- Vaginal secretions>pH 4.5.
- Amine test positive (fishy amine smell present when vaginal secretions mixed with potassium hydroxide).
- Clue cells present on microscopic examination.

Diagnosis is a contentious area – microscopic examination of vaginal smears for 'clue cells' is highly specific for BV, although not critical. Clue cells are epithelial cells that have large numbers of Gram-variable bacilli attached (*G. vaginalis* and *Mobiluncus* spp.). Although a Gram film is recognized as the most appropriate microscopic technique, acridine orange staining offers the advantage of providing screening for both 'clue cells' and *Trichomonas vaginalis*. Gram staining, however, allows both Gram variability and reduction in lactobacilli to be assessed easily and is required if Nugent's or Hay's criteria are used for BV diagnosis.

Key Point

The diagnosis of bacterial vaginosis is still controversial and not standardized throughout microbiology departments. There are two criteria for diagnosing BV (Nugent's and Hay's) and the reader is referred to both publications to see how divisions exist in diagnosis (see Reference list at the end of the book).

Lancefield Group B *Streptococcus* is a transient vaginal commensal. During pregnancy, however, the organism may infect the amnion which potentially can cause sepsis and meningitis in the neonate. Similarly, vertical transmission can occur at birth due to vaginal colonization. Testing for carriage tends to follow local policy and often involves screening introital and rectal swabs. Subsequent treatment during pregnancy and/or childbirth should follow both national and local policy. The presence of Lancefield Group A streptococci in HVS swabs during pregnancy is now quite uncommon but was the scourge of previous generations as many pregnancies resulted in **puerperal sepsis** and subsequent death in the mother either during or within days of delivery. Although uncommon, the significance of *Streptococcus* Group A in an HVS sample shouldn't be underestimated.

Normally, the isolation of *S. aureus* from a vaginal swab may be of doubtful significance, but the isolation of toxin-producing *S. aureus* from women of child-bearing age can be hugely significant, as it has been associated with the condition **toxic shock syndrome** (TSS). TSS has been linked to certain factors, particularly tampon usage, and is characterized by pyrexia, erythema, and hypotension. To produce toxin, *S. aureus* firstly requires a protein-rich environment. This is initially provided by the menstrual blood flow. In addition, both a neutral vaginal pH and increased oxygen levels are necessary; menstruation causes a drop in vaginal pH, whilst an inserted tampon alters the normally anaerobic vaginal environment.

Vaginal swabs from cases of suspected listeriosis, women who have experienced intrauterine death, miscarriage, or post-mortem foetal tissue should be investigated for the presence of

CASE STUDY 7.2 *Toxic shock syndrome*

The late 1970s saw the introduction of a new range of tampons in the US, driven mainly by demand from American women for increased absorbency. Procter and Gamble subsequently launched the 'Rely Superabsorbant' brand which appeared to contain the entire menstrual flow without leakage or constant replacement. However, in 1980 epidemiologists noted a rise in numbers of a newly described condition, TSS, mainly in menstruating women. Although other highly absorbent tampons were also later implicated, the Rely brand, consisting of carboxymethyl-

cellulose and polyester, appeared to filter the toxin produced by *S. aureus* and significantly increase the risk of TSS. These products and materials are no longer used in tampons and, consequently, rates of TSS in women using tampons have fallen dramatically.

1. What samples would have been taken?

2. How would these samples have been processed?

3. What would the role of the reference laboratory be?

Listeria monocytogenes. It has been shown to be the cause of maternal septicaemia and serious morbidity and mortality to the foetus. Other samples warranting investigation include products of conception (POC), placental tissue/swabs, and neonatal screens.

Intrauterine contraceptive devices (IUCDs) or coils have been associated with cases of PID, sometimes as a result of a polymicrobial infection. If signs and symptoms point to PID and/or an inflammatory response in an IUCD-wearing female, the organism *Actinomyces israelii* should also be considered. The removed IUCD should be inspected macroscopically for 'sulphur granules' – small, hard 'growths' on the surface of the coil that are essentially clumps of organisms. They do not actually contain any sulphur, but are yellow and sulphur-like in appearance. These can be crushed between two glass slides and Gram stained. *Actinomyces* species appear as branching Gram-positive bacilli. Extended anaerobic culture up to 10 or 14 days is essential for the recovery of this pathogen on primary isolation. Metronidazole can be added to specific culture media, as they are intrinsically resistant, unlike anaerobes. Unfortunately, differentiation from *Propionibacterium* spp. is still an issue, although the rapid indole test helps.

Other infections of the female genital tract include cervicitis, endometritis, salpingitis, PID, and Bartholinitis (infection of the secretory Bartholin's glands on the vaginal wall). Generally, most of the organisms discussed in this section could cause any of these conditions, sometimes as complications and sequelae of vaginitis. In addition, it is important to remember that ascending infection during pregnancy can have adverse effects on the unborn child, as well as the mother.

Infections of the male genitourinary tract include prostitis, orchitis, epididymitis, and **balanitis** (inflammation of the prepuce). In addition to *N. gonorrhoeae*, causative agents include *C. trachomatis*, coliforms, and *Pseudomonas*, β-HS, and *S. aureus*. *Candida* species are capable of causing penile candidiasis, although this is less common than vaginal thrush.

7.8 *Neisseria gonorrhoeae*: virulence factors

Although *N. gonorrhoeae* does not produce toxins, the organism has a wide range of virulence factors enabling it to cause disease, including three outer membrane proteins (PI, PII, and PIII).

Initially, the bacterium will adhere to microvilli of non-ciliated columnar epithelial cells (of the cervix). Adherence is accomplished using fimbrae and specific proteins (PII or Opa); penetration of the cells and multiplication of the organism then follows.

The porin protein, PI (Por), is believed to mediate penetration of host cells – the organisms enter cells by **endocytosis**, are delivered to the base of the cells via vacuoles and leave by **exocytosis**. Bacteria are then able to progress to subepithelial tissue. PI is also believed to help gonococci survive post-phagocytosis. The PI proteins are antigenic and each strain of N. gonorrhoeae exhibits only one type of PI; a trait used by laboratories to help confirm the identity of N. gonorrheae. Antibodies to a further membrane protein, PIII or Rmp, are believed to block the natural immune response.

Cross reference
See Chapter 15.

Within the Gram-negative cell wall, N. gonorrhoeae exhibits large amounts of **lipooligosaccaharide** (LOS) which is believed to play a key role in pathogenesis. It is able to stimulate the production of TNF (tumour necrosis factor) which causes cell damage (e.g. to fallopian tubes) and can induce the production of proteases and phospholipases that are thought to help cause disease. Its presence is also known to cause a significant inflammatory response and is believed to be responsible for many of the symptoms of gonorrhoea. The organism is also capable of extracting iron from its host which is crucial for growth, multiplication, and cellular invasion.

7.9 **Sample processing**

Samples specifically for *Chlamydia* and viral investigations incorporating appropriate transport media are submitted to the microbiology laboratory, but are not considered in detail in this section. In most laboratories these are forwarded to reference laboratories for processing, generally using molecular detection methods.

Processing of genital specimens for bacteriology will vary according to local policy. Variables such as clinical details and age will dictate how specimens are investigated and are therefore critical for accurate diagnosis. Generally, all genital specimens being screened for STIs are cultured for *Candida* species and N. gonorrhoeae. Selective media are advisable for the isolation of yeasts and gonococci to help suppress the growth of commensal organisms. Sabouraud dextrose agar and gonococci (GC) selective media containing an antifungal agent are usually employed, respectively. Gonococci are fastidious organisms and require an incubation temperature of 35–37 °C supplemented with 5–10% CO_2 to grow and may take 48 h. Figure 7.9 shows the characteristic Gram-negative diplococci of N. gonorrhoeae in a urethral smear. Note how many of the organisms are intracellular.

Nucleic acid amplification testing (NAAT) is available that detects both C. trachomatis and N. gonorrhoeae from one sample. As mentioned previously, the sensitivity of C. trachomatis detection has increased with the introduction of molecular techniques. Likewise these

FIGURE 7.9

Photomicrograph of a urethral discharge showing intracellular Gram-negative diplococci characteristic of N. gonorrhoeae.

Source: Courtesy of CDC/Brenda Novak.

techniques appear to be particularly sensitive for the detection of *N. gonorrhoeae* and can detect extremely low bacterial loads. It is accepted that occasional strains of *N. gonorrhoeae* may be inhibited by concentrations of vancomycin present in GC selective media. Infection with these strains may therefore produce discrepant results between culture and NAAT testing and need further investigating, including the use of enriched non-selective media. NAAT testing has now been validated for rectal and pharyngeal swabs, which makes detection of *N. gonorrhoeae* from these specimen types more likely due to the drawbacks in using selective media , especially from sites with high numbers of bacterial flora, especially other commensal *Neisseria* spp. An important drawback in the application of NAAT testing, however, is currently its inability to produce susceptibility test results. As a result, a positive NAAT for *N. gonorrhoeae* will often result in a swab taken for susceptibility testing. Remember antibiotic resistance in gonococci is on the increase.

In addition, whilst some laboratories examine all HVS samples for TV (either by microscopy or by culture), others rely on specific clinical requesting, which could lead to either underreporting or at least delayed detection. All female specimens should be examined microscopically for BV. Specimens of urethral discharge should also be Gram stained for Gram-negative cocci.

Any postoperative samples should be examined for pathogens. All male genital specimens should be cultured to media that will also support the growth of staphylococci, β-HS, coliforms, *Pseudomonas*, and anaerobes. Similarly, swabs from prepubescent, postmenopausal or pregnant women should be cultured in this way, as should those detailing PID or other complications discussed earlier. Swabs from cases of vaginitis in young girls should be investigated for *H. influenzae* using chocolate agar.

Enrichment, selective and/or differential media may be employed for the isolation of:

* Lancefield Group B streptococci in appropriate swabs from pregnant women.
* *Actinomyces* species from IUCDs.
* *Listeria* species from intrauterine death, miscarriage or suspected listeriosis.
* *Haemophilus ducreyi*, although usually clinically diagnosed.

Susceptibility testing of significant isolates, such as *N. gonorrhoeae*, assists with the treatment of patients, but also may help determine resistance surveillance. Each year the HPA Sexually Transmitted Diseases Reference Laboratory (STBRL) in Colindale, London, collects isolates of *N. gonorrhoeae* over a 3-month period from sentinel sites across the UK (Gonococcal Resistance to Antimicrobials Surveillance Programme – GRASP). Trends in antimicrobial resistance are published and distributed to appropriate UK health departments annually. At present, due to their rarity, any isolate of *N. gonorrhoeae* exhibiting resistance to antimicrobials such as azithromycin or cefixime should be forwarded to this reference facility for confirmation of the result.

7.10 **Medicolegal issues**

Specimens are sometimes collected that may have medicolegal implications. These include genital specimens from victims of alleged rape and sexual abuse. Local policies apply, but specimens of this type usually undergo a 'chain-of-evidence' procedure, where signatories are required at every stage of the process from collection of the specimen through to reporting of results, including transport. Final results are signed by registered biomedical scientists and then counter-signed by a more senior member of staff. Traceability of these samples is essential, and helps ensure tampering of specimens and results is impossible, as serious legal proceedings may follow. Lot numbers and expiry dates of culture media, kit reagents, and other consumables are also recorded to help validate test results.

All possible pathogens are considered, but the following describes the investigation of *N. gonorrhoeae*.

Due to the delicate nature of the infection, precise identification of *N. gonorrhoeae* is critical in all patients, not just medicolegal cases, and so laboratories often follow the same protocols for identification of *N. gonorrhoeae* as is required by law.

N. gonorrhoeae should grow as colonially typical (grey, translucent) colonies on GC selective media. The bacteria should be oxidase-positive, Gram-negative cocci. Furthermore, they should be confirmed using two identification methods. Typically, laboratories firstly employ biochemical methods, including fermentation testing of glucose, maltose, and lactose and/or the detection of preformed enzymes. A second test, usually antigenic, is employed to detect surface proteins (e.g. PI) as they are highly specific. Cultural methods of detection and subsequent identification have always been regarded as the 'gold standard', both for gonococci and *Chlamydia*. At present, molecular detection of *N. gonorrhoeae* is untested fully and hence is not accepted in the court of law.

SELF-CHECK 7.12

Can you describe the methods available for the laboratory diagnosis of gonorrhoea?

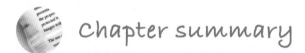

Chapter summary

After reading this chapter you should know and understand:

- Most organisms associated with the skin are commensals.
- The skin and mucosal surfaces form an effective barrier, but breaching can lead to infection.
- Skin infections include cellulitis, folliculitis, boils, abscesses, and ulceration.
- The most common causes of skin infections include *S. aureus*, β-haemolytic streptococci, and anaerobes.
- The Gram stain can provide important information to clinicians, but can sometimes mislead.
- Selective media need to be used to allow the target pathogen to be isolated from a mixture of 'normal flora'.
- A variety of virulence factors and toxins are produced by pathogens to produce infection.
- Mucosal infections include conjunctivitis, otitis media, and pharyngitis.
- The importance of *H. influenzae*, *S. pneumonia*, and Lancefield Group A streptococci.
- Selection of the correct media is critical in the isolation of pathogens. This will sometimes involve the use of selective media, e.g. for *N. gonorrhoeae*.

- Genital infections include gonorrhoea, *Chlamydia*, and syphilis.
- Specimen quality and choice of site can be critical for accurate diagnosis of STIs.

 Further reading

- **Bowler PG, Duerden BI, Armstrong DG. Wound microbiology and associated approaches to wound management.** *Clinical Microbiology Reviews* 2001; **14**: 244–269.

  Excellent text for information on microbiological aspects of wound and soft tissue infections.

- **Hall GS. Molecular diagnostic methods for the detection of *Neisseria gonorrhoeae* and *Chlamydia trachomatis*.** *Reviews in Medical Microbiology* 2005; **16**: 69–78.

  Review article describing the current methodologies for the diagnosis of important STDs.

- **Pellati D, Mylonakis I, Bertoloni G, Fiore C, Andrisani A, Ambrosini G, Armanini D. Genital tract infections and infertility.** *European Journal of Obstetrics, Gynaecology and Reproductive Biology* 2008; **140**: 3–11.

  Article showing how infection of the genital tract can be associated with infertility and other complications.

- **Goering RV, Dockrell H, Zuckerman M, Roitt I, Chiodini PL.** *Mims' Medical Microbiology*, **5th edition. Saunders, 2012.**

  Excellent text on infectious diseases and the process by which organisms mediate infection and insight into their pathogenic properties.

- **Ison CA, Alexander S. Antimicrobial resistance in *Neisseria gonorrhoeae* in the UK: surveillance and management.** *Expert Review of Anti-infective Therapy.* 2011; **9**(10): 867–876.

  Very good review of resistance in gonococci by one of the leading UK experts in the field.

- **Centre for Disease Control and Prevention (CDC). www.cdc.gov/std/.**

  Excellent resource for reports and other publications related to human health.

 Discussion questions

7.1 Do you think only molecular methods should now be used to detect the presence of *N. gonorrhoeae* in clinical samples? If not why not?

7.2 Why is *S. aureus* such a common occurrence in an infected wound?

7.3 Why are selective media so commonly used when isolating pathogens from wound and genital swabs?

7.4 Do you think there should only be one laboratory method for the diagnosis of bacterial vaginosis? Explain your reasoning.

8

Examination of cerebrospinal fluid and fluids from sterile sites

Derek Law

Although there are many body sites that are not sterile, such as the respiratory tract, genital tract, and intestinal tract, there are also various internal body sites that are considered microbiologically sterile. These sites can become infected by bacteria or viruses via various routes causing overt clinical symptoms. However, other factors, such as trauma, inflammation, and carcinoma, may also cause similar symptoms. These sites are frequently sampled for microbiological and other investigations. This chapter will describe the various fluids commonly received in the laboratory and describe the methods for processing these. The fluids to be considered in this chapter are cerebrospinal fluids, synovial, pleural, ascitic, pericardial, and peritoneal dialysis fluids.

Learning objectives

After studying this chapter you should be able to:

- Understand the different fluids received in the laboratory.
- Know how to safely handle the samples.
- Understand the role of cell counts in processing and diagnosis.
- Know the appropriate culture methods for fluids.
- Know the common pathogens isolated from different fluids.
- Recognize when further or other investigations are required.

8.1 Investigation of cerebrospinal fluids

The meninges are a system of membranes that envelope and protect the central nervous system (brain and spinal column). They consist of three layers: the dura mater, the arachnoid mater, and the pia mater. Cerebrospinal fluid (CSF) is a clear fluid that is found in the space between the pia mater and the arachnoid mater and is found in the ventricles of the brain and surrounding the spinal cord. Its main function is to protect the brain by acting as a cushion against shock.

Figure 8.1 shows the relationship between the various membrane layers and the brain and the skull. The pia mater is attached to the brain and follows the contours of the brain; the dura mater is attached to the skull. Cerebrospinal fluid is found in the gap between the pia mater and the arachnoid mater – the subarachnoid space.

Inflammation of the meninges is known as **meningitis**. Meningitis can be caused by bacteria, viruses, or fungi and is an extremely serious condition owing to the proximity of the infection and inflammation to the brain and spinal cord. The potential for serious neurological damage or death requires prompt medical attention and the laboratory plays an important role in helping to establish or refute a diagnosis of meningitis. Various other conditions can mimic meningitis, particularly neurological conditions such as stroke and **subarachnoid haemorrhage**, and these must be differentiated from meningitis as the management of the patient is quite different in these cases.

We will first consider the signs and symptoms of the different types of meningitis as this can provide information on the possible cause of the infection.

Key Point

Inflammation of the meninges is called meningitis; meningitis can be caused by infection with bacteria, viruses, or fungi. Meningitis is an extremely serious illness and requires prompt medical attention.

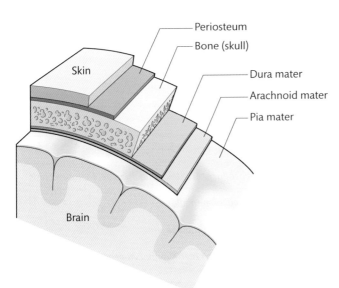

Periosteum
Bone (skull)
Skin
Dura mater
Arachnoid mater
Pia mater
Brain

FIGURE 8.1
Diagrammatic cross section of the skull showing the arrangement of the protective coverings of the brain. The meninges consist of three layers, the dura mater, arachnoid mater, and pia mater. Cerebrospinal fluid is found between the arachnoid mater and the pia mater – the subarachnoid space.
Source: Courtesy of D. Law.

8.1.1 Bacterial meningitis

Although bacterial meningitis can be caused by many different organisms, the vast majority of cases are caused by a small number of bacterial species; Table 8.1 shows the bacterial species most commonly found in cases of meningitis. The patient populations affected by the different species of bacteria are also shown as there are clear differences in infecting organism based on patient age.

Bacterial meningitis is usually much more severe than viral meningitis and without urgent antibacterial treatment carries a high mortality; however, even with antibiotic therapy the patient may survive with various neurological disorders such as deafness or **cerebral palsy**.

The symptoms of meningitis can be variable; initially the disease may start as a flu-like illness and further symptoms develop over the course of a few days, although they can have a very sudden onset. The main symptoms are severe headache, fever, **photophobia**, neck stiffness, pyrexia, and in some cases a rash, and there is often drowsiness and a decreased level of consciousness. One of the most common causes of meningitis is *Neisseria meningitidis* (meningococci). Meningococcal septicaemia may accompany meningococcal meningitis and occurs when bacteria enter the bloodstream and multiply uncontrollably.

Endotoxin is released which initiates various organ dysfunctions and disturbances of blood clotting.

Blood leaks from capillaries into the skin causing a **purpuric rash**. Meningitis and septicaemia often occur together but meningitis can occur without septicaemia and septicaemia can occur without meningitis.

Meningococci colonize the oropharynx of a small proportion of healthy people; in this situation the patient remains healthy but can act as a carrier and transmit the organism to others. In an individual, transition from carrier state to disease can occur; the factors responsible for the switch from carrier to invasive disease are not known. Spread of organisms from person to person is favoured by overcrowding and is more frequent in people living in close proximity, such as students and army recruits. Infections are also most common in these groups. Infections also occur more frequently in patients who have had their spleen removed (**splenectomy**).

Meningococcal septicaemia can occur with meningitis or it can occur on its own. It is a very serious illness; a purpuric rash is one of the most common symptoms. The release of

Cross reference
Septicaemia is described in Chapter 5, Blood cultures.

photophobia
Photophobia is a dislike of bright lights.

endotoxin
Endotoxin is a component of Gram-negative bacterial cell walls. When released into the bloodstream it causes fever.

purpuric rash
Purpuric rash is the appearance of red or purple discolorations on the skin, caused by bleeding underneath the skin

splenectomy
Splenectomy is removal of the spleen. Because the spleen is involved with the immune system, splenectomy patients are more susceptible to certain types of infection including meningitis.

TABLE 8.1 Common CSF pathogens according to patient type.

Age/type of patient	Common organisms
Neonates	Group B streptococci, *E. coli*, *Listeria monocytogenes*
Infants	*N. meningitidis*, *H. influenzae*, *Strep. pneumoniae*, *M. tuberculosis*
Children	*N. meningitidis*, *Strep. pneumoniae*
Adults	*N. meningitidis*, *Strep. pneumoniae*
Immunosuppressed patients	*Cryptococcus neoformans*, *Listeria monocytogenes*. Potentially other organisms

endotoxin from the meningococcus results in disorders of blood clotting. This can lead to death of tissue on extremities, which in severe cases can eventually lead to **gangrene**.

Streptococcus pneumoniae (pneumococcal) meningitis can occur in any age group. In many cases the meninges are infected by spread from an ear infection. Pneumococcal meningitis is more common in patients who have had a splenectomy or who have a **complement** deficiency.

Group B streptococcal infection occurs principally in babies and two distinct forms exist: early onset and late onset. The early-onset form is acquired during birth (the organism is usually acquired from the mother's vagina during birth) and symptoms develop in the first few days of life. The late-onset form develops weeks to months later and infection is acquired from other sources. In both cases pneumonia and septicaemia are common.

Other causes of meningitis include *M. tuberculosis*; meningitis with this organism is rare in some countries but should be considered in patients from high-risk areas. It has a slow onset and signs and symptoms are not as clear cut as those of more typical, acute bacterial meningitis.

complement

Complement is a series of proteins found in blood; when activated the proteins have an antibacterial action and help the body to fight infection.

> ### Key Point
>
> Meningitis can affect all age groups; however, different bacterial pathogens are isolated from cases of meningitis in different age groups.

SELF-CHECK 8.1

What are the commonest causes of bacterial meningitis?

8.1.2 Viral meningitis

Viral meningitis is a relatively benign illness and is more common than bacterial meningitis. Many different viruses can cause meningitis; the most common are the enteroviruses and mumps virus. The illness is often mild, with the patient feeling unwell, developing flu-like symptoms and a headache. Many cases are not severe enough for medical attention and go unrecognized. In more severe cases where neck stiffness and other meningitis symptoms such as photophobia develop, the patient may seek medical attention and be referred to hospital. Most patients with viral meningitis make a full recovery, although some may be left with residual side effects.

> ### Key Point
>
> Compared with bacterial meningitis, viral meningitis is a milder illness and many cases do not require medical attention.

8.1.3 Cryptococcal meningitis

Cryptococcal meningitis caused by the fungus *Cryptococcus neoformans* is found mainly in patients with HIV infection. It also occurs in patients not infected with HIV but who have other cell-mediated immune defects.

8.1.4 Processing of CSF samples

Diagnosis of meningitis is a medical emergency and samples must be processed without delay and results reported back to the ward as soon as they are available. This section deals with how a CSF sample is processed. In a patient with suspected meningitis it is necessary to obtain a sample of CSF for analysis by **lumber puncture**. CSF samples are taken by inserting a needle between the third and fourth lower vertebrae and capturing some of the fluid. Figure 8.2 shows a diagram of a CSF sample being withdrawn. Notice that the needle is inserted between the vertebrae and pierces the lining of the spinal column to withdraw the CSF around the spinal cord. Samples for bacteriology are normally taken first and the sample is often split into three separate samples for reasons described later. Samples should be labelled 1, 2, and 3 if this is the case. Other samples are often taken for immunological investigation and biochemical investigations – glucose and protein measurements are important in helping differentiate different forms of meningitis. Samples should be transported to the laboratory without delay and once in the laboratory should be processed with urgency.

lumbar puncture

Lumbar puncture is the procedure used to obtain a CSF sample from a patient.

Key Point

CSF analysis by biochemistry, immunology, and cytology departments plays an important role in the diagnosis of meningitis and other neurological disorders, and the results of these investigations must be examined along with microbiological data.

There are various procedures involved in processing CSF samples all of which are important in arriving at a correct diagnosis and guiding the correct therapy for the patient:

- Appearance of sample.
- Cell count.
- Centrifugation.
- Gram stain.
- Culture.
- Further tests based on microscopy results.

We will now discuss these stages of processing a CSF sample.

Appearance of CSF

The appearance of the sample is important as it gives an early indication of whether a patient has bacterial meningitis and helps in deciding further steps in processing. The sample should be in a clear, clean container and examined for turbidity, coloration, and clots. Normal fluid is clear and colourless; in cases of bacterial meningitis large numbers of white blood cells are present in the CSF giving a turbid appearance. In cases of stroke or subarachnoid haemorrhage (SAH) the fluid may be stained with red cells; in some cases the degree of blood staining may be very heavy and a blood clot may form. Where an SAH occurred several days previously, the CSF may be yellow in appearance due to the presence of lysed red blood cells. This is known as **xanthochromia**; however, an accurate diagnosis of xanthochromia and hence an SAH can only be made by biochemical measurement of the blood pigments in a CSF sample.

xanthochromia

Xanthochromia is the term used to describe the yellow coloration of CSF samples caused by lysed blood. Confirmation of xanthochromia requires biochemical investigations.

Xanthochromia may only be evident after centrifugation of the sample. The presence of a fine spider's web-type clot is often indicative of tubercular meningitis. If three samples are received the appearance of each should be recorded. Occasionally, when a CSF is taken the needle

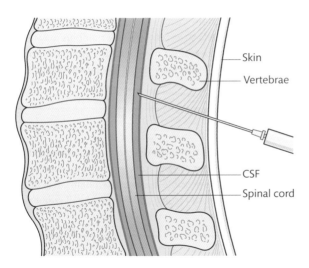

Skin

Vertebrae

CSF

Spinal cord

FIGURE 8.2

Diagram showing how a CSF sample is taken. The needle is inserted between the vertebrae and a sample of the fluid surrounding the spinal cord is aspirated.

nicks a capillary when inserted; this is known as a **traumatic tap**. In such cases the appearance of the three samples differs; the amount of blood in each sample diminishes. If blood is present because of a haemorrhage then each sample will look similar. If it is because of a traumatic tap, then the amount of blood in the first sample is high and less in the second, and so on. This will be determined from the cell count and it is very important to the requesting clinician. This is the main reason that three samples are taken. In some cases of meningitis the presence of blood from a traumatic tap may mask the turbidity due to meningitis. The appearance of the CSF should be recorded and reported.

traumatic tap

Traumatic tap is where a capillary or blood vessel is 'nicked' when a CSF sample is taken. Samples become blood stained. Serial samples can help identify whether the blood is due to a traumatic tap.

> ### Key Point
>
> The appearance of a CSF sample can help in the diagnosis of meningitis and other illnesses. Cloudy fluids indicate a raised white cell count and possible infection. Xanthochromia may indicate a possible stroke. Many CSF samples received in the laboratory are clear and colourless but must still be processed.

Cross reference

See companion volume *Clinical Biochemistry* by Nessar Ahmed for measurement and characterization of xanthochromia.

> ### Key Point
>
> Cell counts on serial CSF samples allow differentiation of blood staining due to a traumatic tap from blood staining due to a stroke or recent subarachnoid haemorrhage. In the case of a traumatic tap the last sample provides the most information as to whether the patient has meningitis.

Cell count

The cell count is the next stage in processing the sample. In this stage we are looking for the total number and type of cells present in a CSF sample. We are interested in counting the numbers of red and white blood cells and in differentiating the white blood cells into polymorphonuclear cells (polymorphs) and lymphocytes. This gives important clues to whether infection is present and what the infecting organism is. Under normal conditions the number of white cells in a CSF sample is very small, typically $<5/mm^3$ in children and adults, and $<20/mm^3$ in neonates.

Cross reference

See Bain, *Blood Cells – A Practical Guide*, in the References section, for morphology and function of the various types of white blood cell.

In cases of bacterial meningitis the white cell count increases dramatically and counts frequently exceed 1000/mm³ although in the very early stages of the illness numbers may be low. The cells are typically polymorphs. In viral and tuberculosis meningitis the white cell count is lower and cells are mainly lymphocytes, although in the early stages of viral meningitis a proportion of the cells may consist of polymorphs.

Key Point

The differential cell count is an important first stage in the diagnosis of meningitis. The number of cells and the type of cells (polymorphs or lymphocytes) are important indicators of whether meningitis is present and the possible cause of meningitis. It is often possible to make a provisional diagnosis on these results, and a normal cell count will often eliminate meningitis as a possible diagnosis.

For accuracy in counting cells, a **haemocytometer** counting chamber is used; a small drop of fluid is placed in the counting chamber which is then examined under a microscope. There are many types of counting chamber, but all have a grid with large and small squares marked on the underside. The grid is set up such that an area encompassing a fixed number of small or large squares is equivalent to a cubic millimetre of fluid. Counting the cells in that area gives the number of cells per cubic millimetre of fluid. It is essential that the user is familiar with the type of counting chamber used in their laboratory. Figure 8.3a shows a typical counting chamber used for counting cells. The fluid is loaded under the coverslip. Figure 8.3b shows a typical grid under the microscope; notice the single and triple lines which mark out distinct areas of the grid. In the sample some red cells can be seen.

Clear or slightly turbid fluids can usually be added directly to the chamber and using a microscope with ×10 and ×40 objectives the cells can be enumerated by counting the number of cells in sufficient marked squares to give the number of cells per cubic millimetre. Red cells and white cells should be enumerated separately. It may also be possible to differentiate the different types of white cells based on the appearance of the nucleus. However, training and experience is necessary to help identify different cell types.

Where the cell count is high (number of cells >200/mm³) or where the sample is turbid or blood stained, samples will often require some dilution in sterile saline before loading into the counting chamber, to get the cell numbers to countable levels. Cell counts then must be multiplied by the dilution factor to arrive at the correct count. In some cases it is possible that several dilutions of the CSF are required to produce a suspension that is countable. Typical dilutions for blood stained samples are 1:20, 1:50, or 1:100. This allows the red cell count to be obtained.

When a sample is blood stained it is also important to determine the ratio of red cells to white cells to determine if the white cell count is raised above normal due to a combination of white cells in the CSF and white cells in the blood . This is achieved by carrying out a separate white cell count, after first destroying the red blood cells. This is achieved by diluting the CSF sample in a white cell counting fluid, consisting of acetic acid and methylene blue. This fluid lyses red cells but does not affect white cells and stains their nuclei blue allowing them to be counted and allowing differentiation of polymorphs and lymphocytes. For white cell counts, typical dilutions of CSF are 1:2 or 1:10. Again, the relevant dilution factor must be taken into consideration when calculating the cell count per cubic millimetre. Typically, the RBC:WBC ratio in normal blood is between 300 and 500 and a lower ratio indicates a raised white cell count.

For CSF samples where serial samples have been received it is necessary to determine the red and white cell counts in each sample to assess any sample to sample variation. However, if the

(a)

Grid area under coverslip

Red blood cells   Grid lines

(b)

FIGURE 8.3
(a) Photograph of a counting chamber used for counting cells in CSF samples.
(b) Photomicrograph of counting chamber with a blood stained CSF sample; the grid lines are clearly visible as are numerous red blood cells.

Source: Courtesy of D. Law.

first sample has no or very few cells then there is little value in counting the remaining samples. However, if the red cell count is high in the first sample the successive samples should be counted: a decreasing count is indicative of a traumatic tap, whereas similar counts indicate that the red cells originated in the CSF.

It is not appropriate to carry out cell counts on heavily blood stained samples which have clotted, as such counts are inaccurate.

Key Point

Counting chambers are used to accurately determine the cell count in CSF samples. Dilution of samples is often required when cell counts are high or when samples are blood stained. The use of red cell lysing fluids is useful for accurate white cell counts in blood stained fluids. Accurate determination of cell counts in blood stained fluids can be time consuming if separate dilutions and counts are required for red and white blood cells.

Why is it important to differentiate between polymorphonuclear cells and lymphocytes in CSF samples?

Centrifugation of CSF

Once the red and white cell counts have been determined, the sample must be centrifuged – this only applies to samples where the volume is >0.5 mL. Centrifugation serves an important function in concentrating organisms into a small volume of fluid, increasing the sensitivity of both culture and Gram stain. Centrifugation should be at 3000 g for at least 10 min. After centrifugation the supernatant should be removed with a sterile pipette to a clean, sterile, labelled container. The appearance of the supernatant should be recorded. The presence of xanthochromia in the supernatant is an indicator of a subarachnoid haemorrhage. The deposit should be resuspended in about 0.5 mL of the supernatant fluid and this is used to perform the next stages of sample processing. All supernatants should be retained and stored at 4°C in case further tests are required, such as viral culture.

HEALTH & SAFETY

Appropriate precautions should be taken when centrifuging samples. Sealed buckets should be used and after centrifugation samples should be opened inside a safety cabinet.

When working with cultures of *Neisseria meningitidis*, work should be carried out in a safety cabinet as there is a risk of contracting meningitis from aerosols formed when performing Gram stains or preparing suspensions for identification or agglutination tests.

Occasionally, samples may be sent from patients with a possible diagnosis of Creutzfeldt–Jakob disease (CJD) or other related illnesses. Such samples should be handled in a safety cabinet, and gloves should be worn during all procedures. All materials should be incinerated after use.

Microscopy

In some laboratories all CSF samples are Gram stained, in others Gram stains are only carried out on samples containing >5 WBC/mm³. Whatever the local protocol, a Gram stain is prepared from the resuspended deposit rather than the fluid itself. It is helpful to mark the slide where the drop is placed to help focus the microscope. If tuberculosis meningitis is suspected a smear for acid–alcohol-fast bacilli (AAFB) staining should be prepared at the same time. To increase sensitivity, a CSF AAFB smear usually has three drops of liquid applied, each added when the others have dried.

Cross reference

Gram staining is described in Chapter 2.

Gram stains and AAFB stains are carried out as described earlier and examined as normal.

Cross reference

AAFB staining is described in Chapter 9.

The Gram stain serves two functions – it stains bacteria present and also helps differentiate white blood cells into polymorphonuclear cells or lymphocytes. Although this can be done during the cell count it is sometimes easier to carry out on a Gram stain as the cellular structure is easier to see. A careful search for bacteria is required; organisms may be intracellular and may be difficult to see. *Haemophilus influenzae* stains poorly with neutral red counterstain and dilute carbol fuchsin is often favoured as a counterstain for CSF samples. Because CSF is a normally sterile liquid the presence of bacteria in a sample is indicative of meningitis. Medical staff should be immediately alerted if bacteria are seen on a Gram stain.

Once microscopy has been carried out, the results of the appearance, cell count and Gram stain can be reported. Because of the urgency of CSF samples, processing time to this stage should be kept to a minimum; samples not requiring dilution, for cell count and Gram stain can often be performed within 30 min of sample receipt.

SELF-CHECK 8.3

Will the biomedical scientist always see bacteria in a Gram stain of an infected CSF?

Culture of CSF

Culture of CSF samples is relatively simple if there are no organisms seen on the Gram stain; a drop of the deposit from the centrifuged sample is inoculated onto a chocolate agar plate incubated in CO_2 for 48 h. Some laboratories inoculate aerobic and anaerobic blood agar plates but anaerobes are extremely rare in CSF samples and in most cases anaerobic plates are not required. Similarly, some laboratories inoculate a portion of the deposit into an enrichment broth. However, the benefits of enrichment culture are not clear. It is rare to isolate a pathogen from an enrichment broth when the culture on agar media is negative, and contamination can be problematic. If organisms are seen on the Gram stain then further media may be inoculated, such as aerobic and anaerobic blood agars. Direct susceptibility tests and key identification tests should also be set up dependent on the identity of the organism on the Gram stain, for example if Gram-positive cocci in pairs are seen then an optochin sensitivity test should be set up to confirm the identity of S. pneumoniae.

Cross reference
See Chapter 4, Section 4.3.

Cross reference
See Chapter 2.

Culture plates should be examined at 24 h and 48 h before being discarded. Enrichment broths should be incubated for at least 48 h and then plated onto chocolate agar incubated in CO_2 and aerobic and anaerobic blood agar.

The pathogens encountered in CSF are dependent on age and immunological status of the patients. Refer to Table 8.1 for a list of the pathogens commonly found in CSF samples.

Key Point

Meningococci and other meningitis pathogens are capsulate, that is they are surrounded by a polysaccharide capsule which makes them virulent. The capsules can be used to identify the organism and they also have a role in vaccination.

HEALTH & SAFETY

Because of the infection risk all work with potential N. meningitidis colonies should be carried out in a Class II safety cabinet. This includes preparing Gram stains from colonies, preparing suspensions for agglutination tests or biochemical identification tests.

8.1.5 Characteristics and identification of common meningitis pathogens

It is essential that the laboratory worker is familiar with the standard methods for identifying the common organisms encountered in CSF.

Tests routinely used in the laboratory are for N. meningitidis, Gram stain, oxidase reaction and fermentation tests of glucose and maltose or various enzymatic tests available in commercial kits. N. meningitidis occurs in several different serogroups based on the polysaccharide capsule which surrounds the bacterial cell. Antisera or latex agglutination kits are also available to identify the capsule type of *N. meningitidis* which can provide further confirmation of the identity. If antisera is not available, isolates should be sent to a reference laboratory as serotype determination is important for epidemiological purposes. The most common serogroup is Group B, which causes approximately 60% of cases, followed by Group C, which causes about 40% of cases. Other serogroups, such as Group A, W135, are rare. This epidemiology can, however, vary considerably between geographical regions.

S. pneumoniae can be identified using Gram and colonial appearance and optochin susceptibility (if typical Gram-positive cocci are seen in the CSF then optochin susceptibility tests should be set up on the direct culture). Polyvalent antisera can be used to confirm the identity.

H. influenzae can be identified by its Gram-stain appearance, its colonial appearance, and the characteristic poor growth on blood agar but good growth on chocolate agar. Dependence on X and V factors is used to establish the identity. Agglutination tests with type b antisera can be used to confirm the serotype. Vaccination of children against *H. influenzae* type b has resulted in a marked decrease in cases of infection with this organism.

Group B streptococci can be identified by colonial appearance and haemolytic reaction. Rapid confirmation can be carried out very quickly using a Lancefield grouping test.

E. coli can be provisionally identified by colonial appearance. Most strains from neonates possess the K1 capsule antigen and can be identified using appropriate antisera. Final confirmation of identity is through use of commercial identification kits.

L. monocytogenes can be identified by typical morphology on Gram stain and haemolysis reaction on blood agar. Further confirmation can be obtained by observing typical tumbling motility in liquid cultures grown at 30°C, a positive esculin reaction and growth on *Listeria* spp. selective media.

It is possible to isolate almost any organism from a CSF sample and an organism must be considered potentially significant until confirmatory tests or clinical information suggest otherwise. In the absence of markers such as a raised CSF white cell count, growth of small numbers of organisms such as coagulase negative staphylococci or some Gram-positive bacilli, especially when isolated from enrichment broths, are usually regarded as contaminants. But each result must be decided on a case by case basis. Contamination of samples may occur when the sample is taken or during processing in the laboratory. CSF is a nutritious growth medium and organisms will readily grow in CSF samples.

In cases of meningitis, blood cultures should also be taken as they may become positive earlier than the CSF sample and help guide antibiotic therapy.

SELF-CHECK 8.4

Why is it important to fully identify the organism infecting the CSF?

8.1.6 Antigen testing

Microscopy and culture are the main means of processing CSF samples and a diagnosis of bacterial meningitis is typically made by a high white cell count with a predominance of polymorphonuclear cells and the presence of bacteria on a Gram stain. However, there are occasions when white cell counts may be raised but bacteria may not be seen; this can occur for several reasons. Firstly, if the patient has meningitis but antibiotics have been given and bacteria may be dead and/or lysed and therefore not detected on microscopy; secondly, in cases of early meningitis organisms may not be present in sufficient numbers to detect on Gram stain. In such cases antigen detection may be a useful test to carry out on samples using commercially available antigen detection kits due to the following:

- Many of the bacterial pathogens that cause meningitis produce capsules – polysaccharide coats around the cell that protect the bacteria from phagocytosis by white blood cells. These capsules are important for virulence of the organism and are highly antigenic.

- Antibodies raised against the organisms are coated onto latex particles. When these particles are mixed with antigen present in CSF or from organisms growing on an agar plate they agglutinate.

- Antigen tests are often positive when microscopy and culture are negative due to previous antibiotic therapy, and can therefore give a positive diagnosis and help guide appropriate therapy.

Key Point

Antigen tests are often positive when microscopy and culture are negative due to previous antibiotic therapy, and can therefore give a positive diagnosis and help guide appropriate therapy.

CLINICAL CORRELATION

Because prompt administration of antibiotics can be life-saving in cases of meningitis, patients may arrive at hospital having received antibiotics. In such cases organisms may be scanty or absent on Gram stain. The use of antigen detection kits in such situations can help identify the causative organism, as sufficient antigen will be present in the sample to give a positive reaction.

8.1.7 Molecular testing

Some laboratories now offer **PCR** tests on CSF samples as a means of rapid diagnosis. These are useful when available to confirm the identity of an organism seen on Gram stain, and also in patients with a strong suspicion of having meningitis but who have received antibiotics and no bacteria can be seen on Gram stain. They are an alternative to antigen detection kits. Specific examples would include detection of meningococcal meningitis on patients receiving antimicrobial therapy or for a range of viral pathogens, such as enterovirus. Normally, such requests would be forwarded to a reference laboratory for analysis. In cases where the CSF (or other important sterile fluid) shows no growth on culture, molecular methods which use PCR amplification and sequencing of 16S ribosomal DNA are now becoming more widely requested. In CSF for example, bacteria that may have perished (due to antibiotics) or cannot be grown on routine culture (due to extreme nutritional requirements) can now be detected. This technique is now considered optimal for patient management where there is a clinical indication of infection but no causative agent can be found.

PCR

Polymerase chain reaction (PCR) is a technique involving amplification of specific DNA sequences which can be used to rapidly identify pathogens.

See Chapter 16.

8.1.8 Viral meningitis

As described earlier, viral meningitis is a milder illness than bacterial meningitis. The typical CSF picture of viral meningitis is shown in Table 8.2. There is an increase in white cells, which are typically lymphocytes, glucose levels are normal and protein levels may be raised. No organisms are seen on Gram stain. If viral meningitis is suspected based on clinical findings and results of CSF analysis, the sample should be sent for virological analysis. This typically involves culture of the sample on a variety of cell lines. The CSF supernatant is suitable for virological analysis and should be transported to the virology laboratory on ice, along with full patient and clinical details. Common viruses isolated from CSF samples include mumps virus, echovirus, and Coxsackie viruses.

8.1.9 Tuberculosis meningitis

Tuberculosis meningitis is a slow chronic illness where the patient complains of headaches and malaise with, eventually, decreasing levels of consciousness. The course of the disease is slow and may take weeks to develop.

TABLE 8.2 CSF parameters in health and disease.

	CSF appearance	CSF protein	CSF glucose	CSF cell count (per mm³)	CSF Gram stain	Additional features
Normal	Clear and colourless	0.2–0.4 g/L (neonate <1.7 g/L)	60–80% of plasma glucose	<20 in neonates and <5 in older children and adults	No organisms	
Bacterial meningitis	Cloudy and turbid (if severe)	Raised >1.5 g/L	Glucose level is <50% of the plasma level	Cell count is high (100 to 1000+) and mostly neutrophils	Organism usually seen, morphology may help identification	Antigen tests are useful if organisms are not seen
Viral/aseptic meningitis	Clear	Raised or high end of normal	Glucose level is usually within normal limits	Cell count is high (100 to 1000+) and mostly lymphocytes	No organisms	Viral culture or PCR should be set up
Tuberculous meningitis	Clear or slightly cloudy, may have a cobweb appearance	Raised >1.5 g/L Protein is high (much higher than bacterial meningitis)	Glucose level is <50% of the plasma level	Cell count is high (100 to 1000+) with mainly lymphocytes	Negative	AFB smear should be carried out or PCR in reference laboratory
Cryptococcus meningitis	Slightly turbid	Raised	Normal to low	Moderate number of lymphocytes	Yeasts	India ink may show capsulate yeasts; cryptococcal antigen positive
Subarachnoid haemorrhage	Blood stained (although not always)	Raised or high end of normal	Glucose level is usually low	High number of RBCs	No organisms	Xanthochromia present
Guillain–Barré syndrome	Clear	Markedly raised	Glucose level is usually low	Normal levels	No organisms	
Multiple sclerosis	Clear	Raised	Glucose level is usually within normal limits	Mild pleocytosis with mononuclear cells	No organisms	

- CSF samples are typically slightly turbid and may contain a clot. The protein levels are markedly raised and glucose levels are low. The cell count is raised and is predominantly lymphocytic. It is sometimes difficult to distinguish tuberculosis meningitis from viral meningitis on the basis of cell count and biochemical data.

- A Ziehl–Neelsen (ZN) stain or auramine stain can be carried out to detect *M. tuberculosis* in the sample, but is not always positive.

- Culture is the most sensitive method of detection and if tuberculosis meningitis is suspected a portion of the deposit should be submitted for culture. Inoculation into liquid media such as Kirchner's medium is preferred as positive results are available earlier than using solid culture media. Further, contamination is not usually a problem.

- There is now growing use of PCR for diagnosis of TB, and CSF samples are highly amenable to PCR as the sample volume is small and inhibitors are generally absent, and because the sample is clean there is no interference with environmental organisms.

- When there is a strong suspicion of tuberculosis meningitis, serial samples may be taken over the course of several days to increase the chances of detection and isolation.

Cross reference

See Chapter 9 for culture methods for TB.

Key Point

Tuberculosis meningitis is a rare form of meningitis. It is difficult to diagnose as the illness is chronic and symptoms are not well defined. Microscopy (AAFB stain) and culture are standard diagnostic techniques, although the sensitivity of microscopy is low. Molecular-based techniques, such as PCR, are being used more often as they can provide rapid, specific and sensitive results.

8.1.10 Cryptococcal meningitis

This is caused by the yeast *Cryptococcus neoformans* and infection typically occurs in immunosuppressed patients or patients with other cell-mediated immunity defects. When meningitis is suspected in an immunosuppressed patient, infection with *C. neoformans* should be considered. Cells of *C. neoformans* are surrounded by a capsule which distinguishes this organism from common yeast pathogens such as *Candida* spp. Capsulate yeasts can be easily recognized using India ink stain. By mixing a sample (either a CSF sample or colony emulsified in saline) with India ink and observing under the microscope it is possible to visualize the yeast cell surrounded by a clear capsule. Look at Figure 8.4; it shows the centrifuged deposit of a sample of CSF from an HIV patient with headache and photophobia. The deposit has been mixed with India ink which stains the background; note the yeast-shaped cells surrounded by a clear halo – the capsule. This highly suggestive of *C. neoformans*.

Diagnosis of cryptococcal meningitis can be made by examining a Gram stain of the CSF deposit for the presence of typical yeast cells, with confirmation using an India ink preparation of the CSF deposit to detect capsulate yeasts.

Additional confirmation can be made by detecting cryptococcal antigen in the CSF. The capsular material is shed from the yeast and can be detected in an agglutination test in a similar way to the detection of bacterial antigens in CSF. The amount of antigen present can be measured in a semiquantitative fashion by diluting CSF in saline and carrying out antigen tests on diluted samples – the highest dilution to show a positive reaction is the titre. This has importance as it has been shown that the titre can be used to monitor the efficacy of therapy.

Cross reference

See Chapter 14 for methods of yeast identification and susceptibility testing.

Yeast cell surrounded by capsule

FIGURE 8.4
Photomicrograph of a CSF deposit from an HIV patient stained with India ink. Yeast cells surrounded by a clear capsule are clearly visible.
Source: Photo kindly provided by CDC/Dr Leanor Haley.

Samples are often taken on a weekly basis during therapy. A falling titre indicates successful therapy, whereas a steady or rising titre suggests a poor response to therapy.

CSF samples from immunosuppressed patients with raised white cell counts should be cultured on Sabouraud's agar incubated at 37°C and 30°C for up to 4 weeks, regardless of whether yeasts are seen. Any yeast isolated from the sample should be fully identified and have susceptibility tests carried out.

CLINICAL CORRELATION

Cryptococcal antigen can be used as a tool for diagnosing infection with *C. neoformans*. It can also be used to monitor therapy – declining antigen titre in CSF indicates successful therapy. Many HIV patients with cryptococcal meningitis take antifungal drugs for life to prevent recurrences of infection.

8.1.11 Neurosurgical patients

Acute bacterial meningitis with the exception of neonates typically occurs in patients in the community and is caused by the bacteria described previously. However, meningitis can occur in hospitalized patients and frequently occurs in patients who have had some form of neurosurgical procedure carried out. Following surgery there are often shunts placed into the CSF to remove fluid; infection is frequently acquired through the shunts.

The microbiology of meningitis in neurological patients may be different to that seen in community patients. Common infecting organisms include *Staphylococcus aureus*, coagulase negative staphylococci, *Pseudomonas aeruginosa*, and members of the Enterobacteriaceae. CSF samples from such patients are commonly blood stained and/or turbid and have raised white cell counts in the absence of infection.

Samples from neurosurgical patients are processed in the same way as other CSFs, in that they have a cell count, centrifugation, microscopy, and culture, but cultural procedures that reflect the different pathogens should be employed. For example, anaerobic cultures may be set up and chromogenic media can be inoculated to help give rapid identification of bacteria. If bacteria are seen on Gram staining then medical staff must be informed immediately. Treatment of infections may require the use of antibiotics injected directly into the CSF – **intrathecal** antibiotics. This produces high local levels of drug and can be more effective at eradicating infection. Often daily samples of fluid are received for analysis – declining white cell counts indicates successful treatment of infection.

Some patients may have a condition known as **hydrocephalus**, in which excess CSF is produced or it is not absorbed; this condition is most common in infants. Treatment is usually by insertion of a shunt which drains CSF away from the brain either into the abdomen or into the heart. Occasionally, the shunt has to be removed because it becomes infected. This can produce meningitis-like symptoms of infection. CSF may be obtained from such patients and processed as described as above. The actual shunt may be removed and a new shunt inserted. The old shunt should be cultured to determine if it is infected. Any obvious pus on the outside of the shunt should be removed with a swab and cultured. The interior of the shunt should be rinsed with sterile saline and the rinse material cultured. Typical pathogens are coagulase-negative staphylococci, *S. aureus*, *P. aeruginosa*, and members of the Enterobacteriaceae.

There are various neurological conditions that may give similar symptoms to meningitis, for example **Guillian–Barré syndrome**, multiple sclerosis, and CVA (stroke). CSF samples may be obtained from such patients; cell counts and biochemical data help distinguish these conditions from infective meningitis.

intrathecal
Intrathecal administration of antibiotics is the administration directly into the CSF. This rapidly produces good levels of drug in the CSF, but toxicity may be a problem.

hydrocephalus
Hydrocephalus means water on the brain. It is a build-up of CSF around the brain and it causes enlargement of the head in neonates.

Key Point

The microbiology of meningitis in neurology/neurosurgical patients differs considerably from that of meningitis in community patients. Hospital pathogens such as staphylococci, Enterobacteriaceae, and *Pseudomonas* spp. are common.

8.1.12 Treatment of meningitis

Meningitis is a serious infection and requires prompt and aggressive therapy. It is recognized that commencing therapy as soon as possible outweighs the need for a microbiological diagnosis. This means that where there is a strong suspicion of meningitis, treatment will commence before a CSF sample can be taken. Treatment is with very high doses of cefotaxime or ceftriaxone given intravenously; these antibiotics are active against the majority of bacteria causing meningitis including penicillin-resistant pneumococci and meningococci. They also penetrate well into the CSF. Treatment may be modified by results of susceptibility tests, and it is important that such tests are carried out on all isolated pathogens.

Close contacts of patients with meningococcal meningitis may be given **prophylactic** antibiotics to reduce the risk of them developing meningitis.

Tuberculosis meningitis and cryptococcal meningitis require long-term treatment with specialized antitubercular or antifungal drugs, respectively.

prophylaxis
Prophylaxis means the administration of antibiotics to prevent disease developing.

SELF-CHECK 8.5

If a patient was suspected of having bacterial meningitis would the clinician wait until susceptibility test results are known before starting treatment?

Cross reference
Antifungal drugs are described in Chapter 14.

8.1.13 Prevention of meningitis – the role of vaccination

Because meningitis is caused by a limited number of bacterial species it is possible to protect against some cases. In several countries, meningococcal meningitis is caused primarily by group B meningococci and the remaining cases are caused by group C meningococci.

vaccination

Vaccination is the administration of material (an antigen) to produce immunity to a disease, usually by production of antibodies.

- **Vaccination** is available against group C meningococci based on the polysaccharide group C capsule antigen. This is given to babies to prevent infection in the early years of life and a booster is often given in the teens as a second peak of infection occurs among students. There is currently no vaccine against group B meningococci, the predominant cause of meningitis in many countries; this is primarily due to the poor immunogenicity of the group B antigen. Intensive efforts are underway to identify antigens that are able to induce antibody to meningococci regardless of the serogroup.

- A vaccine is also available for pneumococcal meningitis which covers many of the serotypes that are associated with meningitis. This is given to babies and gives protection not only against meningitis but against other pneumococcal diseases.

- *H. influenzae* type b (Hib) used to be the most common cause of meningitis in young children; however, the implementation of a vaccination campaign against this organism has seen the number of cases reduced dramatically.

All cultures of *N. meningitidis*, *S. pneumonia*, and *H. influenzae* isolated from CSF or blood should be submitted to a reference laboratory for typing. This identifies the current serotypes in circulation and ensures that current vaccines provide coverage against the common types. The emergence of new types not covered by vaccines may require a change in the vaccine composition.

Education of the public about the signs and symptoms of meningitis is important in ensuring that cases receive urgent medical attention.

Key Point

The antigens used in meningitis vaccines are derived from the capsules of the bacteria. Vaccination only gives immunity to the same capsular type. Group A and C meningococcal vaccines are available but give immunity only against the same serotype. There is currently no vaccine for group B meningococci. Research is ongoing to develop a vaccine which provides immunity against all serogroups of meningococci.

CASE STUDY 8.1 *Meningococcal meningitis*

An 18-year-old student had a 1-day history of feeling unwell with a temperature; he began to develop a headache and went to bed. The next morning his friends tried to wake him but he was unresponsive so they called a doctor. When the doctor arrived he noted an unresponsive patient with pyrexia and purple blotches on his skin. The doctor immediately administered intravenous penicillin and called an ambulance. In the Emergency Department room a sample of CSF was taken which was found to be turbid. In the microbiology laboratory a cell count was performed; results were 1622 WBC/mm³ with 95% polymorphs and 5% lymphocytes. No organisms were seen. Because of the high white cell count but absence of organisms, antigen tests against a panel of bacterial antigens were carried out. The antigen test was positive for meningococcal group C antigen. The patient was started on intravenous ceftriaxone. The CSF was cultured and the following day a light growth of N. meningitidis was isolated. This was found to be group C using appropriate antisera. Identification of the organism was confirmed using commercial kits. The student's flatmates were given prophylactic rifampicin to prevent them developing meningitis. The patient spent a week on the ICU but made an uneventful recovery.

1. Why did the doctor immediately administer penicillin?

2. What other condition is this patient likely to have besides meningitis? What samples would be taken to confirm this and why might they be negative in this patient?

3. What is the relevance of the positive antigen test when the microscopy is negative?

8.2 Other sterile body fluids

There are other body fluids that are typically sterile but which may become infected. This section of the chapter will focus on the microbiology of these fluids. The fluids we are going to consider are synovial fluid, pleural fluid, ascitic (peritoneal) fluid, and pericardial fluid. Processing of all of these samples is very similar and they can be considered together. Processing typically follows the same stages as those used to process CSF samples – a cell count is performed as this gives an indication of the likelihood of infection, the sample is centrifuged, then centrifugation microscopy and culture are performed on the deposit.

8.2.1 Synovial and bursa fluids

The joints of the body are lubricated by synovial fluid, a viscous yellow fluid. Occasionally this can become infected, causing septic **arthritis**. The main symptoms of this are pain, decreased movement in the joint, redness in the skin over a joint and fever. Fluid can be aspirated from the joint via a needle and sent to the laboratory for analysis. Normal fluid is straw coloured and slightly viscous, but in cases of infection and other inflammatory disorders, such as rheumatoid arthritis, it becomes cloudy due to the presence of white blood cells. Bursae are small sacs of fluid that help lubricate ligaments as they pass over bones. They can become inflamed through trauma or by pressure, but they can also become infected. The main symptoms of infected bursae are pain and tenderness in a joint. Common infecting organisms are S. aureus and streptococci.

> **arthritis**
>
> Arthritis is the name used to describe inflammation in a joint. Septic arthritis is the name used to describe inflammation of a joint caused by infection.

8.2.2 Pleural fluid

The lung is surrounded by two membranes – the pleural membranes. Pleural fluid is found between the two membranes, and an increase in the volume of pleural fluid is known as a pleural effusion. Effusions may arise because of infection such as pneumonia, TB or carcinoma, or due to conditions such as heart failure. A collection of pus in the pleural cavity, which occurs as a complication of bacterial infection, is known as an empyema. A wide variety of organisms may be involved in empyema, including anaerobes and other organisms causing lower respiratory tract infections, such as S. pneumoniae. Empyema is commonly a polymicrobial infection.

Fluid can be withdrawn from the effusion, and is sometimes used to assist the patient, as large volumes of effusion may compromise lung function.

The most common organisms found in pleural fluids are S. pneumoniae and S. aureus.

8.2.3 Pericardial fluid

The heart is surrounded by a membrane – the pericardium; inflammation of the pericardium is known as **pericarditis** and results in an increase in the volume of fluid in the pericardial sac. When a pericardial effusion occurs it can compromise cardiac function; aspiration is therefore important in improving cardiac function and allows analysis of fluid for infective causes. The most common infective agents in pericarditis are viruses such as enteroviruses and Coxsackie viruses; bacterial causes of infection include *S. aureus*, *S. pneumoniae*, and *M. tuberculosis*.

8.2.4 Ascitic or peritoneal fluid

Ascites is an accumulation of fluid in the peritoneal cavity. The most common cause of ascites is cirrhosis or liver disease although cancer may be a cause in rarer cases. Bacterial infection is, however, extremely rare.

Fluid is aspirated from the abdomen and sent to the laboratory for analysis.

SELF-CHECK 8.6

What are the common organisms likely to infect sterile sites?

8.2.5 Processing of fluids

The appearance of the fluids can vary enormously. Normal fluids are yellowish in colour and clear; when infected they become turbid because of ingress of white blood cells. Trauma sometimes causes damage and these fluids are frequently blood stained and become clotted.

As well as microbiological investigations such as microscopy and culture, samples may also be sent for other investigations such as histology for malignant cells and biochemistry for a variety of investigations dependent on the sample and likely diagnosis; viral cultures may also be carried out.

Cell count

Although cell counts can be carried out in a quantitative manner using a counting chamber, because of the viscous nature of some of these fluids, semiquantitative counts are carried out in some laboratories.

Quantitative counts are carried out in the same way as for CSF samples; dilution and red cell lysis may be required, depending on the appearance of the sample.

Semiquantitative estimates of cells are carried out on well-mixed, uncentrifuged samples by taking a small (30–50 μL) sample and placing it on a microscope slide, placing a coverslip on top and examining the slide under the microscope using phase contrast. Red and white cells are easily distinguished and the numbers are recorded in a semiquantitative manner, that is +/- , +, ++, +++. In general, a report of + cells represents approximately 10 cells per high power field.

Bacteria are not always detected in such preparations. Following the cell count the fluid must then be centrifuged to concentrate the organisms into a smaller volume of fluid, increasing the sensitivity of the Gram stain and culture. It must be noted that clots can be present, which will make it impossible to provide a quantitation of cells present.

> ### Key Point
> Cell counts may be carried out in a semiquantitative or quantitative manner. Both red and white blood cells should be quantitated.

Microscopy and culture

After centrifugation the supernatant is removed to a clean sterile container, and the deposit is resuspended in a small volume of fluid. The supernatant can be used for biochemical investigations if necessary. The deposit is then used to inoculate culture plates and carry out a Gram stain if required. If any bacteria are seen, they should be immediately reported to a medical microbiologist. If organisms are seen on the Gram stain, additional media and direct sensitivity tests should be set up appropriate to the organisms seen. Typical culture plates for fluids with no organisms seen on Gram stain are a chocolate plate incubated in CO_2 and aerobic and anaerobic blood agar plates. These are incubated for 48 h and discarded if negative. Enrichment cultures using a nutrient-rich broth, such as cooked meat broth or serum broth, can also be inoculated. This can be subcultured onto the chocolate plate in CO_2 and aerobic and anaerobic blood agar plates after 48 h incubation.

Additional tests

There are several additional investigations that may be appropriate for certain sample types, and cytology may be appropriate on pleural fluids as various types of carcinoma may manifest as a pleural effusion.

One of the most common causes of swollen, inflamed joints is gout; this is a metabolic disorder characterized by elevated levels of uric acid in the blood. Crystals of uric acid get deposited in the joints, where they are ingested by white blood cells which burst, releasing their contents which then attack the linings of the joint, bringing about pain and inflammation. In cases of gout, the synovial fluid contains white blood cells and uric acid crystals, which are often present inside the white cells. In some hospitals, rheumatology departments screen for uric acid crystals; in other hospitals it is the microbiology laboratory that carries out this investigation.

Identification of crystals requires specialized microscopic equipment and experience. Identification of uric acid crystals is carried out by placing a drop of a centrifuged deposit of a joint fluid on a microscope slide and examining the slide under dark field microscopy. Crystals appear as bright, regular-shaped objects which can be located extracellularly or they can be intracellular, inside white blood cells. Confirmation of the identity of the crystal is carried out using a polarizing filter – uric acid show as crystals with a particular colour under polarized light. Pyrophosphate crystals, which occur in synovial fluid as a cause of pseudogout, are a different colour under polarized light and can therefore be distinguished from uric acid crystals. Figure 8.5 shows a sample of knee fluid from a patient with gout viewed under polarized light; against the pink background (due to the polarizing filter) the long crystals of uric acid appear blue. Also present in this sample are some red blood cells.

The type and quantity of crystals should be reported. Occasionally, other types of crystal, such as oxalate crystals, may be detected in synovial fluids. These have a different appearance to uric acid or pyrophosphate crystals; their identification can be difficult and samples where the presence or identity of crystals is unclear are best referred to an expert for analysis.

FIGURE 8.5

Photomicrograph of knee fluid from a patient with gout viewed under phase contrast with a polarizing filter. Long crystals are obvious which show blue coloration, indicative of uric acid.

Source: Photo kindly provided by Dr Philip Platt.

Key Point

Gout is a metabolic illness characterized by deposits of uric acid crystals in various joints. Microscopy of aspirated fluid is one of the main methods of diagnosis. In cases of gout, uric acid crystals are seen in the fluid and inside white blood cells. They display a distinct coloration in polarized light, distinct from that observed with pyrophosphate crystals which cause pseudogout.

TB culture

TB culture may be requested on certain samples, particularly pleural fluids. The centrifuged deposit is used to prepare a smear for AAFB and the deposit is sent for TB culture. Microscopy with such samples is not very sensitive and culture should always be performed.

Occasionally, fluids may be received which contain large numbers of white blood cells. Such samples may be better treated as pus samples and additional culture plates set up, for example selective anaerobic plates.

Cross reference
See Chapter 9, Section 9.4.

8.2.6 Continuous ambulatory peritoneal dialysis (CAPD) fluids

Patients with kidney failure are unable to rid their body of the waste products normally eliminated by the kidneys. Dialysis is frequently used as a means of eliminating the waste products. Haemodialysis is the most conventional form of dialysis but requires that the patient is attached to a haemodialysis machine for long periods of time, restricting many of their daily activities.

Continuous ambulatory peritoneal dialysis (CAPD) is an alternative treatment strategy for patients with renal failure, and has many advantages over haemodialysis; patients are mobile and active during dialysis and live a relatively normal life without the requirement for dialysis through a machine. Dialysis takes place by instilling 1–2 litres of fluid into the patient's abdominal cavity via a catheter. Waste products diffuse into the dialysis fluid, which is replaced every 6 h. In this way waste products are removed from the patient's blood.

Although CAPD has many advantages over peritoneal dialysis, it has one main disadvantage, peritonitis – infection of the peritoneal cavity. This is a relatively common problem with CAPD and although not life-threatening causes significant pain and discomfort for the patient, and may necessitate haemodialysis until peritonitis is cured. Most infections arise by contamination of the catheter when fluid is instilled into the peritoneal cavity or when it is drained out. The main symptoms of infection in CAPD patients are abdominal pain and pyrexia; the dialysis fluid, which is normally clear and colourless, becomes cloudy due to the presence of white blood cells. The most common organisms causing CAPD peritonitis are coagulase-negative staphylococci; these are usually derived from the patient's own skin. Other organisms frequently isolated from CAPD are *S. aureus*, members of the Enterobacteriaceae and *Pseudomonas* spp.; however, many different types of organism have been isolated as significant pathogens from CAPD fluids.

Key Point

Dialysis is a method used to get rid of waste products that build up in the blood of patients with kidney (renal) failure. There are two main forms – haemodialysis and continuous ambulatory peritoneal dialysis (CAPD). CAPD has many advantages for patients but peritonitis is the main disadvantage.

Processing CAPD fluid

When a patient on CAPD presents with symptoms of peritonitis, a sample of peritoneal fluid is drained into a sterile container for processing. Care must be taken not to contaminate the sample when it is being taken as common skin organisms such as coagulase-negative staphylococci are also frequent pathogens in CAPD fluids. Processing of CAPD fluids follows the same steps as other fluids: cell count, centrifugation followed by Gram stain and culture.

Cell count

Uninfected CAPD fluids are clear and colourless or with a very faint haziness; infected fluids become very cloudy due to the presence of white blood cells. The first part of the process is to enumerate the cells.

The cell count on a CAPD fluid is carried out in a counting chamber, in the same way as a CSF sample. Occasionally, with exceptionally high white cell counts the sample may require diluting in saline before counting. Occasional red blood cells may be seen and their presence should be recorded. Heavily blood stained samples are sometimes received and the red cells can be counted on a diluted sample and white cells counted on a sample diluted with red cell lysing fluid (see above for CSF processing). Counts of >100 WBCs per mm^3 are usually indicative of infection.

Despite the cloudiness of infected CAPD fluids the number of organisms present is often low; the fluid must therefore be concentrated by centrifugation as described previously. Following centrifugation the pellet should be retained and as much of the supernatant as possible removed and retained.

Gram stain

A small amount of the pellet should be used to prepare a Gram stain. The Gram stain should be examined carefully as the organisms may be scarce and in some cases may be inside the white blood cells. It is not uncommon to find no organisms, even in very turbid samples and in more than 70% of samples no organisms are seen. If organisms are detected in a sample their presence should be reported to medical staff so that appropriate treatment can be started.

> **Key Point**
>
> The Gram stain is positive in only about 30% of cases of CAPD peritonitis.

Culture of CAPD fluid

There is no defined method for culturing CAPD fluids and different techniques are used in different laboratories. Because organisms are often found inside the white cells and either do not grow or grow slowly, techniques are used to lyse the white cells and release the intra cellular organisms. This can be achieved by adding **Triton X** or **saponin** to the deposit; however, addition of a small volume of water to the deposit followed by mixing can bring about lysis of white cells, and is less toxic to fastidious or delicate organisms. Following lysis a drop of the deposit can then be inoculated onto aerobic and anaerobic blood agar plates and a chocolate agar plate incubated in CO_2. The remainder of the sample can be inoculated into an enrichment broth, although some laboratories favour inoculating blood culture bottles, especially if automated detection systems are used as this can speed up detection of infection.

The agar plates should be examined at 24 and 48 h and any enrichment broths subcultured after 48 h. Samples inoculated into blood culture bottles are treated as blood cultures and discarded after 5 days if negative and processed as a positive blood culture when they become positive.

If organisms are seen on Gram stain then appropriate direct sensitivity tests may be inoculated.

> **Key Point**
>
> Improved positivity rates can be obtained by using procedures which lyse cells or enrichment techniques such as inoculation of the deposit into blood culture bottles.

Although culture has a higher positivity rate than microscopy, up to 30% of cultures may be negative in patients with cloudy fluids and signs of infection. If the patient continues to be unwell and fluid is persistently cloudy with an elevated white cell count, additional work can be carried out on samples. Larger volume samples should be obtained and these should be centrifuged and pooled to give more material for further investigations. These could include inoculation of larger volumes into blood culture bottles, culture for yeasts at 37°C and 30°C on Sabourauds agar, prolonged incubation of standard culture plates for fastidious organisms and mycobacterial cultures.

> **Key Point**
>
> Although CAPD fluids may be cloudy and have high white blood cell counts, microscopy is frequently negative and many samples do not yield a pathogen on culture. Where samples have a high white cell count but no organisms are seen, antibiotics will often be administered to the patients. Many culture-negative infections will respond to antibiotics, suggesting that infection is caused by bacteria.

Why are lysis techniques useful for processing CAPD samples?

Treatment of CAPD peritonitis

In the majority of cases infection remains localized to the peritoneal cavity and does not spread to other parts of the body. Treatment is often by administering antibiotics into the peritoneal fluid. Because the majority of infections are caused by Gram-positive organisms, such as coagulase-negative staphylococci or S. aureus, vancomycin, an antibiotic that is active against Gram-positive but not Gram-negative organisms, is commonly used as a treatment. This will often be used even if bacteria are not seen on the Gram stain if the patient has signs of infection and the CAPD fluid is cloudy and contains white cells. If Gram-negative bacteria are seen, gentamicin or tobramycin are used as alternatives. Susceptibility testing of any isolated bacteria should be carried out to provide alternative treatments to vancomycin, gentamicin or tobramycin.

Prevention of CAPD infection

Infection is the most common problem in CAPD patients; the risk of infection can be minimized by strict adherence to correct procedures and the use of aseptic technique. CAPD is best suited to well-motivated patients who understand the procedures and the practices required to minimize infection.

 Chapter summary

After reading this chapter you should know and understand:

- Meningitis and the bacterial pathogens involved.

- Pathogens infecting the CSF differ depending upon patient type.

- The importance of the CSF cell count and the role of other departments in the diagnosis of meningitis.

- How to process CSF samples in the laboratory and the requirement for urgency when processing these samples.

- Why certain antibiotics are used to treat meningitis and why only a limited number are useful.

- The importance of vaccination to protect from meningitis.

- The other sterile body sites and why fluids are taken from these sites.

- Fluid samples require different media to be inoculated depending on the sample site.

- The importance of non-cultural methods such as antigen detection to provide a diagnosis.

Further reading

- **Meningitis Research Foundation.** www.meningitis.org/.

  Educational site which provides information and patient experiences of meningitis.

- **Merck Online Medical Manual.** www.merck.com/mmhe/index.html.

  Excellent general source of medical information, containing much relevant information on meningitis and other neurological conditions.

- **CAPD dialysis.** http://homedialysis.org.au/peritoneal-dialysis/how-does-capd-work/.

  American site providing information and graphics showing the process of CAPD plus other related material.

Discussion questions

8.1   Why are certain CSF pathogens associated with certain patient groups and what can be done to prevent this?

8.2   What is the role of other departments in the diagnosis of meningitis?

8.3   How useful is the Gram stain in providing an initial diagnosis of an infection in a sterile fluid?

9

Investigation of respiratory samples

Louise Hill-King

Respiratory infections are among the most common causes of morbidity. Clinicians send respiratory samples, such as sputum, to the microbiology laboratory in order to identify the causative organisms and to obtain guidance for administering appropriate treatment.

This chapter describes the laboratory investigations that are used for detection of pathogenic organisms in lower respiratory tract samples. Infections of the nose and throat are described in Chapter 7.

Learning objectives

After studying this chapter you should be able to:

- Describe the anatomy of the respiratory tract.
- List the organisms that constitute normal respiratory flora.
- List the common respiratory pathogens.
- Describe the routine tests used for respiratory samples.
- Discuss infections associated with cystic fibrosis.
- Describe the tests used to diagnose tuberculosis (TB).
- Discuss the health and safety issues associated with respiratory samples.

9.1 The respiratory tract

9.1.1 Overview of the respiratory tract

In order to appreciate the impact that respiratory infections have on the body we must first gain an understanding of how the healthy respiratory tract works. Its prime function is to supply oxygen to the body and remove carbon dioxide from it.

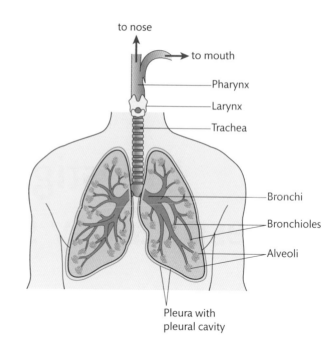

FIGURE 9.1
Schematic illustration of the respiratory tract.

Look at Figure 9.1 to appreciate the anatomy of the lower respiratory tract.

After passing through the nose or throat, air travels through the larynx (voicebox) and trachea (windpipe) into the lower respiratory tract. The rest of the tract is referred to as the bronchial tree because of the way the airways branch into increasingly smaller airways. The smallest branches end in tiny balloon-type sacs called alveoli. This is where the gas exchange of oxygen (into the blood) and carbon dioxide (out of the blood) takes place. A network of capillaries surrounds each alveolus where the membranes are so thin that molecules of oxygen and carbon dioxide can diffuse across them.

9.1.2 Respiratory tract membranes

Each lung is surrounded by a double-layered serous membrane, called the pleura. The two layers are lubricated by the pleural fluid.

There are two features of the respiratory tract lining which are crucial in preventing infection. Firstly, mucous glands produce mucus, a sticky substance which traps dust particles and organisms. Secondly, the motion of **cilia** moves the mucus, along with its trapped particles, upwards to the pharynx where it is swallowed.

Biological methods of removing organisms include the action of antibodies (in mucus), enzymes (e.g. lysozyme) and **macrophages** (in the alveoli).

cilia
Cilia are hair-like beating structures which protrude from respiratory epithelial cells.

macrophage
Macrophages are white blood cells (WBCs) which engulf then digest foreign bodies including organisms.

> **Key Point**
>
> The lower respiratory tract is a branching series of tubes which deliver oxygen to the blood and remove carbon dioxide from it.

9.1.3 Normal flora of the respiratory tract

Many of the body's mucous membranes are covered with colonizing bacteria. Since the respiratory tract is open to the external environment, many organisms are continually entering the
tract. We have already discussed various ways in which the body removes these organisms.
Some, however, manage to **colonize** the inner surface of the tract. We refer to such organisms
as **normal flora** or human microbiotica.

The composition of each person's normal flora varies and is influenced by many factors including
age, sex, nutrition, genetics, and environmental exposure. Typically, normal respiratory flora is a
mixture of non-haemolytic and a **α-haemolytic** streptococci, *Neisseria* spp., *Haemophilus* spp.,
and *Moraxella* spp. Importantly, organisms that are pathogenic for the lower respiratory tract
are often part of the normal flora of the upper respiratory tract.

colonize
Organisms are said to colonize
a body site when they live
without causing harm.

normal flora
Normal flora or human
microbiotica is the collective
term for the organisms
colonizing a given body site.

**α-haemolytic,
β-haemolytic**
Bacterial colonies can be
described as α-haemolytic,
β-haemolytic, or non-
haemolytic depending on
their action on the red blood
cells in the culture medium.

9.1.4 Disruption of the normal flora

The composition of the normal flora can gradually change with time. Some situations, however, cause an abrupt change which may or may not result in disease. Examples of such disruption include:

- Viral infections.
- Antibiotics.
- Injury.
- Invasive instrumentation.

Hospitalization, especially when patients are on antimicrobials and mechanically venti-
lated, tends to result in the replacement of the pre-existing normal flora by Gram-negative
bacilli such as *Escherichia coli*, *Pseudomonas aeruginosa*, *Acinetobacter* spp., and *Enterobacter
cloacae*. Since antibiotics kill much of the normal flora, resistant organisms are able to
flourish.

9.1.5 Infections of the lower respiratory tract

Infections result when organisms cease to merely colonize our cells and manage to invade them, causing damage. Alternatively, infections may occur when a new organism is encountered.

Infections of the lower respiratory tract are generally described according to the region that they affect rather than by the infecting organism. For example:

- Bronchitis: inflammation of the bronchi.
- Bronchiolitis: inflammation of the bronchioles.
- Pneumonia: inflammation of the alveoli.

9.1.6 Common bacterial pathogens

It would be difficult to list every organism that is capable of causing a lower respiratory tract infection (LRTI). Many cases are caused by viruses. In this chapter, we shall concentrate on bacterial causes of LRTI, although we shall also consider the main fungal pathogens.

Let us consider the bacteria that can cause pneumonia. The range of common pathogens varies depending on factors such as:

- Where the pneumonia was acquired: in hospital or in the community.
- Whether the patient has an underlying disease.

Cross reference
See Chapter 13 and Chapter 14.

- The patient's age.

9.1.7 Community-acquired pneumonia

The most common bacterium to cause community-acquired pneumonia is *Streptococccus pneumoniae*. Other frequent culprits are *Haemophilus influenzae*, *Mycoplasma pneumoniae*, *Staphylococcus aureus*, and *Moraxella catarrhalis*. With the exception of *M. pneumoniae*, these organisms are part of the normal upper respiratory flora.

S. aureus is associated with secondary infections following influenza or measles. The viruses responsible for these primary infections damage the respiratory tract lining. This makes the patient more susceptible to infection by bacteria which were previously colonizing the tract.

9.1.8 Typical and atypical pneumonia

M. pneumoniae mainly affects children and young adults. It is the second most common non-viral cause of community-acquired pneumonia. Unlike the typical pneumonia caused by *S. pneumoniae*, *H. influenzae*, *S. aureus*, and *M. catarrhalis*, with acute onset and production of sputum, the pneumonia caused by *M. pneumoniae* is described as **atypical pneumonia** with minimal, if any, sputum production and chronic onset.

Typical and atypical pneumonia are caused by different groups of organisms; atypical pneumonia is associated with **intracellular organisms**, that is, organisms which can only multiply within the cells of their host. In addition to *M. pneumoniae*, causes of atypical pneumonia include:

- *Chlamydophila psittaci* (acquired from parrots, causes psittacosis).
- *Coxiella burnetii* (acquired from farm animals, causes Q fever).
- *Legionella pneumophila* (acquired from water storage systems, often associated with foreign travel, causes Legionnaires' disease).

Typical and atypical pneumonia can be differentiated by non-microbiological techniques such as chest X-rays. As we shall learn later, microbiological testing does not always identify a pathogen so other diagnostic tools are important.

9.1.9 Hospital-acquired pneumonia

Although pneumonia in hospitalized patients may be caused by the same organisms as community-acquired pneumonia, it is often caused by different organisms.

As we saw earlier, the composition of the normal flora is altered by such interventions as antibiotics and invasive instrumentation. Hospitalized patients are more likely to harbour resistant organisms such as methicillin-resistant *S. aureus* (MRSA). Intensive care patients frequently require mechanical ventilation. As a consequence of this, they tend to be colonized with Gram-negative bacilli more usually associated with the intestines. These organisms can then cause pneumonia. If an infection develops more than 48 h after admission to hospital, it is described as **nosocomial infection.**

Nosocomial pneumonia is increasingly caused by bacteria that are resistant to multiple antibiotics. Many of these organisms were previously thought to have low pathogenicity but now cause particular problems in intensive care wards. *Stenotrophomonas maltophilia* and *Acinetobacter baumannii* are examples of such organisms.

Neonates (babies less than 1 month old) with pneumonia are usually infected by organisms from their mother's normal vaginal flora. Examples include *E. coli* and *Streptococcus agalactiae* (Group B *Streptococcus*).

9.1.10 Predisposing factors

Underlying diseases may increase the risk of developing pneumonia. Situations that affect consciousness, such as strokes, seizures, or alcoholism, increase the likelihood of **aspiration pneumonia**. This occurs when the epiglottis fails to cover the larynx during swallowing. Food and saliva, which would normally be directed down the oesophagus, enter the trachea and can lead to pneumonia. This can give rise to infections with organisms normally found in the mouth. Examples are:

- Actinomycosis (caused by *Actinomyces* spp.).
- Mixed anaerobic/streptococcal infections.

A major predisposing factor for respiratory tract infection is the immunological status of the individual. **Immunocompromised** patients are at the greatest risk of infection as they do not possess the necessary mechanisms to resist infection.

In addition to the organisms that can infect immunocompetent individuals, immunocompromised patients can develop pneumonia with organisms that would not ordinarily cause disease. Examples of this include:

- Nocardiosis (caused by *Nocardia* spp.).
- *Mycobacterium avium* complex (MAC) infections.
- *Pneumocystis* pneumonia (PCP), caused by *Pneumocystis jirovecii* (formerly *Pneumocystis carinii*).

MAC organisms will be discussed in Section 9.4. Sometimes the isolation of unusual pathogens from a patient can alert the clinician to immunodeficiencies that were previously undetected.

immunocompromised, immunodeficient, immunosuppressed
Immunocompromised, immunodeficient, and immunosuppressed all refer to cases where the patient's body is unable, or less effectively able, to resist infection. This can result from drug action or disease.

9.1.11 Lung abscesses

Abscesses are pus-filled cavities surrounded by inflamed tissue. They can form in the lungs as a complication of aspiration pneumonia or they can arise from blood-borne spread of organisms from other sites. Lung abscesses can be caused by a mixture of organisms, commonly anaerobes and members of the *Streptococcus anginosis* group (formerly the 'milleri' group). if there are multiple small abscesses the condition is called **necrotizing pneumonia**.

9.1.12 Whooping cough

Whooping cough, or pertussis, is a two-stage disease. The first stage, which lasts around 10 days, is fairly non-specific and symptoms resemble those of a common cold. During this stage, the bacterium *Bordetella pertussis* colonizes the cilia in the upper respiratory tract. It multiplies there and can be spread to other people by coughing or sneezing. The second stage, which is mediated by toxins, is more specific. Patients develop fits of prolonged coughing ending with a characteristic 'whoop'.

A mild form of whooping cough is caused by another bacterium, *Bordetella parapertussis*.

9.1.13 Common fungal pathogens

Cross reference

See Chapter 14.

Fungi are sometimes isolated from lower respiratory tract samples. Fungi are discussed in detail in Chapter 14 but it is worth considering the most common respiratory fungi here. Fungi are divided into two groups: yeasts and moulds.

9.1.14 Yeasts

Yeasts are common components of normal respiratory flora. Since the majority of lower respiratory samples are collected in a way which contaminates them with upper respiratory flora, it is not surprising that many of them are found to contain yeasts, primarily *Candida* spp. It is thought, however, that these merely reflect overgrowth of yeasts in the upper respiratory tract and that genuine candidal pneumonia is rare.

9.1.15 Moulds

The most common types of mould found in the respiratory tract are *Aspergillus* spp. *Aspergillus* spores are inhaled from the air by all of us, probably on a daily basis and do not generally cause disease. However, they can be highly pathogenic for immunosuppressed patients or those with pre-existing lung disease. When *Aspergillus* grows in the lungs it forms a ball of fungus called an **aspergilloma**.

A particular problem in hospitals dealing with immunosuppressed patients is that disturbance of the environment, as occurs with building work, increases the circulation of fungal spores in the air. This increases the likelihood of fungal lung infections.

Key Point: Overgrowth by Candida spp.

Although yeasts commonly colonize the upper respiratory tract they are usually present in relatively low numbers. Some medical interventions disturb the balance of the normal flora and allow the number of yeast cells to markedly increase. The resultant white coating of areas such as the tongue is called oral thrush. Drugs that are commonly associated with this problem include antibiotics (to which they are resistant) and anti-cancer drugs. Apart from being unpleasant, this situation makes interpretation of sputum cultures difficult.

There is a group of fungal respiratory infections that are relatively rare in the UK but need to be considered if patients have a relevant travel history. These include:

- Histoplasmosis.
- Blastomycosis.
- Coccidiomycosis.
- Paracoccidiomycosis.

P. jirovecii is an unusual organism. It is now believed to be a fungus but has previously been classified as a protozoon.

9.1.16 Parasites

Parasitic infections of the respiratory tract are rare in the UK but may be seen in immigrants or returning travellers. Parasites that may pass through the lungs include *Ascaris lumbricoides*, *Strongyloides stercoralis*, and *Paragonimus westermani*. One of the body's responses to parasitic infection is the proliferation of **eosinophils**. Eosinophils are a type of WBC associated with allergy. They may be detected in sputum microscopically. Clinical parasitology is covered in detail in Chapter 11.

Cross reference
See Chapter 11.

Key Point

Lower respiratory tract infections may be caused by viruses, bacteria, fungi, or parasites. Bacterial infections are usually caused by organisms from the upper respiratory tract. Hospital patients tend to be infected with different organisms to those infecting patients from the community.

9.2 Processing of lower respiratory samples

9.2.1 Sample types

The most common respiratory sample received by microbiology laboratories is sputum. The advantage of this sample is the ease with which it can be obtained, especially if the patient has a **productive cough**.

Ideally, patients should rinse their mouth with water prior to providing a sputum sample and should avoid adding saliva to their sputum. Unfortunately, such advice is often lacking and the poor quality of many samples significantly diminishes the validity of the results. Small children are unable to produce sputum so cough swabs are sometimes taken as an alternative.

productive cough
A productive cough results in the expectoration of sputum.

We have already considered the problems associated with the contamination of lower respiratory samples by upper respiratory flora. One approach to solving this problem is to physically bypass the upper tract in order to take a sample directly from the lower tract. Bronchoscopes are used for this purpose.

Key Point: Bronchoscopy samples

A bronchoscope is a thin, flexible, fibre-optic telescope which is passed into the bronchi via the nose, mouth, or an endotracheal tube. Sterile saline is introduced through the bronchoscope and then aspirated into a sterile container to send to the laboratory.

The two most common sample types collected in this way are:

- ■ Bronchial washings – from large airways.
- ■ Bronchoalveolar lavages (BALs) – from small airways.

Pleural fluids are also sent for microbiological investigation. As we learned earlier, the two layers of the pleura are lubricated by the pleural fluid. The volume of this fluid is normally around 15 mL. If it accumulates, either by overproduction or by failure to drain away, we call this a **pleural effusion**. Samples are collected by inserting a needle between the ribs through the back. There are many causes of pleural effusion, including infection. If pus is present in the fluid, the condition is called **empyema**; this is likely to be due to bacterial infection.

In cases of suspected whooping cough, testing can be performed on nasopharyngeal aspirates, nasopharyngeal swabs or **pernasal swabs**. The organism is only present in high numbers during the first 3 weeks of the illness. Later stages of the illness require blood tests for specific antibodies.

empyema

Empyema is a collection of pus and necrotic tissue in a body cavity, e.g. the pleural cavity.

pernasal swab

A pernasal swab is taken by passing a thin, flexible swab through the nose to the back of the throat.

Key Point

The majority of lower respiratory tract samples received by microbiology laboratories are sputum. Cough swabs, bronchial washings, bronchoalveolar lavages, pleural fluids, and lung biopsies are also received.

9.2.2 Sample processing

When sputum is received in the laboratory, its macroscopic appearance is noted. This is to assess how **purulent** the sample is and to note any bloodstaining.

purulent

A purulent sample is a sample containing a lot of pus

Terms used to describe sputa include:

- Purulent (pus-like).
- Mucoid (mucus-like).
- Salivary (saliva-like).
- Mucopurulent (part mucoid, part purulent).
- Mucosalivary (part mucoid, part salivary).
- Bloodstained (in addition to any of the above).

Bloodstained sputum samples are indicative of **haemoptysis**, which may be present in cases of pulmonary TB.

Laboratory policies regarding poor sputum samples vary. Some laboratories do not process salivary samples. Other laboratories are more stringent and do not process mucoid samples either. These decisions reflect the likelihood that such samples originate from the upper respiratory tract. Any organisms that are present merely reflect the patient's normal upper respiratory flora and it would be misleading to imply that they were responsible for causing the lower respiratory symptoms.

Additional information can be obtained by examining sputum microscopically. Gram staining may be used for this. A good sputum sample will contain many WBCs and few epithelial cells. In contrast, a poor sputum sample will contain few WBCs and many epithelial cells. In general >25 epithelial cells per low-power field on microscopy is considered to be an unacceptable sample for culture.

The decision to discard a sputum sample isn't always appropriate. If a patient is immunocompromised, shows signs of atypical pneumonia or is suspected of having TB, then their samples should be processed, regardless of their macroscopic or microscopic appearance.

haemoptysis
Haemoptysis literally means 'the spitting of blood'.

SELF-CHECK 9.1

Why is it inappropriate to consider a mucoid sample from an immunocompromised patient to be unsuitable for culture?

Homogenization of sputum samples

Sputum is viscous due to the presence of pus and mucus. Also, the organisms in sputum are distributed unevenly throughout the sample. In order to overcome these limitations, it is common practice to use digestion agents to liquefy the samples, and agitation to homogenize them. Examples of digestion agents are dithiothreitol (DTT) and *N*-acetyl-L-cysteine (NAC). These compounds do not affect the viability of respiratory pathogens.

Since the number of organisms causing an infection should be significantly higher than the number of contaminating organisms, dilution of the sample is performed. This removes much of the normal flora but retains the significant organisms. The dilution factor used to achieve this is 1 : 1000.

Concentration of lower respiratory samples

In contrast to the dilution of sputum described above, pleural fluids and samples that have been obtained by bronchoscopy, such as BALs, need to be concentrated. Contaminating organisms should not be present in these samples and any pathogens present will have been diluted by the saline used in bronchoscopy.

Concentration is achieved by centrifugation. The supernatant is removed and the deposit is used for microscopy and culture.

Key Point

Respiratory samples, particularly sputum, need to be pretreated before they are suitable for culture.

Why do some lower respiratory samples need to be diluted before testing whilst others need to be concentrated?

9.2.3 Microscopy techniques

A variety of staining techniques are used on lower respiratory samples to visualize organisms and/or blood cells. The most common procedures are:

1. Gram staining.
2. Immunofluorescence for *Legionella* spp.
3. Immunofluorescence or histochemical staining for *P. jirovecii*.
4. Differential staining of WBC for eosinophilia.
5. Acid–alcohol-fast bacilli (AAFB or AFB) staining.

We shall consider AAFB staining in Section 9.4. We shall look at the rest in turn here.

Gram staining

We have already seen how Gram staining can be used to assess the quality of sputum samples. It can also be used diagnostically to predict which organisms are present. This is only presumptive identification and its value depends on the organisms seen. Table 9.1 summarizes the common organisms that cause pneumonia and describes their appearance on a Gram stain.

TABLE 9.1 The Gram stain appearance of common lower respiratory pathogens.

Organism	Gram appearance	Further information
S. pneumoniae	Gram-positive cocci	Diplococci*, lancet-shaped
S. aureus	Gram-positive cocci	Clusters ('bunches of grapes')
M. catarrhalis	Gram-negative cocci	
N. meningitidis	Gram-negative cocci	
H. influenzae	Gram-negative bacilli	Slender bacilli or coccobacilli
Enterobacteriaceae	Gram-negative bacilli	Large
P. aeruginosa	Gram-negative bacilli	Large
S. maltophilia	Gram-negative bacilli	Large
L. pneumophila	Gram-negative bacilli	Stain poorly, pleomorphic†
B. pertussis	Gram-negative bacilli	Coccobacilli‡
Candida spp.	Gram-positive	Large, oval-shaped
M. pneumoniae	No Gram reaction	No cell wall to stain

* pairs of cocci.
† short when young but long when old.
‡ short with rounded ends.

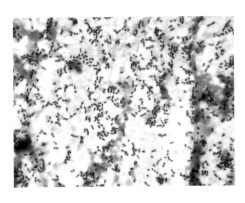

FIGURE 9.2
Gram stain of *S. pneumoniae* showing characteristic Gram-positive cocci in pairs.
Source: Courtesy of Mike Grover.

A useful feature of *S. pneumoniae* is its distinctive appearance on a Gram stain. Remember that this is the most common bacterial cause of community-acquired pneumonia. Its cells are seen as Gram-positive diplococci. If you look at the dark purple cells in Figure 9.2 you can see that the cocci, arranged in pairs, are not spherical but slightly elongated with pointed ends. This appearance is referred to as lanceolate (lancet-shaped). In addition to this characteristic shape, a Gram stain of *S. pneumoniae* can reveal a zone of clearing around each pair of cells. This is the polysaccharide capsule surrounding the cells.

The majority of other bacteria associated with pneumonia are insufficiently distinctive for a Gram stain to have much predictive value; they may look identical or very similar to other organisms which are not pathogenic. Yeast cells are significantly larger than bacterial cells, have an oval shape and appear Gram positive.

We learned earlier that *M. pneumoniae* is the second most common cause of community-acquired bacterial pneumonia. An unusual feature of mycoplasmas is their lack of cell walls. Since Gram staining relies on the dyes binding to the cell wall, mycoplasmas are not detectable by this method.

> **Key Point**
>
> Just because you may see Gram-positive diplococci on a Gram stain, it does not necessarily mean that the patient has a *S. pneumoniae* infection. All you may be seeing is some normal flora. The number of organisms present and the clinical condition of the patient need to be considered in the overall diagnosis.

Microscopy for detection of Legionella spp.

L. pneumophila, which causes Legionnaires' disease, can be detected in lower respiratory samples using immunofluorescence. This technique utilizes specific antibodies which bind to specific *Legionella* antigens in the sample. Bound antibodies are detected by the fluorescence of an attached dye. The two methods used for this are referred to as DFA (direct fluorescent antibody) and IFAT (indirect fluorescent antibody test). However, these tests are associated with a poor predictive value for *Legionella* infection.

FIGURE 9.3

P. jirovecii cysts staining black with methanamine silver stain.
Source: Courtesy CDC/ Dr. Edwin P. Ewing, Jr. (PHIL #960), 1984.

Microscopy for PCP

induced sputum

A sputum sample can be induced by inhaling nebulized saline.

Microscopy is the principal means of diagnosing PCP, as *P. jirovecii* does not grow on routine culture media. The optimal sample types are BAL, **induced sputum**, or lung tissue.

Immunofluorescent microscopy, similar to that used for *Legionella* spp., may be used for *P. jirovecii*. Alternatively, a variety of histochemical stains can be used including:

- Methenamine silver nitrate.
- Calcofluor white.
- Giemsa.

Departments other than microbiology, such as histology, often perform PCP testing. Figure 9.3 shows cells of *P. jirovecii* stained black by methenamine silver stain.

SELF-CHECK 9.3

If PCP testing is requested on a sample, what does this imply about the patient?

Differential staining of WBC (eosinophils)

Cross reference

See Chapter 3.

As their name suggests, eosinophils take up the acidic stain eosin. More specifically, the stain is concentrated within the granules of their cytoplasm, giving them a characteristic granular appearance which differentiates them from other WBCs. Their presence in a respiratory sample indicates an allergic response.

> **Key Point**
>
> Microscopy of lower respiratory samples can be used either to indicate the quality of a sample, to give an indication of likely pathogens or to specifically detect pathogens.

9.2.4 Common isolation media

Cross reference

See Chapter 16.

Most of the bacteria and fungi associated with LRTIs can be isolated using routine culture techniques. The main exception is *M. pneumoniae*. Although isolation media for mycoplasmas exist, they are not commonly used in laboratories; diagnosis of *M. pneumoniae* infection usually relies on serological tests. Reference laboratories offer molecular tests for respiratory samples, where necessary.

The exact selection of culture media varies between laboratories but will always reflect the spectrum of organisms associated with LRTIs. A combination of **selective** and **non-selective** agars is generally necessary.

Commonly, three basic media are used for lower respiratory samples:

- Chocolate agar.
- Blood agar.
- Cysteine lactose electrolyte deficient (CLED) agar or MacConkey agar.

Between them, these support the growth of:

- *S. pneumoniae*.
- *H. influenzae*.
- *S. aureus*.
- *M. catarrhalis*.
- *Enterobacteriaceae*.
- *Pseudomonas* spp.
- *S. maltophilia*.
- *Candida* spp.
- *Aspergillus* spp.

In order to recover *S. pneumoniae* and *H. influenzae* directly from clinical samples, the incubation atmosphere needs to be enriched with carbon dioxide. In this atmosphere *S. pneumoniae* produce characteristic 'draughtsman' like colonies on blood agar; look at Figure 9.4 to see these.

Chocolate agar can be made more selective for *H. influenzae* by adding an antibiotic, bacitracin. Since *H. influenzae* is Gram negative it will grow in the presence of bacitracin, an antibiotic that will kill Gram-positive organisms in the sample and thus aid the growth of *H. influenzae* through lack of competition with other flora

Although *S. aureus*, *Candida* spp., and *Aspergillus* spp. can grow on the media listed previously, selective agar is indicated for immunocompromised patients and those with **bronchiectasis**. Several media that are selective for *S. aureus* are available. Sabouraud's agar is the most common fungal agar for respiratory samples. It contains nutrients which enhance the growth of fungi, and antibiotics to suppress the growth of bacteria. Selective **chromogenic agars** are also available for both *S. aureus* and *Candida* spp. These utilize colour to highlight the organisms of interest.

non-selective, selective
Non-selective agars support the growth of a wide range of organisms; they do not contain inhibitory substances. Selective agars contain substances which inhibit the growth of certain organisms in order to enhance the isolation of others.

bronchiectasis
Bronchiectasis is the irreversible dilation of the bronchi.

Cross reference
See Chapter 3.

FIGURE 9.4
Blood agar plate showing characteristic draughtsman-like colonies of
S. pneumoniae.
Source: Courtesy of Deane Rhone.

If the pathogens grow on the basic isolation media, why are selective agars necessary?

Samples from cystic fibrosis patients need further selective plates; these are discussed later.

If Legionnaires' disease is suspected, or if a patient has signs of atypical pneumonia, then selective agar for *L. pneumophila* is necessary. Buffered charcoal yeast extract (BCYE) agar is available in various formulations, each containing a different cocktail of antimicrobial substances to inhibit the growth of other organisms. Pretreatment of samples by heat or dilution can also remove other organisms. The agars need to contain cysteine and iron salts since these are essential growth requirements for *L. pneumophila*.

Colonies of *L. pneumophila* have a ground glass, iridescent appearance. As *L. pneumophila* is a slow-growing organism, the plates need to be incubated for up to 10 days.

Sometimes, *Legionella* infections are diagnosed by an alternative test: the urinary antigen test (*L. pneumophila* serogroup 1 only). This is as sensitive as culture of respiratory samples, is highly specific and is simpler to perform. A disadvantage of the antigen test is the lack of epidemiological data which culture provides. These data can be valuable in outbreak situations.

Culture of *Bordetella* spp., for cases of suspected whooping cough, requires selective agar containing charcoal and blood. An antibiotic, cephalexin, is incorporated into the agar to inhibit normal respiratory flora. These plates can be made available to nursing staff directly on the ward so they can be inoculated directly as the organism often dies rapidly even on transport swabs. *It must be remembered that uninoculated plates, especially those containing antibiotics, can have a shelf-life of only 1 week.*

A high level of humidity in the incubation atmosphere is important for these organisms and the plates need to be incubated for up to 7 days. Colonies of *B. pertussis* are domed with a pearly appearance.

Key Point

All culture media containing antibiotics should be used when as fresh as possible due to the possible degradation of the antibiotic over time, especially those containing β-lactam antibiotics. If this occurs, the selectivity of the medium is compromised.

We have seen the importance of receiving a good quality sample, we have looked at ways of pretreating the sample and we have considered the range of media used to grow the organisms associated with LRTIs. Despite all of these requirements being satisfied, a significant proportion of samples do not yield a pathogen. Many of these cases are due to viral infection but others may be caused by organisms which we are currently unable to culture or are not yet recognized as pathogens.

Key Point

A combination of selective and non-selective agars is used to culture respiratory samples. Certain clinical details prompt the inclusion of further selective agars.

9.2.5 Confirmatory tests

Experienced biomedical scientists are able to presumptively identify the pathogens isolated from lower respiratory samples by examining the **primary culture plates** visually.

We have already seen how the distinctive microscopic appearance of *S. pneumoniae* is useful. Similarly, its macroscopic appearance can also be distinctive. Colonies of *S. pneumoniae* can undergo **autolysis** which results in the centre of the colony subsiding. These colonies are described as 'draughtsman' colonies and are highly characteristic of *S. pneumoniae*

Most presumptive identifications need to be confirmed, usually by biochemical tests, or increasingly by MALDI-TOF analysis. Some of these can be incorporated into the primary culture step. For example, addition of an **optochin** disc to a primary plate serves to differentiate *S. pneumoniae* from other a-haemolytic colonies.

If you study Table 9.2, you will see some of the other confirmatory tests which may be used for the identification of respiratory pathogens. There is a growing trend for laboratories to use automated instruments which perform identification tests as well as antimicrobial susceptibility tests but these have not yet superseded the need for manual identification techniques entirely.

Key Point: Confirmatory tests used for Haemophilus spp.

Colonies of presumptive *Haemophilus* spp. can be identified as *H. influenzae* by demonstrating their requirement for two growth factors: X factor and V factor. This is shown in Figure 9.5.

Colonies demonstrating requirement for only one of the factors may be another species of *Haemophilus*, e.g. *H. parainfluenzae* requires only V factor. Both X and V factor are available from chocolate agar but only X factor is available from blood agar. The phenomenon of **satellitism** occurs on blood agar, where *H. influenzae* is able to grow around colonies of other organisms producing V factor, e.g. *S. aureus*.

TABLE 9.2 Confirmatory tests for common lower respiratory pathogens.

Organism	Confirmatory tests
S. pneumoniae	Optochin sensitivity, bile solubility, latex agglutination
S. aureus	Latex agglutination, DNase, coagulase, selective agar
M. catarrhalis	Butyl esterase, tributyrin
N. meningitidis	Commercial kit
H. influenzae	X/V dependency
Enterobacteriaceae	Commercial kit
P. aeruginosa	Oxidase, growth at 42°C, commercial kit
S. maltophilia	Oxidase, resistance to imipenem, esculin, commercial kit
L. pneumophila	Subculture to BCYE +/– cysteine, autofluorescence, latex agglutination
B. pertussis	Agglutination with antisera
Candida spp.	Pseudopods, germ tube, selective agar

primary culture plates

Primary culture plates are those onto which the clinical samples are directly inoculated. Organisms from primary plates can be inoculated onto further plates; these secondary plates are called subcultures.

autolysis

Autolysis is where an organism produces enzymes which lead to the breakdown of its own cells.

optochin

Optochin is another name for ethyl hydrocuprein hydrochloride. Most strains of *S. pneumoniae* are sensitive to optochin whilst most other α-haemolytic streptococci are resistant.

Cross reference

See Chapter 2.

Cross reference

See Chapter 2 which describes identification tests in more detail.

FIGURE 9.5

Iso-Sensitest agar showing *H. influenzae* only growing around a disc containing both X and V factor.

Source: Courtesy of Louise Hill-King.

In some instances, identification of the organism to species level may not be necessary. Many laboratories would report a yeast as 'Candida spp.' or a member of the Enterobacteriaceae as a '**coliform**'.

Routine microbiology laboratories can identify common respiratory pathogens to the required level for most situations. Occasionally, further testing by a reference laboratory is necessary. Reasons for this include:

* Outbreaks of infection requiring typing of organisms.
* Unusual antimicrobial susceptibility patterns requiring confirmation.

coliform

Coliform is a loose term used for bacteria which are 'Escherichia coli-like'. They are members of the Enterobacteriaceae family which ferment lactose to produce acid and gas at 35–37°C.

> **Key Point**
>
> Bacteria isolated on culture plates need to be identified to determine if they are pathogens, generally to genus or species level, usually by means of biochemical tests.

9.2.6 Antimicrobial susceptibility testing

Often the most important aspect of a microbiology report is the information regarding antimicrobials. The range of antimicrobials against which an organism is tested is determined by the type of organism. The choice of antimicrobials to include in the report is determined by factors such as:

* The severity of the disease.
* Whether or not the patient is in hospital.
* The patient's age.
* Pregnancy.
* Drug allergies, e.g. penicillin.
* Local factors, e.g. known circulation of resistant strains.

Cross reference

Antimicrobial susceptibility testing methods are discussed in Chapter 4.

As with other infections, patients with an LRTI will frequently be prescribed a 'best guess' antibiotic, based on likely pathogens. Once the results are available, a different antibiotic can be prescribed if appropriate.

The disadvantage of partial identification is that correct interpretation of antimicrobial susceptibility test results often requires species-level identification. Several types of coliform are known to be naturally resistant to aminopenicillins. Ampicillin and amoxycillin, which are aminopenicillins, are commonly prescribed for LRTIs.

Antifungal susceptibility testing is not routinely carried out for respiratory infections so treatment is often empirical. *Candida albicans* is generally sensitive to the antifungal agents that are likely to be prescribed, whereas some other species of *Candida* are resistant. In this situation, the differentiation of '*albicans*' and '*non-albicans*' yeasts is helpful. However, if the patient is immunocompromised, antifungal susceptibility tests are often performed as the infection can be life threatening.

> **Key Point**
>
> Bacteria isolated from lower respiratory samples are challenged with a range of antimicrobial substances in the laboratory. The results of these tests form the basis of recommendations for appropriate treatment.

9.3 **Cystic fibrosis**

Cystic fibrosis (CF) is an inherited disease. CF has such a profound effect on the patient's lungs that they experience respiratory infections which merit special attention. First, let us examine the symptoms that predispose them to these infections.

9.3.1 Symptoms and outcome of CF

CF occurs due to mutation of the CF transmembrane conductance regulator (*CFTR*) gene. This leads to an imbalance of sodium and chloride ions throughout the body, resulting in the dehydration of secretions from affected organs, including the lungs. These thick, dehydrated secretions block passages in the body and lead to the classical CF symptoms.

Earlier, we learned that mucus is continually cleared from the respiratory tract by cilia. In CF patients, the mucus is so thick that the cilia are ineffective, so the mucus collects in the airways. Trapped organisms multiply in this mucus and form biofilms. These biofilms provide a reservoir of organisms which can cause infections. The body mounts an inflammatory response to clear the organisms; this causes further damage. The airways respond to the damage caused by repeated episodes of inflammation by dilating irreversibly. This condition, which is not unique to CF patients, is called bronchiectasis.

With good health care, CF patients can now survive beyond 40 years but eventually the cumulative damage to the lungs culminates in respiratory failure and death. The life of some patients can be prolonged by lung transplantation.

Key Point

Cystic fibrosis is an inherited disease which involves progressive lung damage associated with recurrent infections.

9.3.2 Organisms associated with CF

Initially, pneumonia in CF patients is caused by the same organisms as in the rest of the population. Infections with typical respiratory pathogens, such as *H. influenzae*, tend to be followed by infection with *S. aureus*. Another, more complex, stage then develops which is characterized by *Pseudomonas* spp. including *P. aeruginosa*.

Once *P. aeruginosa* has colonized the CF respiratory tract it adapts well to its environment and starts to produce an **exopolysaccharide** (EPS, also called alginate). This slimy substance provides a matrix for biofilms and helps to anchor the organisms to the respiratory cells. It also serves to protect the organism from internal attack by the body's immune system, and from external attack by antimicrobial substances. When these organisms are cultured in the laboratory, they produce large, mucoid colonies which contrast with typical non-mucoid colonies of *P. aeruginosa*. Multiple strains of mucoid and non-mucoid *P. aeruginosa* can coexist in the CF lung.

Many other bacteria are found to be colonizing the lungs at this stage, including several species that are usually associated with environmental contamination of other samples. Their clinical significance is the subject of debate as they seem to flourish after the patient has been given antipseudomonal drugs. Are they simply filling a niche created by the eradication of other organisms or are they part of the disease process? Examples of these organisms are:

- S. maltophilia.
- Achromobacter xylosoxidans.
- Ralstonia spp.
- Burkholderia gladioli.

There is a group of bacteria that are collectively known as the **Burkholderia cepacia complex** (Bcc). They are not associated with disease in the general population but cause respiratory infections in CF patients, particularly in the advanced stages. Some Bcc organisms seem to be more transmissible and cause more severe, even fatal, infections. Therefore, the importance of detecting and correctly identifying the Bcc organisms has social, as well as physical, implications for the patient.

Cross reference
See Chapter 14, Section 14.6

The presence of Bcc organisms in the CF lung reflects the extensive use of antimicrobial substances throughout the patient's life. Bcc organisms are resistant to a wide range of antimicrobials and are therefore able to survive and multiply when other organisms are eradicated or suppressed. This situation also applies to other multiresistant organisms including atypical *Mycobacterium* spp. and fungi, particularly *Aspergillus* spp. *Mycobacterium* spp. are covered in more detail in Section 9.4.

Key Point

Recurrent respiratory infections are a prominent feature of cystic fibrosis. Specific organisms, such as mucoid strains of *P. aeruginosa* and members of the *B. cepacia* complex (Bcc), are associated with the condition.

9.3.3 Culture of CF samples

Lower respiratory samples from CF patients need to be tested for the same organisms as routine samples but also need additional investigations to detect the organisms which are specifically associated with CF:

- S. aureus.
- Mucoid and non-mucoid *P. aeruginosa*.
- S. maltophilia.
- B. cepacia complex.
- Fungi.

Cross reference
Chapter 3

These organisms are generally sought by adding additional selective agars to the routine culture protocol, for example mannitol salt agar (MSA) or chromogenic agar for *S. aureus*, *Pseudomonas*-selective agar for *P. aeruginosa*, *cepacia*-selective agar for Bcc organisms, and Sabouraud's agar for fungi.

Key Point

A wider range of selective agars needs to be used for cystic fibrosis samples compared with other samples because of the wider range of organisms that can cause infection.

9.3.4 Identification of pathogens from CF samples

Presumptive identifications of colonies growing from CF samples need to be confirmed with biochemical tests, as for other samples. The most common confirmatory tests are shown in Table 9.2 but we need to consider some further tests for CF isolates here.

For colonies of presumptive *Aspergillus* spp., microscopy using lactophenol cotton blue (LPCB) can demonstrate typical microscopic structures.

Resistance to imipenem and the ability to hydrolyse esculin are useful markers for *S. malto-philia*. *S. maltophilia* is intrinsically resistant to imipenem whilst most *Pseudomonas* spp. are sensitive.

Identification of colonies growing on *cepacia*-selective agar can be problematic. Most laboratories use commercial identification kits but they have limited ability to differentiate Bcc organisms from other biochemically similar organisms. It is therefore advisable to refer possible Bcc isolates to a reference laboratory for confirmation.

Cross reference

Microscopy techniques for fungi are described in Chapter 14.

SELF-CHECK 9.5

Why is it so important to correctly identify organisms of the *B. cepacia* complex?

9.3.5 Further identification of Bcc organisms

The *B. cepacia* complex comprises at least 10 types of bacteria with distinct genomic profiles. We refer to these as genomovars to reflect the way in which they are differentiated. Previously, these were biochemically indistinguishable and thought to be a single species which was called *B. cepacia* (formerly *Pseudomonas cepacia*). Each genomovar is designated by a Roman numeral and a name. These are shown in Table 9.3.

All Bcc genomovars have been isolated from the lungs of CF patients but genomovars II (*B. multivorans*) and III (*B. cenocepacia*) are more closely associated with disease. CF clinics are especially interested in genomovar III as it is associated with greater person-to-person transmission and higher virulence than other genomovars.

Genomovar typing is beyond the scope of routine microbiology laboratories so Bcc isolates are referred to a reference laboratory for typing.

Key Point

B. cepacia complex organisms need to be referred to a reference laboratory for genomovar typing.

9.3.6 Antimicrobial susceptibility testing of CF isolates

If the isolates from a CF sample are typical respiratory pathogens, such as *H. influenzae* or *S. aureus*, then antimicrobial susceptibility testing is the same as for any other sample. If, however, the isolates are mucoid *P. aeruginosa*, Bcc organisms, or other CF-associated Gram-negative bacilli then susceptibility testing is more challenging. Difficulties include:

TABLE 9.3 *B. cepacia* complex genomovars.

Bcc genomovar	Name
I	*B. cepacia*
II	*B. multivorans*
III	*B. cenocepacia*
IV	*B. stabilis*
V	*B. vietnamiensis*
VI	*B. dolosa*
VII	*B. ambifaria*
VIII	*B. athina*
IX	*B. pyrrocinia*
X	*B. ubonensis*
XI	*B. latens*
XII	*B. diffusa*
XIII	*B. arboris*
XIV	*B. seminalis*
XV	*B. metallica*
XVI	*B. contaminans*
XVII	*B. lata*

- Mixtures of similar organisms can be difficult to separate.
- Organisms can be slow growing.
- Mucoid organisms can be difficult to manipulate and mask other pathogens.
- Results can be difficult to interpret due to the lack of relevant data.
- False susceptibility is common with disc testing.
- A wide range of antimicrobials needs to be tested.

Key Point

Antimicrobial susceptibility testing of CF isolates is problematic.

9.3.7 Antimicrobial strategies for CF

The treatment of CF patients requires a multidisciplinary approach, one aspect of which is antimicrobial therapy. The risk of infection is lowered by physiotherapy to remove excess mucus from the lungs.

Unfortunately, it is apparent that clinical response to antimicrobials does not correlate well with laboratory results for CF isolates. This is partly related to the complex environment of the CF lung and partly to the combination therapy that patients receive.

There are two reasons for giving antimicrobials to a CF patient. One is for the specific treatment of an active infection. The other is to manage the colonization of the lungs between active infections. The first of these reasons is generally guided by laboratory results but the second tends to be more empirical and based on local policies.

In CF, it is usual practice to prescribe more than one antimicrobial at a time. Ideally, the infecting organism should be tested against these substances in combination but, in practice, such testing is labour intensive and only performed in specialist microbiology laboratories.

nebulized
Nebulized drugs are inhaled using a device which creates a cloud of small particles. High drug concentration in the lung is achieved and minimal systemic absorption reduces toxicity.

If a patient needs intravenous antibiotics then they require hospitalization. This is inconvenient for the patient and costly to the health service. For long-term administration of antimicrobials between active infections, **nebulized antimicrobials** are used to suppress the growth of *P. aeruginosa* (e.g. tobramycin or colistin).

Key Point

Long-term strategies for antimicrobial therapy are necessary for CF patients. Combination therapy and nebulized antimicrobials are widely used.

9.4 Mycobacteria

lipids
Lipids are fat soluble, naturally occurring compounds such as fats, oils, and waxes.

The family of bacteria that are commonly called mycobacteria are sufficiently different from the other bacteria we have described to merit separate discussion. They have distinctive cell walls containing a high concentration of **lipids**.

Mycolic acids
Arabinogalactan
Peptidoglycan
Cytoplasmic membrane

Cytoplasm

FIGURE 9.6
Structure of the mycobacterial cell wall showing the parallel arrangement of mycolic acid molecules.

These lipid-rich cell walls offer a high degree of protection to the cells and account for many of the properties that set mycobacteria apart. For example:

- Resistance to drying and osmotic lysis.
- Resistance to many antibiotics and disinfectants.
- Resistance to acids and alkalis.
- Impermeability to stains.
- Survival within macrophages.

The most notable lipids in the mycobacterial cell wall are **mycolic acids**. These are long **fatty acid** molecules with one long chain and one short chain. If you look at Figure 9.6 you can see how they are arranged in the cell wall, forming a **hydrophobic** (literally 'water-hating') barrier.

One of the mycolic acids in mycobacteria, **cord factor**, promotes the formation of strings of cells which give a cord-like appearance microscopically. This led early workers to liken them to the structures of fungal hyphae, hence the name mycobacteria (literally 'fungus-like bacteria').

> **fatty acids**
> Fatty acids are acids found in fats and oils. They consist of long hydrocarbon chains with a carboxyl acid group at one end.

Key Point
The lipid-rich cell walls of mycobacteria are different from those of other bacteria and give them distinctive properties.

9.4.1 Common mycobacterial types

Tuberculosis (TB) is the most significant mycobacterial disease worldwide and so the mycobacteria are often divided into those that cause TB and those that do not.

The group of organisms that cause TB is known as the *Mycobacterium tuberculosis* (MTB) complex which comprises the following species:

- *M. tuberculosis.*
- *M. bovis.*
- *M. africanum.*
- *M. pinnipedii.*
- *M. microti.*
- *M. caprae.*
- *M. canettii.*

Most human cases of TB are caused by the first three of these.

The mycobacteria that are not part of the MTB complex are grouped together and variously called *non-tuberculous mycobacteria, atypical mycobacteria, and mycobacteria other than tubercle bacilli.*

Mycobacteria are described as **rapid-growing mycobacteria** if they produce visible colonies on solid culture media within 7 days. Those taking longer than 7 days to produce visible colonies are described as **slow-growing mycobacteria**. All of the mycobacteria that cause respiratory infections are slow growers.

Of the non-tuberculous mycobacteria, members of the *M. avium* complex (MAC) cause the majority of respiratory infections. The MAC includes several species, the two most important of which are:

- *M. avium.*
- *M. intracellulare.*

MAC infection is closely associated with immunocompromised patients, particularly those infected by human immunodeficiency virus (HIV).

Key Point

Most respiratory mycobacterial infections in humans are caused by members of the *Mycobacterium tuberculosis* (MTB) complex or the *Mycobacterium avium* complex (MAC).

Key Point: The BCG strain of *M. bovis*

The Bacille Calmette–Guérin (BCG) vaccine contains a live, attenuated strain of *M. bovis.* An isolate of *M. bovis* was subcultured every 3 weeks for 13 years by Calmette and Guérin in Paris. They noted that it had become less virulent in animals over that time and it was first used as a human vaccine in 1921.

Normally, people receiving the vaccine would not develop disease from it. Immunocompromised people, however, can develop active infection with the BCG strain of *M. bovis.*

9.4.2 Microscopy for *Mycobacterium* spp.

Since mycobacteria grow so slowly, microscopy results can be available several weeks before culture results. Positive microscopy results can therefore have a significant impact on patient management. Negative results are less influential; if the clinical presentation of a patient suggests TB then treatment will be given, regardless of negative microscopy results. As we shall see later, microscopy lacks the sensitivity of other tests.

Conventional staining techniques, as used for other bacteria, are of no use with mycobacteria because of their impermeability to dyes.

Fortunately, there are ways of overcoming this impermeability. The two most common staining techniques for mycobacteria both use **phenol**. Phenol (formerly carbolic acid) acts like a detergent; it reduces the hydrophobic effect of the lipids, enabling the dye to penetrate the cell wall.

Phenol

Phenol is a toxic substance. Although toxic by inhalation, its distinctive smell alerts workers to its presence before dangerous quantities are inhaled. Toxicity to skin is more likely to be a problem; there is a risk of burns during the preparation of phenolic stains.

Historically, phenolic disinfectants were widely used for decontamination procedures in TB laboratories. They have now been superseded by less hazardous alternatives.

In the **Ziehl-Neelsen** (ZN) technique, the dye fuchsin is combined with phenol. This mixture is called carbol fuchsin. The use of phenol in the other common technique is more obvious as it is referred to as the **auramine–phenol** stain. Figure 9.7 shows the typical fluorescence of mycobacteria upon staining with a fluorescent dye.

The use of heat can also facilitate dye penetration and this is employed in the ZN technique.

To distinguish mycobacteria from other bacteria we use a further characteristic of the mycobacterial cell wall: resistance to acids. Addition of acid/alcohol mixtures to most stained bacteria would result in the removal of any bound dyes, that is decolorization. However, dyes that are bound to mycobacteria are resistant to acid/alcohol attack so decolorization does not occur. Therefore, we describe these organisms as being **acid-fast** (or acid–alcohol-fast) and mycobacteria are referred to as acid-fast bacilli (AFB) or acid–alcohol-fast bacilli (AAFB).

Key Point: **Non-mycobacterial acid-fast organisms**

Some non-mycobacterial organisms are also acid-fast due to the presence of mycolic acids in their cell walls. In these organisms, the mycolic acids are shorter than those in mycobacteria and they constitute a lower proportion of the cell wall. Consequently such organisms, which include *Nocardia* spp. and *Rhodococcus* spp., tend to be weakly acid-fast.

Since respiratory secretions containing mycobacteria accumulate in the lungs overnight, early morning sputum samples will contain more mycobacteria than those taken later in the day. It is usual practice to collect sputum samples on three consecutive days for mycobacterial testing. Sputum samples can be smeared directly onto a glass slide for staining. Other samples, such as pleural fluids or BALs, require concentration by centrifugation.

FIGURE 9.7

Acridine orange stained *M. tuberculosis* in sputum showing yellow fluorescent bacillus.

Source: Courtesy of Michael Ford.

> ### Key Point
>
> Microscopy techniques for mycobacteria exploit their acid-fast nature. Microscopy results may be available several weeks before culture results so they can influence early patient management.

9.4.3 Conventional culture for mycobacteria

Despite the advantages of simplicity and rapid results, microscopy for AFB requires 5,000–10,000 bacilli/mL of sample. Culture, though slow, is more sensitive, requiring only 10–100 bacilli/mL. In addition, isolation of the causative organism enables full identification, antimicrobial susceptibility testing and typing of the organism to be performed.

The aim of any culture method is to encourage the growth of the target organism(s) and discourage the growth of others. This is especially important for mycobacteria as they grow so slowly relative to other organisms. Although inhibitory substances are incorporated into mycobacterial culture media, they cannot sufficiently inhibit all contaminants; it is therefore necessary to **decontaminate** many samples before adding them to the culture medium.

decontamination

Decontamination of samples involves the killing of organisms other than the target organisms.

There are several methods for decontaminating samples. Unfortunately, all of the methods affect mycobacteria also. Optimizing the process is therefore aimed at killing *most* of the contaminants whilst preserving *most* of the mycobacteria. Some methods include the use of a digestion agent.

SELF-CHECK 9.6

Why are decontamination agents used for sputum samples submitted for TB?

Pleural fluids should not contain any contaminating organisms so do not require a decontamination step.

9.4.4 Solid and liquid culture media for mycobacteria

Three types of media are used for conventional mycobacterial culture:

- Egg-based solid media (e.g. Löwenstein–Jensen medium).
- Agar-based solid media (e.g. Middlebrook agar).
- Liquid media (e.g. Kirchner or Middlebrook broth).

Ideally, a combination of solid and liquid media should be used.

Solid media

In the UK, Löwenstein–Jensen (LJ) medium is the most commonly used solid medium. It includes:

- Glycerol (± pyruvate).
- Malachite green.
- Eggs.

FIGURE 9.8
LJ slope showing colonial growth of *M. tuberculosis*.
Source: Licensed under the Creative Commons Attribution 2.0 Generic license.
© Agarwal *et al.*/BioMed Central Ltd., courtesy of the Biology Image Library/CC-BY-2.0

LJ medium is prepared in bottles, which are heated whilst tilted. The heat dehydrates the egg proteins so the medium solidifies. This process is called **inspissation**. Since a sloping medium is obtained, a large visible surface area is available for inoculation with the sample.

The dye, malachite green, is inhibitory to most bacteria but not to mycobacteria. It is included in the culture medium to prevent the growth of organisms that survive the decontamination step.

Within a couple of weeks of incubation at 35–37°C, typical *M. tuberculosis* appears on LJ medium as irregular, dry colonies which are buff-coloured (beige). They are 'rough, tough and buff'. Other mycobacteria can display different colonial appearances. You can see the typical colonial appearance of mycobacteria in Figure 9.8.

Solid media need to be incubated for 10–12 weeks before they can be deemed negative. Although the MTB complex organisms will grow within a few weeks, some other mycobacteria require this extended incubation period (e.g. *M. xenopi*).

Liquid media

Mycobacteria grow more quickly in liquid culture broths than on solid media. A disadvantage of conventional liquid media is that contaminated or mixed cultures cause difficulties.

Key Point

Conventional culture methods for mycobacteria include solid and liquid media. They have the drawback of being particularly slow as visible colonies can take several weeks to grow.

9.4.5 Automated mycobacterial culture methods

The use of automated systems for mycobacterial culture is now widespread in the UK. Various automated systems are commercially available. They are all based on liquid culture and detect the growth of mycobacteria more rapidly than conventional culture.

Growth of organisms consumes oxygen and produces carbon dioxide. This may be detected by changes in:

- Radioactivity.
- Fluorescence.
- Reflectance.
- Pressure.

The use of radiolabelling is now discouraged due to waste disposal problems. The fully automated systems continuously monitor the culture bottles and flag new positives.

Despite the advantages of automated systems for mycobacterial culture, some disadvantages remain. These include the use of a single incubation temperature and the necessity for supplementary solid media.

Key Point

Automated systems for mycobacterial culture reduce the time to detection but still have limitations.

9.4.6 Identification of *Mycobacterium* spp.

Full identification of mycobacteria is not performed in routine laboratories. Testing is more efficient and more accurate when performed by reference laboratories. Following isolation of presumptive mycobacteria, laboratories issue a report to indicate that a *Mycobacterium* species has been isolated; some may add a comment relating to the likelihood of the isolate being typical *M. tuberculosis* or otherwise. A further report is issued once the organism has been fully identified.

Culture-based identification methods for mycobacteria are slow. They have largely been superseded by molecular techniques.

Cross reference
See Chapter 16.

Some molecular techniques require an amplification step to generate multiple copies of the target sequence. If a technique involves amplification, it is referred to as a nucleic acid amplification test (NAAT).

Key Point: Infection control measures for active MTB infection

Patients with MTB complex infections are infectious whereas other mycobacterial species are not associated with person-to-person transmission. Infection control measures such as patient isolation and contact tracing need to be considered for cases of active MTB infection.

---

genetic probe
A genetic probe is a nucleic acid sequence which is complementary to the target sequence.

An alternative approach for detecting known sequences is the use of **genetic probes**. If a target sequence is present, a labelled probe will hybridize with it. The label on the probe can then be detected.

Current UK guidelines recommend that a NAAT or a hybridization gene probe test should be performed within one working day of isolating MTB.

Key Point

Rapid molecular identification methods for mycobacteria have replaced conventional tests.

9.4.7 Antimicrobial susceptibility testing

TB treatment includes the long-term administration of multiple antimicrobial substances. This is arduous for the patient and expensive for the health service. It is therefore important to obtain accurate and timely information regarding the antimicrobial susceptibility of mycobacteria.

Key Point

Treatment for TB disease involves multiple antibiotics which need to be taken for 6 months.

Antimicrobial susceptibility testing of mycobacteria is generally performed by reference laboratories.

Automated liquid culture systems can be used to detect antimicrobial resistance by adding antimicrobial substances to the culture bottles.

Conventional techniques for detecting resistance to antimycobacterial drugs rely on growth, or inhibition of growth, of the organism. Since resistance arises from genetic mutations, another approach is to detect the mutations themselves. Many mutations associated with resistance have been identified and molecular tests to detect them have been developed.

Key Point: TB treatment in the UK

The antimicrobial treatment of active TB comprises two stages:

1. Initial stage: isoniazid, rifampicin, and pyrazinamide for 2 months.
2. Continuation stage: isoniazid and rifampicin are continued for a further 4 months.

Strains which are resistant to both isoniazid and rifampicin are said to be multidrug resistant (MDR). Treatment of patients with MDRTB involves the use of five drugs.

Rifampicin resistance is used as a marker for possible MDRTB. Recent statistics show that approximately 1% of UK isolates of *M. tuberculosis* are MDR but some other countries have a greater MDRTB problem, particularly in populations with a high HIV prevalence.

Key Point: Antimicrobial susceptibility testing of mycobacteria

The methods for determining antimicrobial susceptibility of mycobacteria include:

1. Absolute concentration method – determines minimum inhibitory concentration (MIC).
2. Resistance ratio method – compares MIC with that of a control strain.
3. Proportion method – determines the proportion of bacterial cells that are resistant.
4. Mycobacteriophage method – uses viruses that infect live mycobacteria but not antibiotic-killed mycobacteria.

> ### Key Point
> Antimycobacterial susceptibility testing can be based on inhibition of growth or detection of genetic mutations. Tests are generally carried out in reference laboratories.

9.4.8 Typing of mycobacteria

All new MTB complex isolates need to be typed. This means using further tests that can discriminate between multiple isolates of the same species. Many typing methods are now based on genomic differences between the isolates (genotyping) rather than on differences in their behaviour (phenotyping).

The typing method that is currently recommended enables comparisons to be made nationally or internationally. It is known as mycobacterial interspersed repetitive units–variable number tandem repeats (MIRU-VNTR) typing and is performed in reference laboratories. A 15-digit profile is obtained and entered onto a national database.

> ### Key Point
> MIRU-VNTR typing is used to discriminate between different strains of *M. tuberculosis*.

9.4.9 Immunodiagnostic tests

cytokine
A cytokine is a regulatory protein, released by cells of the immune system.

Tests that are used for diagnosing latent TB infection do not involve detection of mycobacteria; they assess the host's cell-mediated immune response by detecting a **cytokine**, interferon-gamma (IFN-γ). They are used to detect latent disease in patients who are at risk of developing active disease, that is those whose immune function is diminishing due to disease, immuno-suppressive drugs or age.

Detection of latent TB previously relied solely on the **tuberculin skin test** (TST). The TST involves the subcutaneous inoculation of a purified protein derivative of MTB.

> ### Key Point
> Latent TB can be detected using immunodiagnostic tests that are based on cytokine production.

9.5 Hazardous organisms

Many organisms are capable of causing LRTIs, most of which do not pose great risks to laboratory workers. Some, however, present a greater risk and need to be handled accordingly. *M. tuberculosis* falls into this category.

9.5.1 Classification of hazardous organisms

The Advisory Committee on Dangerous Pathogens (ACDP) is a UK advisory body whose responsibilities include:

- The classification of biological agents into **Hazard Groups**.
- The definition of **Containment Levels** for laboratory work.

Biological agents are assigned to Hazard Groups 1, 2, 3, or 4. Group 4 is the most hazardous. Table 9.4 shows the relevant considerations for each of the groups.

M. tuberculosis, M. bovis, and *M. africanum* are in Hazard Group 3, whilst many other myco-bacteria are in Hazard Group 2, including *M. avium*, *M. intracellulare* and the BCG strain of *M. bovis.*

SELF-CHECK 9.7

Which species of *Mycobacterium* most commonly cause respiratory infections? To which Hazard Groups do they belong?

Key Point

Organisms are classified by the Advisory Committee on Dangerous Pathogens (ACDP) as belonging to Hazard Group 1, 2, 3, or 4.

9.5.2 Containment Levels

The handling of clinical samples requires the use of facilities and working practices that are appropriate for the highest Hazard Group likely to be encountered. The ACDP defines four Containment Levels (1, 2, 3, and 4) for laboratory work; these directly correspond to the four Hazard Groups, for example Hazard Group 3 organisms require Containment Level 3 facilities and working practices. The general requirements for Containment Level 3 are shown next.

TABLE 9.4 Assignment of biological agents to ACDP Hazard Groups.

Hazard Group	Causes human disease?	Hazardous to workers?	Spread to community?	Effective treatment available?
1	Unlikely	No	No	N/A
2	Yes	Possibly	Unlikely	Usually
3	Yes (can be severe)	Yes (can be serious)	Possible	Usually
4	Yes (severe)	Yes (serious)	Likely	Usually not

General requirements of Containment Level 3 are as follows.

Facilities:

1. Spacious, self-contained room.
2. Dedicated equipment.
3. Easily cleanable surfaces.
4. Negative air pressure.
5. Microbiological safety cabinet.
6. High efficiency particulate absorption (HEPA) filtration of extracted air.
7. Sealable room to permit fumigation.
8. Non-opening window.
9. Wash basin near the exit.

Working Practices:

1. High standard of training and close supervision of staff.
2. Dedicated laboratory coats (autoclaved).
3. Disposable gloves must be worn.
4. The use of 'sharps' should be avoided.
5. Manipulations of organisms/samples to be carried out in a microbiological safety cabinet.
6. Documentation of procedures, maintenance records and names of staff using the facility.
7. Clear evacuation procedures in the event of an accident.

Key Point

Containment Levels 1, 2, 3, and 4 prescribe the facilities and working practices that are required for Hazard Group 1, 2, 3, and 4 organisms, respectively.

9.5.3 Microbiological safety cabinets

Containment Level 3 requirements include the use of a microbiological safety cabinet. There are three types of cabinet available: Class I, II, and III.

All three types of cabinet protect the worker from hazardous aerosols by extracting air through a HEPA filter. The greatest protection is offered by Class III cabinets as they are totally enclosed; manipulations are achieved using gloves or gauntlets. In addition to protecting the worker, Class II cabinets protect the sample by recirculating some of the extracted air, creating a downward laminar airflow. Generally, Containment Level 3 work in clinical microbiology laboratories is performed in Class I cabinets.

The airflow patterns for the three classes of cabinet can be understood by studying Figure 9.9. The airflow speed in a safety cabinet must be regularly monitored and recorded. A typical class I safety cabinet is shown in Figure 9.9.

Key Point

Containment Level 3 work is generally performed in Class I microbiological safety cabinets.

FIGURE 9.9
Airflow through microbiological safety cabinets.

9.5.4 Personal protective equipment

Another element of laboratory safety is the use of **personal protective equipment** (PPE). PPE creates a physical barrier between a worker and potential hazards. The most common forms of PPE that are used in microbiology laboratories are:

● Laboratory coats.

● Disposable gloves.

● Eye goggles.

The coats that are required for microbiological work need to fasten to the neck and have elasticated cuffs. Those that are used for Containment Level 3 work must be decontaminated by autoclaving before being washed. Concurrent use of a plastic apron overcomes the problem of laboratory coats not being waterproof.

The use of gloves is advisable, and often desirable, for Containment Level 2 work but is mandatory for Containment Level 3.

For procedures that are performed outside of the cabinet in a Containment Level 3 room, goggles provide eye protection from potential splashes.

> **Key Point**
>
> **Personal protective equipment (PPE) creates a barrier between the worker and potential hazards.**

9.5.5 Spillages

All staff who are authorized to work in a Containment Level 3 laboratory must be familiar with the protocol for spillages.

Small spillages, which are contained within a microbiological safety cabinet, only require decontamination of the surface.

Large spillages require a different course of action. All respiratory samples are treated as potentially harbouring *M. tuberculosis* so large spillages necessitate *evacuation of the room*. Microbiological safety cabinets are decontaminated by **fumigation** with formaldehyde vapour.

Key Point

Large spillages in Containment Level 3 laboratories require evacuation of the room, decontamination of surfaces and fumigation of safety cabinets.

Chapter summary

After reading this chapter you should know and understand:

- The respiratory tract is normally colonized by organisms which do not cause harm.

- The respiratory tract cleanses itself by trapping organisms in mucus and then removing the mucus by the action of cilia.

- Bacterial infections of the lower respiratory tract are usually caused by organisms descending from the upper respiratory tract and are the result of some impairment of the usual defence mechanisms.

- Laboratory investigations of lower respiratory samples (e.g. sputum) include microscopy and culture techniques.

- Interpretation of sputum cultures can be difficult due to the presence of upper respiratory organisms in badly taken samples.

- Cystic fibrosis patients experience recurrent respiratory infections due to the thick secretions resulting from their genetic defect.

- Cystic fibrosis patients are susceptible to infections with organisms that rarely affect other people, e.g. *B. cepacia* and mucoid *P. aeruginosa*.

- Mycobacteria have distinctive cell walls with a high lipid content.

- Microscopy for mycobacteria exploits their acid-fast nature.

- Traditional culture techniques for mycobacteria take several weeks.

- Automated systems for mycobacterial culture are more rapid.

- Identification, susceptibility testing, and typing of mycobacteria mostly rely on molecular techniques at reference laboratories.

- Organisms are categorized into Hazard Groups 1, 2, 3, and 4.

- If samples are likely to contain organisms from Hazard Group 3 then work must be carried out under Containment Level 3 conditions.

Further reading

- Field SK, Fisher D, Jarand JM, Cowie RL **New treatment options for multidrug-resistant tuberculosis.** *Therapeutic Advances in Respiratory Disease* 2012; **6**(5): 255–268.

  Excellent review article on TB and muti-drug resistant tuberculosis strains and impact on global health.

- Meachery G, De Soyza A, Nicholson A, *et al.* **Outcomes of lung transplantation for cystic fibrosis in a large UK cohort.** *Thorax* 2008; **63**: 725–731.

  Article discussing the survival outcomes for patients with CF who have undergone lung transplantation.

- Patel RR, Ryu JH, Vassallo R. **Cigarette smoking and diffuse lung disease.** *Drugs* 2008; **68**: 1511–1527.

  Review article which investigates the complex relationship between cigarette smoking and lung disease.

- Davies DO, Gordon SB, Davies GR. *Clinical Tuberculosis*, 5th edition. CRC Press, 2014.

  Good clinical text describing the management of patients with TB.

Discussion questions

9.1 What happens to the respiratory tract when a person smokes? How does this help bacteria to multiply and cause a chest infection?

9.2 Some of the organisms that cause respiratory tract infections are part of the normal flora. What are the processes involved in changing from normal flora to infection-producing organisms?

9.3 Why do only a very limited number of mycobacteria commonly cause human respiratory tract infections?

9.4 Organisms of the *Burkholderia cepacia* complex only cause infection in a limited range of patients. Why is this so?

10

Investigation of gastrointestinal specimens

Michael Ford and Kathy Nye

One of the most common types of infection, even in the Western world, is a gastrointestinal (GI) infection characterized by diarrhoea and/or vomiting. In the developing world, due to poor sanitation, GI disease is extremely common and associated with significant morbidity and mortality. It has been estimated that between 5 and 6 million people die each year in these areas alone as a result of GI disease. However, in a generally fit and healthy individual the symptoms of GI disease, while severe in the early stages, often resolve themselves over a few days. As a result most patients do not seek medical attention, as the disease is often self-limiting. In developing countries GI disease is more severe due to the health of those infected and the difficulties in obtaining basic therapies such as easy access to clean water for oral rehydration therapy (ORT). In addition, the infection is more likely to spread as sanitation is often less than adequate.

It must be remembered that not all cases of diarrhoea have an infectious cause and it can be due to various forms of bowel disease such as IBD, extremes of dietary intake, or other forms of forms of food contamination such as chemical contamination. Of the infectious causes of GI disease, it is estimated that around 1 in 5 people (approximately 9.5 million people) in England will suffer every year. Of these, only 1 in 7 will go to their doctor and still fewer will have samples sent to a laboratory for examination. Even when the most rigorous techniques are used, no causative microorganism will be detected in half to two-thirds of cases. This may be because there are other infectious causes of gastrointestinal disease which are, as yet, unknown to us, or, perhaps, that known organisms are present in numbers too small to detect.

SELF-CHECK 10.1

Why do you think that only a small number of infected patients seek medical attention and even fewer submit a stool sample?

In this chapter, you will discover how microbiologists detect and identify the major, known, microbiological causes of gastrointestinal disease as well as an insight into their epidemiology, pathogenicity, and clinical management . Despite gastrointestinal samples being most unpleasant to process, most biomedical scientists would agree that enteric microbiology is one of the most interesting and challenging areas to work in.

Learning objectives

After reading this chapter you should be able to:

- Recognize the major microbiological pathogens implicated in gastrointestinal disease.
- Understand the principal techniques available for the detection of these pathogens.
- Describe the main mechanisms involved in the production of disease.
- Outline the methods available for their identification and differentiation.
- List the options for patient management and control of infection.
- Understand the technical limitations of current methods and how to make best use of reference facilities.

10.1 The general principles of the investigation of gastrointestinal disease

Essentially the gastrointestinal tract is just one long tube which starts at the mouth and runs for around 10 metres including the oesophagus, stomach, small, and large intestines, ending at the anus (Figure 10.1). Each part of the gastrointestinal tract has particular mechanisms designed to prevent an infectious process developing.

The pathogen's journey begins when taken into the mouth, most often via food or drink. However, contamination via the hands or inanimate objects can also introduce gastrointestinal pathogens into the mouth. The latter is especially true of young children. Once ingested, they are quickly recognized as alien and various defence systems are triggered. These fall into five different categories; that is pH, the normal microflora, gut motility, immunity, and enzymes.

There are no significant defence mechanisms in the mouth as this is only to assist in the breakdown of food before it reaches the stomach. However, the taste buds can help in the recognition that food is 'off' due to breakdown of the food by spoilage organisms, as a result the food should be ejected from the mouth, which would lessen the chances of developing GI disease. The nose also plays an important role in ensuring food is not consumed as detection of bacterial products and spoilage is possible. Have you noticed how many people smell their food before consuming? This is a good protective mechanism!

The main host defence mechanism is the acidity of the normal stomach which has a pH of <4. The food, churned around in the stomach vessel, is bathed at pH 4. At such a low pH >99.9% of ingested Gram-negative enteric organisms are killed in under 30 minutes and thus play no further role in the initiation of infection. It is worth nothing that if this acidity is reduced such as in patients with achlorhydria or those receiving drugs to reduce gastric acid production, they are more susceptible to GI disease as potential pathogens may not be killed in the stomach.

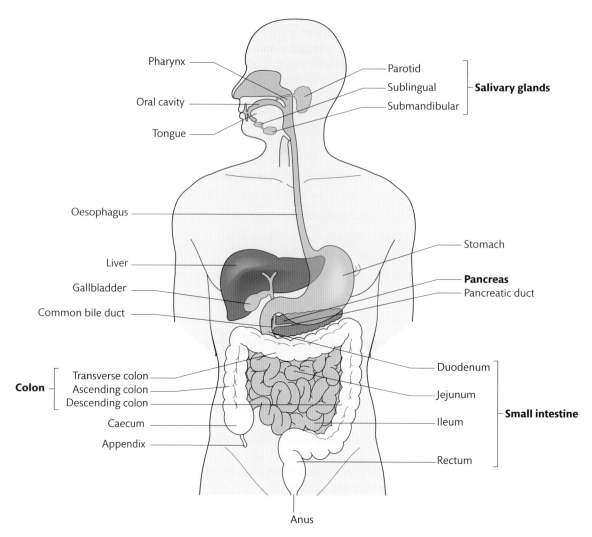

FIGURE 10.1
Diagram of the human gastrointestinal tract.

Phagocytes (white cells) and immunoglobulins (e.g. IgA) are abundant in the lining of the gut and form a further line of defence. In addition, the presence of digestive enzymes which help create a hostile environment, and gut motility (**peristalsis**) keep the intestinal contents moving along so an infectious process is difficult to initiate.

The normal microbial inhabitants of the bowel are also vitally important. These organisms, usually bacteria and protozoa, form a tightly knit and finely balanced community, surviving on the internal surface (**epithelium**) of the gut, along its entire length. By means of complex interactions, which are still poorly understood, they work to prevent harmful microbes from becoming established and boost immunity to disease.

> ### Key Point
> There are numerous host mechanisms to ensure that it is very difficult for a microorganism to initiate gastrointestinal disease.

SELF-CHECK 10.2

What host mechanisms are involved to ensure that harmful microbes don't cause gastrointestinal infections?

This competition with other organisms in the GI tract is best demonstrated if the numbers of competing organisms are considered. In the fluid of the small intestine around a million (mainly Gram-positive bacteria) per millilitre of fluid are observed and more than 10^{11} mixed organisms per gram of faeces in the large bowel. The majority of these are anaerobic bacteria. This is a vast number of organisms and you can see why it is difficult for pathogenic organisms to promote infection especially after they have been bathed in stomach acid first!

The host defences weaken over time through age, illness, drugs, malnutrition etc., and individually or combined can render a person more susceptible to all infectious intestinal diseases. However, the likelihood of individuals developing such disease depends not only upon their own susceptibility, but also on the capacity of the organism to cause illness (its **virulence** and the dose ingested), and upon the opportunity for exposure, that is what the person ate or drank, where they have been and at what time of year. Many gastrointestinal infections have a definite seasonal variation and may be particularly prevalent in specific geographical areas. Most laboratories see an increase in faeces samples in the summer, as foreign holidays and poorly cooked food on barbeques result in an increase in diarrhoeal episodes.

Once the patient is infected, it will take some time before a susceptible person develops signs of illness, which may be hours or days. This time, during which the infection develops, is called the **incubation period** and varies within generally accepted ranges for each pathogen.

The most common symptoms are diarrhoea, nausea and/or vomiting, and abdominal pain, although, in some circumstances, systemic upset such as fever, headache and general malaise may be prominent features. The nature of the diarrhoea (e.g. presence of blood, watery consistency, etc.) may give clues as to the cause.

Although in the developed world most people recover quickly from gastrointestinal infections, severe and sometimes life-threatening infections are still seen, particularly in those who are already vulnerable, for example, the very young, the elderly and those debilitated through illness. Even in the otherwise healthy, this type of infection accounts for many working days lost and consequently major economic losses.

In large parts of the world where nutrition and healthcare are poor, simple intestinal infections are still important causes of death, especially in young children.

virulence

Virulence is the ability of a microorganism to cause disease. Various factors are involved in this such as the ability to adhere to the gastrointestinal tract for example.

incubation period

This is the length of time between exposure to the organism and when symptoms begin.

SELF-CHECK 10.3

How severe are gastrointestinal diseases in the Western world compared to the developing world? What are the reasons for these differences?

When samples, usually of faeces, are submitted to the laboratory for investigation, it will not be possible or practical to attempt to look for all potential causes of infection. For this reason, the microbiologist must decide which causes are most likely, based on any information available. In practice, investigations are selected to cover the most common and severe infections, with additional testing depending upon what is known about the patient and where they have travelled recently.

10.2 Bacterial pathogens associated with gastrointestinal disease

An overview of the main features of infection by the principal bacterial pathogens is provided in Table 10.1.

TABLE 10.1 Clinical features and other factors associated with common bacterial enteric pathogens.

Bacterium		Usual incubation period	Main clinical features	Usual duration of symptoms	Source	Usual infectious dose
Campylobacter spp.		2–5 days	D, AP, F, B	2–7 days	F, W, A	10^2–10^6
Salmonella spp. (excluding enteric fever)		12 h–3 days	D, V, F	2–7 days	F, PP, A	10^5
Shigella spp.		1–7 days	D, B	Up to 2 weeks	F, W, PP	10^1–10^2
Clostridium perfringens		12–18 h	D, AP	24 h	F	10^5
Clostridium difficile		1–7 days	D, B	Highly variable	PP, via contaminated environment	N/A
Escherichia coli (VTEC)		1–6 days	D, B, kidney failure	4–6 days if uncomplicated	F, W, A, PP	$<10^2$
Bacillus cereus	Emetic illness	1–5 h	V, N (D, AP)	24 h	F	N/A
	Diarrhoeal illness	8–16 h	D, N (V & AP)	24 h	F	N/A
Other *Bacillus* spp.		1–15 h	D +/- N, V, AP	24 h	F	N/A
Staphylococcus aureus		2–4 h	V +/- AP/F	12–48 h	F	N/A
Salmonella typhi (enteric fevers)		1–3 weeks	F and general malaise	10–14 days	F, PP	10^5
Vibrio cholerae		2–3 days	D (watery)	1–7 days	F, W	10^8
Other *Vibrio* spp.		12–18 h	D	1–7 days	F	10^8
Yersinia spp.		3–7 days	D, AP, F	1–3 weeks	F, A	10^9

Clinical features key: D, diarrhoea; B, blood in faeces; V, vomiting; AP, abdominal pain; N, nausea; F, fever.
Source key: F, contaminated food; W, contaminated water; PP, person to person (faeco-oral); A, contact with animals.

10.2.1 *Campylobacter* species

Campylobacters are one of the most frequently isolated and characteristic bacteria causing GI disease. They are found in and excreted from the gut of a wide variety of domestic and wild animals and birds, but are particularly common in poultry. As a result, outbreaks have been associated with under-cooked meat, particularly poultry, and increased numbers of infections are seen during the 'barbeque' season. However, the majority of infections are believed to occur sporadically. Although many species exist, most cases of human disease are caused by *C. jejuni* and, to a lesser extent, *C. coli*, which are often associated with eating under-cooked poultry meat or food which has been cross-contaminated from raw meat. Campylobacters are not normally transmitted from person to person. Infection with a pathogenic *Campylobacter* often results in severe abdominal pain and the appearance of blood in the stools. This indicates the individual is more likely to be infected with *Campylobacter* than other bacterial causes, especially if no foreign travel has occurred. Figure 10.2 shows the characteristic 'S' shape of the organism when seen on electron microscopy.

FIGURE 10.2
Electron micrograph of *Campylobacter jejuni*. Note its characteristic 'S' shape.
Source: Courtesy of De Wood, Pooley, USDA, ARS, EMU.

10.2.2 *Salmonella* species

After campylobacters, salmonellae are the next most commonly isolated bacterial cause of infectious intestinal disease. Interestingly, *Salmonella* infection is believed to occur more frequently than *Campylobacter*, but because the symptoms of the latter are more severe it is believed more patients seek medical help resulting in an increased isolation rate for *Campylobacter*. The organisms are found in a wide range of animals and birds, which often carry them without any symptoms. Several thousand different types of *Salmonella* have been identified, but the two most commonly found in the UK are *S. enteritidis* and *S. typhimurium*.

Salmonella disease is often attributed to the consumption of under-cooked or contaminated food, but person-to-person spread is also important. Salmonellae usually cause gastrointestinal infection but some species are said to be 'host-adapted', that is they are able to cause severe, systemic disease in specific animal species. In humans, *S. typhi* and *S. paratyphi* are the agents of typhoid and paratyphoid respectively, known as the enteric fevers. After an incubation period of around 2 weeks they produce a septicaemia with high fever and 'flu-like' symptoms. Diarrhoea may develop but is not the principal feature of the illness and culture from the stool sample may be negative. Infection is acquired from other humans, either by direct person-to-person spread or indirectly via food and water contaminated by human sewage. Naturally, it is a greater problem in areas of the world where sanitation is poor and most cases identified in the UK are acquired abroad.

In vulnerable people, the food-poisoning salmonellae can sometimes cause a typhoid-like illness.

carrier state
A carrier state is where an individual, who is not ill, can harbour an infectious organism which may cause disease if it is passed on.

After infection with any salmonellae, the bacteria can be excreted in faeces for several weeks or months even after clinical recovery. This is described as a **carrier state** and people carrying salmonellae remain a potential source of infection to others unless they pay scrupulous attention to personal hygiene.

10.2.3 *Shigella* species

These bacteria are human pathogens and are not found in animals. A very low infective dose is required for development of disease and they are transmitted easily between people via contaminated food and water. Four species exist, of which only *S. sonnei* is a significant cause of diarrhoeal illness in the UK. *S. sonnei* is the mildest form of shigellosis and tends to cause outbreaks involving young children in nurseries, schools, and mental health facilities where it is difficult to ensure good personal hygiene.

Shigellae cause classical bacillary dysentery, which is diarrhoea characterized by the presence of blood and mucus in the stool, accompanied by fever and abdominal cramps. *S. dysenteriae* causes the most severe disease and in common with *S. flexneri* and *S. boydii*, is usually acquired in parts of the world where sanitation is poor. In the UK, the isolation of one of these *Shigella* types is almost always from patients who have travelled abroad.

Bacillary dysentery can be life threatening, particularly amongst populations already debilitated by malnutrition and illness. It has been said that in several military campaigns of previous centuries, bacillary dysentery killed more people than war-related injuries.

10.2.4 *Escherichia coli*

E. coli forms part of the normal gut flora of man as well as many animals and birds, and whilst generally harmless, several distinct strains can act as human pathogens causing diarrhoeal illness by a variety of mechanisms. Strains recognized as pathogenic include enteropathogenic *E. coli* (EPEC), enterotoxigenic *E. coli* (ETEC), enteroinvasive *E. coli* (EIEC), enteroaggregative *E. coli* (EAEC), and diffusely adherent *E. coli* (DAEC).

Their isolation and characterization is difficult due to their similarity to most *E. coli* strains, which are relatively harmless and as most infections are mild and self-limiting, the majority of laboratories are not equipped to look for them. However, one group of *E. coli* strains is capable of producing a severe illness with bloody diarrhoea and complications include kidney failure and derangement of blood clotting. These are the verocytotoxin-producing *E. coli* or VTEC.

The most common VTEC is identified by its possession of the polysaccharide antigen O157. The infecting dose is very low, less than 100 organisms. VTEC are found in cattle and a number of other food animals. Infection is usually acquired by eating under-cooked or cross-contaminated meat or by direct contact with infected animals or their faeces. Contamination of water and milk may also occur and person-to-person spread is a frequent feature. A number of large, foodborne outbreaks have been described, with a particularly high rate of serious complications in those affected. In June 2011 an outbreak occurred in Germany with a rare serotype O104 with several deaths linked to the outbreak. The source of the outbreak was believed to be beansprouts. Methods used for the identification of *E. coli* O157 would not have worked to detect this strain, but since the disease has characteristic symptoms reference laboratories were able to pinpoint the cause as *E. coli* O104.

10.2.5 *Vibrio* species

Vibrio species are found in surface and sea waters around the world. Several species are capable of producing human disease, the most important being *V. cholerae*, which, as its name suggests, is the cause of cholera.

Cholera is acquired via contaminated water or food and produces a range of illness from a mild gastrointestinal upset to profuse, watery diarrhoea, which, if untreated, may kill the patient in a few hours due to severe fluid and electrolyte loss (Figure 10.3). Some patients, however, may have no symptoms at all, while others may recover and become chronic carriers. In times past, cholera has been responsible for a number of major **pandemics**. Its infective dose is generally far higher than for other gastrointestinal pathogens as it is highly susceptible to acid found in the stomach.

Several variants of *V. cholerae* have been identified, which have subtly different clinical and epidemiological characteristics.

pandemic
A pandemic is an epidemic that occurs over a wide geographical area such as a region or even worldwide.

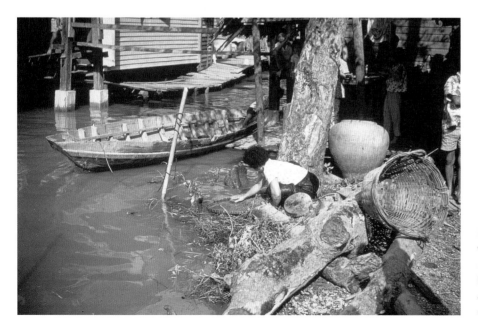

FIGURE 10.3
Image of a contaminated water supply with *V. cholerae*. Note the environment and how easy it is for transmission of the organism to occur under such conditions.

V. parahaemolyticus causes a milder, diarrhoeal illness, as a result of eating raw or under-cooked seafood, or food rinsed by contaminated seawater. A number of other *Vibrio* species have also been implicated in the causation of diarrhoea but their precise role is less well documented.

10.2.6 *Yersinia* species

Y. enterocolitica is the main species associated with human gastrointestinal disease and often gives rise to symptoms similar to those of appendicitis. Only a small number of strains are capable of causing illness and must possess specific virulence factors in order to act as pathogens.

Y. enterocolitica is found in the normal gut flora of many mammals, including pigs, sheep, and cattle, and it is thought that most cases result from eating undercooked meat. A particular feature of infection is its prolonged duration and potential to give rise to chronic, immune-mediated complications such as arthritis.

10.2.7 *Bacillus cereus*

These bacteria are extremely widespread in the environment and are able to form resistant spores to survive adverse conditions. Spores are found on many cereal crops (e.g. rice and wheat).

When the cooking process is insufficient to destroy all spores, for example, when boiling rice, and the food is left unrefrigerated post-cooking, the spores develop into vegetative bacteria, growing quickly to large numbers. During the period of exponential growth, toxins are formed which cannot be denatured by brief re-heating of the food. It is these toxins which cause disease. A classic example of this type of food poisoning occurs when boiled rice, left unrefrigerated overnight, is stir-fried briefly before consumption. The resulting illness is known as 'Chinese restaurant syndrome'. *B. cereus* is the most commonly implicated species and, in this case, two different toxins may be formed. The first, an **emetic toxin**, produces vomiting 1–5 h after ingestion, and the second, a diarrhoeal toxin, produces diarrhoea after 8–16 h.

Both syndromes are unpleasant, but short-lived and rarely cause serious illness, and come to public attention mainly when outbreaks occur rather than sporadic cases.

emetic toxin

This is a toxin which causes severe often projectile vomiting and such a symptom can be characteristic of *B. cereus* food poisoning.

10.2.8 *Staphylococcus aureus*

S. aureus is carried on the skin and in the nose of humans and many animals. Food may contain *S. aureus* for three main reasons: (a) because it was present in the food animal itself; (b) because of contamination from a food handler carrying *S. aureus*; or (c) because of cross-contamination from another source, for example raw to cooked meat. If conditions allow the organism to multiply to high levels in the food, heat-stable enterotoxins are formed which cause the abrupt onset of vomiting a few hours after ingestion. Foods most often implicated in this type of food poisoning are confectionery products, which require a lot of handling, and processed meats.

10.2.9 *Clostridium difficile*

Cross reference
See Chapter 12, Section 12.5.

C. difficile is an anaerobe, which is a normal component of the gut microflora in a proportion of the normal, healthy population, particularly in young children and the elderly. Some strains are capable of producing one or both of two potent toxins, known as toxins A and B, although having the capability to produce toxin does not necessarily mean that the toxins will actually be produced. The toxins can, in predisposed individuals, cause diarrhoea of varying severity, which may be prolonged and difficult to treat.

Predisposed individuals are those with some disturbance of the normal bowel flora, which allows the infection to become established. **Broad-spectrum antibiotics** often cause this disturbance, so it tends to be found most frequently in patients already in health-care settings. Patients with *C. difficile* diarrhoea contaminate their environment widely with resistant spores capable of infecting other susceptible patients via the inanimate environment. These properties make *C. difficile* the foremost cause of hospital-acquired diarrhoea.

Cross reference

Full consideration of *C. difficile* diarrhoea is given in Chapter 12.

Key Point

Not all *C. difficile* strains produce toxins A and B, even though they may have the capacity to do so, however, the majority of strains implicated in disease produce both.

10.2.10 *Clostridium perfringens*

This anaerobic organism makes up part of the normal gut flora of man and many animals. It is able to form highly resistant spores in order to survive under extreme conditions. When large numbers of these bacteria are eaten, they form spores in the adverse environment of the small intestine and, in doing so, release a potent toxin which causes diarrhoea and abdominal pain. Illness is unpleasant, but short-lived and self-limiting.

Thorough cooking at high temperature will kill both vegetative bacteria and spores, problems arise when meat-based foods are subjected to inadequate cooking temperatures and then kept warm for several hours. Warm holding temperatures (e.g. in a bain-marie) allow any surviving spores to develop and multiply quickly to levels sufficient to cause illness.

SELF-CHECK 10.5

Which gastrointestinal infections are seen most in (a) developing countries and (b) developed nations?

10.3 Mechanisms involved in the production of disease by bacterial causes of intestinal infection

Cross reference

See Chapter 15.

There are three principal mechanisms whereby bacteria cause intestinal disease: the first is adhesion by attachment to the gut epithelial cells, invasion of the intestinal epithelial cells and production of toxins. Organisms may utilize one or more of these mechanisms. Many are associated with the possession of specific **transmissible plasmids** coding for the production of virulence factors. For most organisms, mechanisms of pathogenicity are still not completely understood.

- Epithelial adherence: this mechanism is best described in strains of pathogenic *E. coli* where the possession of certain surface antigens, or adhesins, allows the bacterium to attach to the surface of intestinal epithelial cells. Obviously, this gives the bacterium an advantage in terms of ability to colonize the gut, but also brings it into close proximity with

transmissible plasmids

A plasmid is an extra chromosomal DNA particle which can carry genes for antibiotic resistance and virulence factors, e.g. toxins. If they are transmissible then these genes can be acquired by other organisms.

the site of action of its toxins and creates a base from which to invade the deeper layers of the epithelium. Some strains of *E. coli* appear to be able to cause damage to the epithelium at the point of attachment, causing diarrhoea as a result.

- Epithelial invasion: although often accompanied by toxin production, most of the major bacterial causes of gastrointestinal disease, i.e. *Campylobacter*, *Salmonella*, *Shigella*, and *E. coli* are capable of epithelial invasion. This is, again, a plasmid-mediated property and usually depends upon modifications of the 'O' side chain antigens of cell wall lipopolysaccharides.

- Food poisoning salmonellae, like campylobacters, usually invade only the superficial layers of the epithelium lining the small intestine and, to a lesser extent, the colon, where they cause inflammation and an increase in gut motility. It is possible that they also produce toxins, although this has not been firmly established. Occasionally, invading bacteria may reach the bloodstream, causing a bacteraemia carrying infection to other parts of the body.

- In the enteric fevers, bacteria invade deeply via the lymphoid tissue (Peyer's patches) of the small intestine, rapidly leading to bacteraemia rather than diarrhoea.

- Shigellae and some strains of *E. coli* have a particular capacity to burrow into and destroy the superficial layers of the colonic epithelium leading to diarrhoea with blood and mucus, but they rarely penetrate beyond the mucosa, even in severe cases of dysentery.

- Toxin production: toxins produced by bacteria causing gastrointestinal disease fall into three groups: neurotoxins, enterotoxins, and cytotoxins. Production is usually plasmid-mediated and most are polypeptide molecules.

The neurotoxins act on the nervous system of the host to produce symptoms, and, as they are often eaten as pre-formed toxins, have a very short incubation period. Examples of neurotoxins are found in *Staphylococcus aureus* (toxin B) and *Bacillus cereus* (emetic toxin).

adenylate cyclase

This is an intracellular enzyme which catalyses the conversion of ATP to cyclic AMP (cAMP). Increased cAMP results in an outpouring of fluids resulting in diarrhoea and dehydration.

Enterotoxins have a direct effect upon the intestinal epithelium, mainly by causing an irreversible activation of **adenylate cyclase** in the epithelial cells. High levels of cyclic AMP accumulate, causing cell membrane proteins to permit loss of water from the blood into the gut. This fluid loss may be catastrophic, for example in cholera, where death is usually the result of extreme fluid and electrolyte loss.

Apart from *V. cholerae*, other organisms producing varying amounts of enterotoxin are *Shigella dysenteriae*, *C. perfringens*, and *B. cereus*, as well as some strains of pathogenic *E. coli*. *C. difficile* produces two toxins, A and B, of which A is a potent enterotoxin.

Cytotoxins, as their name suggests, actually destroy intestinal epithelial cells causing inflammatory diarrhoea. Perhaps the best known of these is the highly potent Shiga toxin produced by *S. dysenteriae* type 1. *C. perfringens* and verocytotoxin-producing *E. coli* also produce a Shiga-like cytotoxin. *V. parahaemolyticus* and *C. difficile* produce different cytotoxins, although their effects are similar. In the case of *C. difficile*, the cytotoxin is known as toxin B.

A number of other virulence factors are known to exist, including the production of **mucinase**, which presumably aids access to the epithelial cell membrane by breaking down the slimy mucus protecting it, and bacterial motility (e.g. in *V. cholerae*), although there is still a great deal that is not understood about the precise contributions of various mechanisms to the production of disease.

10.4 **Isolation media and how they work**

obligate anaerobes

These are bacteria which only grow when no oxygen is present.

The isolation of pathogenic bacteria from faecal material is extremely difficult. There are around 10^{11} bacteria in every gram of faeces, just over 95% of which are **obligate anaerobes**.

The rest represent a wide variety of organisms, the majority of which are Gram-negative bacilli known collectively as the Enterobacteriaceae. Looking for pathogens, which are often present in relatively small numbers, is, therefore, like looking for needles in haystacks. This is made even more difficult by the fact that some pathogens, for example, *Shigella* spp., are closely related to organisms which are part of the normal intestinal flora, such as *E. coli*. Pathogens such as *Clostridium perfringens* and *Clostridium difficile* whilst recognized as part of the normal bacterial flora, only become pathogenic in certain circumstances. For this reason, it is rarely possible to definitively state than an organism is causing the patient's symptoms simply by isolating colonies of it on an agar plate.

The basic principle of isolation is to encourage the growth of the target organism(s) by exploiting their metabolic characteristics while inhibiting as many other organisms as possible (selection). Some organisms may be present in such low numbers that it would be unlikely, on a purely statistical basis, to have much chance of isolating them from small amounts of faecal material containing vast numbers of 'normal flora' type organisms.

As a result of this, for *Salmonella* in particular it is usual to spend some time attempting to increase their numbers (enrichment), relative to the normal flora, in order to have a better chance of isolating them on selective culture media. In the case of *Salmonella* spp. this is achieved by inoculating an amount of faeces into a 'selective enrichment broth'.

Broth is chosen because it provides ideal conditions for bacterial multiplication. After a few hours of incubation, the broth can be subcultured onto a selective, solid medium. Obviously, simple measures such as aerobic incubation will suppress the growth of all obligate anaerobes, but a thorough knowledge of the action of various antibacterial chemicals and antibiotics is necessary to design a medium which suppresses all but the target organism.

There is no single medium that can select for all enteric pathogens or even all members of the same genus of pathogens. For example some of the many species of salmonellae have sufficiently different characteristics that optimal isolation would only be achieved by using specific media for each.

After enrichment and/or plating onto selective media, there will usually still be a number of 'normal flora' organisms growing alongside any potential pathogens. Isolation media are designed to make it easier to differentiate these two groups by, once again, exploiting their different metabolic characteristics using one or more indicator systems.

Cross reference
See Chapter 3.

Table 10.2 provides a summary of the media most frequently used in the UK for the isolation of enteric pathogens and their methods of identification.

For *Bacillus cereus* and *Clostridium perfringens*, it is important to know roughly how many organisms are present in the faecal material, as both may be found in small numbers in normal, healthy people. Selective media can be used but it is best practice to dilute the faeces and then plate out the dilution in order to estimate the number of bacteria present in the sample. As some organisms may be present as spores, a more reliable estimate of both spores and vegetative bacteria can be obtained by additionally incubating the sample in 95% ethanol before dilutions are made so that vegetative bacteria are destroyed.

Key Point

Spores are resting cells associated with *Bacillus* and *Clostridium* spp. As conditions improve the spores 'generate' into vegetative cells and on media appear as the typical organism.

TABLE 10.2 Guide to the isolation and identification of common bacterial enteric pathogens.

Bacterium	Enrichment (time)	Selective medium	Selective agents	Incubation (atmosphere/ temperature)	Colonial appearance	Identification
Campylobacter	N/A	CCDA (charcoal, cefoperazone desoxycholate) agar	Amphotericin, cefoperazone, sodium desoxycholate	Microaerophilic/ 42°C	Grey, moist, pink or metallic sheen often noted	Typical 'gull wing' appearance on Gram stain
Salmonella	Selenite cysteine or Rappaport-Vassiliadis broth (16–24 h)	XLD (xylose lysine desoxycholate) agar Chromogenic medium such as Harlequin™ Salmonella ABC	Sodium desoxycholate	Aerobic/37°C	Red with black centre. H₂S negative strains red colonies only. Green colonies	Biochemical and serological profiles
Shigella	N/A	XLD (xylose lysine desoxycholate) agar	Sodium desoxycholate	Aerobic/37°C	Red	Biochemical and serological profiles
VTEC	N/A	CT-SMAC (cefixime, tellurite sorbitol MacConkey) agar	Cefixime, potassium tellurite, bile salts	Aerobic/37°C	Colourless	Biochemical profile and agglutination with specific antiserum
V. cholerae V. parahaemolyticus	Alkaline peptone water (5–8 h)	TCBS (thiosulphate, citrate, bile, sucrose) agar	Ox bile, sodium chloride	Aerobic/37°C	Yellow Blue-green	Biochemical profile
Yersinia enterocolitica	N/A for routine culture	CIN (cefsulodin, irgasan, novobiocin) agar	Cefsulodin, irgasan, novobiocin, sodium desoxycholate	Aerobic/30°C	Pale periphery, red centre–'bulls eye' colonies	Biochemical profile
Clostridium perfringens	N/A	Neomycin blood agar	Neomycin sulphate	Anaerobic/37°C	Large, convex, shiny +/- haemolytic	Motility test Nagler reaction Lactose/sucrose utilization
Clostridium difficile	N/A	CCEY (cycloserine, cefoxitin, egg yolk) agar	Cefoxitin, D-cycloserine	Anaerobic/37°C	Yellow, 'ground glass' appearance with serrated edge	Agglutination of colonies with specific antisera
Bacillus cereus	N/A	B. cereus selective agar (PEMBA)	Polymyxin B	Aerobic/37°C	Peacock blue with zone of blue precipitation	Typical appearance on spare/lipid staining

Why are enrichment broths used for the detection of *Salmonella* but not *Shigella* spp. from faeces samples?

10.5 Identification of bacterial pathogens isolated from faeces samples

Presumptive identification of enteric pathogens can be made by examining the characteristics of colonies growing on the selective isolation medium and by performing a few simple tests.

Colonies of bacteria appear very different depending on the culture medium used. For example, on xylose lysine desoxycholate agar (XLD), *Salmonella* and *Shigella* spp. both appear as red colonies. Most *Salmonella* spp. will also have a black centre due to the production of hydrogen sulphide (Figure 10.4). A small number of non-pathogenic bacteria produce identical colonies (e.g. *Proteus* and *Citrobacter freundii*). In order to narrow the identification down further, suspect colonies are tested for the enzyme urease which exists preformed (high levels) in *Proteus* spp. Salmonellae and shigellae do not produce urease, so only negative colonies need to be investigated further. Even at this stage (black colonies which are urease negative), it is still possible that the colonies are not *Salmonella*, although the probability is low.

One of the problems associated with media such as XLD for detection of *Salmonella*, is that it can be quite time consuming to rule out other organisms which look the same on the medium. As a result several chromogenic media have been developed where more specific biochemical properties of the *Salmonella* strain are exploited so plates can be read faster as 'interfering' organisms such as *Proteus* spp. in particular do not resemble colonies of *Salmonella*. A good

FIGURE 10.4
XLD plate showing the typical colonial appearance of *Salmonella typhimurium*. Note the typical black colonies due to the organism producing hydrogen sulphide.
Source: Courtesy of Emma Marrs.

FIGURE 10.5

Harlequin™ Salmonella ABC showing typical green *Salmonella* colonies. These are easy to distinguish from non-pathogens growing on the media which appear most often as black colonies.

Source: Courtesy of M. Ford.

example is Harlequin™ Salmonella ABC medium where presumptive *Salmonella* appear as green colonies and other organisms appear as either black or colourless colonies (Figure 10.5). When used to subculture Selenite enrichment broths, such media can considerably reduce the scientist's workload.

10.5.1 Agglutination tests

All bacteria possess a variety of antigenic compounds on the cell surface, to which specific antisera can be raised in animals. In Gram-negative bacteria, it is usually the polysaccharide **'O' antigen**, forming part of the cell wall that has properties characteristic of the particular strain. By reacting bacterial suspensions with a series of specific antisera, many organisms can be attributed to serogroups and specific serotypes.

flagellae

These are hair-like projections which project from the cell body. Their primary function is locomotion.

If the bacterium possesses **flagellae**, antisera to these 'H' antigens can also be used further to subdivide the strains. For the typing of *Salmonella*, both 'O' and 'H' agglutination tests are used. This involves the use of polyvalent antisera where antibodies to several common *Salmonella* types are contained within one vial. Essentially, if the test organism agglutinates against this, the strongly suspicion is that the organism is a *Salmonella*. Since this antisera is polyvalent the organism can then be agglutinated against individual serotypes. This process can also be performed using polyvalent antisera against the flagella (H antigens) of *Salmonella*. For example, strains agglutinating with 04 antisera are most likely to be *Salmonella typhimurium* and 09 *Salmonella enteritidis*, although the more serious *S. typhi* also agglutinates with 09 antisera.

Key Point

Remember that *Salmonella* strains can have a similar antigenic structure to non-pathogenic Gram-negative rods, so a positive agglutination test must be considered a presumptive identification only. Biochemical tests will provide a more definitive identification than the use of antisera alone.

There are several media available for the isolation of *Campylobacter* spp. from stool samples. The variation is in the choice of selective supplement. Generally the supplement consists of an antifungal agent such as amphotericin B, and both Gram-negative and Gram-positive selective agents. A selective broth is available for enrichment of small numbers of organisms.

Since these organisms are **microaerophilles** it is essential that the plates are incubated in this environment as soon as possible. Following 24–48 h incubation, characteristic effuse wet colonies are seen often with a pink or metallic sheen. Selectivity can be increased by incubation at 42 °C.

Confirmation is by characteristic curved or 'S' shaped appearance (Figure 10.2) on a Gram stain. Human pathogenic *Campylobacter* spp. such as C. *jejuni* are typically oxidase and hippurate positive. As MALDI-TOF instruments are now being used routinely, the identification of many pathogens associated with GI disease has become faster, more reliable, and far less labour-intensive.

Sorbitol MacConkey's agar is used for the selective isolation of E. *coli* O157 strains. Commonly the medium is supplemented with cefixime and potassium tellurite to improve selectivity for E. *coli* O157 strains generally. Cefixime is an antibiotic to which Gram-negative strains in particular are susceptible, however, E. *coli* O157 strains are quite resistant to it. Differentiation of E. *coli* O157 strains is achieved because they generally fail to ferment the sorbitol in the medium, in contrast to other 'normal flora' E. *coli* strains. As a result E. *coli* O157 strains appear as 'pale colonies' on Sorbitol MacConkey agar. Confirmation is through the use of serological tests (agglutination with antisera) and/or biochemical/MALDI-TOF identification. Generally, if the isolate is suspected of being an E. *coli* O157 it would be forwarded to a reference laboratory to confirm the presence of toxin genes.

The medium thiosulphate, citrate, bile, sucrose (TCBS) agar is used for the selective isolation of pathogenic vibrios. The medium has a high alkaline pH and this helps to improve selectivity as most enteric organisms will only grow well around neutral pH. Typically V. *cholera* strains are isolated as large yellow colonies due to the fermentation of sucrose and the acidity causing a change in the indicator from blue to yellow. Other vibrios such as V. *vulnificus* and V. *parahae-molyticus* appear as blue–green colonies due to lack of sucrose fermentation. Confirmation would be biochemically and/or with MALDI-TOF.

Table 10.1 provides a guide to the isolation and identification of common bacterial enteric pathogens together with typical colonial characteristics.

Once a pathogen is suspected on the isolation medium, the biomedical scientist can now proceed to fully identify the organism using more complex tests, generally based on the metabolic and biochemical properties of the suspected pathogen. Each organism has a well-established metabolic and biochemical profile which will enable confident identification in the majority of cases. These are often performed using kit systems (e.g. API). In many laboratories identification is moving away from using biochemical tests to the use of MALDI-TOF systems, which can provide and identification in minutes rather than overnight incubation. This is important for epidemiological control.

microaerophillic

Microaerophillic is a term applied to organisms such as *Campylobacter* spp. whereby the organisms require an environment containing a reduced oxygen level for optimal growth. Many microphiles also require an elevated concentration of carbon dioxide (>5%).

Cross reference
See Chapter 2.

SELF-CHECK 10.7

If a colony is red on XLD with a black centre does it mean it is a *Salmonella*? If not why not?

For food poisoning salmonellae and shigellae, the exact speciesis confirmed by serological testing. Suspensions of the organism are mixed with a series of specific antisera raised against characteristic antigens. According to the agglutination patterns detected, species or, in the case of *Salmonella enterica*, serovars can be identified.

For salmonellae, a complex serotyping scheme has been developed over the years, which is known as the **Kauffmann–White scheme**. This scheme is dependent upon the reactions of suspensions of salmonellae with crude antisera raised against other strains. By painstaking comparisons, different antigenic groups were identified and designated as *Salmonella* 'species'. It was discovered later that the *Salmonella* antigens were derived from three sources: the 'O' polysaccharide component of the bacterial cell wall, the 'H' flagellar antigens, present in most strains and the 'Vi' virulence antigen which is a specialized polysaccharide, capsular antigen, present mainly, but not exclusively, in *S. typhi*.

Kauffmann–White's original scheme developed with specific antisera raised against these three antigenic structures. It was found that each strain could possess several 'O' determinants and, on this basis, they could be attributed to a particular 'O' group; for example, group A salmonellae such as *S. paratyphi* possess 'O' antigen 2 as their major determinant. Further subdivision can be achieved on the basis of the flagellar 'H' antigens.

Although initially treated as separate species, of which there are currently well over 1,500, these strains are now recognized as serovars of *Salmonella enterica* and are named as such, for example *S. enterica* var. *typhimurium*. Most clinical laboratories stock only a limited number of specific antisera with which to help identify the most commonly isolated strains. Those unable to be identified are routinely sent to a reference laboratory where a wider range of antisera can be applied.

Cross reference

For a full description of identification tests the reader is referred to Chapter 2.

Key Point

It must be remembered that other Gram-negative organisms can have similar antigens to those of *Salmonella* and *Shigella*, so cross reactions and false-positive reactions can occur when performing agglutination tests on part of the colony. This is the reason why biochemical or other properties are used to confirm the organism is a pathogen.

10.5.2 Non-cultural methods for the detection of bacterial causes of gastrointestinal disease

In most cases of bacterial gastrointestinal disease, it is appropriate to use culture techniques in order fully to characterize the causative organism. However, this is a time-consuming method and may not always be sensitive enough to detect small numbers of pathogens. Two newer methods of improving isolation rates and detection times are outlined next.

Immunomagnetic separation (IMS)

Effectively a selective enrichment technique, this process has been used in the detection of several enteric pathogens, principally salmonellae. Specific antibodies are bound to latex beads which are then mixed with a suspension of faecal material. The beads are washed to remove the faecal debris, leaving any salmonellae bound to the antibody-coated beads which are then cultured in the usual way. Salmonellae present in the sample are thus concentrated and contaminating organisms are removed, allowing a significantly higher isolation rate to be achieved.

While IMS improves isolation rates for the selected pathogen, in most clinical situations, a range of organisms needs to be sought, as the cause is unknown. The additional cost of this technique and the fact that only limited, selected organisms can be detected, render it of doubtful cost-effectiveness in routine clinical bacteriology.

Molecular bacteriology

DNA probes are available for the detection of some species (pathogenic *E. coli*). 'Signature' DNA sequences characteristic of the target organism are sought by incubating a preparation of the sample with a complementary oligonucleotide segment which binds to the target site. This section of hybridized DNA is then repeatedly replicated or amplified until it reaches levels able to be detected.

This technique is very sensitive but is expensive and demands considerable technical expertise. Once again, its specificity often renders it unsuitable for screening clinical samples where a number of different pathogens may be involved. Similarly, it does not result in the isolation of an organism which can easily be fully characterized (e.g. susceptibility tests) and so far has failed to find a place in the routine diagnosis of bacterial GI disease. As techniques and cost-effectiveness improve, this technology may become more generally useful in the future. So far molecular techniques have found a role for detecting viral GI disease and the toxin genes of *C. difficile* in some laboratories.

Molecular techniques are used by reference laboratories in the detection of genes coding for toxin production, for example VTEC and *S. aureus*.

10.5.3 Bacterial toxin detection

The detection of toxins in faecal material is not straightforward. This is because the faeces sample itself contains many millions of bacteria, food debris, and toxic chemicals resulting from food breakdown or direct ingestion. Just think of how many chemicals are contained in the GI tract. Any one of these can interfere with the detection of a toxin.

Suspected infection with *C. difficile* is the only circumstance in which toxins are routinely sought directly from faeces. This is generally performed using enzyme immunoassay. Culture of the organism is used only when it is important to know whether infecting strains are related, for example, in outbreaks, or to establish carriage of the organism.

Some diseases, as we have discovered earlier in the chapter, are toxin mediated. This means the living bacterium doesn't need to be present as it could have been destroyed by cooking but the toxin remains to initiate illness. For other toxin-mediated diseases, the microbiologist will attempt to detect toxins either present in food implicated in the illness or produced by bacteria isolated from faeces or food. In certain circumstances, for example infection with VTEC and *S. aureus*, it is possible, using DNA probes, to demonstrate that the organism possesses genes coding for toxin production even if the toxin itself is not detected.

The following methods are used for toxin detection.

Tissue culture

Cytotoxins, such as *C. difficile* toxin B and Shiga toxin, destroy epithelial cells and some of the earliest tests for these molecules were performed on living animals. A popular model was to use an isolated loop of rabbit ileum, into which the suspect sample was instilled. Cytotoxins would rapidly cause severe damage to the epithelium associated with bleeding and fluid secretion. As you can imagine this was not the most pleasant of tests to perform routinely!

This technique was developed into a tissue culture method; it became possible to grow a thin layer of cells on the inside surface of a clear bottle, bathed in a supporting fluid. When an extract containing suspected cytotoxin was added to the cell layer, any effects could be observed directly by low-power magnification. Toxin-affected cells would shrivel up into balls and die.

For many years, this detection method was accepted as the 'gold standard' for detecting *C. difficile* toxin B. However, faeces may contain chemicals that cause a cytotoxic effect as well as other toxin-producing bacteria. The test can be made more specific by retesting after the addition of an antitoxin, which neutralizes the effect of toxin B. Toxin B is unstable and any delay in transport to the laboratory or failure to keep the sample cool may result in false-negative results. Although some laboratories still use tissue culture, it is labour-intensive, time consuming and does not detect toxin A, which is more important in the causation of diarrhoea. Since *C. difficile* is an extremely important cause of morbidity and mortality the number of requests for examination for *C. difficile* is growing rapidly. As a result, less labour-intensive methods have superseded cell culture.

Cross reference
See Chapter 12, Section 12.5.

Enzyme immunoassay

In this technique, specific antibodies to *C. difficile* toxins are conjugated with an enzyme capable of breaking down an indicator molecule (substrate). In a simple example, purified toxin is used to coat the wells of a microtitre tray. A suspension of the sample is added to the well, followed by a dilute preparation containing the antibody–enzyme conjugate. In a control well, the sample is replaced by distilled water or saline.

The conjugate will bind with any toxin present, that is both in the liquid in the well and on the tray surface. In the control well, it will only bind at the surface. The wells are then washed and a detector substrate added – usually a colour indicator or fluorescent compound. In the control well, a very strong signal will be detected, as all the conjugate would have bound to the surface. In the test well, the signal will be less as much of the conjugate would have bound to the toxin present in the sample.

Cross reference
See Chapter 13, Section 13.5.

Various modifications of this test are used in the detection of *C. difficile* toxins A and B, *S. aureus* enterotoxin, and *B. cereus*, *C. perfringens*, and VTEC toxins, although only tests for *C. difficile* are used in routine microbiology laboratories.

SELF-CHECK 10.8

What are the advantages and disadvantages of using cell culture for detection of *C. difficile* toxins?

10.5.4 Typing techniques

Although the major bacterial species responsible for infectious intestinal disease have been known for many years, it was quickly realized that it would be helpful to find ways of differentiating apparently identical organisms in order to track their **epidemiology** and to clarify their role in human illness.

epidemiology
Epidemiology is the study of disease origin and spread.

Serotyping

Serotyping is used in the differentiation of *Campylobacter* spp. (Lior and Penner types), *E. coli*, *Shigella* spp., *Yersinia* spp., *V. cholerae*, *B. cereus*, *C. perfringens*, and as previously explained *Salmonella* spp.

Unfortunately, related bacteria share many surface antigens associated with enteric pathogens, for example *Shigella* spp. share many common antigens with non-pathogenic *E. coli*, so it is vitally important to ensure full biochemical identification is secure before proceeding to serotyping.

Phage typing

Bacteriophages are viruses that attack bacteria, causing them to burst or lyse. They will usually attack only a certain range of bacteria, so, if a selection of lytic bacteriophages is applied to a culture of a particular bacterium, the pattern of lysis is fairly specific to that strain. Phage typing can be used further to subdivide bacterial serotypes or to type those species which are too homogeneous for serotyping to be of much use. This technique is used to differentiate strains of *S. aureus* and VTEC and to further subdivide *S. sonnei*, *S. enterica* serovars *enteritidis*, *typhimurium*, *Virchow*, and *hadar*. Phage typing is now only performed in reference laboratories.

PCR ribotyping

This technique analyses strain-to-strain variations in particular regions of bacterial ribosomal RNA. It can be used to try to differentiate many bacteria but is particularly useful in identifying distinct strains of *C. difficile*.

SELF-CHECK 10.9

Which would you consider to be the most definitive for the identification of a *Salmonella* or *Shigella* – serotyping or biochemical/MALDI-TOF identification?

10.6 Patient management and control of infection

Any patient with diarrhoea and/or vomiting should be treated as potentially infectious until the cause of the illness is determined. Person-to-person spread occurs via the faeco-oral route, that is, faecal contamination of hands, food, water, or the environment, followed by ingestion.

For the toxin-mediated food poisonings associated with *S. aureus*, *B. cereus*, and *C. perfringens*, person-to-person spread does not occur. With the exception of *Campylobacter* spp., where person-to-person spread is rare. For most other bacterial causes the likelihood of spread depends on the infectious dose and the susceptibility of the person exposed. VTEC and *Shigella* spp. are highly infectious due to their low infective dose (Table 10.1).

C. difficile is a special case, as the patient's environment quickly becomes heavily contaminated with resistant spores, exposing vulnerable people to infection via inanimate objects.

It is important that, in health-care settings, patients are isolated as quickly as possible. They should have separate toilet facilities and all those attending them should observe scrupulous hand hygiene and wear disposable gloves and aprons to protect themselves. Enhanced cleaning of the environment, especially 'touch points' (e.g. door handles) should be carried out using an appropriate disinfectant. Visiting must be restricted to the minimum. Patients must remain isolated for at least 48 h after cessation of all symptoms.

Although many may continue to excrete the causative organism for some time after clinical recovery, with good personal hygiene there is much less risk of transmission at this time.

SELF-CHECK 10.10

Would you wait for the culture results to be positive before you would isolate the patient? If not, why not?

10.7 Therapeutic regimes

For most common gastrointestinal pathogens, no specific treatment is required, other than supportive measures to ensure that the patient remains well hydrated and in electrolyte balance. Simple pain relief for abdominal cramps and sponging with tepid water to reduce fever are usually all that is necessary.

Antibiotic treatment is not usually needed and may, in fact, prolong carriage of the pathogen. Widespread overuse of antibiotics for such infections has resulted in major problems with bacterial resistance and, for seriously ill patients, it is now essential to check antibiotic susceptibilities. Antibiotics are indicated for the enteric fevers, severe cases of *Salmonella* food poisoning and shigellosis, although their use takes second place to the correction of fluid and electrolyte depletion. For VTEC, the role of antibiotics is unclear but there is evidence that they may actually make the illness worse.

SELF-CHECK 10.11

Why would a patient be prescribed antibiotics for an enteric fever but generally not for diarrhoea and vomiting?

10.8 Non-bacterial causes of gastrointestinal disease

Cross reference

See Chapter 11.

Apart from the bacterial causes outlined above, three other groups of organisms cause infectious intestinal diseases, these are viruses, protozoa, and worms (**helminths**). The latter two will be discussed in greater detail in Chapter 11. However, it is important to be aware that symptoms similar to those of infectious intestinal diseases may be caused by a number of other factors.

Structural or functional abnormalities of the gut, including surgical procedures, cancers, **malabsorptive states** and diverticular disease can all cause diarrhoea, abdominal pain and/or vomiting. Many medicines can have similar effects, as can dietary factors; for example, patients receiving **nasogastric feeds** often develop diarrhoea. It is important that patients with unexplained and persistent symptoms are fully investigated by a specialist.

10.8.1 Viral pathogens

Most cases of gastroenteritis caused by viruses are mild and short-lived, lasting only 1 to 2 days and rarely cause the person to seek medical attention. Transmission is principally person-to-person, but can also be via the inhalation of airborne droplets, which are produced during explosive vomiting. Food-borne outbreaks occur and usually result from contamination during food preparation by an infected food handler, or from food contamination by sewage.

Two of the most important enteric viruses are rotavirus and norovirus. Both are highly infectious and occur most frequently in the winter months, although cases can occur at any time.

- Rotaviruses (Figure 10.6) affect mainly children under 2 years of age, spreading rapidly in nurseries and playgroups. Older children are less often affected as they have usually acquired immunity by the age of 3.

- Norovirus affects all age groups and, due to its very low infective dose (<100 particles), its capacity to spread via aerosols and ability to survive for long periods in the environment, causes many thousands of infections each year.

- Numerous norovirus serotypes are recognized and immunity after infection lasts only 3 to 4 months for each, so repeated infection is common. Outbreaks are particularly common where people are in close proximity, e.g. schools, hospitals, nursing homes, hotels, and even cruise liners.

- Caliciviruses are similar, yet distinct, and sometimes cause outbreaks of diarrhoea in young children. They are not a common cause of diarrhoea.

- Adenoviruses usually cause respiratory infections, but certain strains of subgenus F cause gastrointestinal symptoms. Infections tend to occur in nursery and primary school children and occur throughout the year.

- Astroviruses are infrequent causes of gastroenteritis, the peak incidence being in winter and early spring. Children are mainly affected. A number of different serotypes have been described.

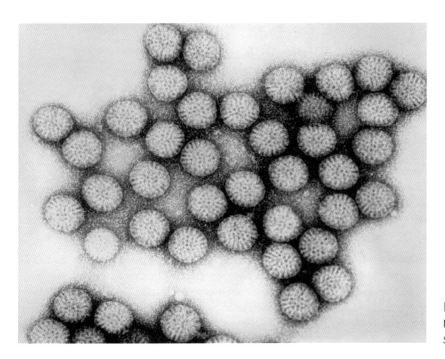

FIGURE 10.6
Electron micrograph of a rotavirus.
Source: Courtesy of CDC/Dr Erskine Palmer.

Laboratory detection

Electron microscopy was once the only method of detecting enteric viruses. Although it is expensive, slow and relatively insensitive, it allowed visualization of the viral particles, hence the names of some of the first to be detected, for example rota (wheel-like) and astro (star-shaped) viruses.

Latex agglutination and enzyme immunoassay techniques were then developed for the more common viruses, although only selected serotypes could be detected.

More recently, a variety of PCR-based methods have largely superseded these tests. However, in most laboratories, viral detection is only used in specific circumstances, such as outbreaks or during recognized seasonal increases.

SELF-CHECK 10.12

Why do most laboratories only look for viral pathogens in specific circumstances?

Patient management and infection control

There is no specific treatment for any of the viral infections discussed and, for the most part, due to the relatively mild and short-lived nature of the illness, only hydration, rest, and simple analgesia are required.

Infection control is the main problem as, even in previously fit people, the onset of symptoms can be surprisingly abrupt, with vomiting a prominent feature, resulting in infectious aerosol formation and contamination of the environment. Patients should stay at home, or, in the health-care setting, be isolated until 48h after the symptoms have completely resolved. Rigorous cleaning with a chlorine-based disinfectant is essential, concentrating on 'touch points'. As alcohol hand rubs are not **virucidal**, thorough hand washing with soap and water is most important.

10.8.2 Parasitic infections

These are described in greater detail in Chapter 11.

Protozoa

Protozoa are single-celled organisms which, when ingested, can, in some cases, cause gastro-intestinal disease. Worldwide, they are major causes of morbidity and mortality but in the UK they are much less common than bacterial or viral infections. The three most important are *Cryptosporidium parvum* (Figure 10.7), *Giardia intestinalis*, and *Entamoeba histolytica*. They can survive well in the environment – *Giardia* and *Entamoeba* forming resilient cysts – and often contaminate surface waters. They are resistant to chlorine and so may survive even in treated tap water.

Cryptosporidium affects animals as well as humans and can be acquired by direct contact as well as via contaminated water. It causes an unpleasant, sometimes prolonged but self-limiting diarrhoea. However, in immunocompromised people, especially those with HIV infection, it may be severe and life threatening. There is no specific treatment, although several drugs, including gamma interferon, have been tried in an attempt to enhance the immune response. For *Cryptosporidium parvum* a smear of faecal material is made on a glass slide and, after

FIGURE 10.7

Immunofluorescence of *Cryptosporidium parvum* oocysts from a stool sample.

Source: Courtesy of EPA/H.D.A. Lindquist.

allowing it to dry at room temperature, it is generally stained using either a fluorescent stain or a modified **Ziehl–Neelsen** technique. For all other parasites, a concentration method using differential centrifugation (formol–ether separation) is used in order to increase the chances of finding cysts and ova. A wet preparation of the supernatant is placed under a cover slip and examined by low-power light microscopy. A 10% solution of iodine can be used to enhance the features of the organisms. Great expertise and experience is needed to make an accurate examination as many non-pathogenic protozoa and food debris such as plant cells can be mistaken for clinically important parasites.

- Giardia is usually acquired from water contaminated by sewage, but also spreads person-to-person. It may be entirely **asymptomatic** but, in some cases, diarrhoea may persist and damage to the gut mucosa leads to malabsorption and weight loss. Treatment, if needed, is usually with metronidazole or tinidazole.

- Several species of *Entamoeba* live as part of the normal human gut microflora, but only *E. histolytica* causes disease. Some strains appear to be more virulent than others, but in its full-blown form it causes amoebic dysentery, in which amoebae invade the colonic mucosa forming shallow ulcers. Diarrhoea is severe, with blood and mucus. Amoebae may spread to other organs, usually the liver, via the bloodstream and form abscesses. Treatment is with **metronidazole**, but patients should also receive a course of diloxanide furoate to eradicate cysts, which may remain. Cysts of *E. histolytica* are identical to those of the non-pathogenic *Entamoeba dispar*. The diagnosis of amoebiasis therefore rests on the examination of freshly passed, 'hot' stool, in order to see motile trophozoites, which, characteristically, ingest red blood cells.

asymptomatic

Asymptomatic indicates the presence of the organism but without symptoms developing.

Although faeco-oral spread may occur, good sanitation and clean water are, as usual, the best preventive measures.

A number of methods are available for the detection of parasites in stool samples, the most common of which is the parasite concentration method. Briefly, the sample is mixed with formalin to kill any harmful organisms and it is then mixed with an organic solvent such as ethyl acetate. This solvent extracts fat and debris from the faeces sample in order to ensure the 'cleanest' possible preparation is produced. Following centrifugation the parasites are concentrated at the bottom of the tube and a drop is examined by light microscopy.

Cross reference

See Chapter 11.

A variety of treatments are available for all the helminthic infections, although some are more successful than others. Apart from the simplest infections, patients are generally referred to specialist infectious disease physicians for treatment.

SELF-CHECK 10.13

What are the common treatments for diarrhoea? Is it appropriate to treat gastrointestinal infections with antibiotics? If not, why not?

10.9 The role of the reference laboratory

Most developed countries have one or two highly specialized laboratories which have the capability to give a definitive verdict on the identification and nature of microorganisms implicated in disease. In order to be able to do this work, a large proportion of their effort is spent in developing and evaluating new methods, some of which may, eventually, find their way into routine use.

There are four situations in which samples or isolates are sent to the reference laboratory:

- To confirm the result obtained by the initial testing laboratory.
- To give a definitive identification where preliminary results are inconclusive.
- To characterize an organism fully, including typing which is unavailable routinely.
- To perform tests that are either too complex for routine use or so infrequently performed in individual laboratories that staff have insufficient expertise to render the test reliable.

In addition, the reference laboratory can collect data on all isolates referred, in order to detect regional and national patterns of disease, which may not always be obvious at the local level. Finally, experts are able to act in an advisory capacity to assist staff in local laboratories in their management of individual patients and outbreaks.

 CASE STUDY 10.1 *An outbreak of gastroenteritis in a residential care home*

The manager of a residential home for the elderly telephones the environmental health department of the local authority to report a suspected outbreak of food poisoning.

Over a 24-h period, 18 out of 80 residents and three members of staff have become ill, the main symptoms being vomiting, diarrhoea, headache, and feeling feverish. Two residents have had to be admitted to hospital. All the affected residents and staff had attended a birthday celebration at the home around 18h before the first resident developed symptoms. No one who was not at the party had become ill. Food for the party was prepared in the kitchen of the home by a catering assistant with help from an untrained member of staff. Egg mayonnaise, ham, and cheese sandwiches had been served as well as a homemade trifle. The kitchens were noticeably untidy, with poor separation of preparation areas and utensils for raw and cooked food. There was only one sink, which was used for washing large utensils and food, as well for hand washing.

1. What samples would you suggest are taken?

2. How would you process such samples?

3. What possible causes would you suggest for the outbreak?

4. What would be the role of the Environmental Health Office and Health Protection Unit (HPU)?

5. If a *Salmonella* was isolated how would you confirm its identity, what else would you do with the organism?

6. What action would be required at the residential home?

CASE STUDY 10.2 *Profuse watery diarrhoea*

A 33-year-old woman was in a UN hospital in Africa and was found to be barely conscious. Her companion indicated she was well 48 hours ago and then rapidly deteriorated with no other symptoms apart from profuse watery diarrhoea and muscle cramps.

1. What would be your initial diagnosis of the problem?

2. What treatment options would be considered?

3. Would you send samples to the laboratory? If so what samples and what tests would you request?

Her companion had collected all 12 L of diarrhoeal excretions believing that if they could be put back into her she would be 'cured' as all of her nutrients were contained within it and this was why she was so ill. Within the hospital there are several other patients with exactly the same type of illness.

After the administration of isotonic NaCl and isotonic bicarbonate in significant volumes the patient slowly started to recover.

4. Why did these solutions cause the patient to recover?

5. Since there are other patients with the same symptoms would any agencies need to be informed and why?

CASE STUDY 10.3 *Profuse vomiting and diarrhoea*

On Christmas day a large family gathered for a traditional lunch. Seven out of the 12 family members who attended experienced profuse vomiting and diarrhoea 16 hours after consuming the meal. They symptoms lasted only 36 hours but sadly the two most elderly family members (76 and 71 years) required hospitalization.

1. What would you suggest as the cause of the D+V to be?

2. Why did only two people require hospitalization?

3. What measures would the hospital take on admission of the two patients?

4. What tests (if any) would be required to confirm the diagnosis?

Upon further investigation one of the family members had been ill 3 days earlier with severe D+V but since it had resolved she continued to prepare for the Christmas celebrations.

5. Could this D+V outbreak have been prevented and if so how?

Chapter summary

After reading this chapter you should know and understand:

- How common gastrointestinal diseases are throughout the world.

- The importance of the various host defences to ensure gastrointestinal pathogens do not initiate infection.

- The wide range of bacterial gastrointestinal pathogens and why some are associated more with developing nations.

- Culture is still the gold standard for detection of most common bacterial pathogens and the range of culture media available for their isolation.

- The basic principles of such culture media and how they are used to isolate and detect bacterial pathogens.

- The complex mechanisms by which bacterial pathogens can evade the host defences and initiate infection.

- The role of toxins A and B in the promotion of *C. difficile* infection and the national significance of this organism.

- Important viral pathogens and the significance of norovirus outbreaks.

- How the reference laboratory can be used to identify suspect isolates and confirm the presence of toxin genes, etc., and the role this plays in outbreak analysis.

- The potential control of infection issues for both hospitalized and community patients when a gastrointestinal pathogen is detected.

- The role of environmental health officers and Health Protection Units in the investigation of outbreaks.

Further reading

- **World Health Organization. www.who.int.**

  Numerous publications on infectious diseases and current global programmes.

- **Centers for Disease Control (CDC). www.cdc.gov.**

  Excellent resource for all aspects of health care and an excellent image bank.

- **Health Protection Agency. Infectious diseases. www.hpa.org.uk/Topics/Infectious Diseases/InfectionsAZ/ (accessed 14 August, 2013).**

  Extensive library of information on infectious diseases and many other health-care related topics.

- **American Society for Microbiology. www.asm.org.**

  One of the largest and oldest microbiology worldwide resource.

Discussion questions

10.1 Are all cases of bacterial gastroenteritis confirmed by culture? If not why not?

10.2 Do you believe that commonly used culture media for the isolation of bacterial pathogens from stool samples are sensitive and specific enough?

10.3 What measures would you use to try to ensure gastrointestinal infections are eradicated worldwide?

10.4 What GI pathogens would you look for with the following clinical details?

  a. Diarrhoea in a child < 2 years.

  b. A 68-year-old male, post-surgery being treated with ciprofloxacin.

  c. Chronic diarrhoea in a student following a gap year in Nepal.

  d. Profuse watery diarrhoea in an aid worker who has recently returned from Somalia.

11

Clinical parasitology

Tony Worthington

You had no right to be born; for you make no use of life. Instead of living for, in, and with yourself as a reasonable being ought, you seek only to fasten your feebleness on some other person's strength.

Charlotte Bronte (1847)

Parasitology may be defined as the biological science of parasites, their hosts, and the relationship between them. Typically, the discipline encompasses the study of both ectoparasites: parasites which live on or in the skin of an organism, e.g. ticks; and endoparasites: parasites which live within another organism, e.g. tapeworms.

Clinical parasitology is an important sub-discipline of pure parasitology and may be defined as the study of human infections caused by ecto- and endoparasites. In the twenty-first century, parasites now contribute to an ever-increasing number of human blood, tissue, and gastrointestinal infections which are often associated with important risk factors including immunosuppression e.g. HIV infection, which is now widespread in both developed and developing nations, and poor hygiene/sanitation which is typically linked to developing areas of the world.

Clinical parasitology is without doubt a vast subject and outside the realms of a single chapter within this book. This chapter will therefore focus primarily upon some clinically important parasitic infections which may be acquired through the faecal–oral route and have gastrointestinal or subsequent extraintestinal clinical manifestations. Aspects including epidemiology life cycles, symptoms, diagnosis, and treatment of these medically important parasitic infections will be considered.

Cross reference

See companion volume *Haematology* by Gary Moore, Gavin Knight, and Andrew Blann for more on blood parasites.

Learning objectives

After studying this chapter you should be able to:

- Define a parasite.
- Understand the difference between protozoa, nematodes, cestodes, and trematodes.
- List the parasites commonly acquired via the faecal–oral route.
- Describe the life cycles of selected gastrointestinal parasites.
- Describe the clinical manifestations of parasitic infections.
- Describe common laboratory approaches for diagnosing parasitic infections.

■ Describe characteristic morphological features used to identify parasites acquired through the faecal-oral route.

■ List the common antiparasitic agents.

11.1 **What are parasites?**

Prior to considering parasites and the diseases they cause, it is important to understand what parasites are. The word parasite is derived from a combination of the Greek words '*para*' which means 'beside', and '*sitos*' which means 'food'; in order to survive and replicate or reproduce, a parasite must obtain its food from another living creature or its host, for example: mammals, birds, fish, and crustaceans. A parasite offers nothing to the relationship with its host, thus creating an association which may be neutral or harmful, but never positive; this differentiates parasitism from commensalism and mutualism.

As parasites depend upon their host for a constant nutritional supply over a long period of time a well-adapted or 'good' parasite should not kill its host. By strict definition, microorganisms including viruses, some bacteria, and prions may be considered parasitic, however, this chapter will be restricted to gastrointestinal **protozoa** and **helminths**.

An overview of parasites and their general features is given here:

- They are eukaryotic organisms comprising membrane-bound organelles.
- They may be unicellular (e.g. protozoa) or multicellular (helminths: worms). Protozoa replicate primarily through asexual reproduction (however, some undergo stages of sexual reproduction within their life cycle).
- Some helminths may be dioecious, requiring both male and female forms to reproduce, whilst some may be hermaphroditic, thus containing all reproductive organs normally associated with both male and female sexes.
- They utilize either one host (the **definitive host**) or more (**intermediate hosts**) to replicate or reproduce, and eventually reach maturity.
- They are usually smaller than their host, thus differentiating them from predators.
- They offer nothing positive to the host–parasite relationship but will exploit the host for nutrition and the purpose of remaining viable.
- They may be transmitted to their host through a variety of routes: vectors (e.g. mosquitos); zoonotic transmission (animal–human); direct contact (e.g. sexual intercourse, skin penetration); congenital transmission; faecal-oral: (a) consumption of contaminated food and water, (b) poor hygiene and contaminated hands. In this chapter, the gastrointestinal/faecal-oral route is considered.

protozoa

Protozoa are unicellular, eukaryotic microorganisms possessing typical eukaryotic organelles, e.g. a membrane-bound nucleus containing chromosomes and mitochondria.

helminth

Helminths are worm-like parasites. Clinically important helminths are broadly separated according to their external structure: roundworms (nematodes), tapeworms (cestodes), and flukes (trematodes).

definitive host

The host in which a mature parasite resides and replicates/reproduces.

intermediate host

The host in which parasitic larval stages reside or non-sexual reproduction occurs.

SELF-CHECK 11.1

What are the main features of parasites?

11.2 **Clinical parasitology in the twenty-first century**

In the twenty-first century, parasitic infections are a significant cause of morbidity and mortality worldwide. In the industrialized world, we rarely consider gastrointestinal (GI) parasitic infections a major problem; indeed, GIs are mainly associated with viruses and bacteria. However, in developing regions, parasites are endemic and continue to cause substantial problems which are reflected in human illness, especially in children, and constitute significant economic losses related to health and agriculture.

Parasites are no respecters of dignity, social class, background, or sexuality and anyone can acquire a parasitic infection given the right circumstances. However, the late twentieth and twenty-first centuries have brought with them various behavioural changes and practices, particularly in developed nations, which predispose people to parasitic infection:

- *Importation of foodstuffs*. There is an increase in the importation of foodstuffs from nations without robust sanitary facilities or environmental health inspection systems and where parasitic infections are endemic. Raw vegetables are relatively safe if peeled before consumption, however, it is particularly difficult to rid of parasitic eggs and cysts from leafy vegetables.

- *Travel/immigration and the dissemination of infection*. International travel has increased exponentially over the past few decades and this includes travel to/and immigration from parts of the world (e.g. areas of India, Asia, and sub-Saharan Africa) where parasitic infections are widespread. Many parasitic infections are acquired through the consumption of contaminated food and water in endemic regions of the world. Drinking untreated water or brushing teeth with contaminated water can be particularly hazardous. As many parasites can withstand freezing, consumption of ice is as equally dangerous.

- *Modern lifestyles*. There is now a trend to consume lightly cooked or undercooked meat and fish, for example, sushi, steak tartar, and raw sausage which may predispose people to gastrointestinal infections including those caused by parasites. Consumption of raw or undercooked meat and fish can lead to infection with a wide range of parasites; some of which will be considered in this chapter.

- *Ageing population*. We are an ageing population and this brings with it an ageing immune system which may not be able to effectively deal with pathogenic microorganisms, including parasites.

- *Immunosuppression/immunodeficiency*. On a global scale, there are now an ever-expanding number of people with immunosuppression e.g. those infected with human immunodeficiency virus (HIV) or those with congenital immunodeficiencies. Patients with underlying immune disorders are at risk from infection due to a whole range of infectious agents, including parasites.

- *Global warming*. It is predicted that there will be an increase of 1°C to 3.5°C in the world during the twenty-first century. In countries with a temperate climate the following may occur: (a) mild winters and warmer summers; (b) increased sea levels associated with polar ice melting and other factors; (c) migration of insect vectors which may carry disease. These predicted changes may influence the geographical range and incidence of vector-borne parasitic infections such as malaria and also water-borne infections including a range of infections due to intestinal protozoa and helminths. In addition, global warming may also increase faecal–oral infections as warmer, wetter conditions may extend the survival of parasitic soil stages which may be subsequently consumed by humans.

Many different species of protozoa and helminths live in the gastrointestinal tract of humans and they infect approximately 3–4 billion people worldwide. Indeed, in many developing nations, gastrointestinal parasitism is accepted as a normal part of life and a high number of people are infected, however, only a relatively low percentage of infected cases progress to serious illness. The major impact of parasitic infection in developing areas is on an economic level, with infections preventing the ability of many people to work. If clinical manifestations of parasitic infection do present in patients, they span the clinical spectrum of symptoms ranging from very mild intestinal disturbances, to acute or chronic diarrhoea, life-threatening infections associated with extraintestinal migration into organs and tissues, and possibly death.

In both the Western and developing world, what are the risk factors associated with acquisition of parasitic infections?

11.3 **Protozoa**

A considerable number of human gastrointestinal infections and those associated with the faecal-oral route are caused by pathogenic protozoa (Table 11.1). These infections are important, not only because they cause human disease and suffering, but also because they may have an impact in the world of agriculture. In the twenty-first century, on a global scale, there has been an increase in protozoan infections possibly due to their association with immunosuppressed

TABLE 11.1 Some medically important protozoan infections associated with the gastrointestinal tract.

Protozoan	Mode of transmission	Symptoms	Importance
AMOEBAE			
Entamoeba histolytica	Faecal-oral; contaminated food and water	Amoebic dysentery characterized by blood and mucus in stool, weight loss, malaise	Extraintestinal invasion may occur (liver, spleen, lungs)
FLAGELLATES			
Giardia intestinalis	Faecal-oral; contaminated food and water	Gut inflammation and reduced absorptive capacity, diarrhoea, malaise, flatulence	Important cause of 'travellers' diarrhoea', 'beaver fever', and 'hikers' diarrhoea'
APICOMPLEXANS			
Cryptosporidium species (C. parvum; C. hominis)	Faecal-oral; contaminated food and water; shellfish	Diarrhoea, abdominal cramps, flatulence	Life threatening in AIDS patients; common in children
Toxoplasma gondii	Faecal-oral; ingestion of undercooked pork, lamb, beef	Often asymptomatic; glandular fever syndrome, birth defects and encephalitis in neonates	Congenital transmission, 30% of AIDS-related deaths (meningitis); seroprevalence 16–80%
Cyclospora cayetanensis	Faecal-oral; contaminated food and water	Diarrhoea, abdominal cramps, flatulence, anorexia	Worldwide distribution; severe infections in AIDS patients
Isospora belli	Faecal-oral	Diarrhoea, abdominal cramps, weight loss	Worldwide distribution; severe infections in AIDS patients
CILIATES			
Balantidium coli	Faecal-oral; contaminated water	Asymptomatic, diarrhoea with blood and pus, abdominal pain	Worldwide distribution; common pathogen of pigs; mucosal ulceration and invasive infection may occur

Trophozoite (active, feeding pathogenic stage)
- Parasitic stage competing with host for nutrients
- Asexual reproduction
- Causes symptoms of infection
- Extraluminal invasion may occur

EXCYSTMENT
- Occurs in intestine following exposure to moisture and nutrients
- Release of active stage

ENCYSTMENT
- Occurs in unfavourable conditions
- Loss of water from trophozoite
- Protective cyst membrane develops

Cyst (infective resistant stage)
- Excreted in faces and survives environmental extremes
- Dormant, resting stage
- Contaminates food and water
- Ingested by host

FIGURE 11.1
Generalized life cycle of gastrointestinal protozoan parasites (e.g. *Giardia*) acquired by the faecal–oral route.
Source: Courtesy of Tony Worthington.

Members of the apicomplexans protozoans, eg. *Cryptosporidium* species and *Toxoplasma gondii* have more complicated life cycles which incorporate both asexual and sexual stages of reproduction. This results in the release of infective oocysts in the faeces of the host.

or compromised patients, e.g. HIV, or those who have deficiencies, e.g. immune/nutritional, especially in the developing nations.

heterotroph
Heterotrophs obtain organic material which originates from other living organisms for use as nutrients and energy.

Medically important protozoa are small (approx. 10–200 µm), **heterotrophic** microorganisms. Some protozoa have well-defined shapes whilst others constantly change their shape e.g. amoeba. In addition, they are broadly separated into four major groups depending upon their method of motility: amoebae (pseudopodia), flagellates (flagella), ciliates (cilia), and apicomplexans (lack locomotor processes). Protozoa that are transmitted by the faecal–oral route often have similar life cycles, with the exception of a few, and modes of transmission and tend to exist in two stages (Figure 11.1):

- An active, feeding stage (e.g. trophozoite) which is associated with human disease and symptoms.

- An infective, resistant stage (e.g. cyst, oocyst) which exists outside the host and is able to withstand environmental extremes for extended periods of time. The cyst or oocyst is ingested by a host through contaminated food and water.

11.3.1 Amoebae

Entamoeba histolytica

Entamoeba histolytica is a gastrointestinal protozoan which is transmitted via the faecal–oral route through the ingestion of its cysts on contaminated food or in faecally contaminated

FIGURE 11.2
Microscopic image of *E. hystolytica* cysts.
Source: Courtesy of T. Carroll.

water (Figure 11.2). *E. histolytica* is the second leading parasitic cause of death and the estimated worldwide prevalence is around 500 million, however, it is primarily associated with subtropical and tropical regions including South East Asia and Africa. In these regions, transmission of infective cysts to foodstuffs through vectors including flies and cockroaches is a major problem. In the UK, approximately 100–200 cases are reported per annum, which are usually associated with travel to endemic regions or immigration from endemic regions into the UK. In the Western world, *E. histolytica* is also seen in mental health facilities, prisons, and orphanages where poor hygiene and overcrowding are key risk factors for transmission. Furthermore, a higher prevalence is observed in men who have sex with men (MSM).

The symptoms associated with *E. histolytica* infection are caused by the active trophozoite following encystment and they span the clinical spectrum; most patients (approx. 90%), especially in endemic regions are asymptomatic and are reservoirs of infection.

Key Point

The majority of patients with *E. histolytica* infection are asymptomatic but still serve as reservoirs of infection.

The remaining 10% or so of patients experience ulceration of colonic epithelium and symptoms of amoebic dysentery which is characterized by frequent stools containing mucus and blood. In addition, extraintestinal amoebiasis may occur when the actively motile and feeding trophozoites penetrate through the lumen of the colon and disseminate through the bloodstream to vital organs including the liver where amoebic abscess may develop. Haematogenous spread of the trophozoites to other organs including the brain and lungs are rare but cases have been reported. In MSM, perianal and genital ulcerative lesions may occur following sexual contact however, again this is relatively rare.

11.3.2 Flagellates

Giardia intestinalis

Giardia intestinalis (also known as *G. lamblia*, *G. duodenalis*) is one of the most common protozoan infections worldwide with an estimated prevalence of 200 million. This protozoan is able to infect a large range of animals and **zoonotic transmission** is possible but not widely reported. *G. intestinalis* is also commonly associated with lakes and streams which are inhabited by beavers and as a consequence, giardiasis is often referred to as 'beaver fever' or 'hikers'

zoonotic transmission
Zoonosis is a disease that normally exists in animals but can be transmitted to humans.

FIGURE 11.3
Microscopic image of *G. lamblia* cyst.
Source: Courtesy of T. Carroll.

diarrhoea' as hikers and backpackers may acquire the infection through drinking water from streams contaminated with animal faeces. In the UK, there are around 2,000 to 4,000 reported cases of giardiasis per annum. Again, *G. in testinalis* exhibits a typical faecal–oral life cycle though which humans become infected through consumption of water and food contaminated with the resistant cysts of *G. intestinalis* and as this protozoan is highly infectious, only a few cysts (10–100) are required to initiate infection. Furthermore, cysts of *G. intestinalis* are able to withstand the normal concentrations of chlorine used routinely in drinking water and recreational swimming pools.

Giardiasis is spread through a number of routes including: consumption of contaminated domestic, recreational, and natural water supplies; consumption of food, e.g. blackberries contaminated with cysts of *G. intestinalis;* and through touching contaminated surfaces, e.g. children's nurseries. Symptoms of giardiasis are caused by the active trophozoite and range from asymptomatic, to self-limiting diarrhoea, through to nutritional disorders including weight loss. The diarrhoea experienced by infected patients is often characteristic of *G. intestinalis* infection and is typically explosive, foul smelling, and contains a high level of fat which is demonstrated by the faeces floating on the surface of the toilet water.

The trophozoite of *G. intestinalis* has a unique morphology and exhibits a typical pear-shape or tear-drop bilateral symmetry ranging from 12–15 μm by 5–10 μm wide. Characteristic features include four pairs of flagella, median bodies, and axonemes. In addition, the trophozoite has a unique concave adhesive (sucking, ventral) disc which allows for the organism to attach to the intestinal epithelium preventing the patient from absorbing carbohydrates and fat which are subsequently excreted. The infective cysts of *G. intestinalis* are oval shaped ranging from 10–15 μm by 5–10 μm wide and cytoplasm of the cyst is retracted from the wall (Figure 11.3). These characterize features of *G. intestinalis* aid in simple recognition of the flagellate in clinical samples.

11.3.3 Apicomplexans

Cryptosporidium species

Cryptosporidium parvum and *C. hominis* are apicomplexan parasites that cause human infection and are distributed worldwide with an estimated 400 million cases per annum. Cryptosporidia species have complicated life cycles which include both asexual and sexual stages of reproduction in the same host which results in the formation of **oocysts**. Oocysts of cryptosporidia excreted in the faeces of the host are the infective stage of the parasite surviving in harsh conditions including brackish, fresh, and salt water for several months. Infection with cryptosporidia occurs through the typical faecal–oral route via consumption of water

oocyst
An encysted zygote of apicomplexan protozoans that undergoes sporogony to produce infective sporozoites.

which is contaminated with oocysts of *Cryptosporidium* species. Foodstuffs, including fruit and vegetables, that have been washed with contaminated water, and shellfish, including oysters, have also been reported as a vector for transmission of infection. Infections with *C. parvum* may also occur following contact with cattle and cattle faeces. The most common clinical presentation of cryptosporidiosis is mild to severe diarrhoea which is generally self-limiting. Additional symptoms including abdominal pain, vomiting and weight loss may also occur. Cryptosporidiosis is more severe and potentially life-threatening in patients with AIDS and other immune disorders. The diarrhoea in this group of patients is profuse and several litres of fluid may be passed per day. Extensive rehydration therapy is frequently required as a life-saving measure, however, the mortality rate in severe cases is high.

11.3.4 *Toxoplasma gondii*

Toxoplasma gondii has a worldwide distribution and is probably the most widespread of all protozoan parasites. It is estimated that around one-third of the world's population is chronically infected with *T. gondii*, however the infection is kept under control in patients with effective immune systems. Based on serological data, it is estimated that 16–40% of people in developed countries are infected whilst the seroprevalence in underdeveloped areas of Central and South America is 50–80%.

Key Point

Many people worldwide are infected with *T. gondii* and an effective immune system is essential for keeping the infection under control. With the increase in immunosuppressed individuals worldwide, the number of cases of reactivation is likely to increase.

Whilst *T. gondii* is found in a wide range of warm-blooded vertebrates the definitive hosts are the felids including domestic and feral cats. The life cycle of *T. gondii* is complex and comprises phases in the both the intestine and tissue (Figure 11.4).

As with other apicomplexan protozoans, the life cycle of *T. gondii* includes both sexual and asexual stages of reproduction. The sexual stage occurs in the definitive host, the felid, and several million infective oocysts are released per day in the faeces of the cat. Asexual reproduction occurs in the intermediate host, of which many exist including birds, mice, sheep, cattle, and pork and these become infected by consuming the oocysts which are ubiquitous in the environment. As *T. gondii* cannot undergo sexual reproduction in the intestine of the intermediate host, **tachyzoites** are released from the oocysts which localize in muscle and neural tissue where they form latent tissue cysts. Humans are accidental hosts and transmission occurs through several routes: consumption of food, unwashed vegetables, and water contaminated with oocysts from cat faeces; consumption of undercooked meat of an intermediate host (e.g. pigs, lamb, cattle) containing tissue cysts; and vertically through congenital transmission. Most patients with *T. gondii* infection are asymptomatic or experience a mild glandular fever-like illness upon contact. As with the intermediate host, both muscle and neural cysts of *T. gondii* develop in humans, however, these are kept under control by an active and effective immune system. In immuocompromised hosts, primary mycocarditis, retinitis, and meningoencephalitis may occur.

tachyzoite
A rapidly multiplying stage in development of the tissue phase of *T. gondii* infection.

Toxoplasmosis has long been regarded as an opportunistic infection as reactivation of neural and muscle cysts associated with latent, chronic infections occur in patients due to

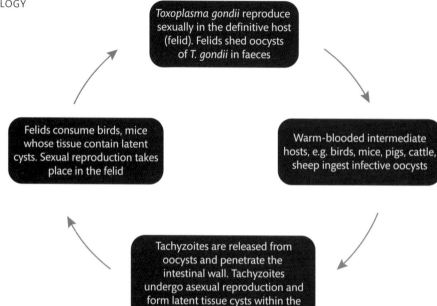

FIGURE 11.4

Generalized life cycle of
Toxoplasma gondii.
Source: Courtesy of Tony
Worthington.

immunosuppression-associated organ transplantation and cancer chemotherapy. In addition, toxoplasmosis is well recognized as a common complication associated with AIDS patients with up to 50% of patients with CD4 cell counts of <100 mm^3 experiencing encephalitis which is characterized by personality swings, schizophrenia, behavioural changes, convulsions, fever, seizures, and other sensory and neuropsychiatric disorders. In AIDS patients, *T. gondii* accounts for approximately 25% of AIDS-related deaths. Toxoplasmosis can also be transmitted congenitally if the mother becomes infected during pregnancy. The symptoms of congenital toxoplasmosis are often severe and include hydrocephalus, retardation, visual defects, and intracerebral calcification. Spontaneous abortion and premature birth may also occur.

11.3.5 Ciliates

Balantidium coli

Balantidium coli is the largest protozoan parasite of humans and the only ciliate which is pathogenic to man. *B. coli* has a worldwide distribution but tends to be more common in tropical regions, e.g. Papua New Guinea. Like several other protozoa, *B. coli* infects a wide range of mammals but is commonly found in pigs and cattle. Infection is transmitted via the faecal–oral route through consumption of food and water contaminated with swine and cattle faeces which contain the infectious cysts. In addition, occasional outbreaks of balantidiasis have been reported following contamination of water supplies. Person-to-person spread through the faecal–oral route has also been documented in people with poor hygiene or following oral–anal contact. It is the active, motile trophozoite of *B. coli* that is associated with symptoms of infection. Whilst many patients infected with *B. coli* are asymptomatic, those demonstrating symptoms often have intermittent diarrhoea containing blood and pus, weight loss, and abdominal pain.

SELF-CHECK 11.3

What is meant by the 'active' and 'infective' stages in the life cycle of a gastrointestinal protozoa?

Which protozoan infections acquired via the faecal–oral route have life cycles comprising both asexual and sexual stages? Of these parasites, which one utilizes an intermediate host in which to undertake its asexual phase of reproduction?

11.4 Helminths

Helminth is a general term meaning 'worm' or 'worm-like' parasite. Gastrointestinal helminths and those acquired by the faecal–oral route are one of the most prevalent forms of parasitic infection and approximately one-quarter of the world's population is infected; however, these infections are generally more common in warm climates and developing nations with poor sanitation. Infections with helminths via the faecal–oral route may be acquired through:

- Consumption of contaminated water and food (including food washed with contaminated water).
- Consumption of raw or undercooked meat and fish.
- Poor hygiene and fingers contaminated with faeces.

Helminths are eukaryotic, multicellular organisms characterized by elongated, flat or round bodies. Their external features comprise either a **cuticle** or **tegument**. They also contain attachment structures which enable them to attach to a host, simple digestive systems (or lack digestive systems), they have rudimentary nervous systems, and are either **dioecious** or **hermaphroditic**. Helminths of medical importance are split into two major groups: nemathelminths (roundworms) and platyhelminths (flatworms). The flatworms are further subdivided into two groups: cestodes (tapeworms) and trematodes (flukes). Helminth growth and development occurs through three stages:

- Egg (ovum); released by a sexually mature adult which resides in a definitive host.
- Larval (young/juvenile) stage; often highly motile, aggressive forms of the helminth; often requires one or more intermediate hosts for full development through to its adult stage.
- Adult helminth (roundworm/tapeworm/fluke); sexually active producing and releasing eggs.

To understand the epidemiology and pathogenicity of helminth infections, the parasitologist requires a thorough understanding of each of these different stages. In addition, it is important to have a sound knowledge of their key morphological features and characteristics in order to establish an accurate laboratory diagnosis which will guide appropriate and effective anti-helminth treatment in infected patients. The key characteristics of some helminths are summarized in Table 11.2

cuticle
Flexible, tough, outer coverings of the nematodes that provides protection. The cuticle is secreted by the epidermis.

tegument
Protective outer body covering of the flatworms that has both secretive and absorptive functions.

dioecious
Separate male and female organisms are required for sexual reproduction.

hermaphroditic
Male and female reproductive systems contained within a single organism.

11.4.1 Nematodes (roundworms)

There are around 16,000 to 20,000 species of nematodes, however only approximately 6,000 are parasitic to vertebrates. Nematodes of clinical importance vary in size and range from 2 mm to 1 m. Nematodes have a generalized structure comprising a cuticle, epidermis, digestive tract, long muscles which run longitudinally, dorsal and ventral nerves, and excretory canals. Adult nematodes demonstrate a sluggish movement and the male is usually smaller than the female. The developmental process in nematodes involves an egg, four larval stages (termed L1, L2, L3, L4), and adult stages. Each of the four larval stages is followed by a moult

TABLE 11.2 Characteristics of some clinically important helminths.

Characteristic	Nematodes (roundworms)	Cestodes (tapeworms)	Trematodes (flukes)
Shape	Cylindrical, non-segmented	Elongated, flat, segmented	Leaf shaped, flat, non-segmented
External structure	Cuticle	Tegument	Tegument
Attachment organs	Lips, 'teeth'	Suckers, rostellum with hooks	Oral and ventral suckers
Internal body cavity with digestive system	Yes	No	Primitive
Reproduction	Dioecious	Hermaphroditic	Hermaphroditic
Pathogenic stage	Adult, larvae	Adult, larvae	Adult, larvae, egg
Some helminths of clinical importance	*Ascaris lumbricoides* (giant roundworm) *Enterobius vermicularis* (pinworm) *Ancylostoma duodenale* (hookworm) *Trichuris trichuria* (whipworm) *Dracunculus medinensis* (Guinea worm) *Loa loa* (African eye worm) *Anisakis simplex* *Strongyloides stercoralis*	*Taenia solium* *Taenia saginata* *Echinococcus granulosus* *Diphyllobothrium latum*	*Fasciola hepatica* *Paragonimus westermanii*

whereby the cuticle is shed. L3 and L4 stages are aggressive larval stages and are parasitic to man. Whilst most nematodes undertake this generalized life cycle, it should be noted that some nematodes utilize an intermediate host in which the larval stages develop e.g. *Anisakis simplex*. This group of worms and their ova are some of the most commonly seen in a routine diagnostic laboratory. Four of the most common are described next.

11.4.2 *Ascaris lumbricoides* (Giant roundworm)

Ascaris lumbricoides is the most common helminth infection worldwide with a prevalence of around 800 million, however it is more prevalent in areas where sanitation is poor (e.g. parts of India and Sub-Saharan Africa) and where untreated human faeces is used as fertilizer. Eggs of *A. lumbricoides* can survive in the environment for several months and humans become infected through consumption of food and water which is contaminated by eggs and through poor personal hygiene. Whilst the life cycle of *A. lumbricoides* is similar to the generalized nematode cycle outlined in Figure 11.5 the L3 larval stage of *A. lumbriocides* undertakes an additional migratory stage to the lungs via the portal and systemic circulation where they undergo further maturation (10–14 days). Mature larval stages penetrate the trachea where they are eventually coughed up and swallowed. Surviving mature larvae then develop into adults in the lumen of the small intestine where they reside for 1–2 years. Many patients with *Ascaris* infection present with no symptoms, especially if the helminth load is low (5–10 worms). However,

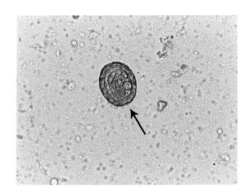

FIGURE 11.5
Microscopic image of an *Ascaris lumbricoides* egg in a concentrated faeces sample.
Source: Courtesy of T. Carroll.

patients showing symptoms may demonstrate intestinal blockage, weight loss, abdominal pain, and distension. In addition, migrating adults or 'wandering worms' (often in response to anti-helminthic treatment) may also obstruct the bile duct, gall bladder, and liver. Patients may also present with pneumonitis and eosinophilia following migration of the L3 larval stages through the lungs.

11.4.3 *Trichuris trichiura* (whipworm)

Trichuris trichiura is more commonly known as the whipworm because of the worm's characteristic shape resembling a whip. The actual worm is 4.5–5 mm long and infection is acquired by ingesting the eggs from the ground which have been excreted from a host. Over a few weeks in the soil the eggs embryonate, from which the adult worm matures inside the host. Once embedded in the host the worms cause significant damage with symptoms of severe abdominal cramps, and if a high level of infection occurs, anaemia due to blood loss. Since both the worm itself and eggs are highly characteristic, lab diagnosis is fairly easy. The egg has the appearance of a tea-tray and is one of the most recognizable structures in parasitology. An image of the egg is shown in Figure 11.6.

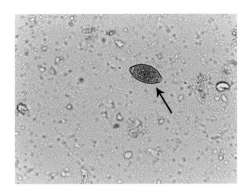

FIGURE 11.6
Egg of a *Tricuris trichuria* – note the characteristic tea-tray shape.
Source: Courtesy of T. Carroll.

11.4.4 *Enterobius vermicularis* (pinworm/threadworm)

Also known as the pinworm due to a characteristic point on the tail, the parasite is believed to be one of the most common parasitic infections in humans, especially children. The parasite has quite an unusual life cycle in that the adult worm migrates down the colon and deposits

FIGURE 11.7
Enterobius **egg from a wet prep obtained**
from the perianal area of a child.
Source: Courtesy of T. Carroll.

the eggs outside the anus on the perianal skin. The female worm then travels back into the colon. The presence of these eggs on the perianal skin causes itching and if this occurs, the eggs transfer to the hands and under the fingernails. Subsequent food consumption re-infects the host or transfers to another host. Secondary bacterial infection can occur due to breaks in the skin. Diagnosis is fairly easy since the eggs are present on the perianal skin, a swab dipped in saline can be rubbed on the area and sent to the laboratory for analysis. This is more convenient for the patient than having to submit a faeces sample. Alternately a piece of sticky tape can be touched onto the perianal skin and then placed onto a slide for direct examination under a microscope. The characteristic eggs can easily be seen. Laboratory staff must remember not to touch the sticky tape as the number of eggs on it can be significant and easily aerosolized. An egg of *Enterobius vermicularis* are shown in Figure 11.7.

11.4.5 *Anisakis simplex*

Infection of humans with the nematode *Anisakis simplex* is a fairly recently recognized infection which was first described in the 1960s following consumption of raw or undercooked fish.

In comparison to more well-recognized and documented gastrointestinal nematodes including hookworm, whipworm, pinworm, and guinea worm, *A. simplex* generally receives less attention, hence its place in this chapter. Anisakiasis has a worldwide distribution but tends to be more prevalent in Japan, USA, Netherlands, Germany, France, Spain, Belgium, and areas with large marine mammal populations. In Japan, there are approximately 2,000 cases reported per annum and in the USA there are around 10 annual cases. However, it is likely that many cases are not reported so these figures are likely to be an underestimation. *A. simplex* is a member of the family Anisakidae and is also known as the whaleworm as its definitive hosts include whales, dolphins, and porpoises.

urticaria
Skin rash characterized by pale red, raised, itchy bumps; often associated with an allergic response.

anaphylaxis
Serious allergic reaction that is rapid in onset. Symptoms include itchy rash, throat swelling, and low blood pressure. May result in death.

Unlike many other gastrointestinal nematode infections *A. simplex* has a fairly complex life cycle which includes planktonic crustaceans, intermediate hosts including fish (e.g. mackerel, salmon, cod, halibut, sardine) and cephalopods (e.g. squid), see Figure 11.8. Humans are accidental hosts following the consumption of L3 larval stages in the undercooked or raw flesh of fish and cephalopods. Foods including smoked herring, sushi, sashimi, and pickled anchovies are all considered high risk. As humans are accidental hosts, *A. simplex* larvae are unable to complete their life cycle and develop through to sexual maturity so they burrow into the intestinal wall. Within 2–5 hours of consuming L3 larvae approximately 97% of people experience gastrointestinal disturbances including abdominal pain, nausea, and vomiting. In around 3% of patients, the larvae migrate to the lungs, liver, and other tissues causing tissue damage that may result in acute allergic manifestations including **urticaria** and **anaphylaxis**.

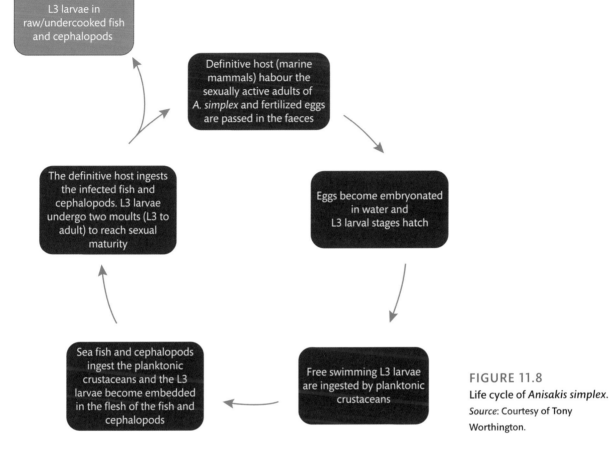

FIGURE 11.8
Life cycle of *Anisakis simplex*.
Source: Courtesy of Tony Worthington.

A. simplex is a gastrointestinal nematode which is dangerous both dead and alive. During the 1990s it was recognized that the consumption of dead worms in fish, which is properly cooked and considered safe, can still cause severe hypersensitivity reactions and that these may in fact be more common than the direct infection itself. It is now well recognized that *A. simplex* produces thermostable allergens that are able to withstand adequate cooking, microwaving, and freezing procedures. Allergic and anaphylactic symptoms may therefore arise from direct infection by the parasites ('gastroallergic anisakiasis'), and also occur following exposure to allergens from dead worms in properly cooked fish and cephalopods.

An effective control measure to prevent direct infection with *A. simplex* is to raise public awareness of anisakiasis and the potential hazards associated with eating raw or lightly cooked fish, however, these measures would not prevent allergic reactions due to thermostable allergens in cooked fish products.

Key Point

Thermostable allergens in *A. simplex* cannot be removed through normal cooking and freezing processes. Some people who state that they are allergic to 'fish' are actually allergic to the thermostable allergens of *A. simplex* present within the fish.

Why do you think *Enterobius* infections are more common in children?

Which morphological characteristics differentiate the nematodes from the cestodes and trematodes?

11.5 Cestodes (tapeworms)

Tapeworms which are important parasites of humans are called cyclophyllidean cestodes and they have a flat, segmented, ribbon-shaped body. The cestodes lack respiratory and digestive systems, nutrients are absorbed through a tegument which covers the body. The anterior end of the cestode comprises a scolex (head) consisting of four suckers and a double ring of hooks (rostellum) which are used for attachment purposes. The body (strobila) of the cestode is made up of segments (proglottids), each of which contains both male and female reproductive organs. Directly beneath the scolex lies immature proglottids whilst the middle section of the cestode contains sexually mature proglottids. The posterior end of the cestode comprises pregnant (gravid) proglottids which contain thousands of eggs. Gravid proglottids either burst, or are shed, in the faeces of the definitive host. Eggs contain the first stage larval form called an oncosphere or hexacanth. Most tapeworms have complicated life cycles including one or more intermediate hosts.

11.5.1 *Taenia saginata* (beef tapeworm) and *Taenia solium* (pork tapeworm)

Taenia saginata has a worldwide distribution, however, it is more common in Central Asia and Central/Eastern Africa and parts of the United States. Humans are the definitive host and become infected through consumption of larval stages (**cysticerci**) in undercooked beef. *Taenia solium* is common in Africa, India, Southeast Asia, and Central America. There are an estimated 50 million people infected with *Taenia* species worldwide. Human taeniasis occurs through consumption of cysticerci in undercooked pork and also through the accidental consumption of *T. solium* eggs on contaminated food, e.g. vegetation or through autoinfection associated with poor personal hygiene; this results in a condition called human cysticercosis. Adult worms remain in the jejunum for up to 25 years and reach a length of approximately 10 m. The egg of a *Taenia* sp. is shown in Figure 11.9. Although *Taenia* spp. are cosmopolitan, modern sanitary facilities and animal husbandry practices in developed countries have significantly reduced the risk of infection. In the UK, there are approximately 50–100 confirmed cases of *T. saginata* infection per year. There have been no reports of *T. solium* infection for some time.

The clinical symptoms associated with taeniasis due to *T. saginata* and *T. solium* are similar: many patients are asymptomatic whilst some present with abdominal pain, indigestion, weight loss, and **pruritis ani**. The complications associated with cysticercosis, however, may be more severe. Patients present with cysticerci in non-vital areas may be asymptomatic but serious complications may follow in patients with brain, eye, and heart involvement where hydrocephalus, meningitis, visual defects, and arrhythmias may result. It is estimated that approximately 1% of the population in endemic countries suffer from cysticercosis and 50,000 patients die per annum.

cysticeri

Larval form of *Taenia* species, consisting of a single scolex enclosed in a bladder-like cyst. Hexacanths, released from eggs, develop into cysticeri in the muscle of the intermediate host over a period of 3–4 months.

pruritis ani

Irritation of the skin of the anus causing patients to scratch.

FIGURE 11.9

Egg of a *Taenia* species.

Source: Courtesy of T. Carroll.

11.5.2 *Echinococcus granulosus*

Echinococcus granulsosus is the smallest medically important tapeworm measuring 2–5 mm in length and comprising three proglottids (immature, mature, gravid). *E. granulosus* is the cause of hydatid disease and has a worldwide distribution; however, it is more common in Europe, Africa, Asia, North and South America, Australia, and New Zealand. Human infection is directly associated with farming and raising sheep. Like many helminth infections, *E. granulosus* has a relatively complicated life cycle including an intermediate host. Humans act as accidental hosts in the life cycle. The definitive host for *E. granulosus* are canines (fox, dog, wolf, jackal, coyote, and dingo) which shed eggs in their faeces and contaminate the environment. The eggs are consumed by herbivores including sheep, cattle, deer, swine, and elk; after which the aggressive hexacanth larvae penetrate the intestinal wall and form hydatid cysts containing protoscolices (young heads) of *E. granulosus* in tissue, liver, and lungs of the intermediate host. Human infection occurs following consumption of water and vegetation which are contaminated with infective eggs or through hand-to-mouth transmission of canine faeces. Clinical symptoms of infection may not be apparent for up to 20 years following consumption of the infective eggs. The first symptom of infection is usually internal pressure within organs (liver, lungs) as the hydatid cyst expands. This may result in generalized pain, bile duct blockage, chest pain, and cough. If the cyst ruptures, fever, urticaria, anaphylactic shock, and death may result. In addition, rupture of hydatid cysts results in systemic dissemination of thousands of protoscolices which may infect other vital organs including the brain. Serological tests can be used to diagnose the disease but can take a long time for results to be available. Usually the surgical team on finding the cyst can remove it, although with extreme caution as leakage of the cyst fluid is very harmful to the patients. The presence of **hydatid sand** confirms the diagnosis. When examined microscopically the characteristic hooks and protoscolices (Figure 11.10) can be seen.

SELF-CHECK 11.7

With regards to the infection process how does human cysticercosis differ from human taeniasis?

Key Point

Whilst humans are considered 'accidental hosts' in the life cycles of *E. granulosus* and *T. solium* (cysticersosis), they 'accidentally' take the place of the true intermediate host in both life cycles.

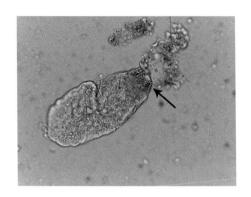

FIGURE 11.10
Scolices of *Echinococcus granulosus* – note the characteristic hooklets.
Source: Courtesy of T. Carroll.

Key Point

Hydatid sand is the scolices of *Echinococcus* contained within the cyst fluid.

11.5.3 Trematodes

Trematodes (flukes) are flat, leaf-shaped worms with an unusual physiology. Trematodes have two suckers, oral and ventral, which are used for consumption of food and attachment respectively, an incomplete digestive system, and are generally hermaphroditic with the exception of *Schistosoma* species. Trematodes have complicated life cycles which require intermediate hosts, the first of which is without exception, molluscs. Some trematodes require additional intermediate hosts to complete their life cycle. The eggs of the trematodes are usually large and with the exception of *Schistosoma* species are equipped with an **operculum**. Other trematodes of medical importance include *Fasciola* species, *Opisthorchis sinensis*, and *Paragonimus westermani* and their generalized life cycle is shown in Figure 11.11.

11.5.4 *Fasciola hepatica*

Fasciola hepatica, commonly called the 'sheep liver fluke', is a parasite of humans and herbivores (sheep, cattle). It has a worldwide distribution and estimated prevalence of 1–2 million and is common in South America, Cuba, North Africa, and parts of Europe. Human infection with *F. hepatica* occurs following consumption of water contaminated with metacercariae or contaminated vegetation, in particular, watercress and dandelion leaves. Following ingestion, the **metacercariae** excyst in the small intestine and migrate through the duodenal wall and across the peritoneal cavity. The larval flukes eventually penetrate the liver and enter the bile ducts where they develop into adult trematodes where hermaphroditic reproduction takes place. Clinical manifestations of infection can be broadly split into those associated with the invasive (acute) phase and the obstructive (chronic) phase. The invasive phase is associated with mechanical destruction of hepatic tissue due to migrating juvenile flukes and symptoms include; allergic reaction, fever, abdominal pain, hepatomegaly, ascites, and jaundice. The obstructive phase occurs months (or years) after initial infection and is characterized by epigastric pain, food intolerance, jaundice, nausea, and biliary obstruction. In severe infection

operculum
A 'lid' at the top of many trematode eggs which allows release of larval trematodes. A useful distinguishing feature when attempting to identify the egg.

metacercariae
Resistant, encysted final stage larval forms of some trematodes.

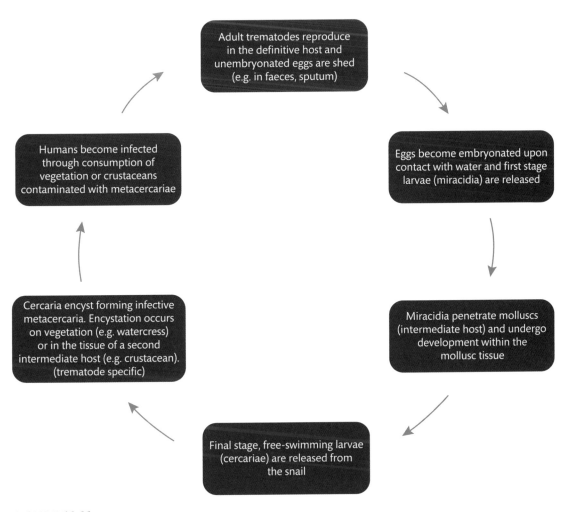

FIGURE 11.11
Generalized life cycle of the trematodes (*Fasciola, Opisthorchis, Paragonimus*).
Source: Courtesy of Tony Worthington.

a secondary bacterial infection may occur. Laboratory diagnosis is through detection of the large ova, approximately 140×80 nm from a stool sample around 2 months after the worm has matured in the host (Figure 11.12).

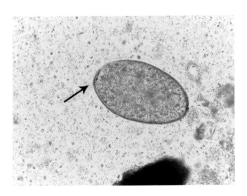

FIGURE 11.12
Ova of *Fasciola hepatica* – note the characteristic operculum (or lid) which can often be difficult to see with microscopy.
Source: Courtesy of T. Carroll.

11.5.5 *Paragonimus westermani*

Paragonimus westermani, commonly called the 'lung fluke' is just one of several species of *Paragonimus* to infect humans and cause the disease paragonimiasis. The infection occurs in several parts of the world but is more common in Asia, Africa, Latin America, and India and it is estimated that around 3 million people are infected. Whilst the general life cycle of *P. westermani* is similar to that of *F. hepatica*, this fluke requires a second intermediate host in which the infective metacercariae form. The second intermediate host in the life cycle of *P. westermani* is the crustacean. Human infection is directly associated with the consumption of metacercariae which is present in the tissue of raw or undercooked crustaceans, particularly freshwater crabs and crayfish. As a result, paragonimiasis is commonly linked with the consumption of pickled crustacean dishes including the Chinese delicacy 'drunken crab', as pickling is ineffective at destroying metacercariae of *P. westermani*. The clinical manifestations of paragonimiaisis are associated initially with the migration of fluke larvae and include eosinophilia, temperature, and rigors. Lung infection with the adult stage results in sputum production, cough with blood-stained sputum, and chest pain. In some patients, fibrosis of lung tissue may occur. Larval stages of *P. westermani* may also migrate to other vital organs including the liver and also brain where severe neurological disease (convulsions, visual defects, motor neuron disorders) may result as cerebral paragonimiasis.

11.6 Diagnosis of gastrointestinal parasitic infections acquired through the gastrointestinal tract

The rapid and accurate diagnosis of parasitic infection is essential to ensure that appropriate antiparasitic treatment is administered. However, a clinical diagnosis of parasitic infection associated with the gastrointestinal tract is difficult as symptoms are often non-specific and the clinician must therefore consider a detailed patient's history including: travel and leisure activities, diet and consumption of various foodstuffs and contact with animals to raise suspicion of parasitic infection. An accurate laboratory diagnosis is therefore always required to confirm a clinical suspicion of parasitic infection, however, a precise diagnosis is influenced by several factors including: collection of appropriate clinical samples, and timely transport to the laboratory, good laboratory practice ensures the appropriate tests are employed and the parasitic agent is accurately identified by an experienced microbiologist, and the results are accurately reported to the clinician in order that the correct anti-parasitic treatment is delivered.

Several laboratory procedures for the diagnosis of parasitic infection have been described and are widely used in clinical practice, these include: macroscopic examination of helminths, usually nematodes or proglottids of cestodes which are eliminated from the patient, microscopic examination of clinical material (duodenal aspirates and biopsies, fresh faeces, faecal concentrates) for ova, cysts, and parasites, serological examination for detection of antibody or parasitic antigens and molecular techniques including nucleic acid hybridization. Whilst several of these methods are useful in detecting a wide range of protozoa and helminths, some, in particular serological assays and molecular methods, aid in diagnosis of specific parasitic infections. Collection of the appropriate clinical sample and utilization of the correct diagnostic procedure cannot be over emphasized in facilitating an accurate diagnosis and these are summarized in Table 11.3 for the parasites described in this chapter.

TABLE 11.3 Clinical samples required and diagnostic procedures for parasitic infections acquired through the gastrointestinal tract.

Parasite	Clinical samples	Common diagnostic procedures
Entamoeba histolytica	Fresh and preserved faeces Serum, liver abscess aspirate	Microscopy (C,P), antigen detection serology (antibody)
Giardia intestinalis	Fresh and preserved faeces. Serum	Microscopy (C,P), antigen detection serology (antibody)
Cryptosporidium species	Fresh and preserved faeces	Microscopy (oocysts); permanent stain
Toxoplasma gondii	Serum	Serology (antibody)
Balantidium coli	Fresh and preserved faeces	Microscopy (C,P)
Ascaris lumbricoides	Preserved faeces. Whole nematode	Microscopy. Macroscopic examination
Anisakis simplex	Whole nematode. Immunological testing	Macroscopic examination. Specific IgE to *A. simplex*
Taenia saginata/solium	Preserved faeces. Serum. Proglottids	Microscopy (O). Serology (antibody to *T. solium*). Macroscopic examination (India ink)
Echinococcus granulosus	Sputum, hydatid cyst contents Serum	Microscopy (cestode hooklets) Serology (antibody)
Fasciola hepatica	Fresh and preserved faeces	Microscopy (O)
Paragonimus westermani	Sputum, fresh and preserved faeces	Microscopy (O)

Key: O: ova, C: cysts, P: parasites

11.7 Examination of faeces for ova, cysts, and parasites (O,C,P)

Microscopic examination of faeces is by far the most common diagnostic test employed by routine clinical microbiology laboratories for identifying parasitic infections and both fresh (hot) faeces and unpreserved formed faeces may be received in the laboratory. Fresh (hot) faeces are required for the detection of motile protozoan trophozoites, in particular *E. histolytica* and *G. intestinalis*. Fresh faeces should arrive in the laboratory within 30 minutes and be examined immediately as trophozoites disintegrate rapidly after defecation and do not encyst.

Unpreserved formed faeces should arrive in the laboratory within 2 hours following passage, and these samples are generally used for faecal concentration of ova, cysts, and parasites, which may be present in the sample.

Key Point

The optimal clinical sample for diagnosis of parasitic infection associated with the gastrointestinal tract is liquid or soft faeces. Some laboratories may reject formed faeces as this may compromise an accurate laboratory diagnosis as a negative result is likely to be obtained.

If there is likely to be a delay in examination of the faecal sample, it should be fixed in an appropriate preservative, for example, 10% formalin-saline is widely used: this serves to preserve any parasitic structures and also to kill any other enteric pathogens which may be present in the sample. However, several other preservatives are available for use including low viscosity polyvinyl alcohol (LV-PVA), merthiolate-iodine-formaldehyde, sodium acetate-acetic acid-formalin (SAF), and Schaudinn's fixative. The number of faecal specimens required to establish a precise diagnosis is influenced by several factors including parasitic load in the patient, sample quality, and accuracy of the diagnostic test. However, under routine circumstances, three faecal samples are generally requested. Once a sample of faeces is received in the clinical microbiology laboratory, a number of techniques can be employed to examine the sample.

1. **Macroscopic examination** of the faecal sample for the direct detection of adult helminths and proglottids of cestodes.

2. **Microscopic examination** of the faecal sample using the X10 or X40 objective. Ideally, three types of preparation should be made for liquid or soft faecal samples:

    a. **Wet preparation**

    For detection of motile trophozoites, cysts, oocysts, helminth eggs, and larvae. However, this technique is particularly useful for identification of active trophozoites thus facilitating the diagnosis of infections due to E. histolytica, G. intestinalis, and B. coli. Patches of blood or mucus within the faecal sample should be selected for direct examination as they may be derived from ulcers or purulent abscesses where large numbers of active amoebic trophozoites may be present.

    b. **Faecal concentration**

    As ova, cysts, and parasites are often in low numbers in clinical samples, concentration techniques are useful in improving the sensitivity of detection. Several techniques are available for faeces concentration, however, the two most commonly used methods are flotation and sedimentation. Flotation techniques incorporate solutions, e.g. zinc sulphate, which have a higher specific gravity than certain parasites which 'float' to the top of the solution whilst faeces debris sinks to the bottom This technique may be used for detection of Ascaris eggs and cysts of G. intestinalis. Another technique is Sheather's flotation which incorporates a concentrated sucrose solution for recovery of Cryptosporidium oocysts in faecal samples. Sedimentation techniques are more commonly used in clinical practice, for example, the formalin-ether concentration (FEC) method which is useful for detecting a wide range of ova, cysts, and parasites. The disadvantage of this method is that potentially hazardous reagents are used (formalin, ethyl acetate) and detection of parasitic structures may be compromised due to large amounts of faecal debris present in the sediment. The faecal concentrate may be stained with iodine to improve detection. This technique facilitates the diagnosis of a wide range of parasitic infections including those due to E. histolytica, G. intestinais, B. coli, A. lumbricoides, Taenia species, F. hepatica, and P. westermani. In most laboratories sedimentation techniques are performed using a kit system as such tests can be quite complex to perform.

    c. **Permanent stained smears**

    Faecal smears and concentrates may be stained with a variety of permanent stains; however, two commonly used stains include the trichrome stain and the iron-haematoxylin stain which enhance the detection and identification of E. histolytica and G. intestinalis. Additional permanent stains widely used in clinical microbiology include the modified Zeihl-Neelson stain for the detection of oocysts of Cryptosporidium species which stain red against a blue-green background. Fluorescent stains including auramine may also be used for the detection of these oocysts. It is generally accepted that the latter is more sensitive for detection of Cryptpsporidia oocysts. Finally, fluorescent antibody stains are also being incorporated for use in some laboratories; these utilize monoclonal antibodies directed against surface antigens of Cryptosporidium species and G. intestinalis.

TABLE 11.4 Characteristic morphological features of parasites used for laboratory identification purposes.

Parasite	Structure	General morphological features
Entamoeba histolytica	Cyst	**Microscopy:** 8–22 µm, circular, up to 4 nuclei, chromatoid bodies
	Trophozoite	**Microscopy:** 12–25 µm, pseudopod, ingested red blood cells, single nucleus
Giardia intestinalis	Cyst	**Microscopy:** 6–17 µm, 4 nuclei, oval
	Trophozoite	**Microscopy:** 10–15 µm, two nuclei, 4 pairs of flagella, axostyle, typical 'African-shield' appearance
Cryptosporidium species	Oocyst	**Microscopy:** 4–7 µm; circular, ZN positive, auramine positive
Balantidium coli	Cyst	**Microscopy**: 43–66 µm, micro and macro nucleus, double cyst wall, contractile vacuole
	Trophozoite	**Microscopy:** 20–150 µm;oval, micro and macro nucleus, cytostome
Ascaris lumbricoides	Ovum	**Microscopy:** 45–90 µm, oval, thick transparent hyaline triple layer shell, brown in colour
	Nematode	**Macroscopy:** 15–35 cm, smooth cuticle (unlike striated earthworm), 3 lips
Anisakis simplex	Nematode	**Macrosocpy:** 2 cm helminths, 'coiled watch-spring' appearance
Taenia saginata/solium	Ovum	**Microscopy:** 30–45 µm, spherical, thick shell with radial striations, three pairs of hooklets
	Proglottids	**Macroscopy:** *T. solium*=<13 uterine branches; *T. saginata*=>13 uterine branches
Echinococcus granulosus	Ovum	**Microscopy:** 30–45 µm, spherical, thick shell with radial striations
	Protoscolices and hooklets	**Microscopy:** protoscolices approximately 100 µm, 'monks-head' appearance, hooklets have typical rose-thorn appearance
Fasciola hepatica	Ovum	**Microscopy:** 150–90 µm, ovoid, opeculum
Paragonimus westermani	Ovum	**Microscopy:** 120–70 µm, ovoid, thick shell, opeculum

Characteristic morphological features of parasites described within this chapter identified through microscopy and macroscopy are shown in Table 11.4.

SELF-CHECK 11.8

Which microscopy techniques may be used for detection and identification of ova, cysts, and parasites in faeces?

SELF-CHECK 11.9

What is the optimal clinical sample for the detection of active parasitic trophozoites?

As the accurate diagnosis of parasitic infection by microscopy requires the microbiologist to identify and measure key structures and morphological features which are present within ova, cysts, and parasites, it is essential that the eyepiece graticule within the microscope objective is accurately calibrated.

11.7.1 Eyepiece calibration

Eyepiece graticule (Figure 11.13). The eyepiece graticule is a glass disc which is inserted into eyepiece of the microscope. The graticule contains a fine scale of 100 eyepiece units (EPU).

Stage unit/micrometer (SU). This is a microscope slide, in the centre of which is an engraved scale containing a series of divisions, each of which is 10 μm.

METHOD

- Start with the lowest power objective on the microscope. Align with the scales of the eyepiece graticule and stage micrometer and take a reading from the scales. The reading is then used to calculate the calibration factor for the objective lens. Example:
  - 100 EPU = 40 SU divisions
  - 1 EPU = 4 SU divisions
  - 1 EPU = 40 μm

SELF-CHECK 11.10

If 100 EPU on the eyepiece graticule measures 63 SU divisions, what does 1 EPU measure?

Microscopy

Eyepiece calibration

STAGE scale
100 units (1 unit = 10 μm)

EYEPIECE scale (100 units)

FIGURE 11.13
Example of eyepiece calibration for measurement of ova, cysts, and parasites.
Source: **Courtesy of Tony Worthington.**

100 EPU = 40 SU
100 EPU = 400 μm
1 EPU = 4 μm

11.8 **Immunological techniques**

In addition to microscopy techniques for the examination of clinical samples, serological assays for detecting parasitic antigens or antibodies to parasites are now being adopted by many diagnostic laboratories. Techniques include agglutination assays, immunofluorescence, enzyme immunoassay (EIA), and complement fixation. Detecting antibodies in serum is a useful adjunct to microscopy and aids in facilitating the diagnosis of parasitic infections due to *E. histolytica*, *T. gondii*, *T. solium*, and *E. granulosus*. However, as circulating antibodies to parasites may be detected in serum for several years following infection, detection of parasitic antigen in clinical samples including serum and faeces may be more appropriate as an indicator of active parasitic infection. A commonly used technique for antigen detection is EIA and is adopted for the diagnosis of infections due to *Cryptosporidium* species, *G. intestinalis*, and *E. histolytica*.

Cross reference
See Chapter 13.

11.9 **Molecular techniques**

Traditionally, parasites have been detected and identified by simple microscopy and serological techniques as outlined previously, However, in the modern world, molecular techniques including nucleic acid hybridization, polymerase chain reaction (PCR), random amplified polymorphic DNA (RAPD), amplified fragment length polymorphism (RFLP), and real-time PCR (RT-PCR) for diagnosis of parasitic infections are becoming more widely considered and available. Molecular diagnostic assays are advantageous in that they are able to both detect parasitic nucleic acid in clinical samples and also differentiate between different infecting parasites and strains of parasites depending upon the nucleic acid probe utilized in the assay. Molecular approaches of this nature also have advantages over serological techniques to detect raised antibody in patients as an active and effective immune response is not necessary to establish a diagnosis. As several parasitic infections are associated with immunocompromised patients including those with nutritional defects and HIV, molecular approaches offer a useful adjunct in diagnosis, however, they are often expensive compared with other techniques. PCR assays for diagnosis of parasitic infections, in particular those associated with *E. histolytica*, were recognized in the early 1990s and have been endorsed by the WHO (World Health Organization). Molecular methods of this nature which target 18S rDNA can be used for detecting and identifying *E. histolytica* from a variety of clinical samples including tissue, liver abscess aspirates, and faeces whilst also differentiating the organism from *E. dispar*. In addition, PCR methods demonstrate a similar performance to ELISA with respect to assay sensitivity and specificity. Despite these advantages, the major disadvantage is that they continue to be expensive and time consuming. A significant development within this area has been RT-PCR which allows quantification of parasitic nucleic acid from clinical and environmental samples as well as estimating the parasitic load and viability of parasites; however, again, cost remains an issue. Nonetheless, these methods have been utilized to study parasitic infections including those associated with *Giardia intestinalis*, *Cryptosporidia* species, and *Toxoplasma gondii*. Many studies have demonstrated that molecular approaches are effective and sensitive for the diagnosis of parasitic infection in humans, yet they continue to be disadvantaged by cost and the traditional 'back to basics' approach including antigen/antibody detection, microscopy, and an experienced eye for identifying parasitic stages which often prevails in the diagnosis of parasitic infection in many routine clinical microbiology laboratories.

11.10 **Treatment of parasitic infections acquired through the gastrointestinal tract**

Appropriate and adequate treatment of parasitic infections associated with the gastrointestinal tract is directly related to accurate diagnosis in the laboratory. It is important to adequately treat these infections for several reasons:

1. To directly eliminate the infection and restore human health.
2. To prevent carriage and subsequent transmission of the infection to further hosts.
3. To prevent further complications associated with the infection – some of which may be fatal.

TABLE 11.5 Antiparasitic agents and modes of action.

Antiparasitic agent	Mode of action	Treatment
Emetine	Interrupts cell division by inhibiting protein synthesis	Severe *E. histolytica* infections and amoebic liver abscess; active against trophozoites
Albendazole/ mebendazole	Inhibits glucose uptake in nematodes and cestodes; energy deprivation	Intestinal nematode and cestode infections; minimally absorbed; high gut concentrations achieved. Treatment of *A. lumbricoides*, *Taenia* infections, *A. simplex*; *E. granulosus* (in combination with surgery for removal of hydatid cysts)
Metronidazole (flagyl)	Superoxide derivatives of metronidazole breakdown interfere with DNA formation and protein synthesis	
Niclosamide	Interrupts oxidative phosphorylation in cestodes. Scolex detachment, muscular paralysis, and cestode disintegration results	Invasive *E. histolytica* infections, *G. intestinalis*, *Cryptosporidium species*, *B. coli*
Praziquantel	Increased membrane permeability to calcium. Muscular paralysis, detachment, and disintegration result	*Taenia infections*
Pyrantel pamoate	Cholinergic antagonist; irreversible contracture in muscle	*Taenia infections* including *cysticercosis*; *F. hepatica*; *P. westermani*
Nitazoxanide	Interference with the pyruvate:ferredoxin oxidoreductase (PFOR) enzyme-dependent electron transfer reaction which is essential to anaerobic energy metabolism	*A. lumbricoides* *Cryptosporidium* species
Pyrimethamine in combination with sulphadiazine	Pyrimethamine interferes with tetrahydrofolic acid synthesis from folic acid by inhibiting the enzyme dihydrofolate reductase which is needed for DNA and RNA synthesis. Sulphadiazine is a competitive inhibitor of bacterial para-aminobenzoic acid, a substrate of the enzyme dihydropteroate synthetase. Synthesis of folic acid is inhibited	Tachyzoites of *T. gondii*

Infections that occur directly in the gastrointestinal tract are treated with drugs that are poorly absorbed therefore high concentrations are achieved where needed, for example, in heavy helminth infections. Drugs that are easily absorbed are required for treatment of invasive parasitic infections, for example, those associated with migrating larvae or extraintestinal amoebiasis.

The summary of commonly used antiparasitic drugs for the parasites outlined in this chapter, along with their mode of action, is shown in Table 11.5.

SELF-CHECK 11.11

Which antiparasitic agents may be used for the treatment of nematode infections?

Chapter summary

After reading this chapter you should know and understand.

- On a worldwide basis, parasitic infections associated with the gastrointestinal tract are a significant cause of human suffering, however, in the UK cases are relatively few in comparison.

- Several protozoa, nematodes, cestodes, and trematodes can cause direct infection of the gastrointestinal tract and also extraintestinal complications.

- A wide range of risk factors can predispose humans to infection.

- Several foodstuffs are implicated in transmission of parasitic infection.

- The spectrum of clinical manifestations include asymptomatic, acute, chronic, and death.

- Parasites require one or more hosts to complete its life cycle and progression to maturity cannot be reached in intermediate hosts.

- Microscopy is the gold standard for diagnosis of parasitic infection and a detailed knowledge of parasitic morphology and characteristics (especially size) is required to establish an accurate diagnosis.

- Several antiparasitic agents are available for treatment of infection.

Further reading

- **Doyle E. *Foodborne Parasites: A Review of the Scientific Literature*. FRI Briefings** 2003. http://fri.wisc.edu/docs/pdf/parasites.pdf (accessed 14 August, 2013).

- **Murray PR, Rosenthal KS, Pfaller MA. *Medical Microbiology*, 6th edition. Mosby, 2009.**

- Winn W, Allen S, Janda W, Koneman E, Procop G, Schreckeberger P, Woods G. *Koneman's Colour Atlas and Textbook of Diagnostic Microbiology*, 6th edition. Lippincott Williams and Wilkins, 2006.

- Zeibig E. *Clinical Parasitology: A Practical Approach*, 2nd edition. Saunders, 2012.

 Discussion questions

11.1 What would be the main measures you would implement in a bid to reduce the number of parasite infections worldwide?

11.2 Many parasitic infections acquired though the gastrointestinal tract give rise to symptoms including diarrhoea, abdominal pain, or perhaps no symptoms at all. Which significant subsequent complications may arise from these relatively mild initial infections?

11.3 Can the detailed knowledge of parasitic life cycles lead to effective infection control?

12

Infection prevention and control

Sheila Morgan and Michael Ford

Infection prevention and control has always been a major priority within any healthcare environment. As an increasing range of organisms are causing outbreaks of infection, the importance of infection prevention and control has never been higher. Whilst several high-profile outbreaks of methicillin-resistant *Staphylococcus aureus* (MRSA) and C. *difficile* have focused attention of the governments and media, other organisms can be equally as important. As a result, the infection prevention and control team has a very varied role in both preventing and controlling the spread of infection.

Learning objectives

Upon reading this chapter the reader will have an understanding of the vital role of the laboratory as part of the infection prevention and control team. This will include:

- Procedures for the isolation and detection of MRSA.
- Procedures for the isolation and detection of vancomycin-resistant enterococci (VRE) strains.
- Pathogens requiring the laboratory to instigate a screening protocol.
- Types of isolation media used for infection prevention and control samples.
- Presumptive identification of these pathogens.
- Use of typing systems.
- Importance of C. *difficile* in hospital outbreaks.
- Use of rapid techniques, e.g. rapid PCR.
- Future problem organisms.

Upon reading this chapter the student will have an understanding of why infection prevention and control is important and the various strategies involved in its implementation. These include:

- Ward-based protocols – hand washing etc.
- Barrier nursing, management of cohorts.

- Current guidelines governing air quality in theatres.
- Disinfection policies used in a hospital.
- Disposal policy used in the hospital.
- Monitoring of air quality in theatres.
- Techniques to check the microbial cleanliness of the hospital environment and equipment.
- Policies for eradication.

12.1 What is infection prevention and control?

This can be simply defined as the attempt to stop the spread of an infectious agent (bacterial, fungal or viral) from contaminating or infecting another individual. Most commonly, this takes place in a hospital environment.

Cross reference

See Chapter 5.

Infection prevention and control has now become very high profile with headlines appearing in national newspapers almost on a daily basis. At present this is due mainly to methicillin-resistant *Staphylococcus aureus*, more commonly known as MRSA. This is a strain of *S. aureus* that has developed the ability to break down a very commonly used antibiotic – methicillin. In addition, most MRSA strains express resistance to a number of other commonly used antibiotics. This has made MRSA a particular problem, as infection with MRSA causes the same life-threatening illnesses as *S. aureus* but it is very difficult to treat – especially if it enters the patient's bloodstream. Hospitals care for patients whose immunity is compromised, or who have IV lines *in situ* or other breaks to the skin – so preventing MRSA getting into such sites is of paramount importance. Once the patient develops an initial focus of infection, or becomes **colonized**, it is not a huge step for the organism to spread into the bloodstream and produce life-threatening septicaemia. Typically, hospitals examine staff and patients as part of an overall screening strategy to detect the presence of MRSA.

colonization

Colonization is where the patient carries an organism on or in a particular body site but it is not doing them any harm. With MRSA it is often the nose that is colonized.

12.2 MRSA screening

MRSA screening is very different from most other samples sent to microbiology laboratories. This is because the patient may have no signs of infection. Indeed it is not just patients who are examined but staff also. The reason for screening is to detect the MRSA and hopefully eradicate it before it spreads to other individuals.

12.2.1 Consequences of MRSA colonization

Often MRSA colonization can go undetected. The MRSA is often not doing the patient or staff member any harm. It is the consequences of its spread that are the most apparent – particularly in a hospital environment.

Historically, the various approaches to MRSA screening have been somewhat haphazard and at times poorly organized. This has allowed some infected/colonized patients onto the wards with their MRSA status unknown. Similarly, staff who are colonized may have commenced work before having swabs taken and this can inadvertently lead to infection of patients on the unit.

A new screening regime called Search and Destroy is becoming popular. This is where all staff and patients are screened on admission and discharge, and in some larger hospitals results in nearly half a million swabs sent to the laboratory per annum.

12.2.2 Justification for MRSA screening

Overall MRSA screening is linked to many government targets to reduce the number of cases of MRSA bacteraemia (bloodstream infection). The main consequence of MRSA bacteraemia is the very high associated patient morbidity and mortality. The second reason is that failing to reduce the numbers of MRSA bacteraemia to within government targets can result in so-called hit squads being called into the hospital from the Department of Health, for example to make recommendations and insist standards of hygiene and techniques are improved. Naturally, this is seen as a failure of the infection prevention and control process and even the management of the hospital in general.

Key Point

Would you want to go or send a relative into a hospital knowing that it was failing in its hygiene standards?

One of the problems most hospitals face in complying with MRSA bacteraemia targets is the transfer of patients from other hospitals and nursing homes. These people may already be infected or colonized with MRSA when they arrive in the hospital. If they develop an MRSA bacteraemia where does the accountability lie? This would count as a bacteraemia for the hospital they are currently in which is argued as unfair. Hence, Search and Destroy programmes have arisen. By screening all patients on admission and discharge it can be proved that they either arrived with MRSA or acquired it during their hospital stay. This type of screening programme helps determine the possible cause when the number of cases of MRSA bacteraemia is examined.

12.2.3 Sample types and collection

The sample types and their collection can vary between hospitals but, generally, swabs are taken from inside the nose and the throat of staff and patients, plus swabs from any lesions (e.g. wounds). The commonest source of carriage of MRSA is the nose. The practice, however, may differ slightly in hospitals depending upon local policy; perineum (near the anus) and axilla (armpit) swabs are taken in some hospitals in addition to the previous. The swabs are then correctly labelled and sent to the laboratory for processing.

SELF-CHECK 12.1

Why are nasal swabs almost always sent for MRSA screening?

12.2.4 Sample processing

There are several different strategies for how MRSA is detected from screening swabs. The most common are enrichment culture, selective agars, chromogenic agar and molecular methods (PCR). We will examine each of these in turn.

Enrichment culture

Since there may only be a few cells of MRSA on a screening swab, finding them can be as difficult as finding a needle in a haystack. Some experts argue that a few cells are hardly going to be responsible for a hospital outbreak and may represent **transient colonization**. Opinion is still divided on how important small numbers of organisms are; however, several different enrichment methods have developed. These generally take the form of a broth culture containing antibiotics which suppresses other competing organisms, allowing the MRSA strains to multiply to high numbers so they are more easily detected.

MRSA selective broth is an example of a selective enrichment medium that is commercially available. It is a medium containing several antibiotics to inhibit methicillin-sensitive *S. aureus* as well as other organisms. The medium is based on the ability of the surviving MRSA strains to ferment mannitol and change the pH indicator from red to yellow due to acid being produced from the fermentation of mannitol.

It is important to understand how the microbiology department receives, processes, and reports results from MRSA screening tests and Figure 12.1 illustrates an example of the process which could be used from receipt of swab to issuing a report. Note how many stages are involved and how labour intensive the processes can be.

Whilst showing excellent sensitivity and specificity from nasal swabs, false-positive results from other sites are common. This is because swabs may contain high numbers of other organisms that may not be totally inhibited by the antibiotics present. As a result the carbohydrate can be fermented and a false-positive result obtained. Perineum swabs may contain high numbers of 'faecal organisms' and it is common for false-positive results to be obtained from such swabs using the broth enrichment method.

The major disadvantage of broth enrichment is that confirmed results may take 48 h to become available. As you can imagine this will have an impact on controlling the spread of MRSA if the patient or staff member is infected/colonized for 2 days before it is detected.

As a result there is a demand for more rapid methods, and newer chromogenic methods in particular can achieve excellent results in 18–24 h. A reduction from 48 to 24 h for the detection of MRSA may be hugely important in limiting its spread and reducing the chances of a patient subsequently developing MRSA bacteraemia. Despite broth enrichment having an advantage in detecting small numbers of MRSA in screening swabs, the method is being superseded because of a demand for more rapid methods.

Key Point

Can you imagine how far an infectious organism such as MRSA can spread if a result is not obtained for 48 h?

Selective media (non-chromogenic)

Most commonly this involves the use of a solid medium (similar principle to MRSA broth) which utilizes the fermentation of mannitol as the method of MRSA colony detection. The medium, mannitol salt agar, contains the antibiotic oxacillin (structurally similar to methicillin) and has a high salt concentration to suppress other bacteria which may interfere with the recognition of MRSA colonies. (MRSA strains survive well in high salt concentrations.) These agents give the medium its selectivity for MRSA. Unfortunately, like so many selective agars

---

transient colonization
Studies have shown that nurses at the start of a shift can be free of MRSA but the organism may be detected in nasal swabs in very low numbers later on. At the start of the next shift the MRSA strain may not be detected. This is an example of transient colonization.

Nasal swab

Place into
transport media

Label swab
and send to
laboratory

Inoculate
culture media

Incubate O/N at 37°C

Examine for typical colonies

(discard and report as negative
if no growth or negative growth)

Perform coagulase test
on typical colonies

Coagulase +ve

Coagulase –ve

Inform
Infection Prevention
+ Control Team

May need to confirm
suspect colonies
by other method
e.g. Mec A

Perform
susceptibility test

Confirmed
susceptibility pattern

FIGURE 12.1

Example of an algorithm for processing MRSA screening swabs.
Source: **Courtesy of M. Ford.**

which contain carbohydrates, the acidity released from fermentation diffuses through the agar, making the individual colonies of MRSA difficult to detect, particularly in mixed culture. This is shown in Figure 12.2. Some authors have demonstrated its limited sensitivity and selectivity for the direct isolation of MRSA from clinical samples and screening swabs. Despite these drawbacks the medium is still used for isolation of MRSA.

FIGURE 12.2

Growth of MRSA on mannitol salt agar. Note the diffusion of acidity away from the colonies.

Source: Courtesy of M. Ford.

Cross reference

See Chapter 3, Section 3.6.

FIGURE 12.3

Photograph of MRSA colonies growing on MRSA ID agar (bioMérieux). Note the difference between this medium and the mannitol salt agar (Figure 12.2) in the appearance of the colonies and the colour of the surrounding medium.

Source: Courtesy of M. Ford.

Another commonly used, non-chromogenic, selective MRSA agar is Baird Parker agar containing ciprofloxacin and potassium tellurite as the selective agents. MRSA strains are seen on the medium as black colonies due to the ability of *S. aureus* (and MRSA strains) to reduce the potassium tellurite and produce black coloration. As with any medium the colonies must be confirmed by a positive coagulase test.

Use of the medium is now dwindling due to several MRSA strains being susceptible to ciprofloxacin. This means the MRSA which is being sought may not grow on the medium, limiting its use.

Selective media (chromogenic)

These media are now well established as the routine method of choice in MRSA screening due to both high sensitivity and selectivity when compared to broth enrichment and other selective MRSA media. The results are available in 18–24 h, thus aiding the infection prevention and control infrastructure in its fight to contain and eradicate MRSA as quickly as possible. These media contain cefoxitin, to which MRSA strains are resistant. You may ask why methicillin is not used as the selective antibiotic in MRSA media. This is difficult to explain within the context of this chapter but it appears the structurally similar cefoxitin is better at inducing resistance in MRSA strains than methicillin.

Detection of the MRSA colonies is through hydrolysis of a chromogenic substrate. The principles of these substrates have been described in Chapter 3.

Key Point

Cefoxitin is a cephalosporin-type antibiotic which is structurally similar to penicillin. Studies have shown that this antibiotic induces *S. aureus* strains to express methicillin resistance better than methicillin itself.

Briefly, the colonies of MRSA which grow on the medium produce enzyme(s) which hydrolyse or 'break down' the colourless chromogenic substrate in the medium. Upon substrate hydrolysis, a rapid reaction with atmospheric oxygen occurs and a coloured compound is produced, as you can see in Figure 12.3. These coloured products are hydrophobic and stick to the surface of the colony. Each MRSA colony is therefore easily recognized, even in mixed culture. Several types of MRSA chromogenic media are available from a variety of commercial companies.

SELF-CHECK 12.2

Why are individual MRSA colonies in mixed culture more easy to spot on a chromogenic plate than on mannitol salt agar?

Molecular methods

Molecular methods would be expected to be ideal in the ever increasing demand for rapid MRSA results showing even higher sensitivity and specificity for MRSA screening when compared to culture methods. However, whilst promising to revolutionize MRSA screening, molecular methods have still not been widely adopted. The possible reasons are high cost, reduced sensitivity for samples other than nasal swabs, non-validation for swabs other than

1

Insert swab into
Sample Reagent vial
and break

2

Vortex and dispense
Sample into
Specimen Port

3

Insert cartridge and
start assay

FIGURE 12.4
Sample protocol for detection of MRSA in nasal swabs using the Cepheid Xpert™ MRSA system.

Source: Courtesy of Cepheid.

nasal and low throughput compared with conventional culture methods. In addition, it is generally perceived that specialist staff are required to perform molecular assays. However, systems such as the Cepheid Xpert™ (Cepheid, Sunnyvale, CA, USA) for MRSA and other assays (e.g. for *C. difficile* and *M. tuberculosis*) are extremely easy to use and can even be taken out of the laboratory setting and used as a point of care test (POCT) by medical and nursing staff at ward level. The assay can generate results in 1 h, which may be highly advantageous in certain clinical situations.

The Cepheid Xpert™ for MRSA combines a user friendly sample preparation system with real-time PCR amplification, with the process being fully automated (Figure 12.4). In trials, the positive predictive value was shown to be 80.5% and the negative predictive value (NPV) 96.6% for nasal swabs. This is higher than results achieved using chromogenic agars.

The cost of MRSA screening using molecular methods is, however, significantly higher in comparison to the costs of selective agars but it is important to always consider the 'bigger picture' in that significant savings may be achievable elsewhere due to operations not being cancelled because of the rapidity of such results, antibiotics may be avoided, spread of MRSA may not occur, etc. In the US, over $2.5 billion excess health-care costs have been attributed to MRSA infection.

Key Point
Remember that health care is a business and everything has to be paid for.

Certainly, reducing the screening time to an hour instead of overnight incubation would be expected to have significant benefits. This could save the patient requiring barrier nursing or having an operation cancelled. However, there are studies which have shown that following introduction of molecular methods costs rose significantly but there was little reduction in the number of MRSA cases.

SELF-CHECK 12.3

What are the benefits of molecular over cultural methods? What are the disadvantages of these methods and, having considered this, what single method would you recommend for MRSA screening in your institution?

Laboratories have been screening for MRSA for a number of years now and yet cases of MRSA bacteraemia are still high. Is screening the only answer?

12.3 Vancomycin-resistant enterococci (VRE)

Enterococci are part of the normal flora of the gastrointestinal tract. As you have seen in previous chapters they cause a wide variety of infections, most commonly urinary tract infections, which can develop into more serious conditions such as septicaemia. Generally, treatment of these infections is relatively straightforward using antimicrobials such as amoxicillin, which generally give a high concentration in the urine under standard dosage regimes.

Cross reference

See Chapter 4.

One of the most important groups of antibiotics are the glycopeptides, particularly vancomycin. As you can see in Chapter 4, vancomycin has very good activity against all commonly encountered Gram-positive pathogens (e.g. *S. aureus*, β-haemolytic streptococci, and enterococci) as resistance to the antibiotic is very rare. Therefore, if a patient is admitted with a suspected Gram-positive infection, clinicians can generally be safe in the knowledge that the patient should respond to vancomycin. This may not be true in all institutions as different geographical regions can have very different patterns of resistance. However, whilst resistance is still extremely rare in staphylococci, more and more infections with VRE strains are being reported, particularly in *Enterococcus faecium*, as you can see in Tables 12.1 and 12.2.

phenotype

A phenotype is a typical characteristic of an organism. This could be seen as its colonial appearance or biochemical properties. A typical *E. coli*, for example, may show different biochemical properties but it is still an *E. coli*.

VRE strains show various levels of resistance. Those expressing a Van A **phenotype** are classed as high-level resistant to both vancomycin and teicoplanin, another commonly used glycopeptide. Such VRE strains have an MIC of >128 mg/L and would show little or no response to treatment with vancomycin. In addition, VRE strains also carry resistance mechanisms to other antimicrobials making them truly multidrug resistant. Naturally, having VRE strains commonly isolated in a hospital environment would have a huge impact on the management of patients. For example, if glycopeptides could no longer be relied upon for treating severely ill patients suspected of having Gram-positive bacteraemia or other serious conditions what else could be used? Some VRE strains can be resistant to all penicillins, aminoglycosides and now glycopeptides, thus severely limiting therapeutic options.

Key Point

It is thought that VRE first developed through the misuse of antibiotics in animal feedstuffs and these resistant organisms transferred to humans through the food chain.

12.3.1 Sample processing

Because resistance to such key groups of antibiotics is extremely important, screening strategies have been developed to detect these in the hospital environment. Similar to MRSA screening there are several different methodologies: selective media, enrichment broth, and molecular methods.

TABLE 12.1 EARSS data on the percentage of invasive infections (blood culture isolates) caused by glycopeptides-resistant *E. faecium* in the EU in 2007.

Country	Invasive infections (%)
Greece	37
Ireland	33
Portugal	29
Cyprus	25
Israel	24
United Kingdom	21
Germany	15
Italy	11
Turkey	8
Czech Republic	6
Slovenia	5
Spain	2
Croatia	2
Austria	2
France	1
Denmark	1
Finland	1
The Netherlands	0

EARSS: European Antimicrobial Resistance Surveillance System.

TABLE 12.2 EARSS data on the percentage of invasive infections (blood culture isolates) caused by glycopeptides-resistant *E. faecalis* in the EU in 2007.

Country	Invasive infections (%)
Greece	6.7
Portugal	3.6
Ireland	2.6
United Kingdom	2.5
Italy	1.8
Czech Republic	1.4
Belgium	1.0
Germany	0.8
Denmark	0.5
Israel	0.5
Austria	0.3
Turkey	0.3
Spain	0.1

SELF-CHECK 12.5

Why is controlling the spread of VRE so important?

Selective media

Since enterococci are part of the gastrointestinal tract it is sensible to obtain samples from sites most likely to detect carriage of VRE in patients. Commonly, rectal swabs are sent, although faeces samples can be sent. The former is generally more acceptable to patients and staff, particularly those on Intensive Care Units (ICUs). These samples may contain high numbers of other bacterial types so culture media contain additional selective agents to remove these competing organisms.

FIGURE 12.5

Growth of *E. faecium* on BEAV agar showing typical black colonies due to the organism's ability to hydrolyse esculin.

There are several different media that have been used to isolate VRE strains from both clinical and environmental samples, all of which contain vancomycin as the selective agent. These media have varied from simple blood agar plus 4 mg/L vancomycin to bile esculin azide vancomycin (BEAV) agar which utilizes sodium azide and vancomycin as the selective agents (Figure 12.5). The latter has the advantage of utilizing esculin which is hydrolysed by enterococci to produce black colonies making detecting VRE strains easier. This medium, however, does not differentiate between species of enterococci and further tests are required to identify the vancomycin resistant strain.

Key Point

Remember other Gram-positive bacteria can be resistant to vancomycin – so just because an organism grows on the medium doesn't mean it is always a VRE!

Chromogenic VRE media

Media such as BEAV are now being superseded by chromogenic media (e.g. chromID VRE agar from bioMérieux). This medium has the advantage of allowing differentiation between the commonest enterococcal strain types, *E. faecalis*, and *E. faecium*, based on the colour of the colony obtained (Figure 12.6). Studies have shown improved recovery of VRE from stool samples over BEAV agar in 24 h. Chromogenic media are gradually superseding conventional media for the isolation of VRE strains, such as those based on esculin. These allow differentiation of *E. faecium* and *E. faecalis* directly. In addition, these organisms grow as discreet colonies with no diffusion of the reaction products into the surrounding medium.

FIGURE 12.6

Growth of *E. faecium* (violet) and *E. faecalis* on chromID VRE agar. Note both the differential aspects of the medium and the localization of the chromogen on the colonies, and lack of diffusion into the surrounding medium.

Source: Courtesy of bioMérieux.

Enrichment culture

Again similar to some MRSA screening strategies, low numbers of VRE in a sample can be enriched to high numbers by the use of broth enrichment. Bile esculin broth (BEB) plus vancomycin at a concentration of 15 mg/L has been compared with BEAV and led to significantly more VRE strains being detected than direct culture. Whilst detection is enhanced it takes a further 24 h for a result to be available compared with direct plating. The enrichment broth is also differential in that the broth turning black indicates the presence of a VRE.

Key Point

Hydrolysis of esculin by bacteria results in the formation of a diffusible black pigment.

12.4 Detection of pathogens that require initiation of a screening programme

In theory the patient-to-patient transmission of any pathogen could prompt the laboratory to initiate a screening programme. Alternatively, this could be from staff to patients or vice versa or even amongst a group of staff. In general, a screening programme would be initiated following detection of a multidrug-resistant bacterium or a significant organism such as a Group A *Streptococcus*. It is important that pathogenic organisms are monitored in highly important clinical areas, such as ICUs, special care baby units (SCBU), or sterile theatres, as the transmission of pathogenic organisms in such environments is likely to have serious consequences and outbreaks could occur. In addition, fungal pathogens can cause significant morbidity and mortality and finding them may also trigger a screening programme.

The laboratory would have to adapt to whatever the problem organism is and develop a plan for its isolation and identification. Good communication with the infection prevention and control team is essential to plan which samples are to arrive and when. In addition, it is imperative to relay the laboratory results back to the team as soon as possible.

Technically, you would need to determine the resistance pattern of the potential outbreak strain as this would be important in determining which media could be used for its selective isolation. You would also need to consider the organism's growth pattern and the atmospheric conditions it is best suited to for optimal isolation. In addition, you will need to consider which enrichment media to use should the situation warrant its use. As you can imagine there are hundreds of possibilities based on the nature of the outbreak strain. Finally, consider the staff resources which may be necessary.

12.5 Importance of *Clostridium difficile* (*C. difficile*) in hospital environments

C. difficile is the major cause of antibiotic-associated diarrhoea (AAD) and **pseudomembranous colitis** throughout the world. In many instances the organism is carried harmlessly as part of the normal human gastrointestinal flora. Indeed it is estimated that over half of all healthy neonates carry the organism asymptomatically. So how does an organism which exists harmlessly in the gastrointestinal tract initiate the disease process?

C. difficile is a Gram-positive anaerobic rod which is carried as a harmless commensal in the gastrointestinal tract of many individuals. Strains can produce one or both of two toxins, A and B. These are large protein toxins. Toxin A is an **enterotoxin** and toxin B is a **cytotoxin**. Toxin A appears to be most important in pseudomembranous colitis. The organism becomes a problem when it can multiply in the gastrointestinal tract and is no longer kept in check by the high numbers of other bacteria in the gastrointestinal tract. Such a proliferation of *C. difficile* can occur when the patient has had, or is undergoing, a course of antibiotics. The antibiotics wipe out the other competing bacterial flora and allow *C. difficile* to multiply. Patients in hospital are often on antibiotics and this tends to increase in the winter months when colds and other viruses trigger off respiratory infections. Since *C. difficile* strains produce a highly cell-damaging toxin, pseudomembranous colitis (Figure 12.7) can develop which is a life-threatening condition, especially in the elderly. This can be even more severe if patients are receiving agents which reduce or stop gut motility, as this prevents the organism and toxin from being excreted.

C. difficile has developed a very high profile as an organism capable of causing significant morbidity and mortality, especially in the elderly. Reduction in the number of *C. difficile* infections is a high government priority. Outbreaks have occurred worldwide, which have resulted in numerous patient deaths and raised the awareness of standards of cleanliness in hospitals generally. Therefore the rapid detection, containment, and treatment of patients with *C. difficile* infection are important targets for both governments and hospitals. In the USA, it is estimated that each case of *C. difficile* infection results in additional costs of over $15,000.

pseudomembranous colitis

Pseudomembranous colitis is an infection of the colon, the symptoms of which are severe diarrhoea, abdominal pain, and fever. The disease can often be fatal, particularly in elderly patients.

enterotoxin

An enterotoxin is a toxin released by an organism in the intestine. It is a protein and frequently cytotoxic, killing the host cells.

cytotoxin

A cytotoxin is a toxin that kills cells.

FIGURE 12.7

Section of the large intestine showing *C. difficile* infection. Pseudomembrane (comprising fibrin, red blood cells, epithelial debris, and mucus) overlies dilated crypts in which epithelium is largely lost.
Source: Reproduced by kind permission of Professor Alan Patterson.

Whilst *C. difficile* infection rates in the vulnerable over 65-year-old group are starting to fall, the UK Health Protection Agency reported that there were 2,704 deaths from *C. difficile* between 2009 and 2010. It is in this age group that most of the deaths due to *C. difficile* occur, with an increase in cases noted in the winter months.

SELF-CHECK 12.6

Why do *C. difficile* infection rates increase in the winter months?

12.5.1 Laboratory diagnosis of *C. difficile*

The accepted gold standard for the detection of *C. difficile* is a cytotoxin assay which utilizes cell culture. Essentially, this is to demonstrate that a faeces supernatant can kill a monolayer of cells, and this effect is lost if an antibody is added which reacts with the toxin and thus protects the cells from damage. Some laboratories use an alternative gold standard (cytotoxigenic culture) where *C. difficile* strains are grown from the sample followed by cell culture to determine toxin production. The latter is used to detect *C. difficile* strains which have the capacity to produce toxin, rather than detecting the presence of toxin in a sample. These assays, however, suffer from the drawbacks of maintenance of cell lines, high turnaround times and being quite labour intensive to perform. As a result the detection of toxins using automated platforms has become widespread.

Other methods are available for the detection of *C. difficile* disease and a single test strategy is no longer deemed appropriate. In the past most laboratories routinely used a single ELISA method to detect toxin in the stool sample. These ELISA tests are relatively simple to perform as they are usually available on automated platforms. These initially superseded the use of cell culture methods which are quite labour intensive with contamination of cell lines a particular problem. The ELISA method takes around 90 min to produce a result, which is then given to both clinicians and infection prevention and control staff so a patient positive for *C. difficile* toxin can be managed appropriately. These patients are often **barrier nursed** in an attempt to contain the organism and stop any potential spread of infection.

However, several studies have shown that the sensitivity and specificity of many ELISA tests are too low for use as a diagnostic test alone. Some studies have highlighted false-negative rates as high as 50%. As a result the latest guidance form the UK Department of Health is to use a first line screening test followed by a sensitive toxin ELISA to confirm the presence of toxin in the sample.

barrier nursing

Barrier nursing involves putting the patient in a side room or with other individuals with exactly the same infection in the same room. The nursing staff wear disposable aprons and gloves when dealing with these patients to minimize any spread of the infection to other patients.

The first-line screening test most favoured is the glutamate dehydrogenase test (GDH) to detect an enzyme which is produced by both toxigenic and non-toxigenic strains of *C. difficile*. It is produced in large amounts and is therefore a useful antigenic marker for the organism. GDH in some studies has a negative predictive value of >99%; thus samples can be screened using a GDH assay and if negative, results can be reported in under 1 h. GDH, however, does not distinguish between toxin-positive and toxin-negative strains. As a result positive samples need to be tested for toxin A + B by a sensitive ELISA method before being reported as positive. Since *C. difficile* is a life-threatening disease, the faster the disease is diagnosed the better for both management of the patient and reduction of spread of the infection.

As an alternative to using GDH as a first-line screening test a rapid molecular method (NAAT) could be used which can detect the presence of toxin-producing *C. difficile* in less than 1 h. Compared with the gold standard of cell culture the sensitivity of molecular assays was shown to be 100% with a specificity of 93%. Since GDH is a low-cost method in comparison to NAAT, most algorithms for the detection of *C. difficile* disease use GDH rather than molecular tests as the first-line screening method. Molecular assays are being developed so they can be ward-based, which removes any potential delays in transportation to the laboratory. It is vital, however, that the infection prevention and control team knows the results generated at ward level from such assays.

The organism can also be cultured on solid media like any other organism. Unfortunately, the colonies smell of horse manure so it is not a particularly pleasant job! The organism has a typical colonial appearance, under anaerobic conditions. It generally takes 48 h to grow the organism, and only then can it be tested to determine if it produces toxin(s). This is a more lengthy process than simply testing the stool sample for toxin. Some algorithms are recommending the use of cultures in certain situations in an attempt to detect patients who are secretors of *C. difficile*. However, culture can be useful to determine if the organism causing the infection is exactly the same as that infecting other patients on the same ward or environment. The process used is that of **ribotyping** which involves extraction of RNA from isolated *C. difficile* cells and comparison with that of other *C. difficile* ribotypes. In the UK, the common ribotypes are 001, 016, and 019; however, an outbreak strain which caused significant mortality in Canada was shown to be ribotype 027. The significance of this strain is high due to its ability to produce much more toxin than other *C. difficile* ribotypes. This 027 strain is known as a hyper toxin producing strain.

ribotyping
Ribotyping is the process of trying to 'fingerprint' an organism by detection of specific genomic DNA.

In severe cases of *C. difficile* infection, the patient would be started on either metronidazole or oral vancomycin for 10 to 14 days. In mild cases, due to antibiotic use, it is usually enough to withdraw the offending drug, allowing diarrhoea to settle within a few days. Since many patients may be frail it is particularly important to correct dietary deficiencies, especially where they are low in protein. In severe cases, the bowel may distend greatly and perforate, leading to peritonitis, in which case urgent surgery is needed.

Key Point

No single laboratory method alone is suitable for the optimal detection of *C. difficile* infection.

SELF-CHECK 12.7

What would you consider to be the best algorithm for the laboratory detection of *C. difficile* infection? What are your reasons?

12.6 **Gram-negative outbreaks**

Whilst considerable attention has focused on transmission and control of Gram-positive pathogens such as MRSA and *C. difficile*, the importance of Gram-negative pathogens in the healthcare environment must not be underestimated. In the past there have been major healthcare problems associated with strains of *Pseudomonas aeruginosa* and *Serratia marcescens* in particular, not because they possess the wide range of virulence properties associated with Gram-positive pathogens as shown earlier, but often because they possess antibiotic resistance traits which can select out for them, allowing them to dominate in particular situations e.g. in the wounds of burns patients and those on ventilators. If we look over the last few years there is a trend developing which shows that multi-antibiotic resistant bacteria are being isolated more frequently. Examples of this include the extended spectrum β-lactamases (ESBL) seen in some Gram-negative bacteria such as *E. coli* and *Klebsiella* spp. These strains have caused outbreaks in some hospitals and in the community. It is reported that their general prevalence is increasing, leading to significant morbidity and mortality.

Of growing concern is the appearance of multi-drug resistant (MDR) strains of *Acinetobacter baumanii*, which of all of the antibiotics in our armoury, some strains are only susceptible *in vivo*, to colistin and tigecycline. These strains have often entered the environment from patients who have been admitted following travel or injury abroad and transported back to the UK for treatment. It is the rapidity with which some organisms can develop such resistance and spread which is causing the greatest concern for future public health.

carbapenemase

Carbapenemase is an enzyme which hydrolyses not only penicillins but also cephalosporins, monobactams, and carbapenems. Strains that produce these enzymes are highly drug resistant.

One of the major concerns with these organisms is their ability to produce an enzyme (**carbapenemase**) which breaks down a group of antibiotics including meropenem and ertapenem. Resistance to carbapenems can also be associated with a cell change which hinders the antibiotic entering the cell. Resistance to carbapenem antibiotics is of serious concern as they are one of the most important antibiotics of choice, particularly for patients with a serious, systemic Gram-negative infection. It is likely that such strains will be encountered more frequently and strategies will need to be developed for their detection. Carbapenemases are intrinsic (found naturally) in some clinically significant bacteria. These include *Stenotrophomonas maltophilia* and *Aeromonas* spp. *Acinetobacter baumannii* posesses a gene for an intrinsic carbapenemase (OXA-51-like), which confers reduced susceptibility or resistance to carbapenems when expressed.

Acquired carbapenemases are diverse and include members of three of the four β-lactamase families:

- *Class A enzymes*: They are probably the most important KPC enzymes, which are endemic in many parts of the world including parts of the USA, Greece, Italy, Israel, and China. These organisms, worryingly, are now being encountered elsewhere, including the UK;

- *Class B enzymes*: These enzymes are known as metallo-β-lactamases (MBLs) or metallo-carbapenemases. The major MBL families encountered in the UK are the NDM and VIM types;

- *Class D enzymes*: This class of enzymes comprises many diverse enzymes, few of which are carbapenemases. Important carbapenemases within the family include OXA-23, -40, -51, and -58 and their variants from *Acinetobacter species*, OXA-48 and related enzymes in Enterobacteriaceae.

To combat carbapenemase-producing Gram-negatives it is essential to understand their epidemiology. Rapid laboratory diagnosis and surveillance based on risk assessments are essential. Patients who are deemed at high risk need to have a rectal swab taken for screening. This would be inoculated onto a selective medium containing a carbapenem. Every healthcare facility must have rigid infection prevention and control procedures in place to manage one of the greatest risks to public health in decades.

SELF-CHECK 12.8

How many antibiotics active against Gram-negative organisms can you think of, and which of them would be effective in treating a MDR *Acinetobacter baumanii*?

Highly pathogenic and MDR organisms require a worldwide strategy for dealing with their spread. This could include the stockpiling of antimicrobial/antiviral drugs, involvement of local and national organizations and dissemination of information to both the public and health-care workers. The infection prevention and control teams need to assess each situation on an individual basis and develop policies and procedures to manage a multitude of different scenarios. Close links therefore with microbiology staff are essential.

12.6.1 Panton–Valentine leukocidin-producing *S. aureus*

S. aureus strains producing a toxin called Panton–Valentine leukocidin (PVL) have been implicated in outbreaks of severe disease in the community. PVL is a toxin produced by *S. aureus* which can kill white cells. Fortunately, it is only produced by a minority of strains at present but infections with such strains are severe, leading to significant morbidity and mortality. Most notably the toxin can be produced by MRSA strains which show susceptibility to ciprofloxacin.

Think back to what you have read so far and if it could be problematic to isolate these strains from screening swabs.

12.7 Other resistance screening and media

New media are becoming commercially available every year and are targeted at resistant organisms or organisms that are currently difficult to isolate using currently available media. Most of the new media arriving on the market contain chromogenic substrates as these make target colonies much easier to detect. However, as a biomedical scientist you may be placed in a position where there are no commercially available media available which will meet your needs. In an emergency situation where you may be required to screen for an organism which is causing IPC issues in your healthcare facility, you may need to make your own. In such situations you need to consider the resistance spectrum of the target organism and also what other selective agents you could add to the medium to suppress competing organisms. For example, incorporating vancomycin is generally a good selective agent for Gram-negative strains in media as the majority of Gram-positive organisms are susceptible to it. Aztreonam will inhibit the growth of many Gram-negative strains and is an excellent selective agent for the majority of Gram-positive pathogens. It is important that the biomedical scientist is aware of any new developments in microbiology so that the best possible media and techniques can be applied for the benefit of patients.

12.8 Infection prevention and control

It is estimated that at any one time, over 1.4 million people worldwide are suffering from infections acquired in hospital and between 5 and 10% of patients admitted to modern hospitals in the developed world acquire one or more infections. As a result, the emphasis on infection prevention and control has never been greater.

Infection prevention and control has always been at the cornerstone of all clinical practices. Since 2000, however, it has assumed new political significance and taken centre stage in government policy. National Audit Office Reports in the UK identified that there needed to be a cultural shift towards infection prevention as well as control as the cost of hospital acquired infection (HAI) to the UK NHS was stated to be as much as £1 billion per year, with 9% of patients acquiring an infection as a result of an inpatient episode, resulting in 5,000 deaths per year. It was estimated that 15% of HAIs could be prevented, releasing circa £150 million back into the NHS.

Since then there have been many national strategies put in place to reduce the incidence of HAIs. These include:

mandatory reporting

Mandatory reporting is the obligatory reporting of a particular condition to local or national authorities. This often applies to communicable disease. Reporting of MRSA bacteraemia and *C. difficile* infection is mandatory in the UK.

- Audit and financing improvements in decontamination facilities.
- **Mandatory reporting** of MRSA bacteraemia.
- Mandatory reporting of VRE bacteraemia.
- Nationally and locally agreed targets for MRSA bacteraemia.
- Recording incidences of *Clostridium difficile*-associated diarrhoea.
- New post of Director for infection prevention and control.

All these strategies have culminated in The Health Act 2006: Code of Practice for the Prevention and Control of Health Care Associated Infections in the UK. This document is statute and therefore compliance with the elements of the Act is mandatory. The Health Act sets out the criteria for senior managers of each NHS organization 'to ensure that patients are cared for in a clean environment, and the risks of Health Care Associated Infections are kept as low as possible'. The Care Quality Commission is responsible for auditing compliance with these criteria. Failure to comply could result in significant consequences for the NHS organization involved. Some of the topics discussed next are encompassed within The Health Act 2006.

12.8.1 Hand hygiene

resident organisms

Resident organisms are also known as normal flora or commensals. These are deeply seated within the epidermis in skin crevices, hair follicles, sebaceous glands, and beneath fingernails. Their purpose is protecting the skin against colonization by transient organisms. They are not readily removed by hand washing.

If hand hygiene is carried out properly then it is the single most important and cost effective method of preventing the transfer of organisms from the environment or patient to another patient and thereby preventing potential infections occurring. However, it is often performed ineffectively and infrequently. Various campaigns and initiatives have been tried in a bid to improve hand washing compliance. One of these, the '5 moments for Hand Hygiene', has been launched to show ward staff in particular that hands must be washed five times in the whole period of patient contact (Figure 12.8).

Hand hygiene consists of two main methods: (a) hand washing and (b) application of alcohol-based hand disinfectants. Both methods disinfect the hands; that is, the processes involved *reduce* the number of potentially harmful organisms on the skin. Organisms found on the skin can be **resident** or transient.

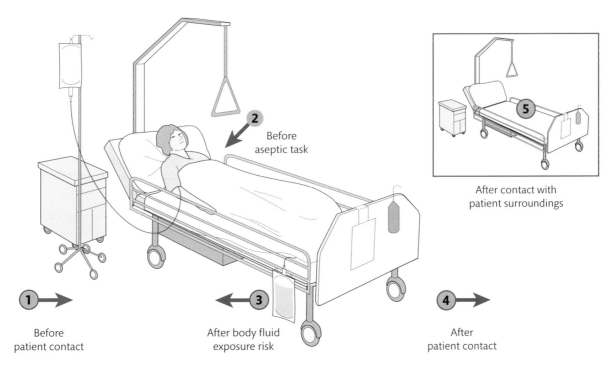

FIGURE 12.8
Image showing the five moments of hand hygiene, used as an educational aid to health-care workers.

The type of soap used will depend upon the nature of the task or procedure that is to be undertaken and the susceptibility of the patient. There are three methods of rendering hands safe: social, disinfectant, and surgical hand wash.

Social hand washing involves the use of soap and water and is used in most activities such as washing hands upon leaving a toilet facility, handling soiled nappies, and preparing food. In general, washing hands for 10–15 seconds with simple liquid soap will suffice for these tasks. This process removes transient organisms.

Liquid disinfectant soaps with greater antimicrobial activity are used for many hand washing practices in hospitals, as patients are more vulnerable to infection. These products remove and destroy transient organisms and remove some detachable resident organisms. Some products, such as chlorhexidine gluconate, have a residual effect.

Surgical hand washes are used prior to theatre procedures and their purpose is to further reduce the number of resident organisms on the skin of the operator/clinician to a safe level to prevent potential infection of the surgical site.

In September 2004, the National Patient Safety Agency issued a Patient Safety Alert to all acute trusts in England instructing that alcohol-based hand gels (AHBG) should be installed at all points of use, for example at ends of beds and bedside lockers, by April 2005 in order to improve hand hygiene compliance to reduce the incidence of **hospital-acquired infections**.

Alcohol-based hand disinfectants have good activity against most organisms save spores. These products should only be used on clean hands, as they are known to be less effective in the presence of soiling and dirt. They do not have any residual antimicrobial activity.

hospital-acquired infection

Hospital-acquired infection is also called nosocomial infection. It is an infection which appears more than 48 h after a patient has been admitted to hospital or other health-care facility.

Do you think ABHG would be useful to eliminate *C. difficile* from the ward environment?

12.8.2 Standard Precautions

Universal Precautions were a set of clinical actions initially introduced in the USA during the 1980s by the Centers for Disease Control (CDC) mainly to address the rising incidence of blood-borne viral infections (e.g. hepatitis B and human immunodeficiency virus) in health-care workers; it was noted that many of these individuals had suffered skin contamination with blood from patients or received sharps injuries.

The main principle of these precautions was to prevent parenteral, mucous membrane, and non-intact skin exposures of health-care workers to blood-borne pathogens through sharps injuries and body fluid splashes/exposure whilst protecting patients from cross-infection. Since then, these principles have been adopted by other national health-care providers and are referred to as Standard Precautions.

Key Point

Sharps injuries often occur from contaminated needles which have been used to take blood and not discarded properly. This situation is totally avoidable!

Standard Precautions involve identifying high-risk procedures rather than high-risk individuals and also have the benefit of preventing patient discrimination. Health-care staff should consider all blood and body fluids (including semen, vaginal secretions, cerebrospinal fluid, amniotic fluid, peritoneal fluid, pericardial fluid, pleural, and synovial fluids) as high risk, that is potentially infective, whether visibly blood-stained or not and wear the appropriate personal protective equipment (PPE) – masks, goggles, gloves, aprons, gowns, etc.

Other essential elements apart from PPE that comprise Standard Precautions are:

- Good standards of hand hygiene.
- Use of gloves (sterile or non-sterile as appropriate).
- Safe disposal of sharps and single use/disposable equipment.
- Management of used and soiled laundry.
- Decontamination of equipment.

12.8.3 Isolation nursing

Patients who are known to have, or are suspected of having, certain serious and potentially communicable (transmissible) infections require isolation precautions and management in order to prevent cross infection. Equally, patients who are particularly vulnerable to infection may also require isolation accommodation.

Ordinarily, the patient is managed in single room accommodation, with an ante-room/lobby, and ideally with en-suite facilities. All doors are kept shut at all times. Sometimes it is necessary to restrict the number of relatives and visitors to the patient depending upon their clinical condition and in some circumstances this can last for several weeks. As you can imagine these facilities are expensive to build and therefore their numbers are limited.

There are two main classes of isolation:

- Source – for known or suspected infectious patients.
- Protective – for patients who are rendered highly susceptible to infection by their disease or therapy.

The common means of transmission of infection are by:

- Airborne route.
- Faecal–oral route.
- Direct contact.

Source isolation

This class of isolation can be divided into three main categories:

- Strict – for highly transmissible or dangerous diseases such as viral haemorrhagic fevers (VHF), e.g. Lassa, Ebola, and Marburg. Currently there are only two of these highly specialized Category 4 units in the United Kingdom sited in Newcastle and London.
- Respiratory – for diseases where the main route of transmission is airborne, e.g. pulmonary tuberculosis, measles, mumps, rubella.
- Standard – for most other communicable disease, e.g. MRSA, viral gastroenteritis, *Clostridium difficile*-associated diarrhoea.

Protective isolation

As patient susceptibility to infection varies considerably, depending upon the patient's disease and/or therapy, so does the isolation requirement for these particular patients. Patients with extensive burns, neutropenia, and those receiving immunosuppressive therapy such as transplant recipients would require protective isolation nursing and management.

12.8.4 Management of cohorts

Due to diseases such as seasonal viral gastroenteritis, for example, it is not always possible to isolate all affected and symptomatic patients due to the shortages and greater demand made upon single room accommodation during such outbreaks. However, whenever possible it is best practice to find appropriate single room accommodation. Where and when this is not possible patients are managed in 'cohorts'. In circumstances such as these, patients who have had contact with the **index patient** are kept together and managed as a group. This prevents potential spreading of the causative organism to patients who have not been exposed to the index carrier thereby minimizing the numbers of patients affected.

index patient
An index patient is the individual who first shows signs of the disease.

SELF-CHECK 12.10

Why are cohorts managed together, generally in the same room, rather than isolated individually?

Underpinning and common to all these types of isolation management, with the exception of Strict Isolation (where additional specialized equipment and procedures are used), are good standards of hand hygiene prior to entering and leaving the facilities, safe disposal of sharps, decontamination of equipment, appropriate waste disposal, management of used laundry, good standards of daily environmental cleanliness, and thorough terminal cleaning of the facility once the patient has been discharged.

12.8.5 Disinfection policy

Every institution must have a disinfection policy to ensure the environment is clean and safe for staff, patients, and visitors. This policy will include several processes by which this is achieved – these are described next. It must be remembered that disinfection does not bring about the same level of reduction in microbial contamination as sterilization.

Sterilization

This is a process used to render an object free from all viable microorganisms, including viruses and spores. For example this process is used for theatre instruments and for instrumentation that enters a sterile body site such as needles and cannulae which are used to access the bloodstream.

It is essential to emphasize that prior to either process being employed, a thorough physical cleaning must be the first step to ensure that all dirt/soiling and organic matter is removed. Hand-hot water and detergent are usually all that is needed for cleaning processes; however, it is prudent to check with manufacturers of equipment to ensure that they are compatible with such.

Disinfectants and alcohol-based products are not effective in the presence of dirt and organic matter and therefore small but significant numbers of potentially pathogenic microorganisms may remain and pose an infection risk to subsequent patients.

Ward routine

Daily dusting and cleaning of the ward environment with hot water and detergent is a daily process and an essential part of ward routine. Occasionally, chlorine-releasing solutions are used to achieve a higher level of disinfection especially during outbreaks of viral gastroenteritis, for example. Should the clinical environment not be subject to high standards of cleanliness it can play a significant part in contributing to the acquisition of health-care associated infections such as *Clostridium difficile*-associated diarrhoea, as highlighted in the UK Healthcare Commission's Report concerning Maidstone and Tunbridge Wells NHS Trust.

Commonly used pieces of equipment, such as stethoscopes and commodes for example, that are used between patients, should also be subject to regular cleaning between each use. Wherever possible adequate numbers of frequently used equipment should be sought so that one particular piece of equipment is not in constant use, preventing cleaning and causing disinfection practices to fall by the wayside, thereby putting vulnerable patients at risk of potential cross infection.

It may be more prudent and cost effective to adopt a policy of single-use disposable equipment than spending valuable nursing expertise cleaning equipment but this would need to be discussed and agreed locally. Regular visual checks and audits of cleaning and disinfection policies and practice will identify if cleanliness standards are being well maintained.

Other departments/units

More formal disinfection processes take place outside of wards in departments such as endoscopy and bronchoscopy units. The equipment used in these areas are usually constructed with materials that allow them to be very flexible and as such are made from heat-labile materials and therefore cannot be subjected to heat disinfection processes. They are thoroughly decontaminated in the first instance by staff wearing appropriate PPE and then processed in stand-alone automated cold chemical washer disinfectors (WD) which are subject to regular disinfection programmes and monitoring of rinse water quality to ensure that the processes function optimally and that the machine does not pose a potential infection risk to subsequent instruments and patients.

Additionally, in departments such as sterile service units, surgical instrumentation undergoes heat disinfection processes in non-chemical WDs. These machines are monitored more closely via process assurance controls. If the system fails to provide water of an adequate temperature, for instance, the cycle will stop and the WD will require fixing and revalidation prior to being put back into operation. These machines utilize controlled programmes of 'time over temperature' processes and are therefore more efficient in killing bacteria and viruses than cold chemical processes or hand decontamination methods.

12.8.6 Waste management

Health-care waste comprises any waste that is produced by and/or is a consequence of health-care activities. Health-care facilities have a legal requirement (Duty of Care) to ensure that the disposal of all categories of waste (e.g. medical, chemical, radioactive, microbiological) occurs in an appropriate manner that does not pose a potential hazard to the public and the environment. Some healthcare institutions have received some adverse publicity for poor waste disposal and leaving clinical waste in non-designated areas. Each healthcare facility must have policies for disposal of all waste and to ensure that these waste streams are followed and adhered to.

CASE STUDY 12.1 *Postoperative infection*

It has been noted that two patients postoperatively have developed sternal wound infections following cardiac surgery. The patients are now pyrexial and the wound is showing a green exudate. A third patient operated on 3 days later has now developed a wound infection.

1. What samples would you take and from which health-care worker? What investigations would you request?

2. Who would you involve in this process?

3. What media would you use in sample processing?

4. What nursing procedures would be implemented?

After 24 h incubation all three patients' wound swabs grew a presumptive *Staphylococcus aureus*. Susceptibility tests show resistance to cefoxitin, erythromycin, trimethoprim, and ciprofloxacin.

5. What are your conclusions about the organism involved?

6. What further tests would you perform on the isolate?

A total of 150 swabs were received at the request of the infection prevention and control team from all staff involved with the patient. It was shown that the nasal swab from the surgeon performing the operations on all three patients was heavily colonized with a presumptive *S. aureus*. Susceptibility tests show the organism has an identical susceptibility pattern.

7. What further tests would you perform on the isolate?

8. What control of infection procedures would be implemented?

9. Would any therapeutic regimes be considered?

CASE STUDY 12.2 Outbreak of a Gram-negative pathogen

Two babies on your hospital's neonatal unit have developed sepsis. The blood cultures show a Gram-negative rod and the bottles have been plated onto conventional culture media together with direct susceptibility tests. A visit to the neonatal unit from the IPC team shows normal practices are being followed although there is small leak in the roof and one of the taps where water is used to wash the patients appears to be dripping. In both cases the estates department have been informed to repair.

1. What would you suggest is the cause of the sepsis and why?

2. What would you recommend happens on the unit next?

The organism growing in both positive blood cultures is confirmed as a Gram-negative rod, which is a strict aerobe and is oxidase-positive. Incidentally two more patients on the unit also have positive blood cultures with a Gram-negative rod.

3. What organism is the likely cause of the sepsis?

4. What is your action plan and report into the outbreak?

CASE STUDY 12.3 Multi-drug resistant organisms

A war casualty from the Middle East was air-lifted to your hospital and whilst in a stable condition had multiple trauma wounds.

1. What screening samples would you suggest on admission?

2. On what media would you process these samples on?

3. What nursing procedures would be implemented and why?

After 24 hours' incubation, only white colonies were seen on the chromogenic MRSA screening plates and on CLED agar a heavy growth of a non-lactose fermenting Gram-negative (rod/coccobacillus), was noted.

4. What are your indications of the patient's MRSA status?

5. Suggest some possible identities for the non-lactose fermenting Gram-negative rod/coccobacillus.

6. How would you proceed with the Gram-negative organism and what further investigations would you perform on it?

It is been demonstrated that other patients on the same unit are growing a very similar looking organism from wound cultures and one patient has developed the organism in his respiratory tract. The organism has been confirmed as an *Acinetobacter* and appears to be resistant to all first-line antibiotics tested.

7. What further antibiotics would you suggest are tested?

8. You are required to prepare some selective media to allow screening swabs etc. to be sent from all patients on the unit. What would your suggestions be as to the selective agents to include and your reasons for this?

9. What nursing procedures need to be in place?

10. Should the public be informed? If so how?

Chapter summary

After reading this chapter you should know and understand:

- The importance and role of the infection prevention and control team within the hospital.

- The significance of MRSA and the impact it has on staff, patients, and hospital resources.

- How MRSA screening is conducted and the laboratory methods used to isolate the organism.

- The importance of *C. difficile* infection and its impact on patients, staff, and health resources.

- Methods used for the detection of *C. difficile* toxins.

- The importance of VRE and methods used for detection.

- The importance of Gram-negative organisms in causing outbreaks.

- The importance of MDR strains.

- Consideration of other organisms which can cause problems in hospitals and strategies for their detection.

- Hand hygiene and its importance in reduction of HCAI.

- Disinfection strategies.

- Management of cohorts and barrier nursing.

- Monitoring air quality in theatres.

- Importance of waste management in the hospital environment.

Further reading

- **Centers for Disease Control (CDC). www.cdc.gov/index.htm.**

  US website dealing with all aspects of infectious disease. Excellent resource for infectious disease information.

- **Finch RG, *Greenwood D, Norrby SR, Whitley RJ* (eds). *Antibiotic and Chemotherapy: Anti-Infective Agents and their use in Therapy*, 8th edition. Churchill Livingstone, 2003.**

  Excellent text for use of antimicrobial agents in clinical practice.

- **Gould D, Brooker C. *Infection Prevention and Control: Applied Microbiology for Healthcare*, 2nd edition. Palgrave Macmillan, 2008.**

  Useful text describing the many aspects and problems associated with infection prevention and control.

- **Murray PR, Rosenthal KS, Pfaller MA. *Medical Microbiology*, 7th edition. Saunders, 2012.**

  Excellent text on infectious diseases and the process by which organisms initiate and spread infection.

Discussion questions

12.1   Why do you think MRSA has become so prevalent in many hospital environments?

12.2   What do you think is making the biggest impact in the battle to reduce health-care-acquired infection and why?

12.3   Why do you think *C. difficile* has become a problem for both the hospital and community? How can infection rates be reduced?

12.4   What are the next major challenges for Infection Prevention and Control teams?

13

Laboratory investigations of viral infections

Jayne Harwood

Viral infections are among the most common and important causes of human disease. The word 'virus' comes from the Latin meaning 'a poison'. A virus is a microscopic organism, consisting mainly of nucleic acid in a protein coat. Viral infections affect every life form, from bacteria, fungi, and plants, to animals and man. Viruses cause a wide range of illnesses ranging from the common cold to the lethal rabies in man.

Viruses are metabolically inert, making them totally dependent upon living cells for replication and their existence. This means that until they enter a host cell capable of supporting their replication, they exist as inactive particles.

Learning objectives

After studying this chapter you should be able to:

- Describe the basic organization, size range, and structure of viruses.
- Describe procedures used in the routine virology laboratory for the diagnosis of viral infections.
- Describe the specimens required for the diagnosis of viral infections.
- List viruses commonly isolated from pathological specimens.
- Have a basic knowledge of antiviral therapy.

13.1 General properties and structure of viruses

Viruses differ from other common infectious agents in a number of ways:

- Viruses are very small, measured in nanometres (nm), that is, 10^{-9} of a metre. Viruses range from about 20–300 nm in diameter and this means they are not visible unless microscopy is used. Whilst conventional microscopes are used to visualize bacterial cells, viruses (apart from the largest viruses, e.g. poxviruses) can only be seen using specialized electron microscopes.

- Viral genomes consist only of DNA or RNA but not both.

The structure of viruses is important in their identification. Viruses are made up from the following basic components, which you can see in Figure 13.1:

- Capsid – protein coat or outer shell enclosing the nucleic acid. The role of the capsid is to aid entry into the host cell and to protect the viral nucleic acid.

- Capsomere – morphological subunit of which the capsid is composed, consisting of a small number of protein molecules.

- Nucleocapsid – the capsid together with the enclosed nucleic acid core.

- Envelope – a lipoprotein membrane which surrounds certain viruses and is acquired during the final stages of viral maturation by a process of budding through the host cell's outer cell membrane.

Whilst some viruses possess enzymes of their own they cannot reproduce and amplify the information in their genomes without the assistance of the host cellular components.

> **Key Point**
>
> **Viruses are totally dependent upon living cells, either eukaryotic or prokaryotic, for replication and existence.**

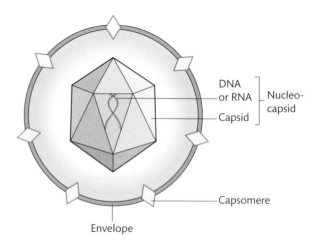

FIGURE 13.1
Structure of a virus.
Source: Courtesy of J. Harwood.

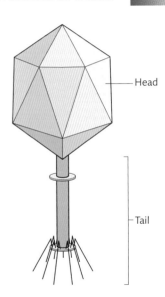

FIGURE 13.2
Structure of a helical virus.
Source: Courtesy of J. Harwood.

FIGURE 13.3
**Structure of a complex virus
(bacteriophage).**
Source: Courtesy of J. Harwood.

13.1.1 Viral morphology

Viral structure shows that they tend to be simplistic and symmetrical in design because of the limited number of proteins available for their configuration. There are three distinct shapes:

- Helical viruses (Figure 13.2).
- Cubic or isometric (icosahedral) viruses.
- Complex viruses (Figure 13.3).

13.1.2 Viral classification

The following criteria are used to classify viruses:

- The type of nucleic acid, i.e. DNA or RNA.
- The number of strands of nucleic acid and their physical construction, i.e. single-stranded, linear, circular, circular with breaks, segmented.
- Polarity of the viral genome, i.e. positive or negative stranded.
- The symmetry of the nucleocapsid.
- The presence or absence of a lipid envelope.

For example, herpes simplex, which causes cold sores, is a DNA virus, because it only contains DNA whereas the influenza virus only contains RNA and is therefore an RNA virus.

Key Point

Viruses, unlike bacteria, possess only one type of nucleic acid, either DNA or RNA.

What are the main differences between a virus and a bacterium?

13.2 **Viral pathogenesis**

The consequences to the patient of a viral infection depend on a number of viral and host factors that affect the development of disease. Viral infection was long thought only to produce acute clinical disease (e.g. mumps); however, viruses can also cause chronic disease, such as liver cirrhosis as a result of hepatitis B infection. Other results of viral infection can include induction of various cancers, progressive neurological disorders and endocrine diseases such as diabetes.

13.2.1 Host cellular response to viral infection

Host cells can respond to a viral infection in three different ways:

1. No effect on the host cell – asymptomatic infection, e.g. **cytomegalovirus** (CMV) infection.
2. Cytopathic effect (CPE) and death – this is a morphological change in host cells as a result of the virus growing inside them.
3. Loss of control of cell replication – this can result in the formation of tumours. This can occur with **Epstein–Barr virus** (EBV) infection which can cause **lymphoma**.

In a host, viruses can cause three basic patterns of infection: localized, **disseminated**, and no apparent disease. In localized viral infection, replication remains localized near the site of entry, for example the skin or respiratory tract. Disseminated (that is systemic) infections usually take place through several steps:

1. Entry of virus into the body.
2. Spread via the bloodstream (**viraemia**) to regional lymph nodes.
3. Further spread to other susceptible organs such as liver or spleen.

> *Key Point*
>
> **Viraemia is the presence of virus in the bloodstream.**

Many viral infections do not necessarily result in viral replication and cell death within the host. Instead following a primary infection, the viral genome enters into a latent state where it is maintained within the host cell in a repressed state which is compatible with the continued survival and normal functioning of that cell. Essentially the virus is 'hiding' in the host cell waiting for a trigger to 'awaken' (reactivate) it.

The virus can be reactivated, allowing active viral replication to occur and the production of numerous infectious virus particles. The events that trigger this reactivation of the **latent virus** include strong sunshine (UV light), trauma, and immunosuppression. For example a patient can develop recurrent cold sores caused by the herpes simplex virus during the summer months as a result of exposure to sunshine.

What is meant by the terms latency and reactivation in viral disease? Can you give an example?

13.3 Samples required for the diagnosis of viral infection

It is imperative that the clinicians know the correct samples required for the diagnosis of viral infections. In addition, it is essential that the samples are submitted in the required container, and transported in the appropriate manner.

The site and timing of specimens are possibly the most important factors for successful virus diagnosis. In general, specimens should be taken from the site of symptoms and as close to the onset of illness as possible.

Specimens for **cell culture** should be transported to the laboratory as soon as possible after being taken. Swabs should be put into a vial containing viral transport medium. There are various formulations of viral transport media but all of them generally contain: (a) a salt solution to ensure correct ionic concentrations; (b) a buffer to maintain pH; (c) a source of protein; and (d) antibiotics and antifungals to prevent overgrowth by bacteria and fungi which may be present in the sample. Bodily fluids and tissues should be placed in a sterile container. If delays of more than an hour are anticipated specimens are best stored at 4°C.

All specimens should be placed in secure transport containers and labelled in accordance with local policy. It is essential that the request form contains relevant clinical information. Such details must include the date of onset of illness, clinical signs and suspected diagnosis.

The specimen used for direct detection and virus isolation is very important. A positive result from the site of the disease would be of much greater diagnostic significance than those from other sites. For example, in the case of herpes simplex (HSV) encephalitis, a positive result from the cerebral spinal fluid (CSF) or the brain would be of much greater significance than a positive result from a cold sore, since as we have seen previously, reactivation of cold sores can occur during times of stress.

Table 13.1 summarizes the specimen types required for a range of viral infections.

TABLE 13.1 Specimen types required for a range of viral diseases.

Disease	Specimen
Respiratory infection	Nasal or throat swabs, postnasal washing, BAL
Gastrointestinal infection	Faeces (rectal swab not satisfactory)
Vesicular rash	Vesicle swab, throat swab, faeces
Hepatitis	Clotted blood, faeces
Central nervous system	CSF, throat swab, faeces
AIDS, lymphadenopathy	Clotted blood

SELF-CHECK 13.3

Why is it important for viral transport media to contain antibacterial and antifungal agents?

13.3.1 Swabs

The use of wooden stick swabs is not advised for the isolation of viruses as this material has been implicated as a source of cell culture toxicity. Plastic swab sticks are the required swabs for isolation of viruses. The amount of material collected must be adequate for testing. Throat and skin swabs must be taken fairly vigorously to capture as many virus-infected cells as possible. After sampling, the tip of the swab is broken off, placed into viral transport medium, and forwarded as soon as possible to the laboratory.

13.3.2 Respiratory samples

Respiratory samples include nasopharyngeal aspirates, swabs, washes, broncheoalveolar lavages (BAL), throat swabs and sputum are the samples of choice for diagnosing viral respiratory infections. Nasopharyngeal samples are extremely useful in the diagnosis of upper respiratory tract infections in young children (e.g. RSV). Respiratory samples are collected in sterile containers.

13.3.3 Cerebrospinal fluid (CSF)

Cross reference
See Chapter 8, Section 8.1.

CSF is often submitted to eliminate viral infection as a cause of aseptic meningitis or encephalitis. Other than collecting an adequate volume into a sterile container and prompt transport to the laboratory, no other special procedures are required.

13.3.4 Vesicle fluid

Vesicle fluid for **electron microscopy** (EM) is collected on the tip of a scalpel blade, spread over an area of about 3-4 mm in diameter on an ordinary microscope slide and allowed to dry. Vesicle fluid for polymerase chain reaction (PCR) is taken in the same way but put into a vial containing viral transport medium.

13.3.5 Faeces

Cross reference
See Chapter 10.

Faeces should be placed in a dry, sterile container. Such samples are particularly useful for the diagnosis of enteroviruses and rotavirus.

13.3.6 Clotted blood

As a general rule, 5–10 mL of blood is taken. Clotted blood is used for serological tests.

13.3.7 EDTA blood

Blood is collected into EDTA blood tubes for any PCR work. Heparin tubes should be avoided for molecular work as the heparin can interfere with some assays.

13.4 Diagnostic methods in virology

13.4.1 Overview of diagnostic methods

In general, diagnostic tests can be grouped into three categories:

1. Direct detection.
2. Indirect examination (virus isolation).
3. Serology.

In direct detection, the clinical specimen is examined directly for the presence of virus particles, viral antigen or viral nucleic acids. This is performed by PCR, electron microscopy and immuno-fluorescence. For indirect examination, the specimen is inoculated into egg or animal **cell lines**, in an attempt to grow the virus: this is called virus isolation. Serology constitutes by far the bulk of the work of any virology laboratory. A serological diagnosis can be made by the detection of rising titres of antibody between acute and convalescent stages of infection, or the detection of **immunoglobulin M** (IgM). In general, the majority of common viral infections can be diagnosed by serology. Serology is also useful for determining the immune status of patients to viruses by detection of **immunoglobulin G** (IgG). For example determining the rubella (German measles) immune status of pregnant women as lack of immunity can lead to serious complications for the foetus if the mother comes into contact with the virus whilst pregnant.

Most serology is carried out using automated analysers, much like those used in Blood Science Laboratories.

SELF-CHECK 13.4

Why do you think that serology is most commonly used for the diagnosis of viral infection?

13.4.2 Direct detection of viruses

Direct detection methods are often called rapid diagnostic methods because a rapid result is required for clinical management. For example respiratory syncytial virus (RSV) can spread rapidly through paediatric wards and the affected individual(s) should be barrier nursed to stop the spread of infection. However, it is important to realize that not all direct examination methods are rapid, and, conversely, virus isolation and serological methods may sometimes give a more rapid result. Rapid diagnostic methods such as PCR have played a very important role in the diagnosis of the swine flu pandemic so patients and contacts can be given antiviral drugs in a bid to contain the severity and spread of the disease.

13.4.3 Electron microscopy (EM) morphology/immune EM

Virus particles can be detected and identified on the basis of morphology, that is how they appear under the electron microscope. A magnification of around 50,000 is normally used to visualize the virus. EM is now mainly used for the diagnosis of viral gastroenteritis by detecting viruses in faeces, for example rotavirus (Figure 13.4), adenovirus, astrovirus, calcivirus, and Norwalk-like viruses (turn back to Figure 10.5). EM has been used widely in the past to visualize viruses and determine their complex structures. An excellent example of this is the influenza virus A (Figure 13.5) showing spikes radiating from its surface. These are the major

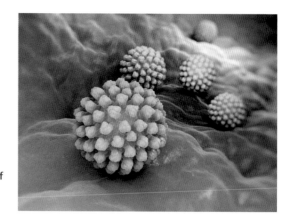

FIGURE 13.4
Electron micrograph of rotavirus, note the distinctive ring of radiating capsomeres.
Source: Courtesy of Istock.

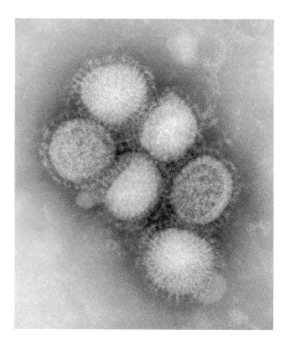

FIGURE 13.5
Electron micrograph of influenza A (H1N1) virus (swine flu virus).
Source: Courtesy of CDC/C.S. Goldsmith and A. Balish.

glycoprotein antigens of haemagglutinin and neuraminidase and are major virulence factors. Occasionally, it may be used for the detection of viruses in **vesicles** and other skin lesions, such as herpes viruses and papillomaviruses. The sensitivity and specificity of EM may be enhanced by immune EM, whereby virus-specific antibody is used to agglutinate virus particles together, thus making them easier to recognize, or to capture virus particles onto the EM grid. The main problem with EM is the expense involved in purchasing the equipment and maintaining the facility. In addition, the sensitivity of EM is often poor, with at least 10^5 to 10^6 virus particles/ millilitre in the sample required for visualization. As a result of reliable antigen detection and molecular methods for the detection of viruses associated with viral gastroenteritis, EM is becoming less widely used as a diagnostic aid.

13.4.4 Histopathological appearance

Replicating viruses often produce histological changes in infected cells. These changes may be characteristic or non-specific. Viral inclusion bodies are basically collections of replicating virus

FIGURE 13.6
Micrograph of Negri bodies found in a patient with rabies encephalitis.
Source: Courtesy of CDC/Dr Daniel P. Perl.

particles either in the nucleus or in cytoplasm of the host cell. Examples of inclusion bodies include the **Negri bodies** (Figure 13.6) and **cytomegalic inclusion bodies** found in rabies and cytomegalovirus (CMV) infections, respectively. Although not sensitive or specific, histology nevertheless serves as a useful adjunct in the diagnosis of certain viral infections.

13.4.5 Antigen detection

Examples of antigen detection include immunofluorescence testing of nasopharyngeal aspirates for respiratory viruses, for example RSV (Figure 13.7), influenza A, influenza B, detection of rotavirus antigen in faeces, and detection of varicella zoster virus in skin scrapings. The main advantage of these assays is that they are rapid, with the result being available within a few hours. However, the technique is often tedious and labour intensive and the result can be difficult to interpret with often low sensitivity and specificity. The quality of the specimen obtained is of utmost importance in order for the test to yield good diagnostic results.

SELF-CHECK 13.5

What are the advantages and disadvantages of rapid detection methods for viral disease?

13.4.6 Molecular techniques for the detection of viral genomes

Methods for the detection of the viral genome are most commonly molecular methods. Molecular methods are now well established as the gold standard in non-clinical diagnosis of

FIGURE 13.7
Photomicrograph of detection of respiratory syncytial virus (RSV) using an indirect immunofluorescence technique.
Source: Courtesy of CDC/Dr H. Craig Lyerla.

viral disease. However, in practice, although the use of molecular methods is widespread, the number of molecular tests is still low compared to serological tests.

Classical molecular techniques, such as dot blot and **Southern blot**, depend on the use of specific DNA/RNA probes for hybridization. The specificity of the reaction depends on the conditions used for hybridization. These techniques may allow for the quantification of DNA/RNA present in the specimen. However, it is often found that the sensitivity of these techniques is comparable with other viral diagnostic methods such as serology.

Newer molecular techniques, such as the polymerase chain reaction (PCR), ligase chain reaction (LCR), nucleic acid-based amplification (NASBA), and branched DNA (bDNA), depend on some form of amplification, either the target nucleic acid or the signal itself.

PCR is the only amplification technique which is in routine diagnostic use. PCR is an extremely sensitive technique; it is possible to achieve a sensitivity of one DNA molecule in a clinical specimen. However, PCR has many problems, most notably contamination, since only a very small amount of contaminating nucleic acid is needed to generate a false-positive result. In addition, because PCR is so sensitive compared to other techniques, a positive PCR result is often difficult to interpret as it does not necessarily indicate the presence of disease. This is a problem of particular concern in the detection of latent viruses such as CMV, since latent CMV genomes may be amplified from the blood of healthy individuals. Despite these drawbacks, PCR is widely used for viral diagnosis, especially as the assays are becoming less expensive and the availability of highly automated systems is readily available, for example real-time PCR and Cobas Amplicor systems (Roche, Basel, Switzerland).

Cross reference
See Chapter 16.

Other amplification techniques (such as LCR and NASBA) are just as susceptible to contamination as PCR but this is eliminated greatly by the use of proprietary closed systems. It is unlikely that other amplification techniques will challenge the dominance of PCR since it is much easier to set up an in-house PCR assay than other assays.

SELF-CHECK 13.6

Why have molecular methods largely replaced other direct detection methods?

13.4.7 Indirect examination

Typically, indirect examination is performed using the following three methods:

1. Cell culture.
2. Fertile hens' eggs.
3. Animals.

Cell cultures, eggs, and animals may be used for isolation of viruses from clinical samples. However, eggs and animals are difficult to handle and most viral diagnostic laboratories depend on cell culture only. To prepare cell cultures, tissue fragments are first dissociated, usually with the aid of trypsin or collagenase. The cell suspension is then placed in a flat-bottomed glass or plastic container together with a suitable liquid medium (e.g. Eagle's) and animal serum. After a variable lag phase, the cells will attach and spread on the bottom of the container and then start dividing, giving rise to a **primary culture**. Attachment to a solid support is essential for the growth of normal cells. Primary cultures are maintained by changing the fluid two or three times a week. When the cultures become too crowded, the cells are detached from the vessel wall either trypsin by or EDTA, and portions are used to initiate secondary cultures. In both primary and secondary cultures, the cells retain some of the characteristics of the tissue from which they are derived. Cells from primary cultures can often be transferred serially a number of times. The cells may then continue to multiply at a constant rate over many successive transfers. Eventually, after a number of transfers, the cells undergo culture **senescence** and cannot be transferred any longer. For human diploid cell cultures, the growth rate declines after about 50 duplications. During the multiplication of the cell strain, some cells become altered in that they acquire a different morphology, grow faster and become able to start a cell culture from a smaller number of cells. These cells are immortalized and have an unlimited life-span. However, they retain contact inhibition.

senescence
The process of growing old and showing effects of increasing age.

There are three types of cell culture:

- Primary cells, e.g. monkey kidney. These are essentially normal cells obtained from freshly killed adult animals. These cells can only be passaged once or twice.

- Semicontinuous cells, e.g. human embryonic kidney and skin fibroblasts. These are cells taken from embryonic tissue, and may be passaged up to 50 times.

- Continuous cells, e.g. HeLa (derived from the cervical cancer cells of an American woman named Henrietta Lacks), Vero (isolated from kidney epithelial cells), BGM (derived from African Green Monkey kidney cells). These are immortalized cells, i.e. tumour cell lines which may be passaged indefinitely.

Key Point

Cell cultures vary greatly in their susceptibility to different viruses. It is extremely important that the most sensitive cell cultures are used for a particular suspected virus.

Upon receipt, the specimen is inoculated into several different types of cell culture depending on the nature of the specimen and the clinical presentation. The maintenance media should be changed after 1 h or, if that is not practicable, the next morning. The inoculated tubes should be incubated at 35–37°C in a rotating drum. Rotation is optimal for the isolation of respiratory viruses and results in an earlier appearance of the CPE for many viruses. If stationary tubes are used, it is essential that the culture tubes be positioned so that the cell **monolayer** is bathed in nutrient medium.

The inoculated tubes should be read at least every other day for the presence of CPE. Certain specimens, such as urine and faeces, may be toxic to cell cultures and may produce a CPE-like effect. If toxic effects are extensive, it may be necessary to passage the inoculated cells. Passaging (also known as subculture or splitting cells) involves transferring a small number of cells into a new vessel. Cell cultures that are contaminated with bacteria should be either reinoculated or passed through a bacterial filter. Cell cultures should be kept for at least 1 to 2 weeks (longer in the case of CMV). Cell cultures should be re-fed with fresh maintenance medium at regular intervals or should the culture medium become too acidic or alkaline. When CPE is seen, it may be advisable to passage infected culture fluid into a fresh culture of the same cell type. For cell-associated viruses such as CMV and VZV, it is necessary to trypsinize and passage intact infected cells. Other viruses such as adenovirus can be **subcultured** after freezing and thawing infected cells.

Primary cell culture is widely acknowledged as the best cell culture system available since it supports the widest range of viruses. However, it is very expensive and it is often difficult to obtain a reliable supply. Continuous cells are the most easy to handle but the range of viruses supported is often limited.

The presence of growing virus is usually detected by:

- Cytopathic effect (CPE) – may be specific or non-specific, e.g. HSV and CMV produce a specific CPE, whereas enteroviruses do not.
- **Haemadsorption** – cultured cells acquire the ability to stick to mammalian red blood cells. Haemadsorption is mainly used for the detection of influenza and parainfluenza viruses. The haemadsorption inhibition test is performed in cell cultures. After adding the tested serum to the cell culture infected with influenza virus and after subsequent adding of red blood cells, the antibodies in the serum protect the haemadsorption effect.

Confirmation of the identity of the virus may be carried out using neutralization, haemadsorption-inhibition, immunofluorescence, or molecular tests.

The main problem with cell culture is the long period (up to 4 weeks) required for a result to be available. Also, the sensitivity is often poor and depends on many factors, such as the condition of the specimen and the condition of the cell sheet. Cell cultures are also very susceptible to bacterial contamination and toxic substances in the specimen. Finally, many viruses will not grow in cell culture at all, including hepatitis B (HBV) and C (HCV), diarrhoeal viruses, and parvovirus.

Rapid culture techniques are available whereby viral antigens are detected 2 to 4 days after the inoculation. Examples of rapid culture techniques include the CMV DEAFF test. In this test, the cell sheet (human embryonic fibroblasts – the most common cells of connective tissue in animals) is grown on individual cover slips in a plastic bottle. After inoculation, the bottle is spun at a low speed for 1 h (to speed up the adsorption of the virus) and then incubated for 2 to 4 days. The cover slip is then taken out and examined for the presence of CMV early antigens by immunofluorescence.

The role of cell culture in the diagnosis of viral infections is being increasingly challenged by rapid diagnostic methods. Therefore, the role of cell culture is expected to decline and is likely to be restricted to large central reference laboratories.

SELF-CHECK 13.7

Why is cell culture still used when there are so many more rapid diagnostic methods available?

13.5 **Serology**

Serology is the mainstay of viral diagnosis in many routine diagnostic laboratories. Following exposure to a virus, antibodies will start to appear in most patients, the first of which to appear is immunoglobulin M IgM (Figure 13.8). This is followed over time by production of immunoglobulin G IgG. Levels of IgG are often higher than those seen with IgM. The detection of these immunoglobulins is most often how the viral infection is diagnosed.

> ### Key Point
> Using serology techniques it must be remembered that it is not the virus that is detected but the patient's immune response to it in the majority of cases.

For serological investigations serum is used which is produced by the centrifugation of a clotted blood sample. For diagnosis of acute infection samples should be taken during the first few days

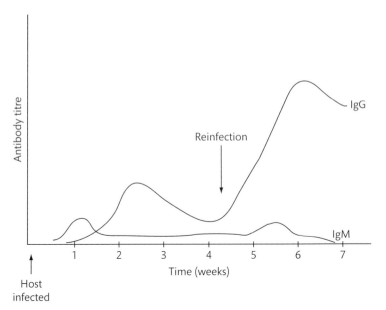

FIGURE 13.8
Serological events following primary infection and reinfection. Note that in reinfection, IgM may be absent or only present transiently at a low level.
Source: Courtesy of J. Harwood.

of symptoms. This is in order to detect an IgM antibody response which occurs during an acute phase of the disease. However, some assays cannot detect the presence of IgM and other methods need to be used. This is often the case in the diagnosis of influenza and some other respiratory infections using the **complement fixation test** (CFT). In such cases a sample should be taken at the time the symptoms appear (acute sample) and again after 10–14 days (**convalescent** sample). This is to demonstrate a rise in IgG levels and hence diagnose the infection.

We will now look at the techniques used for diagnosing viral infections.

13.5.1 Complement fixation test

The complement fixation test is used for the diagnosis of certain respiratory infections where IgM is difficult to detect and as such a rise in the IgG response is used to diagnose the infection using an acute and convalescent serum.

Although CFT is considered to be a relatively simple test, it is a very exacting procedure because five variables are involved, as you can see in Figure 13.9. In essence, the test consists of two antigen–antibody reactions, one of which is the indicator system. The first reaction, between a known virus antigen and a specific antibody, takes place in the presence of a predetermined amount of complement – a group of proteins present in blood plasma and tissue fluid, which combine with an antigen–antibody complex to bring about the lysis of foreign cells. The complement is removed or 'fixed' by the antigen–antibody complex. The second antigen–antibody reaction consists of reacting sheep red blood cells with haemolysin. When this indicator system is added to the reactants, the sensitized red blood cells will only lyse in the presence of free complement. In order for the CFT to perform correctly, the optimal concentration of haemolytic serum, complement and antigen must be determined in advance. The antigens used for CFT tend to be group antigens rather than type-specific antigens. For example, influenza A antigens are antigens from many different strains of the virus. This allows for the diagnostic capacity of the test to be maximized.

The advantage of CFT is the ability to screen against a large number of viral (and bacterial) antigens at the same time. The tests are also relatively inexpensive to perform. The disadvantages

convalescent
Convalescent means the patient has often recovered from the infection or is showing an improvement in the condition. A convalescent sample is taken to demonstrate a rise in antibody levels.

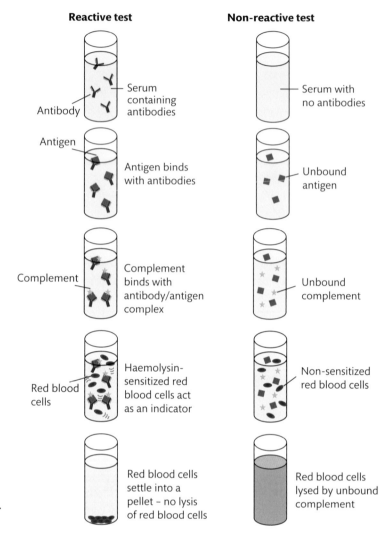

Reactive test

Non-reactive test

Antibody — Serum containing antibodies

Serum with no antibodies

Antigen

Antigen binds with antibodies

Unbound antigen

Complement

Complement binds with antibody/antigen complex

Unbound complement

Red blood cells

Haemolysin-sensitized red blood cells act as an indicator

Non-sensitized red blood cells

Red blood cells settle into a pellet – no lysis of red blood cells

Red blood cells lysed by unbound complement

FIGURE 13.9

Steps of the complement fixation test.

Source: Courtesy of J. Harwood.

are that the test has a low sensitivity and it is highly labour intensive to perform. The test can also be non-specific, for example cross-reactions can occur between the viral antigens used in the test.

> ### Key Point
>
> Many laboratories no longer offer a CFT service due to limitations of the test and the fact that many patients fail to submit a convalescent sample since they have recovered from the infection.

13.5.2 Detection of IgM

Several methods are available for the detection of IgM in serum. These include immunoassays using enzyme (EIA) or radiolabelled substrates (RIA). Immunofluorescence (IF) can also be used to detect IgM. These tests offer a rapid means of diagnosis and are routinely used for detection of IgM produced against viruses such as mumps and EBV. However, there are many problems associated with IgM assays, such as interference by rheumatoid factor, re-infection by the virus, and unexplained persistence of IgM years after the primary infection. Obvious safety issues associated with the use of radiolabelled substrates have rendered these assays unsuitable as a routine test. IF is relatively time consuming to perform and is generally only performed for virus detection in specialist reference centres. EIA is the most widely used method of IgM detection and is performed on highly automated platforms.

13.5.3 Enzyme-linked immunosorbent assay (ELISA)

ELISA was developed in 1970 and became rapidly accepted as the method of choice for the detection of IgG and IgM in serum samples for the diagnosis of viral infection. The principle of this test is that an antigen (or antibody) can be immobilized onto a solid-phase carrier, such as microtitre plates or beads, and then used to separate its **homologous antibody** (or antigen). This complex can be detected by an enzyme-mediated colour change (look at Figure 13.10 to see a diagram of the stages). In general the procedure is as follows:

homologous antibody

Homologous antibody is an antibody derived from an animal of the same species.

- An antigen (or antibody) is linked to a solid phase surface, usually the wells of a 96-well microtitre tray, or on the surface of a polystyrene microparticle (usually a bead).

- This 'sensitized' solid phase surface captures its corresponding antibody (or antigen) if present in the specimen. This surface is washed to remove any unbound material.

- An enzyme-labelled antispecies antibody (conjugate) attaches to the bound antigen–antibody complex. This is again washed to remove any unbound conjugate.

- The attachment of the enzyme labelled conjugate can be detected by a colour change resulting from the hydrolysis of an added enzyme-specific substrate.

- The optical density of the colour reaction is directly proportional to the amount of unknown antibody (or antigen) in the test solution. The result is usually expressed as a quantitative optical density (OD) measurement.

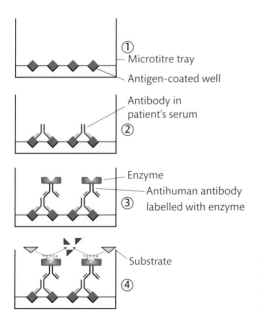

① Microtitre tray
— Antigen-coated well

Antibody in patient's serum ②

— Enzyme
— Antihuman antibody
③ labelled with enzyme

— Substrate
④

FIGURE 13.10

Example of an ELISA. The antigen to the antibody which is being tested for in the patient's serum is coated onto the well (1). The antibody in the serum will bind to the antigen (2). An antihuman antibody labelled with an enzyme is added (3). The substrate is added and will hydrolyse if the reaction has taken place (4) resulting in a colour change.

Source: Courtesy of J. Harwood.

Why is it important for various washing steps to be performed in an ELISA test?

A wide variety of assay principles can be used in ELISA techniques. The most important of these are described in the following sections.

Competitive methods

The competitive ELISA is generally used to detect antibodies and is a quantitative assay over a narrow range. Unlike non-competitive methods, where the test serum is removed before adding the enzyme conjugate by washing (see previously), the enzyme is in direct contact with antibodies in the serum. The method is simple, has only one incubation and wash step, does not **prozone** in the presence of high titre antibody concentrations and is particularly useful for detecting low-affinity antibodies. If antibodies in the test serum compete with the conjugate they block binding sites and prevent the hydrolysis of substrate, reducing the colour change. This lack of colour change indicates a positive reaction.

prozone

Prozone is the phenomenon exhibited by some sera, in which agglutination or precipitation occurs at higher dilution ranges, but is not visible at lower dilutions or when undiluted.

> ### Key Point
>
> A quantitative assay measures the exact amount of antibody present in the sample.

Sandwich methods

Indirect non-competitive ELISA is normally used to detect antibody. The antigen is coated onto the solid phase and incubated with the test serum. If homologous antibody is present, it will bind to the antigen. After washing, the conjugate (an antihuman IgG antibody covalently bound to the enzyme) is added and after incubation the plate is again washed. Substrate is added, the reaction stopped after a specific time period and the OD read at a specific wavelength defined by the substrate.

The double antibody sandwich is normally used to detect antigen, as shown in Figure 13.11. Specific antibody is bound to the solid phase and incubated with the test serum. If homologous antigen is present it will bind to the solid phase antibody. The conjugate is an enzyme linked to a specific IgG antibody homologous for the antigen being detected. Substrate is

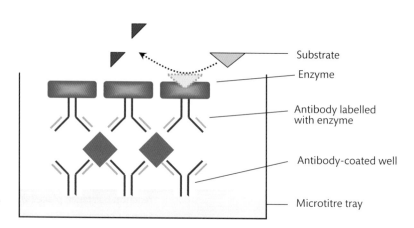

FIGURE 13.11

Sandwich method for ELISA.

Source: Courtesy of J. Harwood.

Substrate
Enzyme
Antibody labelled with enzyme
Antibody-coated well
Microtitre tray

added and the reaction stopped after a specific time period. The OD is determined at a wavelength defined by the substrate.

Antibody capture method

This method requires that the solid phase is coated with antibody to whichever class of immunoglobulin is being sought. For example, if IgM antibodies are to be detected, the solid phase is coated with anti-IgM to which any test IgM will bind. After washing, specific antigen is added followed by conjugate. The conjugate will only bind if the antigen is present which can itself only bind if the homologous IgM was present and captured to the solid phase. **Heterologous** IgM may be bound by capture to the solid phase, but will not bind antigen and therefore not react with the conjugate. Once again, coloration is indicative of a positive reaction which can be accurately assayed spectrophotometrically.

heterologous
Heterologous antibody is derived from an individual of a different species.

13.5.4 Assay characteristics

The use of monoclonal antibodies has led to many improvements in ELISA systems.

- Higher sensitivity – either by selection of antibodies with an extremely high affinity, or by reduction of the height and variability of the background reaction, which makes very low concentrations of analyte more readily detectable.

- Higher specificity – by avoiding the presence of any antibody in the assay system with specific reactivity against non-analyte **epitopes**, and by selecting combinations of monoclonal antibodies which may further increase specificity.

- Higher practicality – by introducing simultaneous incubation of label, solid phase, and sample without risk of prozone effect.

- The enzyme label – most of the assays employ horseradish peroxidase, alkaline phosphatase, or β-D-galactosidase. The most interesting recent developments have been in new methods to detect these enzymes rather than the use of new enzyme labels. Fluorimeters are used to detect alkaline phosphatase and β-D-galactosidase. Methods available for the detection of horseradish peroxidase are by means of **chemiluminescence**.

- Seroconversion – this is defined as changing from a previously antibody negative state to a positive state, e.g. seroconversion against human immunodeficiency virus (HIV) following a needle-stick injury, or against rubella following contact with a known case.

- A single high titre of IgG (or total antibody) – this is a very unreliable means of serological diagnosis since the cut-off is very difficult to define. This is because if the IgG level in the patient against the virus is unknown it is impossible to determine if the antibody titre has risen.

13.5.5 Criteria used for diagnosing a re-infection/ re-activation

It is often very difficult to differentiate re-infection/re-activation from a primary infection. Under most circumstances, it is not important to differentiate between a primary infection and re-infection. However, it is very important under certain situations, such as rubella infection in the first trimester of pregnancy; primary infection is associated with a high risk of foetal damage whereas re-infection is not. In general, a sharp, large rise in antibody titres is found in re-infection whereas IgM is usually low or absent in cases of re-infection/re-activation.

13.5.6 Limitations of serological diagnosis

How useful a serological result is depends on the patient's immune response to an individual virus. For viruses such as rubella and hepatitis A, the onset of clinical symptoms coincides with the development of antibodies in the patient. The detection of IgM in the serum of the patient would be indicative of acute infection. Alternatively, rising titres of IgG in the serum of a patient who has previously been IgG positive would indicate re-activation or re-infection.

Many viruses often produce clinical disease well before the appearance of antibodies, such as respiratory and diarrhoeal viruses. In such instances, any serological diagnosis would be retrospective and therefore would not be of major clinical use. However, the diagnosis may well be useful for epidemiological purposes.

There are many viruses that produce clinical disease months or years after seroconversion (e.g. HIV and rabies). In the case of these viruses, the mere presence of antibody is sufficient to make a definitive diagnosis.

SELF-CHECK 13.9

Why are antibodies detected against HIV enough to make a definitive diagnosis?

Whilst a serological diagnosis is the mainstay in the diagnosis of viral infections, there are a number of problems associated with the serological diagnosis of infection. These problems are:

- The length of time required for diagnosis for paired acute and convalescent sera often results in the convalescent sample not being submitted as the patient may well have made a full recovery.

- Mild, local infections such as HSV genitalis (genital herpes) may not produce a detectable **humoral immune response** as antibodies may not be produced. A better sample would be a swab in viral transport media of the lesion.

- Extensive antigenic cross-reactivity between related viruses, e.g. HSV and VZV, may lead to false-positive results.

- Immunocompromised patients (e.g. transplant recipients) often give a reduced or absent humoral immune response. As such the antibody response may be too weak to detect.

- Patients with infectious mononucleosis (glandular fever) and those with connective tissue disease such as systemic lupus erythematosus (SLE) may react non-specifically, giving a false-positive result.

- Patients given blood or blood products may give a false-positive result due to the transfer of antibody from the donor blood sample to the patient. This is particularly problematic for diagnosis of CMV. Samples from babies are also often problematic as IgG antibodies will cross the placenta from the mother and will give positive results in IgG assays in the baby's sample.

SELF-CHECK 13.10

Why would swabs from a lesion be a better sample than a serum in the diagnosis of HSV genitalis?

13.6 Antiviral chemotherapy

Similar to antimicrobial chemotherapy, there are a number of agents available for the treatment of patients with viral infections. However, since most viral infections are mild and self-limiting they are not as widely used as antibiotics.

Since antiviral agents are required to penetrate into host cells and viruses in general are capable of mutations, designing non-toxic agents is very difficult. As such, only a limited number of antiviral drugs are available and suitable for human use. There are few restrictions on the types of molecules that inhibit virus replication. These vary greatly in complexity and include natural products of plants, synthetic oligonucleotides, oligosaccharides, simple inorganic and organic compounds and nucleoside analogues. Many early antivirals were discovered by screening large numbers of compounds for their activity against viruses. However, this has been largely replaced by designing drugs to act upon the stages of viral replication. Examples of antiviral compounds in current use include:

- Nucleoside analogues – thousands of analogues of naturally occurring nucleosides have now been synthesized and tested in the laboratory. They act by interfering with the synthesis of viral nucleic acids, initially they were used as herpes virus inhibitors (e.g. aciclovir) but now they are used as anti-HIV agents (e.g. azidothymidine (AZT)).

- Non-nucleoside inhibitors of reverse transcription – these target different sites in the reverse transcriptase to those targeted by the nucleoside analogues (e.g. nevirapine).

- Neuraminidase inhibitors – neuraminidase is a surface protein found on influenza A and plays a role in the budding of the virus particles from the infected cell. Inhibiting this enzyme stops the viral particles from being released. Oseltamivir is such a drug which has been used to treat patients in the recent swine flu epidemic.

- Pyrophosphate analogues – foscarnet is an example of a pyrophosphate analogue. This specifically inhibits herpesvirus DNA polymerase at the pyrophosphate binding sites and it also has anti-HIV activity.

- Amantidine molecules – amantidine is licensed for the treatment of influenza A infection.

Only relatively recently have notable successes on a large scale been achieved with antiviral drugs such as aciclovir and AZT. No antiviral compound tested has been able to inhibit completely the replication of any virus and a proportion of viral particles always seem to be able to circumvent the drug-induced blockade.

13.6.1 Resistance of viruses to inhibitors

A disappointing feature of antiviral chemotherapy has been the failure so far of any antiviral molecule to inhibit virus replication completely. Antiviral activity tends to produce a 100- to 1,000-fold reduction in viral load which still allows some infective particles to survive. Viruses, especially RNA viruses, have the ability to mutate at high frequencies, meaning that genotypes encoding for drug resistance can arise rapidly.

When antiviral agents to HIV are used alone, resistance can develop rapidly, usually seen as an increase in the patient's viral load. To counter this, HIV treatment consists of a combination of drugs, such as a protease inhibitor and two reverse transcriptase inhibitors. These drugs attack different sites of the viral replication cycle and therefore make it much more difficult for the virus to mutate and develop resistance. This may have important consequences in immunocompromised patients who may be unable to eradicate any residual virus by way of their immune response.

TABLE 13.2 Common antiviral drugs showing the target and virus affected.

Target	Drug	Virus affected
Penetration and uncoating	Amantadine Rimantadine	Influenza A
Viral nucleic acid synthesis	Aciclovir Ganciclovir Ribavirin Lamivudine Zidovudine Foscarnet	Herpes simplex Varicella CMV Hepatitis C Hepatitis B HIV-1 Herpes simplex and HIV-1
Binding to intact virus particle	Disoxaril	Rhinovirus
Virus release	Oseltamivir Nefinavir	Influenza A and B HIV

13.6.2 Site of action of common antiviral agents

The sites of action for common antiviral drugs can be seen in Table 13.2. These include:

- Interference with virus adsorption or attachment to the receptor-binding site on the cell wall. These drugs prevent the entry of the virus into the cell.
- Inhibition of virus uncoating. This drug will not allow the release of nucleic acid from the inside of the virus and so will not allow the reproduction of the virus.
- Inhibition of viral nucleic acid transcription and replication.
- Interference with cellular processing of viral polypeptides.
- Prevention of virus budding or maturation.

13.7 Common viral infections

13.7.1 Respiratory tract

Adenoviruses: these viruses were first isolated from human adenoids (a mass of lymphatic tissue situated posterior to the nasal cavity), hence their name. They give rise to about 5–10% of respiratory tract infections (RTIs). RTIs caused by adenovirus are mostly mild and require no therapy or only symptomatic treatment. Antigen detection, polymerase chain reaction assay and virus isolation can be used to identify adenovirus infections.

Rhinoviruses: usual cause of the 'common cold'. Symptoms involve nasal congestion, sneezing, sore throat and cough. Usually diagnosis from samples is not necessary. There are specific antibody tests available but these are not generally used.

Influenza: there are three genera: influenza A, B, and C. Influenza C is much less important in human disease. Influenza B is almost exclusively a disease of humans. Influenza A viruses have been designated on the basis of the antigenic relationships of the external spike **haemagglutinin** (HA) and **neuraminidase** (NA) proteins. These are numbered sequentially H1-H15 and N1-N9. Of these, H1, H2, and H3, and N1 and N2 are known to infect humans and cause serious outbreaks. Symptoms include shivering, malaise, headache, aching in limbs, and high temperature. In general, the severity of influenza is proportional to age.

In 2009, a new strain of influenza A, H1N1, was found to be spreading rapidly in Mexico and causing serious infection. The disease rapidly spread around the world and on 11 June 2009, the World Health Organization (WHO) raised the worldwide pandemic alert level to Phase 6 in response to an on-going global spread of the influenza A (H1N1) virus. A Phase 6 designation indicates that a global pandemic is underway. More than 70 countries reported cases of human infection with novel H1N1 flu. A pandemic is an epidemic of infectious disease that has spread through human populations across a large region. The 1918 flu pandemic (January 1918 – December 1920) was an unusually deadly influenza pandemic which infected 500 million people across the world, including remote Pacific islands and the Arctic, killing 20–50 million individuals – 1–3% of the world's population at that time, making it one of the deadliest natural disasters in human history.

Diagnosis of influenza A and B is usually by the complement fixation test, however, in severe cases PCR on respiratory samples can be performed. As with the latter test, a result can often be obtained within 24 hours.

13.7.2 Childhood disease

Measles: this is an acute, highly infectious viral illness transmitted via droplet infection. Almost all who are infected develop symptoms. In temperate countries measles is a comparatively mild infection and serious complications are rare. Before the rash appears there is a prodromal stage which lasts for about 2–3 days, with running nose and eyes, cough and moderate fever. During this time, Koplik spots, which resemble grains of salt, can be seen in the buccal mucous membrane. The rash first appears on the face and spreads to the trunk and limbs within a couple of days. Within 2–3 days of onset, the rash will fade, the temperature will decrease and the child will feel better.

Cross reference

See Chapter 10, Section 10.8.

Measles is usually diagnosed by looking for specific IgM antibodies in the patient's serum. Vaccination is available as a preventative measure. The vaccine is one of the components of MMR vaccine which is given in the national immunization programme at 12–15 months and at 3–5 years of age.

Mumps: this is an acute viral illness transmitted by direct contact with saliva or droplets from the saliva of an infected person. Humans are the only known host of the mumps virus. The onset is marked by malaise and fever followed within 24 h by a painful enlargement of one or both parotid glands. In most cases the swelling subsides within a few days and recovery is uneventful. Diagnosis is usually based on clinical symptoms but confirmation of the diagnosis can be made by looking for the IgM antibodies in the serum. As with measles, vaccination is available.

Respiratory syncytial virus (RSV): causes a highly contagious infection of the respiratory tract found particularly in infants, causing bronchiolitis. In the Northern hemisphere, outbreaks occur in the winter months. The illness usually starts like a common cold but the infant can rapidly deteriorate with respiratory distress. Severe illness carries a high mortality. Diagnosis is by performing PCR on nasopharyngeal washings.

13.7.3 Common viral gastroenteritis

Rotavirus: this primarily infects young children; babies under the age of 2 years are the main victims. The symptoms are mainly diarrhoea, vomiting, and fever. Dehydration is a major problem and must be treated promptly. In the developing world, dehydration resulting from rotavirus infections cause many millions of deaths in young children annually.

Adenovirus: enteric adenoviruses 40 and 41 cause gastroenteritis, usually in children. Most of the adenoviruses identified in stool specimens are not typed.

Norovirus: the most common cause of infectious gastroenteritis (diarrhoea and vomiting) in England and Wales. The illness is generally mild and people usually recover fully within 2–3 days; there are no long-term effects resulting from infection. Infections can occur at any age because immunity is not long lasting.

Several other viruses can cause gastrointestinal infection including astrovirus and calcivirus.

13.7.4 Herpesviruses

The herpesviruses form a large and important group of infective agents. They cause a wide range of syndromes, varying from trivial mucocotaneous lesions to life-threatening infections. An important property of herpesviruses is their ability to cause latent infections that may subsequently become reactivated.

Herpes simplex (HSV): HSV-1 and HSV-2 have many features in common but, as a general rule, HSV-1 affects the upper body and HSV-2 is more usually, but not exclusively, the cause of genital infections. HSV can cause cold sores, painful skin lesions, ophthalmic infections, meningitis and **encephalitis**. HSV-2 can cause infections in newborn babies caused by passage through an infected birth canal. HSV can cause severe and persistent infection in immunocompromised hosts. Diagnosis is usually made by PCR on a swab of the lesion.

Varicella zoster virus (VZV, chickenpox): a common childhood infection. The rash is usually the first sign of disease. The rash is usually more pronounced on the trunk than on the limbs, which first appears as flat macules which rapidly become raised into fluid-filled vesicles. Complications are rare but can include bacterial infection of the spots.

In humans, VZV can reactivate, causing an attack of herpes zoster with a characteristic distribution of vesicular lesions along the affected **dermatome**.

Laboratory diagnosis is rarely sought in cases of varicella because a diagnosis can be reliably made on clinical grounds.

Cytomegalovirus (CMV): CMV can affect all ages. CMV is transmissible to the foetus via the placenta, young children can be affected with overt disease, adolescents and young adults can be infected when the infection is spread by kissing. In this age group, individuals can have an infectious mononucleosis-like infection (glandular fever). The last category of patient to be affected by CMV is not age-related but is due to a depleted immune system, either through transplantation or an immune-deficient disease such as AIDS. In these patients the disease can be exogenous, that is deriving from the donor's tissue or blood transfusion, or endogenous, that is reactivation of an existing infection in the recipient. Reactivations are less serious than primary infections (i.e. exogenous) and may result only in mild symptoms. Primary infections in these patients, however, are extremely serious and may result in death if appropriate antiviral therapy is not instigated quickly.

13.7.5 Hepatitis viruses

Hepatitis A (HAV): primarily spread by the faecal–oral route and by ingestion of contaminated water or food (e.g. contaminated shellfish). HAV is a benign and self-limiting illness with an incubation period of 2-6 weeks and does not cause chronic hepatitis or cirrhosis. It is the most common cause of infective hepatitis in the world. The appearance of IgM type anti-HAV antibodies in the serum is used to diagnose the infection. A vaccination is available for those at risk of contracting HAV, for example, those travelling to endemic countries and health-care workers.

Hepatitis B (HBV): a blood-borne viral infection that can be prevented through vaccination. Patterns of infection are variable and are influenced by age, sex, and the state of the immune system. Many people have no symptoms while others experience a flu-like illness. Other symptoms may include nausea and vomiting. Acute infection can be severe causing abdominal discomfort and jaundice. Mortality during the acute phase of infection is less than 1%.

It is common in South-East Asia, the Middle and Far East, southern Europe, and Africa. The World Health Organization estimates that one-third of the world's population has been infected at some time and that there are approximately 350 million people who are infected long term. In Europe, there are estimated to be one million people infected every year.

In the UK, approximately one in 1,000 people are thought to have the virus. In some inner-city areas with a high percentage of people from parts of the world where the virus is common, as many as one in 50 pregnant women may be infected.

Several markers are looked for in the laboratory to distinguish between the different phases of the disease (i.e. acute, resolved or chronic). Hepatitis B is implicated in chronic hepatitis, cirrhosis of the liver and **hepatocellular carcinoma**. HBV is transmitted in blood and other body fluids, and is prevalent in men who have sexual intercourse with other men and intravenous drug abusers (IVDAs). Vaccination is available for at-risk individuals, such as IVDAs and health-care workers (HCW). HBV immunoglobulin can be administered for temporary passive protection from HBV. It is commonly used in babies born to HBV-positive mothers, sexual partners of individuals with acute HBV and unvaccinated health-care workers who sustain a needlestick injury from a patient with HBV.

Individuals with chronic HBV infection should be evaluated for the potential need for treatment. Drugs currently licensed for the treatment of chronic HBV infection include adefovir dipoxil, alpha interferon, and lamivudine.

Hepatitis C (HCV): a major cause of chronic hepatitis, cirrhosis, and hepatocellular carcinoma. Hepatitis C infection affects different people in different ways; many experience no symptoms at all while others experience extreme tiredness and can feel very unwell, with symptoms such as fatigue, weight loss, abdominal pain and jaundice. The incubation period varies from a few weeks to 6 months.

It is estimated that around 15–20% of infected people clear their infections naturally within the first 6 months of infection. For the remainder, hepatitis C is a chronic infection that can span several decades and can be life-long.

Estimates suggest over 250,000 people in the UK have been infected with hepatitis C, but eight out of ten don't know that they have it because they have no symptoms. Approximately, 75% of these people go on to develop a chronic hepatitis, but because it can take years, even decades, for symptoms to appear, many people (possibly 100,000 or more) remain unaware that they have the infection. By the time they become ill and seek help, considerable damage has been done to the liver.

HCV is blood-borne and many infections are transmitted in IVDAs sharing needles. HCV is diagnosed serologically by detecting antibodies specific to the HCV. There is currently no vaccine for HCV. The ability of HCV to mutate is in part the main difficulty in developing an effective vaccine. Prevention of HCV is focused mainly on education in IVDAs (not sharing needles), screening of blood and blood products and effective universal precautions when performing venepuncture. The treatment for individuals with chronic hepatitis C infection is a combination of two drugs: interferon and ribavirin. This combination therapy is successful in clearing virus from the blood of around 40% of those treated; however, not everybody is suitable for treatment or can tolerate it. Factors such as age, sex, duration of infection, the strain of the virus, and the degree of existing liver damage determine the effectiveness of treatment.

13.7.6 Human immunodeficiency virus (HIV)

The number of people living with HIV globally was estimated to be 34.2 million at the end of 2011, with 2.5 million newly infected individuals during that year. Nine out of ten people living with HIV are in the developing world; 60–70% of those are in Sub-Saharan Africa.

HIV continues to be one of the most important communicable diseases in the UK. It is associated with serious morbidity, high costs of treatment and care, significant mortality, and high number of potential years of life lost. Each year, many thousands of individuals are diagnosed with HIV for the first time. HIV infection is still regarded as stigmatizing and has a prolonged 'silent' period during which it often remains undiagnosed.

HIV is a retrovirus containing RNA. It attacks the T lymphocyte cells and other white blood cells with CD4 receptors on their surface. The virus uses the CD4 receptor to bind with and enter the cell, it then integrates itself into the cells nucleic acid, replicates, and releases a new virus.

HIV kills by slowly destroying the immune system. Several weeks after initial infection, flu-like symptoms are experienced. This is called seroconversion illness. Many people, at this point go undiagnosed as they put the illness down to the 'flu'. The immune system activates and the virus mostly 'retreats into hiding' within lymph tissue. The untreated, infected individual can remain healthy for 5–15 years, but the virus continues to replicate in the background, slowly destroying the immune system. Eventually the body is unable to defend itself against infection and succumbs to overwhelming opportunistic infections that rarely affect healthy individuals. Acquired immune deficiency syndrome (AIDS) is the name given to this final stage of HIV infection, and is characterized by multiple, life-threatening illnesses.

Infections commonly seen include *Pneumocystis jirovecii*, *Cryptococcus neoformans*, and CMV. Many infected individuals are only diagnosed at this point with HIV. New British Association for Sexual Health and HIV guidelines have been produced to highlight the illnesses potentially caused by HIV and therefore encourage patient testing and earlier diagnosis.

HIV is found in body fluids, such as blood, semen, vaginal fluid, and breast milk. It can be passed on by penetrative sexual intercourse, oral sex, and sharing contaminated needles. It can also be passed from mother to baby during pregnancy, childbirth, and breastfeeding.

CASE STUDY 13.1 Clinical history

A 28-year-old man attends his GP with a history of weight loss (30 lb in the last few months), poor appetite, night sweats, and intermittent fevers. He admits to having used intravenous drugs in the past and having sexual intercourse with both men and women. On examination, he has enlarged lymph nodes in his neck and groin.

1. What samples would you take and what tests would you request on them?

2. What would be the possible diagnosis for the patient?

On discussion with the patient it is clear that he falls into a high-risk category. The clinician sends a clotted blood sample away for blood-borne viral serology, after the patient was counselled and consented for the tests to be performed.

3. Why does the patient need to be counselled about the samples taken and the investigations performed on them?

His blood test results reveal that he is HIV positive and his CD4+ lymphocyte count is 375 cells/mm^3. He is given a prescription for anti-HIV drugs and is given an appointment for the Infectious Disease Clinic. The patient fails to attend his clinic appointment and does not take the prescribed drugs.

He is next seen 18 months later when he attends the casualty department of the local hospital complaining of shortness of breath. He is admitted to a ward and chest X-rays show bilateral pulmonary infiltrates. He is also found to be very thin, suffering from memory loss and diarrhoea. His CD4+ count is 146 cells/mm^3. Although the patient is treated for his symptoms and infections, he dies the following week.

4. What was the most likely cause of the patient's pneumonia and how would it be treated?

5. What is the likely cause of the diarrhoea?

6. What was the significance of his CD4 count?

7. What are your conclusions about the patient's condition?

Discussion

The patient is in a high-risk category for HIV, and hepatitis B and C. The highest risk patients of contracting HIV are: homosexual or bisexual males, intravenous drug abusers, patients with haemophilia, recipients of blood transfusions, and heterosexual contacts of the aforementioned. On initial diagnosis of HIV, his CD4+ count was not low enough (<200 cells/mm^3) to be given a diagnosis of AIDS, nor did he have documented AIDS-related infections (e.g. *Candida*, toxoplasmosis), tumours (e.g. Kaposi's sarcoma,

B-cell lymphoma) or severe wasting. However, on his second attendance at the casualty department his HIV infection had progressed to AIDS: his CD4+ count was <200 cells/ mm^3 and he had a diagnosis of PCP. The diarrhoea was also probably attributable to an infectious cause such as *Cryptosporidium* spp. or *Salmonella* spp. The memory loss which was witnessed was probably caused by HIV encephalitis resulting in brain atrophy.

In cases of reinfection, the level of specific IgM either remains the same or rises slightly. However, the level of IgG increases rapidly and far more earlier than in a primary response. Many different types of serological tests are available. With some assays such as EIA and RIA, one can look specifically for IgM or IgG, whereas with other assays such as CFT and HAI, one can only detect total antibody, which comprises mainly IgG. Some of these tests are much more sensitive than others: EIAs and RIAs are the most sensitive tests available, whereas CFT and HAI tests are not so sensitive. Newer techniques such as the EIA offer better sensitivity, specificity, and reproducibility than classical techniques such as CFT and HAI. The sensitivity and specificity of the assays depend greatly on the antigen used. Assays that use recombinant protein or synthetic peptide antigens tend to be more specific than those using whole or disrupted virus particles.

CASE STUDY 13.2 Outbreak of D+V

A young child aged 5 years and two neighbouring children have become ill with diarrhoea and vomiting within 12 hours of each other. The first child initially complained of nausea and this was followed by vomiting and multiple episodes of diarrhoea. The child was unable to eat or drink without vomiting. A stool sample was submitted to her GP and the preliminary result was given as 'negative for the usual bacteria'. The two neighbouring children had similar symptoms which had started a few hours earlier than the initial child. Both had returned to school the day after becoming ill. The three children did not play together but had attended a birthday party on the previous day.

Concerns were raised about homemade ice cream that was served at the party. Fifteen more cases of diarrhoea and

vomiting were reported to the environmental health department. On further investigation it was found that the birthday party had been held at a local swimming pool and one of the parents had raised concerns about the cleanliness of the pool.

1. What is the most likely cause of the diarrhoea and vomiting?

2. What samples should be taken to find the likely cause?

Suspicion of the ice cream would point to a bacterial cause, for example *Salmonella*, however, the index cases faeces sample was negative for this. Viral investigation of faeces samples must always be performed when investigating the cause of an outbreak. The most likely cause of this outbreak is norovirus.

Samples of faeces should be collected from affected individuals. Vomit samples may be tested if diarrhoea is not present. PCR is performed on all samples. Samples should also be collected from the likely source of infection. In this case, the ice cream and the swimming pool water should be tested.

The swimming pool water is found to be the cause of the infection. Norovirus is easily killed by chlorinating the water and a deep clean of the swimming pool facilities must be performed.

CASE STUDY 13.3 *Vaccination*

A 5-year-old child presents to his GP with a high fever which has been present over the preceding 3 days. He was lethargic, had a cough, and was showing symptoms of conjunctivitis. His GP told his mother he had a viral illness and told her to give him paracetamol and keep him hydrated. Two days later he developed a rash which started on his face but spread to the extremities. The child's mother took him back to the GP and on examination the GP noticed Koplik spots on the inside of the child's mouth. The mother explained to the GP that she had never had the child vaccinated against anything.

1. What is the most likely diagnosis?

2. What other questions is the GP likely to ask?

3. Why do you think that the child had not been vaccinated?

4. What would be the treatment options?

5. Who would need to be informed of the child's condition?

Most complications of this type of viral infection occur due to the virus suppressing the host's immune responses, resulting in reactivation of latent infections or super infection by a bacterial pathogen. Consequently, pneumonia is the most frequent complication. Other common infectious complications include otitis media, interstitial pneumonitis, bronchopneumonia, croup, diarrhoea, sinusitis, and keratitis. Rare complications include haemorrhagic measles, purpura fulminans, hepatitis, disseminated intravascular coagulation, subacute sclerosing panencephalitis, and pancreatitis.

Chapter summary

After reading this chapter you should know and understand:

- The general properties and structure of viruses.

- Viral pathogenesis and the consequences of a viral infection on the host.

- Samples required for the diagnosis of viral infection.

- The commonly used diagnostic methods in virology and how they are performed.

- The sites and modes of action of antiviral agents.

- The names of common viral infections and how they are diagnosed.

Further reading

- **Fields BN, Knipe DM, Howley PM.** *Field's Virology*, **3rd edition. Lippincott-Raven, 1996.**

  An excellent reference book for any virologist. The book covers just about every family of viruses. The book is structured well and has sections discussing both the epidemiology, molecular biology, and pathology of the viruses contained within the book.

- **Granoff A, Webster RG eds.** *Encyclopaedia of Virology*, **2nd edition. Academic Press, 1999.**

  An excellent reference book which covers all aspects of virology.

- **Timbury MC.** *Notes on Medical Virology*, **11th edition. Churchill Livingstone, 1997.**

  A good basic book for students learning virology.

- **World Health Organization. www.who.int.**

  Website dedicated to health. Monitors disease outbreaks and assesses performances of health systems around the globe.

- **Health Protection Agency. www.hpa.org.uk.**

  Details on viral infections, outbreaks, and diagnostic algorithms can be found on this website

- **Clinical Virology network. www.clinical-virology.org.**

  Website dedicated to virology. News, clinical tests, and current viruses in circulation are all contained within the pages.

- **Kudesia G, Wreghitt T.** *Clinical and Diagnostic Virology* **(Cambridge Clinical Guides). Cambridge University Press, 2009.**

  Highly informative virology text which covers both diagnostic and clinical aspects of virology.

Discussion questions

13.1 Discuss the provision of a diagnostic virology service to a district general hospital.

13.2 'There is no longer a need for diagnostic laboratories to attempt isolation of viruses in tissue culture.' Comment on this statement.

13.3 What factors would you consider before selecting a commercially available diagnostic assay?

13.4 Discuss the quality assurance of serological assays.

14

Clinical mycology

Derek Law

Mycology is the study of fungi and clinical mycology is the study of human infections caused by fungi. Mycology is a small but growing part of the world of clinical microbiology and the laboratory practitioner must be aware of fungal diseases that are commonly encountered in the laboratory. This chapter describes the clinical symptoms and manifestations of fungal infections, the methods used in laboratory diagnosis of infections, and treatment of such infections.

Learning objectives

After studying this chapter you should be able to:

- Describe the difference between bacteria and fungi.
- List the fungi that commonly cause disease in man.
- Describe the different types of fungal infection and the types of patient that are infected.
- Describe the signs and symptoms of fungal infections.
- Describe the isolation and identification of common fungi.
- Discuss antifungal drugs and methods of susceptibility testing of fungi.

14.1 What are fungi?

Before discussing fungi and their diseases it is necessary to first of all consider what fungi are and how they differ from bacteria. It is difficult to produce a simple definition of what a fungus is as there are very many species of fungi and they vary immensely in terms of structure and morphology.

Bacteria are simple prokaryotic cells; fungi are more complex and are classed as eukaryotic, like human cells.

- They have a nucleus, and membrane-bound organelles such as mitochondria and endoplasmic reticulum.
- They exhibit mitosis.

- They have a rigid cell wall (like plants).

- Unlike plants they do not have chlorophyll and therefore do not carry out photosynthesis.

- Fungi are saprophytic (living on dead organic matter) or parasitic (utilizing living tissue).

Fungi are found throughout nature in *many different environments*, most are invisible to the naked eye and live in soil and decaying matter, where they carry out an essential role in decomposing organic material and cycling of nutrients in the environment.

There are estimated to be 1.5 million different fungal species of which about only 70,000 have been described and characterized. Of these only about 200 are known to cause diseases in man and the vast majority of human infections are caused by about 20 species.

Key Point

Fungi play an important role in nature in helping break down organic material such as plants. They also have uses in the baking and brewing industries, in the production of bread, beers, and wines. Fungi also provide us with food – such as mushrooms.

Fungi exist in two main forms: firstly, as a unicellular yeast form that reproduces by simple budding. The most familiar of the yeasts encountered in the microbiology laboratory is *Candida albicans* which we will learn about in detail in a later section. The second form is a filamentous or mould form composed of long thread-like-filaments; these filaments are often known as **hyphae** or mycelia.

Fungi such as mushrooms are just large masses of hyphae packed tightly together. Reproduction in filamentous fungi is by the production of spores or conidia which are produced by specialized structures known as conidiophores.

Look at Figure 14.1a; this shows a stained preparation of *C. albicans*, a common yeast pathogen of man. Note the typical oval shape of the yeast cells, which are about 5 μm in length. Also visible are yeast cells which are reproducing by budding. In Figure 14.1b a filamentous fungus,

hypha

Hypha (plural hyphae) is a long, branching filamentous cell of a fungus. Hyphae are the main mode of vegetative growth, and are collectively called a mycelium.

(a)

(b)

FIGURE 14.1
(a) Photomicrograph of a yeast stained with a fluorescent antibody. Typical ovoid yeast cells and some budding yeasts are highlighted. (b) Photomicrograph of *Aspergillus fumigatus*, showing hyphae, conidiophore with attached conidia, and some free conidia.
Source: (a) Figure kindly provided by CDC/Maxine Jalbert, Dr Leo Kaufman. (b) Figure kindly provided by CDC.

Aspergillus fumigatus, is shown – note the filamentous hyphae and a conidiophore covered in conidia, with numerous free conidia. The conidia disseminate in the same way as plant seeds. Diseases caused by *A. fumigatus* will be described in detail later in this chapter.

As we will learn later, fungal spores are important as a source of infection; their shape and arrangement are also useful identification aids for various types of fungi. Spores are able to resist heat and drying in a similar way to bacterial spores. They are present in air, soil, dust, and water.

The classification of fungi into yeasts and filamentous fungi is not quite so simple, however. Some fungi are known as **dimorphic** (dimorphic – two forms); this means that they can exist in both a yeast form and a hyphal form. In most cases the environmental conditions dictate the form of the fungus. For example *Histoplasma capsulatum* grows as a hyphal form at 25°C but grows as a yeast at 37°C.

Key Point

Most fungi exist in one of two forms – a yeast form or a filamentous or hyphal form. Certain fungi are dimorphic, i.e. they can exist in either a yeast form or a filamentous form depending on environmental conditions.

Cross reference

Culture media are described in Chapter 3.

Although fungi will grow on many types of culture media used in bacteriology, specialized fungal media are available. The most common medium used is Sabouraud's agar; this is a glucose rich medium, which preferentially stimulates growth of fungi. In many fungal media the pH is low (e.g. pH 5); this favours fungal growth whilst suppressing bacterial growth. To make the media even more selective antibacterial antibiotics such as chloramphenicol, tetracycline or gentamicin are frequently added.

SELF-CHECK 14.1

What are the main differences between bacteria and fungi?

14.2 **Clinical mycology in the twenty-first century**

Twenty or thirty years ago laboratory mycologists dealt primarily with two forms of infection which we consider in detail later, namely infections of skin, nails and hair caused by **dermatophytes** and infections of the mucosa caused by the yeast *C. albicans* and other *Candida* spp.

dermatophytes

Dermatophytes are types of fungi that cause infections of skin, nails and hair; they are described in more detail later in this chapter.

Such infections were and still are very common but rarely life threatening. Indeed life-threatening infections caused by fungi were extremely rare, poorly understood, and in many cases often only recognized at post mortem. Therapy was also limited by the paucity of available agents for treatment. It is now widely recognized that the scope of fungal infections goes beyond mild, non-life-threatening infections to encompass a range of more serious infections where fungi invade the tissues of the body, producing infections which carry a high mortality rate despite treatment with antifungal antibiotics. Fortunately, such infections are still rare, occurring primarily in patients with some underlying illness which reduces or compromises the normal host defences. Examples of conditions and illnesses predisposing to systemic fungal infection will be described in detail in later sections of this chapter.

Although severe fungal infections are rare and much less common than severe bacterial infections, their occurrence in selected populations of patients such as transplant patients, cancer patients undergoing chemotherapy, and in patients with HIV infection and AIDS is sufficient that laboratories must be capable of isolating and characterizing fungi from such infections. In addition there are still many cases of minor fungal infections and most laboratories receive samples from such infections on a daily basis. It is therefore essential that anyone working in a microbiology laboratory has a basic understanding of the fungal infections likely to be encountered in the laboratory, how to process the relevant samples, and the organisms likely to be isolated and methods used to identify such organisms. It is also important to have an understanding of the underlying conditions that predispose to fungal infections, and the antifungal drugs that are available to treat both localized and invasive fungal infections.

As mentioned previously, the incidence of serious invasive fungal infections is increasing. There are four main reasons for this:

1. The majority of invasive fungal infections occur in patients who are **immunocompromised/immunosuppressed** or have other underlying conditions that weaken host defences. The number of such patients is rising because of the increasing number of organ transplants carried out, the increase in patients with malignancy undergoing chemotherapy and the increase in numbers of severely ill patients with underlying conditions or treatments that predispose to reduced immunity and compromised host defences. This can be as a result of drug action (e.g. immunosuppressive drugs used for organ transplantation) or disease (e.g. HIV infection or congenital immunodeficiencies).

2. There is now greater awareness among clinicians regarding the occurrence of invasive fungal infections in at-risk patients. This allows suspicion of an infection in high-risk patients to prompt the correct diagnostic procedures to be instituted, allowing early diagnosis of infection.

3. There are now several different safer antibiotic therapies available for treating severe fungal infections – this has spurred on the need for early recognition of fungal diseases and better diagnostic procedures. Antifungal drugs are discussed later in this chapter.

4. In recent years, improvements in diagnostic tools for invasive fungal diseases have occurred. These include clinical procedures such as **computed tomography scans (CT scans)** and radiography, which can in some cases identify signs specific for fungal infections, and bronchoalveolar lavage (BAL), which can provide better samples for analysis. There are now various commercially available, laboratory-based diagnostic tools which detect fungal cell wall components released during fungal growth which can be used for early detection of infection.

immunocompromised and immunosuppressed
A state where the patient's immune function is absent or impaired so the ability to fight infection is reduced.

computed tomography (CT) scan
CT scans are a medical imaging technique which generates a three-dimensional image of the inside of the body.

SELF-CHECK 14.2

What are the main reasons for the increase in fungal infections?

Cross reference
Processing of bronchoalveolar lavages is described in Chapter 9.

CLINICAL CORRELATION

Serious fungal infections

Most serious fungal infections occur in patients with some other underlying illness which reduces immunity to infection. Common underlying conditions include AIDS, cytotoxic therapy for malignancy, the use of steroid therapy, immunosuppression for transplantation, diabetes, and following abdominal surgery.

The vast majority of fungi are safe to work with, and yeasts can be handled quite safely on an open bench. Spore-producing fungi are more problematic; although most fungi have low virulence, inhalation of spores should be avoided. Whenever cultures start to grow filamentous moulds they should be handled and examined in a safety cabinet, and plates should be taped up to prevent spores being released.

Certain fungi are classed as high risk such as *Penicillium marneffii* and the organisms of the endemic mycoses. If these organisms are suspected (patients usually have a history of foreign travel) then specimens should be referred to a reference laboratory.

14.3 Common fungal infections of man

There are many fungi capable of causing infection in man; however, the vast majority of fungal infections are caused by a small number of fungi. Only the fungi seen with any degree of regularity and clinical significance will be discussed in this chapter. For details on other fungi the reader is urged to consult specialized textbooks or websites (for example the website www.doctorfungus.org gives an in-depth account of fungi encountered in human infections, including photographs of cultures to assist in identification). We will learn about three main forms of fungal disease in this chapter; they differ in the types of fungi involved, how they are acquired, the types of patient involved and their severity and outcome. These infections are:

1. Infections of the skin, nails, and hair:
    *   These infections are caused mainly by dermatophyte fungi.
    *   Infection is usually confined to **keratinized** outer layers of skin.
    *   Infection can occur in any age group and in healthy people, although infections are more common in children.
    *   Sources of infection are the environment, animals (pets and farm animals), and infected people.
2. Infections of the mucosa:
    *   These infections are commonly caused by yeasts such as C. *albicans* which occur in small numbers as part of the **normal flora**.
    *   Infections can occur in healthy individuals but commonly require some predisposing factor.
    *   Common predisposing factors include diabetes, extremes of age, abrasion or occlusion of skin, and use of broad-spectrum antibacterial antibiotics.

keratin
Keratin is a protein found in the outer layers of skin. It serves to protect skin.

normal flora
Normal flora is the collective term for organisms colonizing a given body site.

Key Point

The use of broad-spectrum antibiotics removes much of the normal bacterial flora, allowing overgrowth of yeasts at various body sites. This will predispose to infection with yeasts. Antibacterial antibiotics have no effects on fungi.

Fungal infections and diabetes

Fungal infections are common in diabetic patients and are one of the presenting features of diabetes. Patients with recurring fungal infections should be screened for diabetes.

3. Invasive fungal infections:
    - Infection can occur in any organ in the body but the lung is the main site of infection.
    - They typically occur in patients with underlying illness that reduces immunity or host defences.
    - They carry a high mortality rate even when treated with antifungal drugs.
    - A wide range of fungi can be the cause, many of which are acquired from the environment; however, *Candida* spp. and *Aspergillus* spp. are the most commonly encountered organisms.
    - Often the fungi have low **virulence** and are only capable of establishing infection when the immune system of the host is compromised.

virulence
Virulence is the ability of an organism to produce disease – highly virulent organisms are able to produce disease easily.

SELF-CHECK 14.3

What factors predispose to fungal infections? Are these factors different for bacterial infections?

14.4 Infections of the skin, nails, and hair

The first types of fungal infection that we will consider in this chapter are infections of the skin, nails, and hair. Such infections are common all over the world and, although they are rarely severe, they may cause considerable discomfort to the sufferer. Infections of the skin, nails, and hair are caused by a group of fungi known as the dermatophytes. There are three genera of fungi that comprise the dermatophytes: *Trichophyton*, *Microsporum*, and *Epidermophyton*. Look at Table 14.1 for individual species and the main sites of infection. All of the dermatophyte fungi are filamentous fungi and produce spores which can withstand adverse conditions, such as heat and drying, and can remain infective in soil, on floors, and in the environment for long periods of time.

14.4.1 Sources of dermatophyte infection

There are three main sources of dermatophyte infections:

- The environment; some species live in soil where they live on skin and feathers shed by animals and birds.
- From animals such as dogs, cats, and farm animals.
- From other humans; infection is acquired through contact with spores.

There are various terms used to describe fungal infections of skin, nails and hair. The term **tinea** followed by the part of the body is often used to describe an infection, for example, tinea pedis is used to describe infection of the foot, tinea capitis, infection of the scalp.

tinea
Tinea is the name given to a fungal infection of the body and is usually followed by a term to describe the body site, e.g. tinea capitis.

TABLE 14.1 Dermatophyte species and main sites of infection.

Species	Main sites of infection	Comment
Epidermophyton floccosum	Skin and nails	Common cause of tinea cruris
Trichophyton rubrum	Skin, nails, and hair	Most common dermatophyte in UK
Trichophyton mentagrophytes	Skin, nails, and hair	Common cause of nail infections
Trichophyton schoenleinii	Skin, nails, and hair	
Trichophyton violaceum	Skin, nails, and hair	
Trichophyton tonsurans	Skin, nails, and hair	
Microsporum canis	Hair and skin	Often acquired from cats and dogs
Microsporum gypseum	Hair and skin	
Microsporum audouinii	Hair and skin	

The main symptoms of dermatophyte infections of the skin are scaling of the skin with or without redness and itching. Infection is limited to the outer layers of keratinized skin but can occur on any body site.

CLINICAL CORRELATION

Dermatophyte infections of the skin

Only the outer layers of skin contain keratin. Dermatophytes are able to break down keratin and use it as a nutrient. That is why infection is restricted to the outer layer of skin – the epidermis.

The most common site of dermatophyte infection is the foot, leading to the condition athlete's foot. The infection may spread from person to person in communal showers and bathrooms or in other moist areas where infected people walk barefoot. Infection occurs most frequently in the warm, moist areas between the toes, but can spread to involve the entire sole of the foot. Sometimes scaling is severe and cracks or fissures appear, which can become infected by bacteria. Severe cases can be very painful, and the toe nails may also become involved. Infection of the nails is termed **onychomycosis**; in this condition the fungus attacks and grows in the nail which becomes discoloured, thickened and deformed.

onychomycosis

Onychomycosis is the term given to a fungal infection of the toe or fingernails.

Look at Figure 14.2 – it shows the foot of a patient with athlete's foot caused by *T. rubrum*. Notice the flaking skin between the toes, the most common site of infection. Infection can spread to the sole of the feet and the toe nails. Secondary bacterial infections can also occur.

The fingernails can also become infected following infection of the skin of the hands, and can be unsightly.

Infection of the scalp (known as tinea capitis) is primarily caused by *Trichophyton* spp. It is very common among children and can be highly contagious, and outbreaks of infection may occur in schools. The commonest source of infection is often close contact with pet animals or close contact with an infected individual. The symptoms of tinea capitis can vary but usually involve several discrete area of redness, scaling, and hair loss. In chronic cases the infection can spread

FIGURE 14.2

Photograph of the foot of a patient with athlete's foot showing typical lesions between the toes.

Source: Figure kindly provided by CDC/ Dr Lucille K. Georg.

to cover the entire scalp. Some species of fungi are able to penetrate and infect the hair itself. With certain organisms the hair shows fluorescence under **Wood's light**.

Infection of the body is known as tinea corporis – infection can occur anywhere on the body and usually presents as a round itchy area with pink scaly borders. The infection site gets larger if untreated and can spread to other parts of the body. The lesions may heal in the centre whilst the edge spreads outwards. Eventually several concentric rings may become apparent on the skin; this leads to the term **ringworm** which is another common name for tinea corporis. When infection occurs in the groin or genital area it is known as tinea cruris. Infection may be transferred from one area of the body to another by scratching or contact.

Figure 14.3 shows a typical skin lesion caused by a dermatophyte fungus. The lesion is circular and the outer edges of the lesion show the greatest degree of inflammation.

Wood's light

Wood's light is a long-wave ultraviolet light used as a diagnostic tool by dermatologists to distinguish dermatophyte infections from other causes of scalp irritation and hair loss.

ringworm

Ringworm is the common name for fungal infections of the skin and hair.

SELF-CHECK 14.4

Are dermatophytes likely to cause severe infections such as septicaemia? If not why not?

14.4.2 Diagnosis of dermatophyte infections

The symptoms of dermatophyte infections are non-specific and similar symptoms can be caused by other non-infectious dermatological conditions such as eczema, psoriasis, or infections caused by other organisms. It is important to have a confirmed diagnosis of a dermatophyte infection for three reasons:

- Specific antifungal agents can be prescribed to cure dermatophyte infections – but treatment can be prolonged and drugs may have side effects and it is therefore important that only true dermatophyte infections are treated with antifungal drugs.

FIGURE 14.3

Photograph of a skin lesion from a patient with dermatophyte infection, showing a typical circular lesion with inflammation on the periphery.

Source: Figure kindly provided by CDC/Dr Lucille K. Georg.

- It important to have a correct diagnosis for epidemiological purposes so that sources of infection can be identified and cross infection can be eliminated.

- A negative diagnosis of a dermatophyte infection allows other causes of the complaint to be investigated.

Key Point

Fungal infections of the skin are often indistinguishable from other skin conditions. Laboratory testing is required to confirm infection and to ensure appropriate therapy is given, and to allow further investigations in the case of a negative fungal diagnosis.

The first stage in diagnosis of dermatophyte infections is examination of infected skin and hair sites using a Wood's light; fluorescence is a strong indicator of a fungal infection. Dermatologists will often commence treatment on the basis of clinical signs and a positive Wood's light sign. However, not all dermatophyte infections show fluorescence and therefore its absence cannot rule out a dermatophyte infection.

14.4.3 Collection of samples for diagnosis of dermatophyte infection

As we have seen in previous chapters, good quality samples are necessary for diagnosis, and diagnosis of dermatophytes is no exception; poorly taken samples may prevent an accurate diagnosis. A brief description of the type of samples and how they are taken is given next.

Collection of samples requires skill and experience to select the best sites for sampling and to ensure that sufficient quality material is taken. First of all, skin and nail sites should be cleaned with 70% alcohol; this reduces bacterial contamination and helps remove creams and ointments which can interfere with diagnosis. Skin samples are taken from the edges of lesion where the hyphae are usually most prolific. If multiple lesions are present then several of these should be sampled; newer lesions are likely to be more productive than old lesions. When nails are infected, friable, discoloured material can easily be scraped from the surface of the nail with a scalpel.

Potentially infected hairs which are broken or distorted should be removed using forceps. The use of a Wood's light to identify fluorescent hairs, which can then be removed, is useful. All samples should be placed in black absorbent paper – this serves two purposes: the samples dry out which reduces bacterial contamination during culture and also the samples are much easier to visualize and work with when on a black background. Fungi remain viable within skin samples for many weeks, and there is therefore no requirement for urgent transport to the laboratory; however, any undue delays should be avoided as this will delay diagnosis.

Key Point

Good quality skin, nail, and hair material is required to enable the correct diagnostic procedures to be carried out.

14.4.4 Laboratory procedures for diagnosis of dermatophyte infection

When received in the laboratory samples should be opened carefully to ensure that the contents remain intact. It is very easy for paper to flex and bend creating a shower of skin flakes. The use of gloves by the operator is useful to prevent the possibility of cross infection. Two laboratory methods are used for diagnosis – namely microscopy and culture. Microscopy serves as an initial diagnostic tool and, although not sensitive, can provide a rapid diagnosis when fungal hyphae are seen in samples. Culture is the second method and is generally more sensitive than microscopy; however, growth of dermatophytes can be slow and culture and identification can take several weeks. It may therefore take up to a month before results are available. However, negative culture results are usually reported within 2–3 weeks. Both methods are important and the procedures involved in both will be described in detail. If there is insufficient sample for both microscopy and culture then culture should be set up.

Key Point

Laboratory diagnosis involves two separate techniques: microscopy to identify fungal hyphae in the sample and culture to isolate the infecting fungus. Both methods are important.

Microscopy

The purpose of microscopy is to detect the presence of fungal hyphae in the skin, nail, or hair samples. This is a rapid technique, providing a result within a day of sample receipt, allowing early initiation of antifungal therapy when fungi are detected. However, microscopy is not a straightforward technique for several reasons. The quantity of fungal elements present in a sample may be low in relation to the number of skin cells or nail debris and is very dependent on how well the sample was taken. Fungal hyphae may also be difficult to distinguish from cellular material on microscopy. In the Method Box is a brief description of how microscopy is carried out.

Recently, Calcoflour white has been shown to improve the sensitivity of microscopic examination. Calcoflour white is a dye that fluoresces when bound to cellulose or chitin; both are present in fungal cell walls but absent from human cells. Addition of this to KOH preparations and examination under UV light shows up fungal hyphae as bright fluorescing elements. The microscopy results should be reported as either *'fungal elements seen – culture results to follow'* or *'No fungal elements seen – culture results to follow'.*

 METHOD *Microscopy for dermatophytes*

- Place a drop of 30% KOH on a slide.
- Place fragments of skin, nail, or hair in the drop and apply a coverslip.
- Allow time (15–60 min) for KOH to dissolve skin.
- Examine under ×200–400 magnification for fungal hyphae. These show up as slightly greenish, branching threads which contrast with the colourless material of skin or nails.
- Experience is required to distinguish hyphae from skin and nail debris.

Figure 14.4 shows a Calcoflour white preparation of a skin sample from a patient with a dermatophyte infection. Compare the upper picture which shows the view under traditional phase contrast microscopy – fungal hyphae are present but difficult to see because of debris. The lower picture is the same field of view but using UV microscopy – fungal hyphae which have taken up the Calcoflour stain fluoresce white against the dark background of epithelial cells and are clearly much more visible than in the phase contrast view.

(a)

Hyphae

(b)

FIGURE 14.4

Phase contrast (a) and fluorescent microscopy (b) of same optical field of a skin scraping from a patient with a dermatophyte infection. Hyphae are difficult to see in the phase contrast slide because of skin debris, but are visualized very clearly in the fluorescent slide after staining with Calcoflour white which binds to fungal chitin.

Source: Figure kindly provided by Liz Hamer.

Culture for dermatophytes

Culture is the most reliable method for identifying and confirming a fungal skin or nail infection and allows the isolation of the causative organism. However, culture is not infallible and may be negative when microscopy is positive; this may be because of uneven distribution of fungal hyphae throughout the sample or the effects of prior antifungal treatment.

Culture media for dermatophyte isolation are usually prepared in bottles rather than in Petri dishes. Cultures are often kept for up to 4 weeks and the use of bottles prevents dehydration of the media. Also, because samples may contain fungi that produce spores in profusion, contamination may be problematic; using closed bottles prevents spores escaping from the bottle. Specimens should be cultured onto two different mycological media; typically one of the media will contain the antibiotic **cycloheximide** (this antibiotic inhibits the growth of **non-dermatophyte fungi**), and the other will contain no cycloheximide. Media also contain antibacterial antibiotics to suppress growth of bacteria found in skin and nail samples. Typical media that are used include Sabouraud's agar or variations of this medium.

SELF-CHECK 14.5

What advantage does microscopy for dermatophytes have over culture as a diagnostic tool?

Key Point

Use of media with and without cycloheximide helps in the presumptive identification of a dermatophyte isolate, as other fungi are often inhibited by it.

14.4.5 Confirmation of dermatophyte isolation

When fungal growth occurs on both media and fungal elements are seen on microscopy there is a high probability that a dermatophyte is present in the sample. Confirmation of this is needed and this is carried out by examining the colony for distinct morphological structures. Dermatophytes produce two types of conidia, **microconidia** and **macroconidia**; the structures of these are distinct for each genus of dermatophyte. By examining colonies for the presence and shape of both microconidia and macroconidia it is possible to assign a dermatophyte to one of the three genera described earlier in this chapter.

METHOD Culture for dermatophytes

- Moisten the end of a right-angled inoculating wire; use the moistened tip to pick up samples of the material.
- Press the material into the surface of the agar medium to ensure that the fungal elements come into contact with the nutrients and are able to grow. If there is sufficient sample it can be inoculated at multiple sites on the slope.

---

cycloheximide

Cycloheximide is a useful additive to culture media for dermatophytes as it suppresses growth of fungi such as *Aspergillus* and *Penicillium* which are common in the environment and may contaminate skin and nail samples.

non-dermatophyte fungi

Non-dermatophyte fungi are other filamentous fungi that can cause infections. There are several species that can cause infections of nails.

microconidia, macroconidia

Microconidia and macroconidia are the names given to the spores produced by dermatophyte fungi. They differ in size: microconidia are small, often spherical or tear-drop shaped, 2–4 μM in diameter; macroconidia are much larger – their morphology varies between the three genera with slight variations between species in each genus.

- Incubate for 2–3 weeks at 30°C. The optimal temperature for dermatophytes is below 37°C.
- Examine cultures twice weekly for growth – dermatophytes grow as white velvet/fluffy colonies, and growth appears usually after 3–4 days of incubation although this may be much later in partially treated cases or where the amount of fungus in the sample is low. Eventually the colonies grow in size and may become slightly pigmented; some organisms such as *Trichophyton rubrum* produce a red pigment on the underside of the colony.
- If fungal growth occurs on both cycloheximide-containing and cycloheximide-free media, the organism is probably a dermatophyte; if there is only growth on the cycloheximide medium it is likely that the fungus is a non-dermatophyte. Non-dermatophyte fungi may be contaminants from the sample or in some cases may be significant.

METHOD Identification of dermatophytes

lactophenol blue

Lactophenol blue acts as a good background to visualize fungal structures.

- Remove some growth from the culture and emulsify in **lactophenol blue**.
- Examine microscopically for the presence of microconidia and macroconidia.
- If results are inconclusive inoculate isolate onto a medium to encourage sporulation, such as potato dextrose agar.
- Repeat the process when growth occurs.
- The characteristic appearance of macroconidia and microconidia should help allocate the organism to one of the three dermatophyte genera.

Figure 14.5 shows the different morphology of the dermatophyte macroconidia. Note the distinctive shapes which are characteristic of each dermatophyte genus. Also present in the *Trichophyton* photomicrograph (Figure 14.5b) are some smaller microconidia.

Cross reference

See Chapter 2.

Final confirmation of the species identification is complex and requires various biochemical tests including the ability to grow on various media, colonial characteristics and microscopic morphology. However, due to the introduction of MALDI-TOF systems it is now possible to pick off a small part of the colony and identify the dermatophyte following a sample preparation technique. This means that dermatophytes can be identified several days faster than at present, as soon as the colony forms on the culture medium rather than waiting until characteristic structures are produced. This greatly improves the turnaround times for reporting positive results. For laboratories handling few isolates, dermatophyte isolates should be referred to a reference laboratory for identification.

If a colony is isolated with typical dermatophyte morphology which grows on cycloheximide-containing media, a preliminary report should be issued stating that 'Probable dermatophyte isolated – further identification to follow'.

Susceptibility tests are rarely carried out on dermatophytes but may be appropriate in cases of infection refractory to treatment. Such tests are best carried out in a reference laboratory.

(a)

(b)

(c)

FIGURE 14.5
Photomicrographs of lactophenol blue preparations of three genera of dermatophyte;
(a) *Epidermophyton*,
(b) *Trichophyton*, and
(c) *Microsporum*: showing typical macroconidial morphology.
Source: Figures kindly provided by CDC/Dr Libero Ajello (a, b) and Dr Lucille K. Georg (c).

Repeat sampling should always be considered in cases of suspected dermatophyte infection with negative laboratory reports.

Key Point

Identification of dermatophytes is by cultural characteristics of the colony, the ability to grow on cycloheximide-containing media, and the presence and arrangement of conidia.

14.4.6 Non-dermatophyte fungi as a cause of skin infections

Not all skin and nail infections are caused by dermatophyte fungi; there are several infections that can be encountered that the laboratory mycologist should be aware of, such as infection caused by the **lipophilic** yeast *Malasezzia furfur*. This organism causes scaling and darker patches of the skin, particularly on the chest. Under Wood's light the lesions show fluorescence in various colours, leading to the terminology tinea versicolor. Diagnosis is typically carried out by microscopy. Examination of skin scrapings from tinea versicolor typically shows large numbers of yeasts and hyphal fragments, which is characteristic of this condition and is very different from the microscopic picture from lesions caused by dermatophyte fungi. *M. furfur* will not grow on Sabouraud's agar unless it is supplemented with lipids such as olive oil.

lipophilic
Lipophilic means lipid loving – these organisms require a supply of lipid in the growth medium.

FIGURE 14.6

Photomicrograph of a stained skin sample from a patient with tinea versicolor showing abundant yeast and hyphal forms characteristic of infection with *M. furfur*.

Source: Figure kindly provided by CDC/Dr Lucille K. Georg.

Look at Figure 14.6 — it shows a photomicrograph of a stained skin sample from a patient with tinea versicolor. Note the abundant yeasts and hyphae characteristic of *M. furfur*. This is clearly different from the pattern seen in dermatophyte infections (Figure 14.4).

Although many infections of the nail are caused by dermatophytes, several other fungi are capable of causing infection with a similar clinical picture. These fungi include *Scopulariopsis brevicaulis* and *Scytalidium hyalium*. Microscopically such infections are indistinguishable from those of dermatophyte infections. Diagnosis is by culturing the organism and identification. Because such organisms will often fail to grow on cycloheximide-containing media, cyclohex-imide-free media must always be inoculated. Identification is by examining colony appearance and microscopic structures.

Candida spp. can also cause infections of nails; it is common in people whose hands are continually immersed in water. Such infections will often be evident by growth of large numbers of yeast on culture. These should be identified as described next, and their presence reported to clinicians.

14.4.7 Treatment of skin, nail, and hair infections

Infections of small areas of skin such as athlete's foot can usually be treated with the application of topical antifungal creams or powders. Treatment of more extensive lesions and where nail or hair is infected usually requires oral therapy given for weeks or months. Drugs such as griseofulvin, terbinafine, or itraconazole are usually given for periods of 2 weeks to 6 months, depending on the severity and site of infection.

14.5 *Candida* infections of the mucosa

Yeasts of the genus *Candida* form part of the normal flora of the body and can be found on the skin, throughout the alimentary tract and in the female genitalia. Infections can occur in normal healthy individuals. In such cases infection is usually due to an impaired epithelial barrier function, for example occlusion or abrasions of skin, excessive sweating, or disturbance of the normal flora through the use of antibacterial antibiotics which result in overgrowth of yeasts.

candidiasis

Candidiasis is the name given to infections caused by *Candida* spp.

Candidiasis of the mouth and throat are rarely seen in normal individuals but are common in the newborn and elderly; in the latter group they are often related to the presence of dentures. Infections in other individuals are often associated with some form of immunological impairment, for example leukaemia, neutropenia, HIV infection, and diabetes. Prior therapy

FIGURE 14.7

Photograph of oral cavity of an AIDS patient showing white candidal plaques.

Source: Figure kindly provided by CDC/Sol Silverman, Jr, DDS.

with cytotoxic drugs, radiation, or broad-spectrum antibiotics also predispose to infection. Infection presents as discrete, white plaques on the mucosal surfaces of the mouth and throat. Symptoms include pain and burning on swallowing. A severe form of infection, oesophageal candidiasis, is frequently seen in severely immunosuppressed patients. It is a frequent complication of patients receiving cytotoxic therapy and occurs commonly in AIDS patients. Infection involves the oesophagus and the mouth; the main symptoms are difficulty in and a burning pain on swallowing. Clinical diagnosis often requires the use of an endoscope to visualize the plaques in the oesophagus. Figure 14.7 shows the mouth of an HIV patient with oral candidiasis. The discrete white plaques are evident on the mucosa. This is characteristic of *Candida* infections.

Candidiasis of the skin is most frequently seen in the groin, underneath breasts, in the axillae, and the umbilicus. Such infections require some predisposing factors such as occlusion or abrasion of skin, or excessive sweating; such infections are common in the obese, patients with diabetes, and with the use of broad-spectrum antibiotics. Nappy rash seen in infants is commonly caused by *Candida* spp.

Vaginal *Candida* infection is a common infection in women. *Candida* spp. occur in the vagina in low numbers in women of child-bearing age; however, the use of broad-spectrum antibiotics can remove the normal bacterial flora allowing *Candida* spp. to proliferate. Diabetes and the use of oral contraceptives may be contributing factors and infection is common in the third trimester of pregnancy. The most common symptoms include itching and burning with a creamy white vaginal discharge. Infection can also extend to the external genitalia. In a small proportion of women repeated episodes are common, although the reason for this is unclear.

Key Point

Vaginal infections are one of the commonest infections caused by *Candida* spp. and affect a large proportion of women at some point during their life.

CLINICAL CORRELATION

Infection of the skin caused by *Candida* usually requires some underlying condition – e.g. immunosuppression, diabetes, use of broad-spectrum antibiotics, cytotoxic therapy, intravascular lines, or excessive moisture.

14.5.1 Diagnosis of mucosal *Candida* infections

Mucosal infections caused by *Candida* spp. are the most frequently encountered fungal infections in clinical laboratories. Each day most laboratories receive many samples requiring culture for *Candida*. Fortunately, diagnosis of such infections is relatively simple.

Many samples will be swabs from infected skin sites, or samples of vaginal discharge. Along with any bacteriological investigation required, samples for the diagnosis of *Candida* infection are routinely plated onto Sabouraud's agar. Plates are incubated at 35–37°C for 24–48 h and plates examined for growth of *Candida*. *Candida* spp. grow on Sabouraud's agar as creamy white, **butyrous** colonies, with a typical sweet yeasty odour. Colony size after 24 h is typically 2–3 mm diameter but after 48 h colonies are 4–5 mm diameter. The amount of growth is typically recorded as +, ++ or +++; this will help in the interpretation of the result. True *Candida* infections will normally show ++ or +++ growth if samples have been taken correctly. Very small numbers of organisms will often represent colonization of a site rather than infection. Interpretation of results requires both culture and clinical data.

Microscopy is useful for vaginal swabs. The presence of large numbers of yeasts and white blood cells (pus cells) is often indicative of *Candida* infection. This can often be carried out alongside microscopy for other pathogens such as *Trichomonas vaginalis* and *Gardnerella vaginalis*. Various stains, such as a Gram and acridine orange, may be used to visualize yeasts.

Key Point

Candida spp. grow readily on Sabouraud's agar, and the inclusion of antibiotics helps suppress bacterial growth. *Candida* spp. grow as creamy white colonies with a characteristic odour. Quantitation of the growth helps in interpretation of significance.

The majority of human *Candida* infections are caused by the species *Candida albicans*, although other species will occasionally cause disease in similar situations. The other species commonly found are *C. glabrata*, *C. tropicalis*, *C. krusei*, *C. parapsilosis*, and *C. dubliniensis*. Disease caused by these species is indistinguishable from disease caused by *C. albicans*. Some of these species show resistance to various antifungal drugs. In most laboratories identification of yeasts isolated from skin and vaginal swabs is not carried out and the isolation of a yeast with the quantity of growth is reported.

METHOD The germ tube test

- Place a small amount of the colony to test into a small volume of human or horse serum to produce a faintly turbid suspension.
- Incubate at 35–37°C for 2.5–3 h but do not exceed this.
- Remove a small sample of the fluid and examine microscopically.
- Germ tube production is indicated by the presence of a hyphal structure emerging from the cell.

- True germ tubes of *Candida albicans* have parallel walls where they leave the yeast cell; occasionally other species of yeast may show similar structures, but have constrictions at the site where they leave the yeast cell.
- The quantity of germ tubes produced by different *C. albicans* strains varies; some produce many germ tubes, in other strains the number of cells producing germ tubes is low.

Key Point

Candida glabrata is increasingly isolated from clinical samples and is often resistant to azole antifungals such as fluconazole.

Rapid identification of *C. albicans* is possible by carrying out a germ tube test. The germ tube test is an important identification characteristic and is specific for *C. albicans*, the most common yeast in human infections.

Figure 14.8 shows a preparation of *C. albicans* that has been incubated in human serum for 2 h. A yeast cell is producing a structure that protrudes from the cell – this is a germ tube. It is clearly distinct from the other yeast cell which is not producing a germ tube.

Germ tube-negative isolates are typically reported as *Candida* species not *albicans*. Further identification of germ tube negative species can be carried out using commercially available kits or by using chromogenic culture media. Chromogenic media can also be used as a primary isolation medium and are useful in that they can identify mixed infection, that is infections caused by two or more different species of *Candida*. This can be useful as the colonial appearance of *Candida* spp. on Sabouraud's agar, with the exception of *C. krusei*, is very similar. Figure 14.9 shows the typical colonial appearance of various species of *Candida* on a *Candida* chromogenic medium. The common species of *Candida* are easily distinguished and differentiated on such media. Mixtures of two species of *Candida* are relatively common; however, it is very unlikely that all five species will be seen in a clinical sample, as seen on this plate.

Cross reference
See Chapter 3 for information on chromogenic media.

Germ tube   Yeast cell (*C. albicans*)

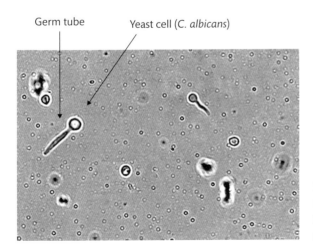

FIGURE 14.8

Photomicrograph of *C. albicans* after 2 h incubation at 37°C in human serum showing production of germ tubes.

Source: Courtesy of bioMérieux.

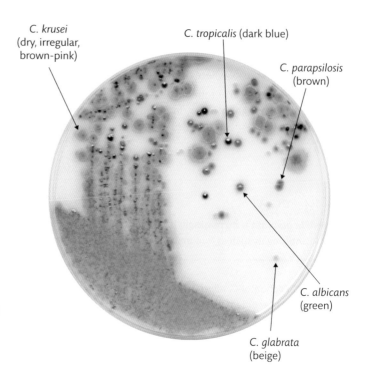

C. krusei
(dry, irregular,
brown-pink)

C. tropicalis (dark blue)

C. parapsilosis
(brown)

C. albicans
(green)

C. glabrata
(beige)

FIGURE 14.9

Photograph of chromogenic *Candida* medium
showing colonial appearance of five common species
of *Candida* after 48 h of incubation.

Source: Photograph copyright of Oxoid, reproduced here
with their permission.

14.5.2 Treatment of mucosal *Candida* infections

Many mucosal infections are self-limiting and can often be cured by removal of the predisposing condition, e.g. reducing obesity or controlling diabetes. Treatment with locally applied
antifungal drugs can often speed up recovery, but unless the underlying conditions are tack-
led infection may recur. Treatment with topical antifungal agents is used in cases of vaginal
candidiasis; however, oral therapy is also effective and has better compliance. Oesophageal
candidiasis is a more serious condition and treatment often requires hospitalization and use
of intravenous antifungal drugs.

Key Point

Candida infections frequently recur after treatment, unless the underlying condition
predisposing to infection is also treated, e.g. stabilization of diabetes or weight loss in
the obese.

14.6 **Invasive fungal infections**

Invasive fungal infections are caused principally by *Candida* spp. and *Aspergillus* spp. but can
also be caused by a variety of other fungi. These are fungal infections of the body which occur
almost exclusively in debilitated patients whose normal defence mechanisms are impaired.
The commonest fungal organisms causing such infections are *Candida* spp. and infections with
these organisms are commonly derived from the patient's own flora.

Invasive infections caused by filamentous fungi such as *Aspergillus* spp. are commonly derived
from the environment. Infection is often acquired through the inhalation of spores and the

lung is the commonest site of infection, although infection can spread (disseminate) to other body sites, including the brain. The organisms that cause such infections often have low intrinsic virulence. With very rare exceptions they are unable to cause infection in the normal healthy host. The increased incidence of these infections is due to the emergence of AIDS, the use of aggressive cytotoxic chemotherapy for malignancy, increased incidence of transplantation requiring immunosuppressive regimes, the widespread use of broad-spectrum antibacterial antibiotics, **cytotoxic agents**, corticosteroids, and surgical and other procedures that result in lowered resistance of the host.

There are several other types of infection caused by fungi, but these are beyond the scope of this book; they include allergic-type reactions to fungal products such as farmer's lung and intoxications caused by fungal-produced toxins found in food. In the USA and other parts of the world there are a group of infections known as the endemic mycoses, caused by several different genera of dimorphic fungi. Although these infections can be severe, they will not be considered here as they are extremely rare in the UK. The types of infection considered in this chapter are described next.

SELF-CHECK 14.6

Why is the respiratory tract the most common site of invasive *Aspergillus* infections?

> ### Key Point
>
> Invasive fungal infections occur mainly in ill patients, particularly those who are immunosuppressed. Such infections carry a high mortality rate – partly because infections are difficult to recognize and because of the underlying status of the patient. Dissemination from an initial infection site is common.

14.6.1 Invasive *Candida* infections

The most common invasive form of *Candida* infection is candidaemia, defined as the presence of *Candida* in the blood. *Candida* is one of the ten most common pathogens isolated from blood cultures; in some centres it may be the fourth or fifth most common pathogen. Predisposing factors include the use of intravenous catheters, surgical procedures (particularly abdominal surgery), burns, parenteral nutrition, chemotherapy-induced damage to the oral or intestinal mucosa, and the use of antibacterial antibiotics. Patients are usually ill but not necessarily immunosuppressed. Infection is initiated on a mucosal surface or following infection of an IV catheter; infection then spreads to the bloodstream and can disseminate to various body organs, causing abscess formation.

There are various other forms of invasive candidiasis, such as gastrointestinal candidiasis; this occurs in patients receiving cytotoxic therapy which damages the mucosa of the intestine. Perforation of the mucosa can lead to spread of organisms to the peritoneum, bloodstream, and other organs such as the liver and spleen.

Invasive candidiasis can occur in babies and neonates, partially because of the immaturity of the immune system, but low birth weight and prematurity are predisposing factors. Organisms often gain access to the bloodstream via intravascular catheters and *C. parapsilosis* is isolated frequently from neonates. Infection may disseminate to cause meningitis and infection in other organs.

Cross reference

See Chapter 6 for information on taking urine samples and interpretation of urine cultures.

Cross reference

Chapter 5 deals with blood culture samples.

One of the most problematic *Candida* infections to diagnose is infection of the urinary tract. Asymptomatic *Candida* infection of the urinary tract occurs mainly in women and occurs following antibiotic or steroid treatment that promotes colonization and growth of *Candida* in the gastrointestinal and genital tracts. Infections of the bladder are also common in diabetic patients and patients with urinary tract abnormalities, especially if the patient is catheterized or receiving antibacterial antibiotics. Infection may spread to the kidney either via the ureters or through haematogenous spread. Diagnosis of renal infection is difficult as isolation of *Candida* from a urine sample may be due to a genuine bladder infection or contamination of a urine sample due to colonization of the genital tract. Samples of urine taken directly from the bladder (suprapubic urine) and blood cultures may help confirm the diagnosis of renal candidiasis.

Diagnosis of invasive candidiasis

Blood cultures are frequently taken to diagnose invasive candidiasis, although they may not always yield *Candida* spp.

Samples can also be taken from other potentially infected body sites, such as the peritoneal cavity, liver and lung, to assist with diagnosis. Isolation of *Candida* spp. from a normally sterile site is indicative of invasive candidiasis. However, isolation of *Candida* from sputum, urine or skin is not conclusive as these sites are frequently colonized in hospitalized patients, particularly if they have been treated with antibacterial antibiotics. Repeated isolation of large numbers of yeasts from a site may be a more reliable diagnostic marker for infection. As yet, there are no reliable markers for diagnosis of systemic infection although PCR tests may become more widespread for detecting and quantitating *Candida* in clinical samples.

empiric therapy

Empiric therapy is the commencement of therapy before it is known what the infective organism is or what its sensitivity is.

Following diagnosis of invasive candidiasis by isolation of yeasts from blood cultures or from another sterile body site in an ill patient, urgent treatment is required. *C. albicans* is usually susceptible to fluconazole, whereas germ tube-negative yeasts such as *C. glabrata* and *C. krusei* are often fluconazole resistant. An **echinocandin** antifungal agent may also be used as they are highly active against most species of *Candida*. In many situations therapy will be started before an organism has been isolated; this is known as **empiric therapy**. It is essential to initiate treatment early because delays can increase mortality. Antibiotic therapy may change when the identity of an organism is known or a susceptibility test is performed.

CASE STUDY 14.1 *Candida septicaemia*

A 60-year-old male diabetic was admitted for colonic surgery. He was given fluconazole prophylaxis as well as antibacterial antibiotic prophylaxis prior to surgery. After surgery he was transferred to the ICU and 3 days later the patient spiked a temperature and felt unwell. Blood cultures were taken and the patient's antibiotics were changed although fluconazole was continued. Then, 24 h later, the patient's condition began to deteriorate, further blood cultures were taken and IV catheters were removed and sent for culture. A further 24 h later, the patient was still febrile, culture results showed that one of the catheters grew +++ yeast, and a germ tube test was carried out and was negative, indicating a non-*albicans Candida*. Because of this fluconazole was discontinued, and an echinocandin drug was given to the patient. Within 12 h the patient's temperature started to fall and his condition improved. Eventually several of the blood cultures became positive and microscopy showed the presence of a yeast. Culture on chromogenic media showed colonies typical of *Candida glabrata*. The yeast isolated from the catheter tip was also identified as *C. glabrata*. The blood culture and catheter isolates were sent to a reference laboratory for susceptibility tests and the MIC to fluconazole was >128 mg/L and to caspofungin was 0.05 mg/L.

1. What are the risk factors in this patient for a *Candida* infection?

2. Why do you think *C. glabrata* was isolated from this patient?

3. What test led to the change in antifungal therapy and why?

14.6.2 Cryptococcal meningitis

Most serious yeast infections are caused by organisms of the *Candida* genus. However, there is one other yeast which can cause severe systemic infection; this is *Cryptococcus neoformans*. *C. neoformans* is a **capsulate** yeast and causes infections of the human respiratory tract and nervous system. Infection is usually acquired by inhalation of desiccated yeast forms or spores and the primary site of infection is the respiratory tract. Infection at this site is often asymptomatic. In patients who are immunosuppressed the organism can disseminate, typically to the nervous system where it causes meningitis. *C. neoformans* is the commonest cause of fungal meningitis and affects up to 10% of AIDS patients. The main symptoms are headache and fever; occasionally, skin lesions may be evident. If left untreated the infection is invariably fatal. Cryptococcal infection should be suspected in any immunosuppressed patient with symptoms of meningitis. Rapid and accurate diagnosis is required so that antifungal therapy can be instituted as soon as possible.

The main samples for diagnosis are CSF samples. Three techniques can be used for diagnosis: microscopy, culture and antigen detection.

The capsule is essential for *C. neoformans* to cause disease, and can be detected and quantified in CSF samples using commercially available kits. Antigen detection can be performed on serial CSF samples to monitor the response to therapy as levels decline with successful therapy.

Samples for *C. neoformans* should be cultured on Sabouraud's agar at 30°C and 37°C. Any yeast isolated from a CSF sample should be examined for the presence of a capsule using an India ink stain, identified to species level, and should have a susceptibility test performed to ensure the correct therapy is given. Treatment of cryptococcal infection often involves combinations of antifungal drugs to maximize the chances of eradication of the organism. Patients often have to remain on therapy for the remainder of their lives to prevent relapse of disease.

capsule

A capsule is a polysaccharide coat that covers some organisms such as *C. neoformans*. Capsules help resist ingestion by white blood cells.

Cross reference

Methods for processing CSF samples are covered in Chapter 8.

Cross reference

Further details on *Cryptococcus* are included in Chapter 8.

Key Point

Cryptococcal meningitis is a frequent complication of AIDS. When meningitis-like symptoms occur in an AIDS patient, the laboratory must be alert for cryptococcal infections.

14.6.3 *Aspergillus* infections

Aspergillus fumigatus and some other species of *Aspergillus*, such as *A. terreus*, *A. flavus*, and *A. niger*, can cause a wide range of infections in man, ranging from mild allergic disease to life-threatening, invasive illness. Next is a list of the common conditions associated with *Aspergillus* spp. Aspergillosis is the term given to an infection caused by an *Aspergillus* spp.

1. Allergic bronchopulmonary aspergillosis (ABPA). This is primarily an allergic reaction to *Aspergillus* antigens. It follows *Aspergillus* colonization of damaged lung tissue although there is no tissue invasion. The main symptoms are wheezing, chest pain, fever, and coughing up brown mucus plugs. It typically occurs in immunocompetent people, but some previous lung damage, for example through cystic fibrosis, heavy smoking, or emphysema, predisposes to this condition.

2. Non-invasive aspergillosis or aspergilloma. This is caused by growth of aspergilli in pre-formed lung cavities, usually secondary to tuberculosis. An aspergilloma may persist for many years without symptoms. The usual symptoms when they occur are a cough with blood-stained sputum.

3. Acute invasive aspergillosis. This is the most serious infection and carries a high mortality rate despite antifungal therapy. The main site of infection is the lung, and it is caused by inhalation of spores from the air. It is a disease of immunosuppressed patients, particularly those who are neutropenic (reduced number of white blood cells). It is most common in leukaemic patients, bone marrow transplant patients, and patients on immunosuppressive or cytotoxic therapy. Symptoms include fever, cough, haemoptysis and pleuritic chest pain and are often non-specific. Lack of response to antibacterial antibiotics often raises suspicion of a fungal infection.

Figure 14.10 is a photomicrograph of a section of a lung infected with *A. fumigatus*. Using a silver stain aspergilli appear black and are easily distinguished against the pink tissue background. A colony of *A. fumigatus* is seen spreading through tissue as the hyphae grow. The spreading nature of the hyphae is responsible for the organism invading adjacent tissue.

In patients who are severely immunosuppressed, the organism may disseminate from the lung to other body sites, including the brain, kidney and bones. Cerebral aspergillosis carries a very high mortality rate. Occasionally, infection will start at a different body site. The nasal sinuses are a common source of infection, again due to inhalation of spores. Infections have frequently been associated with building work in hospitals as this produces dust and disturbs soil, producing large numbers of airborne spores. Other primary sites of infection include the skin; such infections are most commonly seen in patients with severe burns or severe trauma.

For detailed information concerning *Aspergillus* infections (clinical aspects, diagnosis and treatment) the *Aspergillus* website has a wealth of information (www.aspergillus.org.uk).

FIGURE 14.10

Photomicrograph of lung infected with *Aspergillus fumigatus*. The hyphae (stained black) can be seen spreading throughout the tissue.

Source: Thanks to P. Warn for providing the sample.

Key Point

Aspergilloma and ABPA occur in patients who are immunocompetent, disease is localized and there is no invasion of tissue by *Aspergillus*. Invasive aspergillosis typically occurs in patients with compromised immune systems and there is invasion of tissue and dissemination of infection around the body.

Key Point

Aspergillus spp. can cause three main conditions in man: aspergilloma, allergic bronchopulmonary aspergillosis, and finally invasive aspergillosis, which carries a high mortality rate even with treatment.

14.6.4 Diagnosis of ABPA and aspergilloma

In cases of allergic pulmonary aspergillosis and aspergilloma, diagnosis is based mainly on clinical findings such as symptoms, underlying disease, and chest X-rays. The laboratory can play an important role as isolation of *Aspergillus* from sputum can help confirm the diagnosis. Sputum samples may be sent to the laboratory and these should be cultured on standard bacterial media for respiratory bacteriological analysis (including TB if haemoptysis is present) as well as on Sabouraud's agar and incubated for up to 7 days. *Aspergillus* spp. grow as white fluffy colonies 1–2 mm in diameter after 24 h. As the culture is incubated further, colonies grow to 5–10 mm in diameter and change colour as the culture starts to sporulate. *A. fumigatus* typically produces dark green colonies after 2–4 days' incubation; other species of aspergilli may produce colonies of different colours. Figure 14.11 shows the typical colonial appearance

Cross reference

Chapter 9 deals with methods of processing respiratory samples.

(a)   (b)

(c)   (d)

FIGURE 14.11

Appearance of four main species of *Aspergillus* after 3–4 days' growth on Sabouraud's agar; the differences in coloration of the different species are clear. (a) *Aspergillus fumigatus*,
(b) *Aspergillus niger*,
(c) *Aspergillus flavus*,
(d) *Aspergillus terreus*.

of the main *Aspergillus* spp. growing on Sabouraud's agar for 3–4 days. Note the different coloration of the colonies which help in the differentiation of species. The coloration is due to different pigments in the spores or conidia. Some other non-*Aspergillus* fungi can produce colonies that look like aspergilli, and therefore caution is required in identifying a colony solely on the basis of coloration.

The quantity of growth should be recorded in a semiquantitative fashion. It should be noted that because the air contains *Aspergillus* spores, aspergilli are common laboratory contaminants and may be found in the mouth, nose, and sputum of healthy people. The isolation of very small numbers of *Aspergillus* from sputa may not be significant. If there is doubt then repeat samples should be cultured. In the case of aspergilloma sputum samples may yield *Aspergillus* in only 50% of cases.

Blood samples may also be taken to detect antibodies to *Aspergillus* and to measure levels of IgE antibodies. These tests are usually carried out by immunology or mycology reference laboratories.

Treatment for aspergilloma is in most cases conservative – attempts to remove the aspergilloma are dangerous. The main form of treatment of allergic pulmonary aspergillosis is the administration of steroids to suppress the immune response. However, in some instances this can result in invasive aspergillosis. The use of antifungal therapy to reduce the fungal load is being explored and itraconazole has shown promising results.

CLINICAL CORRELATION

Antibodies to *Aspergillus*

High levels of IgE antibodies are indicative of an allergic response. In cases of allergic pulmonary aspergillosis serum contains high levels of total IgE antibodies and high levels of both IgG and IgE to *Aspergillus* antigens. In cases of aspergilloma antibodies to *Aspergillus* are primarily of the IgG class. In cases of invasive aspergillosis because of the poor immune status of the patient the antibody response is very poor.

Key Point

Isolation of *Aspergillus* spp. from a sputum sample is not conclusive evidence of an *Aspergillus* infection. Because *Aspergillus* spores occur in the atmosphere, *Aspergillus* may occur as a contaminant in sputum cultures.

14.6.5 Diagnosis of invasive aspergillosis

Invasive aspergillosis carries a high mortality rate despite treatment with antifungal drugs and numerous studies have shown that the outcome of treatment is influenced by how quickly therapy is administered. Early intervention with antifungal drugs can increase survival rates whereas delayed treatment results in poorer survival rates. Therefore early diagnosis of infection is essential. Clinical diagnosis can be difficult as symptoms are non-specific and may mimic other conditions, including bacterial infections. The main symptoms include fever, cough and pleuritic chest pain. Suspicion of a possible *Aspergillus* infection is raised in patients who are immunosuppressed and where symptoms are not resolved by antibacterial antibiotics.

Chest X-rays and CT scans may be helpful in identifying lung lesions. In high-risk patient groups, such as bone marrow transplant recipients, testing of blood samples by **galactomannan** assay several times each week can help identify potentially infected patients early, allowing further diagnostic procedures to be instituted (galactomannan tests are described later in this section).

Although sputum samples may be produced by patients with invasive aspergillosis, such samples do not always yield *Aspergillus*. Bronchoalveolar lavages and lung biopsies are used to obtain samples deep in the lung and may provide better yields of organisms.

Laboratory diagnosis involves microscopy and culture of samples. BAL samples should be concentrated by centrifugation and examined by microscopy with Gram staining and using KOH preparations similar to dermatophyte microscopy. The presence of branched hyphae in a sample from a patient with supporting clinical symptoms is considered significant. Sputum samples should also be examined microscopically and tissue samples should be sent to a histology laboratory for appropriate processing and staining with special stains such as PAS or methanamine silver to stain fungal structures.

Cross reference
See Bancroft D, Gamble M. *Theory and Practice of Histological Techniques*, listed in the References section, for details of stains suitable for diagnosing fungal infections.

Cultures should also be set up on Sabouraud's agar; colonial appearances are described previously. The identity of any *Aspergillus* isolate should be determined as this can help in selection of appropriate therapy, for example *A. terreus* and *A. flavus* are commonly resistant to **amphotericin B**. Other samples (e.g. skin, pus, or tissue from other sites) should be cultured on standard bacteriological media and Sabouraud's agar and microscopy attempted to identify fungal hyphae in the sample (see relevant earlier sections for how to process the samples).

There is currently a lot of interest in the use of galactomannan and β-glucan detection kits. Galactomannan and β-glucan are fungal cell wall components released into the blood or tissue during fungal growth. Both tests are available as ELISA tests with colorimetric endpoints which measure the levels of the particular component. These can be used as specific diagnostic tests on blood or BAL samples from patients suspected of invasive aspergillosis. Galactomannan and β-glucan have also found utility in monitoring at-risk patients, as they can give a very early indication of infection, often before symptoms develop.

Key Point

Fungal cell walls are composed of an array of carbohydrate polymers such as galactomannan, β-glucan and chitin. These are released from the cell as the fungus grows and galactomannan and β-glucan have found utility in diagnosing fungal disease. The presence of these substances in body fluids is often indicative of a systemic fungal infection.

14.6.6 Treatment of invasive aspergillosis

Early recognition of infection and early treatment are key to successful therapy of invasive aspergillosis (IA). Because safer, less-toxic drugs are available treatment may be instituted before there is a definite diagnosis – this is known as empiric therapy. At the present time voriconazole is the drug of choice for IA, although alternatives such as amphotericin B and the echinocandins are available in cases of voriconazole toxicity, intolerance or treatment failure. There is growing interest in the use of combination therapies involving two or more drugs.

In some units at-risk patients may be given prophylactic antibiotics to prevent infections developing. However, fungal infections do occur in such patients and are more difficult to treat as prophylactic antibiotics may compromise the results of galactomannan and β-glucan tests and therapy of breakthrough infections often requires the use of a different class of drug in case resistance has developed to the prophylactic agent.

Although resistance to antifungal drugs is rare, resistance can develop during therapy, and certain species such as *A. terreus* and *A. flavus* are intrinsically resistant to amphotericin B. Any *Aspergillus* isolate from a case of IA should have a susceptibility test carried out to confirm susceptibility to the drug used initially and to identify alternatives in case a change of therapy is required.

SELF-CHECK 14.7

What are the most common clinical conditions associated with *Aspergillus*?

14.6.7 Other filamentous fungi as a cause of invasive disease

Although the majority of invasive fungal infections are caused by *Candida* spp. and *Aspergillus* spp., a small number of infections are caused by other filamentous fungi. The most common non-*Aspergillus* fungi encountered are listed below. These organisms have low virulence in humans and infections typically occur in severely ill, highly immunocompromised patients. The respiratory tract is the most common site of infection as infection is usually acquired through inhalation of spores, but the organisms can disseminate and infect any body organ. Diagnosis of these infections is based on clinical signs and demonstration of fungi in relevant samples by microscopy and culture. Any fungus isolated from a BAL sample or a tissue sample must be considered potentially significant and should be fully identified and a susceptibility test carried out as many non-*Aspergillus* organisms that are resistant to many of the antifungal agents used.

Organisms that are associated with invasive fungal infections include:

- *Fusarium oxysporum*.
- *Fusarium solani*.
- *Scedosporium prolificans* and *Scedosporium apiospermum*.
- *Absidia corymbifera*.
- *Rhizopus* spp.
- *Mucor* spp.

For details of these organisms you should refer to specialized books or websites such as www.doctorfungus.org.

14.6.8 Fungal infections of the eye

Fungi can cause infections of the eye – fungal **keratitis**. The cornea is the site of infection and typically filamentous fungi such as *Fusarium* spp. are involved. Infection usually follows some trauma to the cornea, although in recent years infections have been seen in contact lens wearers.

Scrapings from the cornea are required to culture the causative organism. Cultures for bacteria and fungi should be set up together and virology may be considered.

Treatment is usually with antibiotic eye drops although in severe cases of infection involving other parts of the eye intravenous antibiotics may also be given.

14.7 Antifungal susceptibility testing

Unlike susceptibility testing of bacteria, susceptibility testing of fungi is a relatively new phenomenon. This is partly due to the small number of available antifungal agents, the complexity of developing a standardized method, and the small numbers of tests required. In this section we will look at the common antifungal agents available, methods of susceptibility testing, and reasons for susceptibility testing.

14.7.1 Antifungal agents

There are many antibacterial antibiotics available but only about 10 clinically useful antifungal drugs, and even less when considering drugs for systemic use for serious infections. The drugs fall into five main classes. The main points on each drug are given in Table 14.2. For more information on antifungal drugs, have a look at the Further reading resources at the end of this chapter.

14.7.2 Methods of susceptibility testing

Susceptibility testing of fungi is more difficult than susceptibility testing of bacteria. It is only in the last 10 years that standardized methods for susceptibility testing have existed. Methods in use include MIC tests, usually in microtitre plates, disc tests, E-tests, and various commercially available kits, some of which are automated. At the present time there are few data to correlate fungal MICs with clinical outcome for certain drugs and breakpoint are only established for several of the azole drugs. However, efforts to develop better susceptibility testing methods and accurate breakpoints are on-going.

The most important question we are faced with in the laboratory is, 'When should susceptibility testing be carried out on fungi?'.

Because of the complex nature and difficulty in carrying out susceptibility tests on fungi, testing is carried out only in limited cases. For dermatophytes and *Candida* spp. isolated from localized infections, susceptibility testing is rarely carried out except in cases of treatment failure. For isolates of fungi from cases of invasive infection or where there is a strong suspicion of invasive infection susceptibility tests should be carried out. In most circumstances clinicians will start therapy before waiting for the susceptibility test result. The test results when available will confirm the correct choice of drug or will on occasion result in a change of antifungal agent.

Because of their specialized nature and the relatively low numbers of fungal susceptibility tests required, it is common practice to refer isolates to specialized centres for testing. This adds extra delays before results are available. In-house testing will give earlier results but if laboratories choose to carry out their own testing, then the methodology chosen must be rigorously tested and controlled. The methods chosen will reflect the number of tests carried out per annum and budgetary considerations. Tests can be time consuming and expensive.

Cross reference

E-tests are discussed in Chapter 4 covering antibiotic susceptibility testing.

Key Point

Fungal susceptibility tests are complex and difficult to perform and are carried out mainly on isolates from invasive infection or in cases of recurrent infection or where there is the possibility of the development of resistance.

TABLE 14.2 Antifungals and clinical uses.

Class	Drugs	Route of administration	Spectrum of activity	Indications	Adverse effects/problems
Polyenes	Nystatin	Oral and topical	Broad-spectrum yeast and moulds	Oral infections and superficial infections	Too toxic for systemic use
	Amphotericin B	IV	Broad-spectrum yeast and moulds	Invasive yeast and mould infections	Nephrotoxic, causes reactions on IV injection
	Lipid formulations of amphotericin B	IV	Broad-spectrum yeast and moulds	Invasive yeast and mould infections	Less toxic than conventional amphotericin B Better tolerated, but expensive
Nucleotide analogues	Flucytosine	Oral and IV	Yeasts only	In combination with other drugs for treatment of cryptococcal meningitis or candidiasis	Toxic at high doses Levels must be monitored regularly
Allylamines	Terbinafine	Oral and topical	Dermatophytes	Treatment of dermatophyte infections Topical treatment for simple local skin infections. Oral therapy for nail and widespread skin/hair infections	Long-term treatment required especially for nail infections (6–12 weeks)
Azoles	Fluconazole	Oral and IV	Yeasts	Treatment of vaginal candidiasis Treatment of systemic candidiasis	Well tolerated. *C. krusei* and *C. glabrata* may be resistant.
	Itraconazole	Oral and IV	Yeast and moulds	Treatment for dermatophyte infections Treatment for invasive yeast and mould infections	Has some effects on liver, interacts with many drugs, oral absorption may be variable. Requirement to measure levels on oral therapy
	Voriconazole	Oral and IV	Yeast and moulds, wider spectrum than itraconazole	Treatment for invasive yeast and moulds	Has side effects, interacts with many drugs. Oral absorption variable Requirement to measure levels.
	Posaconazole	Oral only	Yeast and moulds, wider spectrum than voriconazole	Prophylaxis in high-risk patients Treatment of invasive yeast and mould infections	Can only be given orally, some side effects
Echinocandins	Caspofungin Micafungin Anidulafungin	IV only	Yeast and moulds	Treatment of systemic candidiasis (most species/strains susceptible) Treatment of invasive mould infections	Can only be given by IV route Generally well tolerated, few interactions with other drugs

SELF-CHECK 14.8

Why are antifungal susceptibility tests carried out less frequently than susceptibility tests on bacteria?

14.8 The role of the reference laboratory

Mycology reference laboratories have an important role in mycology, providing a range of useful services. These include:

- Identification of fungi.
- Susceptibility testing of fungi.
- Measurement of antifungal drug levels in blood.
- Other specialized tests such as serological investigations.
- A source of advice for mycological queries, such as significance of isolates, interpretation of test results, and advice on therapy.

The extent to which a laboratory uses a reference laboratory is dependent on the amount of mycology work carried out in the laboratory and the expertise available.

Most laboratories should be able to isolate and identify *Candida* spp. using commercially available kits or chromogenic agars. Whether susceptibility tests should be carried out in house is dependent on the number of strains requiring such tests; where there are sufficient numbers a case could be made for investing and training in some form of testing method such as a commercialized system or E-test. Where only small numbers of isolates are seen it is probably better to refer these to a reference laboratory.

Filamentous fungi isolated from patients with suspected or proven invasive fungal infection should be fully identified and have a susceptibility test performed. As the number of these encountered in a routine laboratory is small and the tests are both complex and time consuming they should be referred to a reference laboratory for testing. Tests for *Aspergillus* antibodies which are useful in the diagnosis of ABPA and aspergilloma are best carried out in a reference laboratory.

For dermatophytes most laboratories should be capable of identifying to genus level the common dermatophytes. Further identification is usually unnecessary; susceptibility testing is not routinely performed on dermatophytes except in cases of treatment failure or development of resistance during therapy.

One important function of the reference laboratory is in the measurement of antifungal drug levels in blood. Unlike antibacterial antibiotics, commercially available automated methods are not available for antifungal drugs. Measurements are carried out using bioassays or HPLC methods; both methods are complex and time consuming, and are probably beyond the capabilities of the average microbiology laboratory. It is therefore common practice to refer antifungal drug level samples to a reference laboratory.

There are several reasons to measure the levels of antifungal drugs:

- To ensure that adequate levels of drugs are achieved; this is particularly important with drugs given orally as absorption may be poor and other medications can both increase and decrease the levels of antifungal drugs.

- In patients receiving long-term therapy measurement ensures that patients are taking the drug and that levels are maintained in the therapeutic range.

- Certain drugs such as flucytosine can be toxic if recommended levels are exceeded; measurement of levels allows alteration of dose to ensure toxic levels are not achieved.

Reference laboratories serve a further function in that they can provide advice across a range of mycological areas and assist both laboratory staff and clinicians in the interpretation of both culture results and test results, and they can suggest alterations in therapy based on both susceptibility test results and drug levels.

Key Point

Reference laboratories serve an important function in identifying and testing unusual fungi, carrying out susceptibility tests on fungi, and acting as a source of advice on fungi, fungal diseases, and therapy.

Chapter summary

After reading this chapter you should know and understand:

- Numerous fungi exist in nature but only a very limited number cause human infections.

- Fungal infections are increasing mainly due to more patients who are immunocompromised.

- Infections of the skin, hair, and nails are caused by dermatophyte fungi and are of low severity.

- The main site of invasive fungal infection in the body is the lung.

- Invasive fungal infections are very serious and are associated with high mortality rates.

- Antifungal susceptibility testing is increasing as better and more standardized methods are used.

- The role of the reference laboratory is very important and is used for expert advice and for a wide range of specialized services such as antifungal drug monitoring.

Further reading

The following websites carry much useful information on antifungal drugs, microscopic and macroscopic appearance of fungi, protocols for identification, and differentiation of fungi.

- **Aspergillus website. www.aspergillus.org.uk (accessed 14 August, 2013).**

  Excellent resource for material regarding all aspect of *Aspergillus* diagnosis, therapy, and laboratory investigations.

- **University of Adelaide Mycology Department. www.mycology.adelaide.edu.au** (accessed 14 August, 2013).

  All round resource for information and photographs related to clinical mycology.

- **Centers for Disease Control, USA. http://phil.cdc.gov/phil/home.asp** (accessed 14 August, 2013).

  Many images of fungi and fungal infections.

- **Kuper KM, Coyle EA, Wanger A. Antifungal susceptibility testing: a primer for clinicians.** *Pharmacotherapy* 2012; **32**(12): 1112–1122.

  Useful text which provides further information on all aspects of antifungal susceptibility testing.

 ## Discussion questions

14.1 Why do you think that most laboratories don't provide a full range of fungal testing services?

14.2 Why do you think it is critical for the laboratory to be as free as possible from *Aspergillus* spores?

14.3 Why do you think fungal infections are on the increase? Is there anything we can do to reverse this trend?

15

Bacterial pathogenesis

Lynn G. Dover

We exist in a microbe-dominated biosphere. In order to do so, our surfaces have evolved to exclude microorganisms from the tissues that lie beneath. Nevertheless millions of us succumb to infections every year, for a whole variety of complex reasons. This chapter aims to illustrate how pathogenic bacteria overcome host barriers and enter their host to cause disease. Key features include the adhesion of the bacteria to epithelial surfaces to secure a foothold from which colonization can be based. Often tissue penetration is a feature of pathogenesis and the protection offered up by the immune system must always be evaded. The ways in which pathogenic bacteria address these challenges will be explored systematically. In this chapter you will see how bacterial products interact with the molecules that direct our own cellular physiology, subverting cellular processes to their own advantage and causing disease as they do so.

Learning objectives

After studying this chapter you should be able to describe characteristics of pathogenic bacteria that allow them to:

- Adhere to epithelial surfaces (adhesins).
- Evade the immune system (evasins and impedins).
- Invade tissues (invasins).
- Damage underlying tissues (toxins).

15.1 **Fundamental themes**

Cross reference

See Chapter 7.

Most of the bacteria that colonize our bodies do so without causing us any harm. The numerous members of our **normal microbial flora** can be described as being in a **mutualistic** relationship with their host, both parties gain some benefit from their interaction. Very few microorganisms are **parasitic** and cause disease; those that do are often described as **pathogens**. The nature of the disease caused is governed by the properties of the microorganism involved and is described as its **pathogenicity**. Various bacteria are pathogenic but the

FIGURE 15.1

Pathogenic organisms vary in virulence. Virulent organisms need only a low lethal dose (LD_{50}) and kill quickly (LT_{50}). Organisms can lose virulence through mutagenesis as exemplified by the production of the BCG vaccine from virulent *Mycobacterium bovis*. They can also gain virulence by mutation and through acquisition of new genes.

severity of their impact upon individual hosts differs, with factors from both sides of the relationship playing a role.

Some bacteria are inherently more damaging than others. Their degree of pathogenicity is described in the term **virulence**. Virulence can be quantified by establishing experimental metrics such as **median lethal dose (LD_{50}**, the number of bacteria that needs to be administered to kill 50% of a subject population) and median to time to death (LT_{50}, the time taken to kill 50% of an infected population). Low scores in these measures indicate a **virulent** bacterium, these would include *Bacillus anthracis* and *Yersinia pestis* for example.

Virulence and pathogenicity are dependent upon the composition of the bacterial genome. Pathogen genomes encode many virulence factors which operate in a concerted fashion to express pathogenicity. These are often secreted (e.g. toxins) or surface-located molecules that influence the outcome of host-pathogen interactions in a variety of ways (e.g. capsule formation). These features will occupy much of this chapter's focus. Sometimes errors of genome replication lead to mutations in these key genes, resulting in a measurable decrease in bacterial virulence. This phenomenon is described as **attenuation** (Figure 15.1).

Key Point: Attenuation of Mycobacterium bovis

A particularly well-known example of attenuation arose from the work of Albert Calmette and Camille Guérin at the Institute Pasteur de Lille. They serially sub-cultured virulent *Mycobacterium bovis* 230 times resulting in an **avirulent** strain, later named Bacille Calmette–Guérin or *M. bovis* BCG. This bacterium had lost its ability to cause tuberculosis in humans. Since 1921, this attenuated organism has been administered as a live vaccine in billions of doses with no reversions to virulence recorded.

The outcome of an infection is clearly also influenced by many host factors. Each infected host sits on a spectrum of susceptibility to that pathogen; some individuals are more resistant to the pathogen than others. The degree of resistance exhibited by an individual relates to the effectiveness of their **innate immunity** and is often heavily influenced by prior experience of that pathogen, either in previous infection or vaccination i.e. their **adaptive immunity**. Some pathogens are described as **opportunists**, only causing disease when these normal host resistance determinants are somehow compromised.

SELF-CHECK 15.1

In relation to the bacterial cell, where do virulence factors carry out their functions?

15.1.1 Important sites of bacterial infection

Bacteria are adept at colonizing surfaces and especially those of animal bodies. Although the human body harbours enormous numbers of microorganisms, infection remains a relatively rare event. Bacteria can infect any tissue if they can gain access to it. Our skin offers an effective barrier to bacteria and infections often arise from breaks in its integrity due to cuts, abrasions, surgical trauma, or insertion of IV catheter lines. Three other bodily sites predominate as sites of infection: the respiratory tract, the gastrointestinal (GI) tract, and the genitourinary (GU) tract. In many respects, these should be considered as external surfaces. This concept might appear more straightforward if we consider that the basic functions of gaseous exchange and digestion/absorption are both carried out by simple fungi at their mycelial surface.

During our evolution our GI tract and lungs have developed as modified surfaces optimized for these specialized individual functions. Their internal location affords these delicate organs physical protection and promotes their efficiency by raising their operating temperature while avoiding their desiccation. However, both of these systems frequently sample our bacterium-rich environment to support our existence. The intestines are adapted to maintain a heavy and diverse bacterial flora that support effective digestion of foodstuffs. In the lung, however, the opposite is true, gaseous exchange across the alveoli would be far less effective if their surfaces were teeming with microbes. Like the gut, the GU tract offers excellent culture environments, the ureter and bladder transporting a nutrient-rich fluid (from the perspective of many nutritionally versatile bacteria); the vagina offers more stable colonization opportunities with its less frequent throughput of materials. At these key surfaces, the contributions of gross anatomy and the innate and adaptive arms of the immune system combine to limit the harmful potential of our metabolically powerful fellow travellers from accessing deeper tissue. As we progress, we will see the various ways pathogenic bacteria use to overcome these.

Elsewhere in this book the local anatomical and histological features that combine to limit the progress of infecting microbes at various body sites is summarized. Elsewhere in the series, the innate and adaptive arms of the immune system that supplement these physical barrier functions are described in greater detail than can be accomplished here.

Cross reference

See Chapter 5.

Only a few bacteria express their pathogenicity from an external location. Enterotoxigenic *E. coli*, *Vibrio cholerae*, and *Corynebacterium diphtheriae* are good examples of microorganisms that produce toxins at a mucosal surface that are almost entirely responsible for their pathogenesis. Most other bacteria attach specifically to a mucosal surface and either (1) multiply there, colonizing the outer surface before eventually invading deeper tissues or (2) invade the epithelium and then colonize the tissue beneath. Resulting infections can remain localized or can spread more widely. **Systemic** infections arise from the broad dissemination of the infecting bacterium via the blood or lymphatic system.

Key Point

Most bacteria invade deeper tissues, few can direct their pathogenicity from mucosal surfaces.

15.2 **Virulence factors**

As we shall see, bacteria express their pathogenicity in a plethora of ways, orchestrating cellular dysfunction in their host via a multitude of virulence factors. Many of these virulence factors are proteins that are active outside of the bacterial cytoplasm. During their export, they can be modified, to ensure they are retained at the surface of the bacterial cell, or they may promote infection independently of the bacterial cell, diffusing locally in a tissue or to distant sites being disseminated broadly via blood or lymph. These virulence factors are the tools through which a bacterium may overcome the challenges our bodies present in establishing an infection. They can be considered in four main classes; **adhesins** that support attachment of bacteria to surfaces to avoid mechanical removal, **invasins** that promote the access of bacteria to sub-mucosal sites, **evasins** that shield the bacterium from immune recognition or damage, **impedins** that interfere with immune processes, and **toxins** that disrupt cellular physiology. These shall be considered in these classes in the coming sections.

One of the most awe-inspiring features of life is its great efficiency. Natural selection demands it! Bacteria are amazing models for ecological study. Pathogens are muscling in on a superb living space (ecological niche) that is highly sought after, teaming with competitors (normal flora) and predators (phagocytes and molecular aspects of immunity such as complement and immunoglobulins). Pathogens need to adapt and multiply quickly in challenging environments. An efficient genome is crucial; every gene counts! It takes time and nutritional resources to reproduce a genome. Imperfections in genome replication can lead to loss-of-function mutations and gene deletions. Genes that do not provide a significant advantage in challenging conditions are eventually lost from a population as individual bacteria that have lost them are not disadvantaged and now require less 'effort' to replicate. As we progress what should become clear is that the genetics of pathogenicity and virulence have been shaped by these selective pressures. Many of the structures or molecules we will meet are multifunctional, epitomize efficiency, and might span two of these classes.

Key Point

Pathogenicity and virulence are usually multifactorial; the coordinated synthesis of many virulence factors is often required.

SELF-CHECK 15.2

Can you identify and briefly define the properties of the main classes of virulence factor?

15.3 Gaining a foothold – early events in infection

15.3.1 Bacterial adhesins

Whether they take a **commensal** or pathogenic approach, bacteria that colonize animals must resist clearance from their bodies by a variety of mechanical processes. For instance, the respiratory tract is equipped with a mucociliary escalator to remove small-inhaled particles; these include any colonizing bacteria. Bacteria can be trapped in the mucus that coats the respiratory tract, which is constantly being moved upwards and away from the sites of gaseous exchange through the beating action of the cilia lining its epithelia. Likewise, the movement of the food bolus and urine through the gastrointestinal and urinary tracts respectively, promotes the physical clearance of bacteria. Pathogens need to get a grip in order to multiply in these

Cross reference

See Chapter 6.

host range

The host range defines the various species in which the pathogen is clinically relevant.

tissue tropism

A tissue tropism relates to a tissue specificity or preference. Both can be defined by adhesin properties.

areas. Once they have adhered to an epithelial surface the interaction is strong, in fact virtually irreversible. It needs to be remembered that a variety of factors can make it easier for potential pathogens to adhere and colonize these surfaces. These include smoking, which has a devastating action on host cilia thus allowing bacteria to multiply without any chance of being cleared. In the urinary tract, the insertion of urinary catheters allows bacteria to evade the natural defences and promote colonization through biofilm production. Patients with long-term indwelling catheters are at a high risk of UTI.

It is now well-established that most bacteria that colonize eukaryotes interact with their cells using a variety of surface-located adhesins. These bind to host macromolecules to secure their foothold. Some bacteria have well-recognized restrictions in their **host range** while others have pronounced **tissue tropisms**. It has been suggested that specific pairings of bacterial adhesins and host receptors might partly explain these phenomena.

Key Point: Tissue-specific adherence

Neisseria gonorrhoeae, which causes the sexually transmitted disease gonorrhoea, colonizes only humans. These bacteria have been shown to preferentially bind to human epithelial cells of the urogenital tract. Key *N. gonorrhoeae* adhesins are the Opacity (Opa) proteins which promote binding to human epithelia. OpaA binds cell surface proteoglycans and promotes bacterial adhesion and entry into epithelial cells. Other Opa proteins promote interactions with neutrophils, suggesting that Opa protein variation might account for tissue tropism displayed by gonococci. Consistent with this idea is the discovery that the various Opa protein variants prefer different members of carcinoembryonic antigen receptors. This family of glycoproteins are differentially expressed in tissues.

In engaging human cells at such close quarters, bacteria risk recognition and triggering a host immune response. Therefore, it is necessary that the bacterial surface possesses an outer layer that both hides and protects the organism from the immune system. This is usually an extensive polysaccharide layer that consists of a secreted capsule and/or the carbohydrate polymers of lipopolysaccharide in Gram-negative bacteria. By definition, adhesins need to protrude beyond this capsule. In doing so, they present themselves as potential targets for the adaptive immune system and many are under consideration as vaccine candidates.

Key Point

The surface presentation of any molecule can lead to immune recognition. In order to promote their colonization of a host, bacteria project specific adhesions beyond their protective layers.

15.3.2 MSCRAMMs

Animal cells are surrounded by an extracellular matrix (ECM). These proteins appear to be preferred targets for bacterial adhesion. The adhesins that bind them are known as MSCRAMMs (microbial surface components recognizing adhesive matrix molecules). Multiple MSCRAMMs are found in many organisms.

These surface components have a complex composition of fibrous proteins and **proteogly-cans** and they function to support and bind together cells and tissues. This function is paramount at mucosal membranes, our interfaces with the microbial world. Here the ECM forms the basement membrane that lies beneath epithelial cells and promotes epithelial integrity. The ECM is composed of four major glycosylated protein classes that are all fibrous in nature: these are collagens, fibronectins, laminins, and elastins. They are woven together via specific interactions to form a complex and ordered matrix. The gaps between them are filled with proteoglycans; these highly glycosylated proteins form a strong hydrated gel that is well suited to supporting tissues.

proteoglycans

Proteoglycans are heavily glycosylated proteins found in ECM. They consist of a protein core decorated with a polymer formed from a repeating disaccharide unit that produces a sugar sequence of an amino sugar followed by a uronic (acidic) sugar.

SELF-CHECK 15.3

Why are ECM proteins useful **ligands** for adhesins?

---

ligand

A ligand is a specific binding partner.

15.3.3 Adhesin structural biology

Bacterial adhesins were first recognized over 100 years ago when it was reported that *E. coli* could aggregate animal cells via appendages protruding from their surface. These appendages were eventually characterized as pili or fimbriae. These names are essentially interchangeable. Both are filamentous multimeric protein structures anchored in the bacterial cell wall that project to the exterior. Over recent years, other classes of adhesins have been described. These include other polymeric surface features like components of Type 3 secretion systems and flagella that contribute to adhesion despite their primary function being related to other aspects of virulence. Other dedicated adhesins are not polymeric like fimbriae but are monomeric or oligomeric in their construction, but these can also feature extended structures that might protrude from the capsular layer.

15.3.4 Fimbrial adhesins of Gram-negative bacteria

Early studies of *E. coli* adhesion revealed that two adhesive properties were exhibited by uropathogenic *E. coli* (UPEC); both were associated with pili of the Chaperone–Usher type. This class of pilus is widely distributed in the Enterobacteriaceae. Figure 15.2 describes their structure; they consist of a very stable rod-shaped structure of about 7 nm in diameter that protrudes from the bacterial surface by 1–2 µm. The rod is composed of non-covalently associated monomers of the protein, pilin. After secretion through the plasma membrane, pilin monomers bind to a chaperone protein in the periplasm that assists their folding and then passes them to an Usher protein in the outer membrane that participates in pilus assembly. The shaft extends by incorporation of new pilin monomers from the base, through a pore in the Usher protein. The distal end of the shaft forms a thinner fibrillum tip that consists of the specific adhesin and a number of accessory proteins. This adhesin protein has two domains; a pilin binding domain attaches it to the protein filament of the pilus shaft, and a **lectin** (carbohydrate-binding) domain that is responsible for the adhesin activity.

SELF-CHECK 15.4

Why are lectins suitable adhesins?

The FimH pilus is present in many *E. coli* strains and mediates interactions with receptor molecules containing mannose-based saccharides. Many are mannosylated glycoproteins

FIGURE 15.2
Chaperone–Usher pili area class of fimbriae of Gram-negative bacteria that present an adhesin at their end, i.e. the adhesion determinant is some distance away from the bacterial cell surface beyond LPS polysaccharide and capsule layers. The characteristics of the adhesin might influence host range or tissue tropism.

including the Tamm–Horsfall protein (loop of Henle) and collagens that promote adhesion to bladder and kidney epithelial cells, buccal cells, erythrocytes, mast cells, macrophages, and neutrophils. The P-pilus system is similar in its construction but is more restricted in its distribution among *E. coli* and is common in UPEC. P-pilus shafts terminate in PapG adhesins, which recognize members of the globoseries of glycosphingolipids (P-antigens) that are found in the membranes of erythrocytes and uroepithelial cell membranes. Three PapG variants exist (PapGI, -II, and –III) with different binding specificities and these appear to partly define the tissue tropism exhibited by UPEC strains. PapGI binds the Gb03 glycolipid which is found in uroepithelial cells. PapGII binds Gb04, which is more abundant in kidney cells and is associated with pyelonephritis. PapGIII binds Gb05 and is mostly associated with cystitis.

Key Point

Many biological surfaces are glycosylated. Consequently many adhesins recognize sugary structures.

Other fimbrial adhesins exist in Gram-negative bacteria but these are less well characterized, among these are the type IV pili. These differ from the Chaperone–Usher pili in being actively polymerized at the outer leaflet of the plasma membrane rather than at the outer membrane. A specific ATPase enzyme is required to power pilus growth. These pili reach and extend from the cell surface passing through an outer membrane protein, secretin. Like the other fimbrial structures, the adhesin is found at the end of the filaments.

In some species (possessing type IVa pili), another 'retraction' ATPase is associated with the structure and this acts as a depolymerase, allowing the pilus to be rapidly remodelled. The

Sortase-directed
wall deposition

Adhesin

Sortase-directed
polymerization

Sortase-bound
Pilin subunits

FIGURE 15.3
Gram-positive pili can be stabilized by covalent bonds between units formed by transpeptidase enzymes known as sortases. Pilus-specific sortases (purple) assemble pili and eventually the structure is attached to newly synthesized peptidoglycan by typical sortases (pink) to secure them in the cell wall.

ability to shorten these pili quickly allows for a type of bacterial locomotion over surfaces known as twitching motility, which has been associated with virulence. In some cases, the shortening of the pilus filaments may simply function to bring the bacterium and epithelial cells into closer contact after their initial engagement.

15.3.5 Fimbrial adhesins of Gram-positive bacteria

Gram-positive bacteria can secure proteins to their surface via a class of transpeptidase enzymes called sortases. In some cases, specialized sortases have evolved that are used to covalently link pilin subunits together to form pilus shafts. Figure 15.3 demonstrates how these filaments are polymerized and eventually secured to the peptidoglycan by a standard 'housekeeping' sortase. Ancillary proteins are included at the base of the pilus and as clusters or single molecules along the length of the pilus shaft. These ancillary proteins are not essential to grow the pilus but can be involved in adhesion. Such structures have now been recognized in several genera including pathogenic members of *Corynebacterium*, *Streptococcus*, and *Enterococcus*. Additionally, variants of Type IV pili have recently been discovered in Gram-positive pathogens including *Corynebacterium diphtheriae* and various pathogenic streptococci.

SELF-CHECK 15.5

What is the function of the sortase enzymes?

15.3.6 Non-fimbrial adhesins

Gram-positive bacteria possess a family of MSCRAMMs that are highly conserved and probably arose from a common ancestral adhesin. They share a modular design and binding domain organization. These proteins are sortase substrates and are covalently attached to peptidoglycan. The **ligand** binding activity of most of these MSCRAMMs is localized to their N-terminal domains.

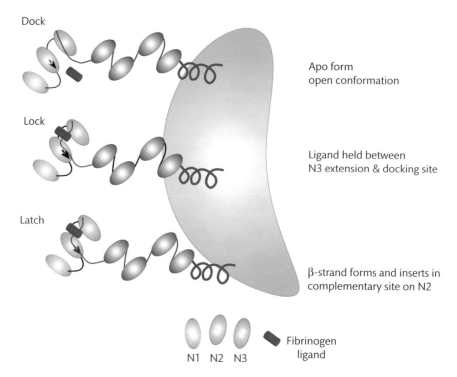

Dock

Apo form
open conformation

Lock

Ligand held between
N3 extension & docking site

Latch

β-strand forms and inserts in
complementary site on N2

N1   N2   N3

Fibrinogen
ligand

FIGURE 15.4

Adhesins often bind very avidly to their ligands or receptors. Indeed, bacterial binding to mucosal surfaces is virtually irreversible. A mechanism that illustrates the avidity of SdrG of ***Staphylococcus epidermidis*** **and fibrinogen has three phases. Firstly, a peptide (part of fibrinogen) interacts with a compatible surface between subdomains N2 and N3. An unstructured (free to move) extension of N3 covers the site to lock the peptide in place and then part of this forms a β-strand that is complementary to a gap in the N2 structure. It stably positions itself there, as if applying a latch to keep the ligand in place.**

The **avidity** (strength) of the interactions of *Staphylococcus epidermidis* SdrG fibrinogen binding protein, the best studied of this class, is explained through a three-stage binding process described as a dock, lock, and latch model that is demonstrated in Figure 15.4. In the docking phase, the adhesin has an open conformation. The initial molecular interactions with the ligand occur at an exposed surface that lies between two subdomains, N2 and N3. Early interactions with fibrinogen induce an unstructured extension of N3 to cover the bound ligand, effectively locking it in place. Then in a final latching process, a part of this N3 extension inserts itself in a pocket on the N2 subdomain and adopts a β-strand conformation that complements the surrounding N2 subdomain β-sheet structure producing a very stable MSCRAMM–ligand complex.

15.3.7 Trimeric autotransporter adhesins

Cross reference

See *Binding host complement inhibitors* in Section 15.5.3 of this chapter.

The trimeric autotransporter adhesins (TAA) form trimers at the inner leaflet of the outer membrane of some Gram-negative bacteria. These proteins have C-terminal transporter domains that combine to form a translocator pore. The N-terminal passenger domains cross the outer membrane to the outside of the cell via the pore formed by the translocator assembly. The best studied of this class are the YadA autotransporter adhesins of *Yersinia enterocolitica* and

Head
adhesin

Stalk

327Å

Anchor

FIGURE 15.5

Trimeric autotransporters offer a non-fimbrial alternative way to present an adhesin beyond the protective exterior layers of the Gram-negative cell. The adhesins traverse the outer membrane through a β-barrel pore made collectively by the autotransporter domains of three monomers. They cover the distance to the outer margins of the cell by the incorporation of a long stalk between the membrane anchor (autotransporter domains) and the adhesin (head).

Source: Image constructed using model coordinates generated by Koretke *et al.* (2008).

Yersinia pseudotuberculosis. Figure 15.5 shows the final head-stalk-anchor architecture that they adopt. The 'head' domains are the adhesins. The stalk not only allows the head to reach over 300 Å from the outer membrane lipid bilayer and interacts with a range of ECM protein ligands including collagen, laminin, and fibronectin. Alongside the extension function of the YadA stalk, it also binds complement factor H which protects the bacterium from this important innate immune system.

15.4 Invasion by bacteria

Very few bacteria direct their pathogenicity from epithelial surfaces. From a bacterial perspective, some form of internal penetration is desirable in order to avoid mechanical clearance and to establish a secure niche for colonization. Figure 15.6 demonstrates the two main ways that bacteria achieve this. Several pathogens of the GI tract, such as *Salmonella*, *Shigella*, and *Yersinia* are adept at invading eukaryotic cells, or to be exact, at inducing their own phagocytosis. These can then cross the epithelium via a paracellular route, i.e. through its cells. Others like *Porphyromonas gingivalis* and *Bacteroides fragilis* take an intercellular or pericellular route. They produce proteolytic toxins that can hydrolyse the proteins that maintain the tight junctions (Occludin), adherens junctions (E-cadherin) between epithelial cells and the cell-extracellular matrix junction (β1-integrin) allowing the bacteria to gain access to the basal lamina and interstitial space that lie beneath. Some, like *P. gingivalis* might then invade cells via their lateral boundaries.

Some pathogens like *S. pneumoniae*, recruit host proteases, rather than their own toxins, to cleave cell junction proteins to promote penetration of epithelial or endothelial barriers. *S. pneumoniae* can be coated with human plasmin, a broad-specificity serine protease and plasminogen its precursor via its MSCRAMMs. Plasminogen enhances adherence to such barriers while the active protease plasmin aids their penetration. E-cadherin, which maintains adherens junctions can be cleaved by active plasmin bound to *S. pneumoniae*. However, as Figure 15.6 shows, adherens junctions lie beneath tight junctions, so you would expect them to be protected from such proteolysis. However, another challenge to mucosal integrity arises when respiratory epithelial cells encounter *S. pneumoniae*. The exposure to the bacteria initiates intracellular signalling cascades that result in the downregulation of the claudin protein components of tight junctions. This weakening of the tight junctions could allow the plasmin-coated bacteria to access the E-cadherin and set about degrading it.

FIGURE 15.6

After colonizing mucosal surfaces, most pathogenic bacteria establish infections by invading deeper structures. They either penetrate the epithelium by a pericellular route (purple bacteria), disrupting cellular junctions (via proteolysis or by interfering with their regulation) or by a paracellular route (blue bacteria), directing their uptake by cells and traversing the epithelium through cells. Some might invade via a non-apical surface after disrupting cellular junctions to gain access to these.

Several bacteria promote their uptake by epithelial cells. Once inside they can avoid the threats posed by binding immune factors such as complement and antibodies and the consequences of their subsequent recognition by macrophage, neutrophils, and cytotoxic T cells. Such paracellular invasion is achieved via one of two ways. Firstly, bacteria can engage their eukaryotic targets by binding of surface receptors. The binding is 'sensed' by the receptor and initiates signalling cascades that promote the internalization of the bacteria. Alternatively, bacteria can directly introduce effector proteins into the target cell cytoplasm via a type III secretion system (T3SS). These effector proteins interact with components of the actin cytoskeleton and its regulatory machinery to subvert their function, driving the cytoskeleton to engulf the bacteria.

Key Point: Bacteria impact mammalian cell biology in diverse ways

Before we explore these mechanisms, it is worth pointing out that regulation of mammalian cellular processes is complex, orchestrated by a bewildering array of regulatory molecules. Often these molecules are controlled by others through mechanisms such as proteolysis, reversible phosphorylation, ligand binding, and complex formation, and combinations of them. As your undergraduate career develops, a deeper understanding of these molecular processes is required; they are often the key to therapies. In the coming sections, some of the signalling pathways that regulate cytoskeletal remodelling and the initiation of the inflammatory response are related in order to understand how bacteria influence host cellular biology during infection. Later we will also see that bacterial toxins sometimes cause pathology by mimicking or interfering with the secondary messenger systems that deliver hormone or neurotransmitter signals within cells. Some molecular detail will be given for two reasons, firstly to give you some insight into the various ways that bacterial effectors interact with host systems, and secondly, to emphasize that the strategies used by bacteria to influence these aspects of mammalian cell biology are often comprehensive and integrated rather than relying on a single molecular interaction. Much more detail lies beneath these illustrations for those who would explore further.

15.4.1 Integrin-mediated invasion

Integrins are a diverse group of cell surface glycoproteins that mediate key cell-cell and cell-ECM interactions. They bind to the ECM components, fibronectin and vitronectin. Figure 15.6 shows that in epithelia, integrins are clustered in important attachment sites known as focal adhesions. Here they anchor the cell to the ECM and also they ensure the integration of cellular attachments with the actin cytoskeleton. Integrins relay information both into and out of the cell. Direct engagement of specific integrin receptors by a bacterial adhesin initiates numerous signalling pathways leading to the activation of cytoskeletal components that direct the engulfment of the bacterium into a vacuole. Pathogenic *Yersinia* use this strategy to enter the **M cells** of **Peyer's patches** in the small intestine.

M cells are unusual in that they express β1-integrins at their apical (free) surfaces, enterocytes do not. A yersinial adhesin protein, invasion, binds to M cell β1 integrins initiating downstream signalling events that lead to the engulfment of the bacteria. After invasion of the M cells, these yersiniae colonize an extracellular niche likely maintained by the binding of YadA autotransporter adhesins to ECM proteins. They then actively inhibit further uptake by phagocytosis by deploying an anti-phagocytic T3SS to which we will return later.

Peyer's patches

Peyer's patches are aggregated lymphoid follicles surrounded by a modified follicle-associated epithelium that forms the interface between this gut-associated lymphoid tissue and the gut lumen. This follicle-associated epithelium contains specialized M cells that transport luminal antigens and bacteria towards the underlying immune cells. There, the immune response can be activated or it might be inhibited, leading to tolerance of that particular bacterium.

Cross reference
See Section 15.5.7.

SELF-CHECK 15.6

Why are M cells able to be targeted by this integrin-mediated invasion strategy?

Some pathogens such as *Streptococcus pyogenes* engage integrins in an indirect way to promote their invasion of epithelial cells. These bacteria exploit the fact that both integrins and their MSCRAMMs bind fibronectin and vitronectin. In essence, they indirectly bind the integrins via an ECM molecule bridge. Although indirect, this interaction is sufficient to trigger the intracellular signalling and cytoskeletal rearrangements that drives invasion.

SELF-CHECK 15.7

Why is this indirect method of binding intergrins able to work?

Other organisms promote invasion by engaging other receptor proteins that can also induce intracellular signalling and engulfment. The P-Pilus associated adhesin of UPECs, FimH, binds uroplakin 1a, a mannosylated glycoprotein. It associates with other uroplakin proteins in plaques that almost entirely cover the luminal epithelium of the bladder to provide an important impermeable barrier. The exposure of bladder cells to FimH also induces intracellular signalling that culminates in bacterial invasion of the bladder epithelium. This invasion process probably establishes a cryptic reservoir of UPEC hidden in the bladder epithelium that is responsible for recurring urinary tract infections, remember that a UTI can lead to life-threatening septicaemia especially those with an altered immune response.

The pathogen, *Listeria monocytogenes*, often associated with serious infection following consumption of cook-chilled meals invades the host through the intestinal epithelium, the blood brain barrier. The foeto-placental barrier is initiated when InlA of its internalin family of adhesins binds the adherens junction protein E-cadherin. Here the bacteria seem not to be attacking the integrity of the tight junctions to access E-cadherin like we saw with *S. pneumoniae* and *P. gingivalis*. Instead they appear to target the systems responsible for upkeep of the epithelium. When senescent cells need to be replaced they are expelled from the epithelium. In order to maintain epithelial continuity, the excluded cell's neighbours must reorganize to form a multicellular junction. During this process, E-cadherin is transiently exposed at the lumenal surface. *L. monocytogenes* takes advantage of this junction remodelling to adhere to the E-cadherin and then invade the epithelium.

Key Point

It is important to remember that the components of biological structures like epithelia have a limited lifespan and are rarely the static entities that might be suggested by textbook illustrations. Biology at all levels, from the macroscopic to the molecular, is incredibly dynamic and opportunities arise for bacteria as a result of this dynamism.

15.4.2 Enterobacterial T3SS promote invasion or intimacy

Type III secretion systems (T3SS) are complex nano-machines devoted to direct secretion of proteins into the cytoplasm of host cells. Fourteen different structural proteins assemble to form a type III needle apparatus or injectisome. The basic structure of a T3SS is shown in Figure 15.7. This complex consists of a basal structure, with components located in both bacterial membranes spanning the periplasm, and an external needle that protrudes from the bacterial surface. The needle is capped by a tip complex. On contact with a host cell, this tip complex forms a pore or translocon in its membrane that acts as a translocation pathway for effector proteins to be delivered into the host cytoplasm. Effector proteins are delivered to the base of the injectisome bound to molecular chaperones, which direct their folding and export. An ATPase complex in the bacterial plasma membrane powers the export of effector proteins through the T3SS needle by disrupting these chaperone-effector complexes. Once in the host cytoplasm, effectors manipulate key cellular processes such as signalling, secretory trafficking, cytoskeletal dynamics, and the inflammatory response to promote the infection and even cellular invasion.

Key Point

Sets of T3SS effectors interfere with host cell biology on multiple fronts in an coordinated manner subverting cellular processes to the advantage of the pathogen.

Salmonella enterica var. typhi (gastroenteritis or systemic typhoid fever) and *Shigella flexneri* (dysentery) both utilize T3SS in order to trigger important changes in the cytoskeleton at the host cell plasma membrane to promote invasion. *S. enterica* serovar Typhimurium produces two T3SS encoded at the SPI-1 and SPI-2 **pathogenicity islands**, areas of the genome related

Effector proteins delivered to host cytoplasm

Host plasma
membrane

Effector proteins delivered to
injectisome by chaperone

FIGURE 15.7

Type 3 secretion systems are complex multi-component nano-machines dedicated to the direct injection of effector proteins in to the host cytoplasm. They span three membranes, the plasma membrane of bacterium and host, as well as the bacterial outer membrane. These sets of effector proteins influence host cell biology in various but integrated ways.

to pathogenicity that have been acquired from external sources by **horizontal gene transfer**. The SPI-2 T3SS is concerned with the establishment of intracellular infection while the SPI-1 T3SS is involved in initial cellular invasion. This *S. enterica* SPI-1 system and its *Shigella* **homologue** both translocate effector proteins that orchestrate temporary actin cytoskeleton rearrangements. In both cases, once invasion is complete the changes induced in the cytoskeleton are allowed to be reversed. In the case of *S. typhimurium* this correcting process is also orchestrated by the microorganism.

Member of the Rho family of small signalling GTPase proteins regulate various aspects of intracellular actin dynamics. Two important members of this family are Cdc42 and Rac1. Between them, they regulate the activities of at least a dozen downstream target proteins. The primary cytoskeletal structures induced by Rac1 activation are lamellipodia, cytoskeletal projections at the edge of the cell formed by actin nucleation. Likewise Cdc42 activation generates filopodia, slender cytoplasmic projections that extend beyond the leading edge of lamellipodia that play roles in sensing and cell-cell interactions.

Rho GTPases, like Rac1 and Cdc42, are essentially molecular switches, they are activated when they bind GTP and are inactive when GDP is bound. Their activities are controlled by their interactions with three classes of proteins. These effectively act as inputs from other signalling pathways to integrate information. Figure 15.8 illustrates activating interactions promoted by guanine nucleotide exchange factor (GEFs). Inhibitory interactions involve GTPase-activating proteins (GAPs) and guanine nucleotide dissociation inhibitors (GDIs). Essentially, GAPs control the ability of the GTPase to hydrolyse GTP to GDP. Although they activate the GTPase, they essentially promote the inactivation of its regulatory function by promoting its GDP-bound state. GEFs reactivate Rho proteins by promoting the exchange of GDP for GTP. Activated Rho

horizontal/lateral gene transfer

Horizontal/lateral gene transfer describes the acquisition of genes via mechanisms unrelated to conventional heredity or vertical transfer. Horizontal transfer can come about through bacterial conjugation and other events involving mobilizable DNA such as bacteriophage integration in bacterial genomes.

homologues

Homologues, in this sense, are evolutionarily related (evidenced through amino acid sequence conservation) entities. These might carry out identical (orthologues) or similar (paralogues) functions.

FIGURE 15.8

Small signalling GTPase proteins are critical to the regulation of the actin cytoskeleton and many other cellular processes. These GTPases are active signallers when GTP is bound (green) but can be inactivated (red forms) by interaction with other proteins. GAPs (light brown) promoted GTPase activity and favour the signalling-inactive GDP-bound form. GDI proteins (pink) bind the GTPase protein in the cytoplasm and inhibit interactions with GEFs (yellow) that promote exchange of GDP for GTP. Bacterial effector proteins can emulate GEFS (yellow box) to promote invasion or GAPs (brown box) and GDIs (pink box) to suppress invasion. YopT of *Yersinia enterocolitica* dysregulates the system and prevents invasion by removing the polyprenyl chain of the GTPase which locates it to the plasma membrane.

proteins are often associated with the plasma membrane but the GDP-bound inactive state leaves the membrane. GDI proteins complex the Rho protein in the cytoplasm, stabilizing its GDP-bound inactive state.

SELF-CHECK 15.8

How does a GAP activate a Rho protein's GTPase activity yet inactivate its signalling capacity?

The T3SS effector proteins direct the formation of a key membrane structure known as a phagocytic cup by mimicking the actions of these regulatory proteins. *S. enterica* SopE and SopE2 operate as GEFs for Cdc42 and Rac1 respectively, promoting their activation and leading to the formation of the membrane extensions required for the uptake of the bacterium. Two other effector proteins, SipC and SipA, modulate actin remodelling in a more direct manner. SipC is a component of the translocon-complex of the T3SS. It forms the pore in host membranes that allows the secretion of effectors into the cytoplasm. SipC also actively drives actin polymerization and the aggregation of actin filaments into bundles. SipA, on the other hand, acts as an inhibitor of two important actin remodelling proteins, cofilin and gelsolin. Cofilin serves to depolymerize actin while gelsolin caps and severs actin filaments. Yet another effector SopB, is an inositol phosphatase. This enzyme serves to deplete the membrane of phosphatidylinositol-4,5-biphosphate (PIP2), an important phospholipid that interacts with many cytoskeleton proteins including cofilin and gelsolin.

SptP is another *S. enterica* effector attempts to return the invaded cell to a normal state. It serves as a GAP for both Cdc42 and Rac1, promoting GTP hydrolysis and the inactivation of the Rho regulator after invasion. Essentially, the half-life in the host cytoplasm of this bacterial GAP is longer than those of the effector GEFs (SopE or SopE2). Therefore, it will remain active longer than the effector GEFs, eventually allowing it to right the regulatory balance toward recovery of the normal cell architecture. Although the *Shigella flexneri* system uses different effectors, they do interact with these eukaryotic regulatory systems using similar principles to achieve the same effect.

SELF-CHECK 15.9

What is the significance of the long half-life of the bacterial GAP SgtP?

Key Point

Bacteria have evolved different solutions to interfere with basic cellular systems. The complexity of the signalling networks of mammalian cells means that the different interventions of bacterial effectors might generate a similar outcome.

Two important *E. coli* **pathotypes**, namely enteropathogenic *E. coli* (EPEC) and enterohaemorrhagic *E. coli* (EHEC) do not invade cells, they direct their pathogenicity from the mucosal surface. However, they orchestrate the process from a characteristic and self-defined location through their manipulation of the actin cytoskeleton. These bacteria induce a characteristic 'attaching and effacing' (A/E) lesion. Both of these *E. coli* pathotypes possess an array of adhesins including the type IV bundle-forming pilus through which they initially adhere to the surface of epithelial cells. The bacteria then induce a localized effacement of the enterocytes' microvilli and an accumulation of cytoskeletal proteins which generate pedestal-like structures; the bacteria sit atop these.

pathotypes
Pathotypes are members of a single species with distinct pathogenicity, i.e. that cause disease in different ways.

The genomic region responsible for this capability is known as the locus of enterocyte effacement (LEE). It encodes a T3SS, its associated effectors, and their molecular chaperones. A particularly interesting effector is known as the translated intimin receptor (Tir). Once injected into the enterocyte, it inserts into the plasma membrane where it serves as the receptor for the LEE-encoded outer membrane adhesin, intimin. Figure 15.9 shows how this unique bacterium-manufactured enterocyte ligand is critical to the formation of the pedestal structures. EPEC Tir can be phosphorylated at a single tyrosine residue by host protein kinases, Fyn and

FIGURE 15.9

Enteropathogenic (EPEC) and enterohaemorrhagic (EHEC) *E. coli* do not invade and stay at the mucosal surface. They subvert the actin cytoskeleton to promote the growth of a pedestal beneath them. In order to achieve this they employ a T3SS to deliver effector proteins to enterocytes. One of these, Tir, is a receptor for their intimin adhesin, which promotes a strong association with the enterocyte. Tir also helps to initiate the actin polymerization that produces the pedestal.

Abl. This modification allows the recruitment of a number of host proteins that form a complex. Firstly, the host adaptor molecule Nck binds to Tir, this complex subsequently recruits N-WASp (a downstream target of Cdc42) and the actin-related protein (ARP) 2/3 complex. Components of ARP2/3 resemble actin and serve as nucleation sites for new actin filaments. Along with other actin-binding proteins α-actinin, talin, and vinculin, these new actin filaments form the characteristic pedestals on which these bacteria sit. The EHEC system varies slightly in terms of composition. EHEC Tir is not phosphorylated and hence does not recruit Nck. Instead other T3SS effectors EspF and EspH act as the adaptor to N-WASp and the ARP2/3 complex.

15.5 **Avoiding the immune response**

Our bodies boast an array of protective mechanisms through which we deal with infecting bacteria. If our mucosal surfaces are breached by any microorganism, our primary defence relies on recognition of the pathogen by the innate immune system. This branch of our immune arsenal then mounts a concerted but generic attack upon the pathogen. Components of this response include restricting iron availability to limit bacterial growth, initiating inflammation, and deploying the complement system. Phagocytes play an important role in engulfing and killing pathogens and also clearing damaged tissue to aid healing. Macrophages, and especially dendritic cells, engulf and digest pathogens. They then interact with T lymphocytes acting as antigen-presenting cells, and therefore represent an important bridge between innate and adaptive immunity. Once adaptive immunity has been successfully invoked, responses to subsequent exposures to the same pathogen can be supplemented by a specific response in the form of antibodies and sometimes cytotoxic T cells.

Key Point

Immune responses are complex and multifactorial and, as we shall see, so are the mechanisms by which bacteria evade them. Such is the threat posed by our sophisticated immune system, it is common for bacteria to deploy multiple evasion strategies. These can be based around modifications to key conserved cell wall components and the production of 'camouflaged surfaces' using **evasins** to avoid detection. Another approach is the production of **impedins** – a subset of virulence factors that modify the activities of immune components to reduce bacterial clearance.

15.5.1 Detection of microbial-associated molecular patterns

Innate immune cells detect pathogens by recognizing common conserved components known as microbial-associated molecular patterns (MAMPs or sometimes pathogen AMPs, PAMPs). These are detected using pattern recognition receptors (PRRs), of which there are various types. Binding of MAMPs by PRRs initiates the innate immune response, leading to inflammation. Many MAMPs are common bacterial cell envelope components including lipopolysaccharide, peptidoglycan, lipoteichoic acids, flagellin, and lipoproteins.

MAMPs are recognized by an array of PRRs. Toll-like receptors (TLR2, TLR4, and TLR5) are transmembrane PRRs expressed in spleen cells, peripheral blood mononuclear cells, dendritic cells, macrophages, and monocytes that are implicated in the detection of peptidoglycan, lipopolysaccharide from Gram-negative bacteria, lipoproteins, lipoteichoic acids from Gram-positive pathogens, and phosphatidylinositol mannosides and lipomannans of mycobacteria. TLR5 recognizes flagellin. TLR9 is another, which is found within endosomes of dendritic cells. This receptor detects unmethylated CpG containing DNA; these cytosine-phosphate-guanine sequences are relatively uncommon in mammalian DNA and are usually methylated at the cytosine. Neither is the case for bacterial DNA, which would be released upon phagocytic killing of a pathogen.

SELF-CHECK 15.10

MAMPs are common bacterial entities with well-conserved structures. Why does innate immunity target them?

TLRs function by transducing signals through the plasma membrane to indicate that their external domain has bound a MAMP. Their intracellular domain reports this binding event through protein–protein interactions, these initiate signalling cascades. One of these leads to gene expression directed by the transcription factor NF-κB, which produces numerous pro-inflammatory cytokines. In addition to NF-κB activation, TLR can also activate signalling cascades controlled by mitogen-activated protein kinases (MAPKs). MAPKs play important roles in cell proliferation, apoptosis, differentiation, and cell migration.

Key Point

MAPK pathways influence which innate immune cells multiply or die, how they develop, and where they go.

The nucleotide oligomerization domain (NOD) and NOD-like proteins are a family of at least 22 intracellular PRRs that respond to diverse triggers. NOD1 and NOD2 sense breakdown products of peptidoglycan known as muropeptides that are transported into phagocytic and epithelial cells. Binding of muropeptides to the receptor domain of these proteins causes NOD proteins to oligomerize and this initiates a series of signalling reactions that also generates an NF-κB-dependent pro-inflammatory response. Other NOD-like receptors form complexes called inflammasomes. These contain caspase-1, a cysteine protease that has dual functions in inflammation. Firstly, it activates the interleukin 1 family of pro-inflammatory cytokines by cleaving their precursor proteins. It also plays a key role in the triggering of cells into apoptosis and pyroptosis, two forms of programmed cell death which might be employed to kill infected cells, limiting the opportunities for growth of invading pathogens. Another PRR class, the C-type lectins (DC-SIGN and mannose receptor) are expressed on dendritic cells and endothelia, their binding of mannose-rich microbial ligands such as glycoproteins and lipomannan from mycobacteria tend to induce signalling pathways that promote phagocytosis.

Although other PRRs, such as the peptidoglycan recognition proteins (PGRP-1-4) and lysozyme, recognize patterns in peptidoglycan, they do not directly induce a signalling cascade to promote an innate immune response. Instead, they act on the bacterium itself, exerting a killing effect. Lysozyme and PGRP-2 are enzymes that hydrolyse peptidoglycan directly. Lysozyme cleaves the glycosidic links of its glycan backbone, while PGRP2 is an amidase that hydrolyses the linkage between backbone N-acetylmuramic acid residues and the stem peptides that cross-link them. The degradation of the exposed peptidoglycan of Gram-positive bacteria would make them less resistant to lysis. The killing activity of PGRP-1, -3, and -4, however, is different; these are antimicrobial peptides that kill by depolarizing the bacterial membrane and generating toxic hydroxyl radicals.

In order to evade recognition (see the summary in Figure 15.10) and avoid the killing mechanisms that can be induced, many bacteria have developed modifications to their peptidoglycan at important positions on both the glycan backbone and the stem peptides. In general, peptidoglycans with glycan chain modifications still elicit a response via NOD receptors but these bacteria are resistant to lysozyme killing. However, modifications to the peptides can help evade recognition by NOD1 leading to a less vigorous inflammatory response.

15.5.2 Opsonization and evasion strategies

Pathogens are targeted for phagocytic clearance by the binding of **opsonins**. These can be specific antibodies or components of the complement system. Complement is a major constituent of the innate immune response. It also enhances the activity of the **humoral** arm of the adaptive immune response, interacting with antibodies to accelerate clearance of opsonized pathogens. Its prime function is in the early recognition and destruction of invading pathogens. Complement is a tightly regulated complex system with numerous receptors and factors circulating in the blood as inactive pro-proteins that can be activated by the initiation of a proteolytic cascade. The cleavage of specific component proteins release peptides that acts as pro-inflammatory cytokines and other fragments drive a cascade of further cleavages resulting in a massive amplification of the response and the formation of a membrane attack complex (MAC) that kills sensitive cells. Important aspects of complement are summarized in Figure 15.11.

humoral

Humoral immunity centres around the properties of antibodies in contrast to cell-mediated immunity.

At least three different activation pathways are recognized, each responding to a different trigger. The availability of multiple pathways maximizes the chances that a non-host cell surface would be recognized and then attacked by the system. There are three major pathways to complement activation. Firstly, there is the classical pathway in which the C1 complex binds to a pathogen via

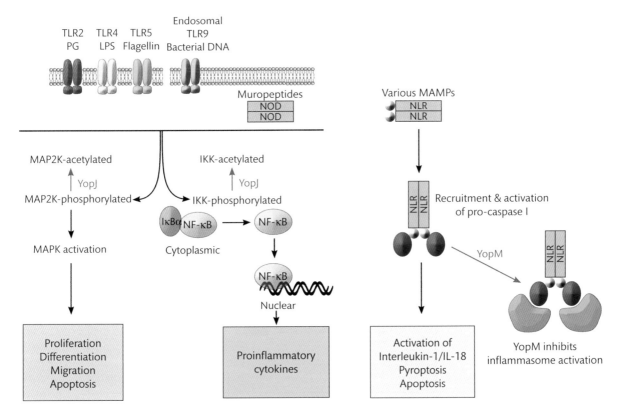

FIGURE 15.10

An array of pattern recognition receptors (PRRs) detects and responds to conserved microbial-associated molecular patterns (MAMPs). Three important signalling routes are illustrated. Various cellular responses arise from MAMPs binding to the nucleotide oligomerization domain (NOD) and Toll-like (TLR) receptors. Some activate signalling via mitogen-activated protein kinases (MAPK) and regulate various cellular events, others release the transcription factor NF-κB to the nucleus to generate pro-inflammatory cytokines. Some NOD-like receptors respond to MAMPs by activating inflammasomes. *Yersinia* effector proteins YopJ and YopM inhibit these routes.

IgG or IgM immunoglobulins. The lectin pathway operates much like the classical pathway but with a different opsonin. Instead of immunoglobulins, mannose-rich microbial surface polysaccharides are recognized by the mannose-binding lectin. Finally, the alternative pathway is triggered via low-level spontaneous cleavage of complement component C3 through an unstable thioester bond. Host cells are able to protect themselves from its activity by recruiting inhibitors (regulators of complement activation, RCA) that circulate in the blood to their surface.

Cross reference
See Chapter 13.

SELF-CHECK 15.11

Why are there several ways to trigger complement?

All of these pathways converge at a common point, each route generates a variant of the protease C3-convertase; these all cleave and activate component C3. The products of this reaction are C3a and C3b. C3a is an anaphylatoxin; it can trigger **degranulation** of endothelial cells, mast cells or phagocytes, raising a local inflammatory response. C3b causes a cascade of further cleavage and activation events. C3b also binds to the surface of pathogens acting as an opsonin and promoting their phagocytosis.

degranulation
Degranulation describes the process by which cells release antimicrobial cytotoxic molecules from secretory vesicles called granules.

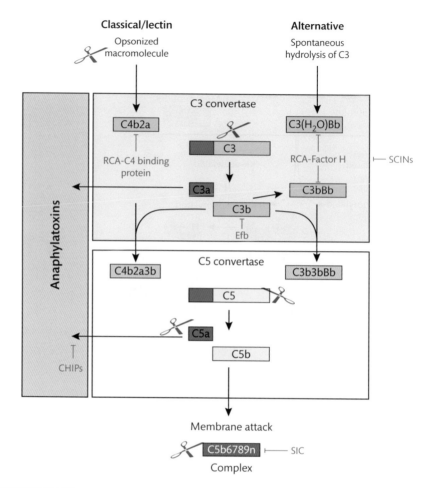

FIGURE 15.11

Complement is a vital component of innate immunity and potentiates adaptive immunity. The classical and lectin pathways are triggered by detection of either antibodies or a mannose-binding lectin, respectively at a bacterial surface. The alternative pathway is spontaneously initiated at a low level. Each pathway produces a C3 convertase (green box) although these have different contributing factors they all cleave component C3 which adapts C3 convertase to a C5 convertase (yellow box). Cleavage of C5 initiates the final even, formation of a membrane attack complex which can puncture and kill some bacterial cells. Cleavage of C3 and C5 by their respective convertases generates 'a' fragments which are anaphylatoxins (red box), they enhance inflammation, and recruit immune cells to the infection. The points at which selected bacterial inhibitors and host regulators of complement activation (RCA) that are recruited by bacteria have influence are indicated. Likewise, targets of bacterial proteases within the system are indicated by the scissor motif.

As well as acting as an opsonin, surface-bound C3b recruits other complement factors to form more C3 convertase, a step which can amplify the response hugely. Covalent binding of C3b-containing complexes can then form the C5 convertase, which cleaves C5 to C5a and C5b. C5a is another potent anaphylatoxin and a very powerful chemotactic signal which attracts phagocytes. C5b, however, recruits C6, C7, C8, and multiple C9 molecules to form the MAC. Once formed, MAC can then create a transmembrane pore in the target cell plasma membrane leading to lysis and death. Although the MAC represents a potent killing mechanism, few bacteria, probably only Gram-negative commensals, are sensitive to it. The greater threat posed by complement lies in opsonization which promotes phagocytic clearance by Kupffer cells in the liver and local macrophage and neutrophils attracted by C5a.

Bacteria have developed three main strategies that they deploy to evade clearance via complement. Either they (1) recruit host regulators of complement activation (RCA), (2) secrete bacterial complement inhibitors, or (3) inactivate complement and immunoglobulins via proteolysis.

SELF-CHECK 15.12

Are all bacteria equally sensitive to the membrane attack complex?

15.5.3 Binding host complement inhibitors

A wide range of bacteria recruit RCAs through binding to surface molecules in order to inhibit the complement cascade on their surface. The strength of this strategy and the likely reason that it is so widely deployed is that RCAs are always available in the blood and as they are structurally related, often a single pathogen protein can recruit multiple host RCAs to the bacteria surface.

Factor H and its homologue Factor H-like protein, are key regulators of the alternative pathway. They compete with factor B for binding to C3b, a critical step in the formation of the alternative pathway C3 convertase (which is composed C3b-Bb). As well as inhibiting the formation of C3 convertase, it also disrupts formed C3 convertase and aids factor I in the degradation of C3b. Likewise another RCA, C4 binding protein, inhibits the classical pathway by aiding factor I in degrading C4b inhibiting the formation of new classical C3 convertase (composed C4b2a), and facilitating the decay of C2a from formed C3 convertase.

Factor H naturally binds to glycosaminoglycans that are not usually present on pathogen surfaces but are to be found on many host cells. In this way it can protect host cells from the random action of the spontaneously degrading C3 that can trigger the alternative pathway. Many pathogens have surface proteins that can bind one or both of these factors.

15.5.4 Bacterial complement inhibitors

Some of the other complex mammalian systems we have explored thus far have been disrupted by multiple bacterial effectors in a variety of different ways. Considering the complexity of the complement cascade, we might expect that bacteria would have evolved impedins that promoted dysfunction at multiple levels. However, very few examples of bacterial complement inhibition have been described. *Borrelia burgdorferi*, the cause of Lyme disease, produces an outer membrane protein that resembles the human CD59 complement inhibitor and binds components C9 and C8 to inhibit MAC formation. The streptococcal inhibitor of complement (SIC) also prevents MAC formation by interfering with the uptake of C5bC6C7 complexes to the bacterial membrane.

Key Point: Staphylococcus aureus complement evasion

Staphylococcus aureus is very well equipped to evade complement. Firstly it produces two proteins that bind immunoglobulins, staphylococcal protein A (SpA) and a second

immunoglobulin-binding protein (Sbi). Both proteins bind antibodies in a manner that blocks the site that C1q would bind during the activation of the classical pathway. Both proteins have multiple anti-immune activities; Sbi also binds the RCA Factor H, while SpA is a B-lymphocyte superantigen which we will explore later.

This organism also produces staphylococcal complement inhibitors (SCINs), small helical molecules that inhibit C3 convertase by stabilizing it in a non-functional dimeric state. This dimerization is critically important as it not only inhibits amplification of the cascade, it also affects the ability of phagocytes to recognize the bound complement and engulf the bacteria. Another staphylococcal protein, the extracellular fibrinogen-binding molecule (Efb) also plays a similar role by binding C3b and blocking its activity as an opsonin and decreasing phagocytosis.

This bacterium produces yet another anti-complement strategy of this type. It employs the impedin *S. aureus* chemotaxis inhibitory protein (CHIPS) which acts as an **antagonist** of the receptor for the chemotactic C5a on neutrophils and other phagocytes, thus decreasing the influx of these phagocytes to the site of infection.

15.5.5 Proteolysis of complement and immunoglobulins

A common strategy deployed by bacteria to evade complement is the hydrolytic inactivation of its components. Pathogen proteases cleave a number of key proteins at various levels of the cascade. These include molecules that are involved in initiation of the classical pathway, such as C1q and immunoglobulins. Others hydrolyse C3, which is crucial for the amplification of the cascade and yet others inactivate C5 and MAC components. A variation on this strategy is used by *Streptococcus agalactiae*, *S. pyogenes*, and *Serratia marcescens*. These target the anaphylatoxin C5a for degradation. In doing so, the chemotactic response that usually accompanies C5 processing and the subsequent local recruitment of phagocytes is limited.

We saw earlier that *Streptococcus pneumoniae* binds plasminogen and plasmin to bring about pericellular invasion at mucosal membranes, here a similar strategy is used by *Staphylococcus aureus* to evade opsonization. The bacterium produces staphylokinase which appears to protect the bacterium by forming two important complexes. Firstly, it binds to α-defensins, bactericidal peptides produced by neutrophils, abolishing their bactericidal properties. Additionally, staphylokinase converts plasminogen bound at the bacterial surface to active plasmin. Not only does its broad-spectrum proteolytic activity assist with tissue penetration but it also degrades C3 and IgG to prevent opsonization. To further emphasize *S. aureus'* genetic investment in immune evasion, it also produces its own C3 metalloprotease, aureolysin.

15.5.6 Antiphagocytic outer polysaccharidic layers

Where present, the bacterial capsule is usually an outer polysaccharide layer but some bacteria use alternate polymers. The anthrax agent, *Bacillus anthracis*, for example, has a poly-D-glutamic acid capsule. Beneath a capsular layer, Gram-negative bacteria also have at least a glycosylated lipooligosaccharide as a major component of the exterior face of their outer membrane; many have a much more extensively glycosylated lipopolysaccharide.

Encapsulation is recognized as an important virulence determinant factor based on its antiphagocytic activity. The capsule of *Streptococcus pneumoniae* is very well studied as a virulence factor. All *S. pneumoniae* clinical isolates that cause invasive disease are encapsulated. Furthermore, *S. pneumoniae* mutants that do not possess capsules are drastically attenuated in animal models of infection. The composition of the capsular polysaccharide is both very varied and important to virulence. Over 90 antigenically distinct capsular serotypes exist; their compositions vary subtly based on the sequence and types of sugars within the main polysaccharide chains and side branches. Bacteria expressing these different capsular serotypes vary in the ability to cause invasive disease.

The capsule may have greater significance at different points in the progress of *S. pneumoniae* invasive disease. Two variants of *S. pneumoniae* are described based on their colony morphology. Opaque phase variants have a thicker capsule than transparent phase variants. It is these opaque phase variants that predominate during invasive phases of infection. However, the transparent phase variants are much more successful in colonizing the nasopharynx. A simple explanation could be that a thinner capsule reveals more adhesins and effectively enhances binding to the epithelial surface.

The external position of the capsule means it is ideally situated to modulate interactions between *S. pneumoniae*, host cells, and proteins. Unencapsulated mutants suffer a greater deposition of complement components on their surface and are more susceptible to phagocytosis by neutrophils. Several plausible mechanisms by which bacterial capsules might inhibit complement exist. Capsules may inhibit recognition of surface antigens by specific antibodies, thereby preventing classical pathway activation. Additionally capsular polysaccharide might prevent binding of complement components with their targets elsewhere in the cell wall. Some bacteria incorporate hyaluronic acid and sialic acid in their capsules and these resemble many host cell surfaces, camouflaging them from the immune system. Broadly similar advantages are also claimed for the possession of the polysaccharide chains (O-antigens) of Gram-negative bacteria.

Key Point

The relative success of opaque and transparent phase variant of *S. pneumoniae* in colonization and invasion demonstrates the point that the human body is a particularly diverse environment for bacteria. Heavy encapsulation serves a purpose in protecting the bacterium from killing mechanisms after invasion but limits its potential to colonize in the nasopharynx. Similarly, long O-antigen chains are advantageous in protecting *Salmonella typhimurium* against various antimicrobial agents it might encounter but reduces its ability to tolerate bile, an important property of a small intestine pathogen.

The biosynthetic system that produce these polysaccharide structures are highly regulated at the genetic level; the regulatory circuits of successful pathogens have generally found the best profiles of gene expression to produce appropriate phenotypes under various conditions that enhance their natural history.

15.5.7 Antiphagocytic and anti-inflammatory action of T3SS effectors

We saw earlier that the enteropathogens *Yersinia enterocolitica* and *Y. pseudotuberculosis* orchestrate their uptake into M cells by binding β1-integrins with their adhesin, invasin. They migrate to the basal lamina where they then occupy an extracellular niche by actively resisting cellular uptake and phagocytosis.

Cross reference

See Section 15.4.1.

Cross reference

See Section 15.4.2.

These bacteria possess the pYV virulence plasmid that encodes the Ysc T3SS, which delivers six effectors (*Yersinia* outer proteins, YopE, YopH, YopJ YopM, YopO, and YopT). Most of their targets are cellular components that influence the host innate immune response. Like the T3SS effectors of *Salmonella enterica* discussed earlier in the context of invasion, several of these anti-phagocytic yersinial effectors also interact with Rac1 and Cdc42 signalling. However, the focus here is inhibitory, to block the cytoskeletal remodelling that leads to phagocytosis. Their functions are indicated in Figure 15.8. YopE is a GAP for RhoA, Rac1, and Cdc42. Its stimulation of GTP hydrolysis essentially deactivates the Rho protein as an activator of the cytoskeleton. Another important aspect of the regulation of the activity of Rho proteins like RhoA, and Rac1 is their membrane anchor. Some Rho proteins have a geranylgeranyl lipid chain, which is added as a post-translational modification near their C-termini. YopT has protease activity and it exerts its anti-phagocytic effect by cleaving the Rho polypeptide just upstream to where the prenyl chain is located. This effectively removes the regulators' membrane anchors meaning that they are not localized correctly and cannot conduct their normal signalling functions.

The C-terminal domain of another effector, YopO interacts with RhoA and Rac1. It mimics a GDI, excluding the Rho proteins from the membrane and inhibiting GTP exchange and activation. However, YopO is a multifunctional effector. Its N-terminal domain is a serine/threonine kinase that is activated by actin. The activated YopO kinase specifically phosphorylates a G protein Gαq, impairing its nucleotide binding and preventing Gαq-dependent cellular processes. There could be many downstream consequences of Gαq inactivation; it is, for instance, responsible for activation of RhoA.

YopH is another effector with anti-phagocytic activity. It has protein tyrosine phosphatase activity that disrupts several signalling pathways. YopH specifically localizes to focal adhesion complexes where it interacts with and dephosphorylates proteins (FAK, Cas, and paxillin). These are involved in the invasin-β1-integrin initiated invasion pathway described earlier for *Y. enterocolitica* and *Y. pseudotuberculosis*.

Earlier, we considered the detection of MAMPs by PRRs as key events in the initiation of MAPK and NF-κB-dependent transcription and the inflammatory response. Figure 15.10 illustrates how our penultimate effector YopJ inhibits multiple NF-κB and MAPK pathways. It achieves this by acetylating key serine and threonine residues in MAP2K and IκB kinase (IKK). These residues would be phosphorylated during normal signalling, their acetylation blocks this key element of the signalling pathway. The inhibition of these two important kinases impacts on pathways we have already seen. MAP2K is a kinase that activates MAPKs, while IKK phosphorylates the inhibitory IκBα protein that binds NF-κB and prevents it from entering the nucleus. Under normal conditions, its phosphorylation dislodges IκBα allowing NF-κB to enter the nucleus and activate the gene expression. The inhibition of these upstream regulators by YopJ effectively blocks pro-inflammatory cytokine production and induces apoptosis in affected macrophages.

As we saw earlier, another important signalling route involved in the activation of a pro-inflammatory response is the assembly of an inflammasome. Figure 15.10 shows that the inflammasome then activates the caspase-1 cascade which promotes the maturation of pro-inflammatory cytokines IL-1β and IL-18 and initiates pyroptosis, an inflammatory cell death program that protects against pathogens by restricting the potential for intracellular growth shielded from the immune system. IL-18 stimulates production of IFNγ and initiates the development of a TH$_1$ response that results in an increase in cytokine levels, which will enhance the inflammation and drive the development of an adaptive immune response. The final effector of this series, YopM directly binds caspase-1 blocking formation of a mature inflammasome and subsequent phagocyte pyroptosis.

15.5.8 *Staphylococcus aureus* produces superantigens that influence lymphocyte populations

Staphylococcus aureus produces a series of impedins that influence distinct populations of B and T lymphocytes. These are termed **superantigens** as they influence a much greater proportion of our B- and T-cell repertoire than a conventional specific antigen would. They achieve this through productively binding B- and T-cell antigen receptors at sites where they express limited structural variability. Simply, their interaction with the receptor initiates normal signalling pathways as if a specific antigen had bound. Receptor paratopes, the conventional antigen binding site, are extremely variable allowing for great diversity in antigen structure that can be sensed and the development of a specific adaptive immune response. Superantigens bind the receptors at sites where far less structural variability occurs than at the paratope. Consequently a higher proportion of B or T cells can be stimulated by this single molecule.

Key Point

Different forms of superantigen are relevant to B and T lymphocytes.

15.5.9 Staphylococcal protein A is a superantigen that kills specialized B lymphocytes

SpA is an abundant surface protein anchored to the bacterial cell wall by sortases. It was initially discovered through its ability to mediate bacterial precipitation of immunoglobulins. Its avid binding of IgG is via their complement C1q binding (Fcγ) region which, as you will see in Figure 15.12, is distant to its antigen binding **paratope**. Binding of IgG via Fcγ on its cell surface is used as a strategy to mask underlying surface antigens and also to limit complement activation by the classical pathway and inhibit phagocytic killing of *S. aureus* by neutrophils.

However, SpA also inhibits the development of humoral immunity to *S. aureus* by acting as a B lymphocyte superantigen. B-cell superantigens can specifically interact with immunoglobulins (Ig) and B-cell antigen receptors (BCR). SpA also binds to some Ig and BCR by their Fab (fragment, antigen binding) region but at a site distinct from their paratope. In humans, there are seven families of the Ig VH genes; these encode the variable portion of Ig heavy chains that are constituents of Fab. SpA specifically binds the largest of these families VH3, which represents ~50% of our antibody repertoire.

If SpA is injected into transgenic mice with humanized antibody genes, a major and rapid depletion of specialized B lymphocytes occurs, specifically of B-1a cells in the peritoneal cavity and VH3 B cells in the marginal zone (MZ) of the spleen. Both of these cell types support innate immunity. B-1 cells produce substantial amounts of IgA and are the major producers of natural antibodies. These secreted Igs are usually germline-encoded, i.e. they are not products of the adaptive immune response. These often recognize epitopes of carbohydrates, which might resemble bacterial antigens, and thus provide early protection against a variety of pathogens. These antibodies can induce the classical competent pathway.

Similarly, splenic MZ B cells are a strategically-located reservoir of B cells in the spleen that can rapidly produce natural antibodies in systemic infection. It seems highly likely that elimination of these B-cell subpopulations that contribute to innate immunity promotes *S. aureus* infection.

FIGURE 15.12

IgG and B-cell receptors are almost identical in structure. Specific antigen recognition determinants are carried on the variable (V_H and V_L) components and form the paratope (indicated by a star). IgG can opsonize a bacterial surface and initiate complement by binding C1q at the Fcγ site of CH3. *Staphylococcus aureus* protein A (SpA) has two immune evasion functions based around its binding to these molecules. Firstly, it inhibits C1q binding and complement activation by occupying Fcγ. It also acts as a superantigen binding to VH3 containing B-cell receptor variants in a way that emulates antigen-binding. As the region of VH3 to which it binds varies less than paratopes, almost 50% of natural antibody producing B cells are susceptible.

15.5.10 Toxic shock syndromes are elicited by T-cell-specific superantigens

A rare but dramatic consequence of *S. aureus* infection is toxic shock syndrome (TSS). Early symptoms include a sunburn-like rash, high fever, hypotension, malaise, and confusion, which can progress rapidly to coma and multiple organ failure. A similar TSS is also caused by *S. pyogenes* which generally arises from skin infections. *S. aureus* TSS is caused by the action of a superantigen toxin (TSS toxin-1, TSST-1) that subverts antigen presentation to T-cell receptors, thereby non-specifically activating T cells. During TSS, approaching 20% of T cells may be activated causing the development of a 'cytokine storm' that promotes the multi-organ disease.

Antigen-presenting cells, such as a macrophage or dendritic cells, generate peptide antigens through the digestive processing of a pathogen. As you can see from Figure 15.13, normal T-cell-mediated immunity is initiated when they present the antigen at its surface within a groove formed by the α and β chains of a class II major histocompatibility complex (MHC). If it is recognized as foreign by a T-cell receptor (TCR), a signalling cascade will induce T-cell proliferation and differentiation. TCRs vary enormously in their antigen binding CDR3 region. The TCR β-chain variable domain (Vβ) has far less structural diversity, with only around 50 variants being expressed in humans and it is here that TSST-1 binds directly, without the need for processing by an antigen-presenting cell. The productive binding of TSST-1 to this region of the TCR results in the activation of many more T cells than during the conventional antigen processing, ultimately driving the development of the 'cytokine storm'.

SELF-CHECK 15.13

How do superantigens influence such high proportions of our T-cell or antibody repertoires?

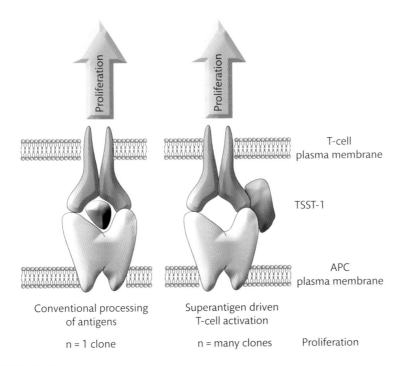

Conventional processing
of antigens

n = 1 clone

Superantigen driven
T-cell activation

n = many clones

T-cell
plasma membrane

TSST-1

APC
plasma membrane

Proliferation

FIGURE 15.13

Phagocytes, particularly dendritic cells, promote the development of adaptive immunity by acting as antigen presenting cells (APC). They degrade bacteria and present potential antigens at their surface using the major histocompatibility complex II (MHCII) (white). This then interacts with T-cell receptors and can lead to T-cell proliferation. Toxic shock syndrome toxin-1 (TSST-1) acts as a superantigen imitating this process. It binds an area of the receptor that varies little and does not define antigen specificity. The signalling responses initiated by this binding leads to inappropriate proliferation of large numbers of T cells.

As we have seen in the previous sections, *Staphylococcus aureus* produces an impressive array of impedins to limit the activities of the immune system. Bearing this in mind, its production of a virulence factor that strongly promotes the activation of the adaptive immune system seems counter-intuitive. However, it is also important to note that *S. aureus* produces a diverse array of at least 23 superantigens, many are implicated in food poisoning. In this scenario, pathogenesis doesn't rely on viable *S. aureus* actually being present in the intestine; the toxins are often produced in contaminated foodstuffs. The possession of such an array of these toxins suggests that they might contribute more broadly to this organism's ecology than in the induction of TSS and certainly food poisoning. Both of the major superantigen producers, *S. aureus* and *S. pyogenes*, colonize the human nasopharynx and many of us possess antibodies that react with these toxins in health. This suggests that superantigens are relevant during minor infections or asymptomatic colonization. It seems likely that the primary roles of these toxins may be in influencing populations of T cells to prolong carriage of superantigen-producing bacteria and to aid their transmission.

Key Point

Although *Staphylococcus aureus* is considered an opportunistic pathogen, it is extremely well equipped with evasins and impedins. These might be necessary to maintain a stable colonization of the nasopharynx.

15.6 **Toxinogenesis**

Many bacteria produce exotoxins that are secreted and damage or destroy host cells or tissues. Exotoxins may exert their effects at sites distant to the producing bacterium. A convenient tripartite classification of bacterial toxins is possible; it describes toxins that (1) act at membrane surfaces by engaging receptors and subverting signalling cascades, (2) disrupt cell membrane integrity, and (3) enter cells and disrupt their metabolism. There are literally hundreds of known bacterial toxins and great diversity in form and function is evident within all of these classes. Illustrative examples of each will be related.

15.6.1 Toxins that subvert membrane receptor signalling

We have just considered an obvious example of this toxin class in *S. aureus* TSST-1. It has traditionally been considered a toxin through its undoubted role in the pathophysiology of the dramatic toxic shock syndrome. It was considered in the earlier section as it is emerging that it might have greater significance in prolonging *S. aureus* colonization than in the pathogenesis of a relatively rare syndrome.

Another well-understood example of this toxin class is the heat-stable enterotoxin (STa) produced by enterotoxigenic *E. coli* (ETEC). This is a toxic peptide that causes acute diarrhoea, primarily in infants and travellers to developing countries – so-called 'travellers' diarrhoea'. STa binds to a receptor located on the mucosal surface of the small intestine and colon that belongs to the membrane-bound guanylate cyclase (GC) family, known as GC-C.

The natural function of this receptor is the detection of the peptide hormones guanylin and uroguanylin. These are synthesized from prepropeptides mainly in gastrointestinal mucosa and are secreted both into intestinal lumen and into the blood in order to regulate sodium and potassium balances. Figure 15.14 shows that when the hormones bind to GC-C, intracellular cyclic GMP levels rise, which activates protein kinase G and protein kinase A. These can both phosphorylate the CFTR chloride ion channel. CFTR actively secretes Cl^- to the intestinal lumen, water, Na^+, K^+, and HCO_3^- follow. Essentially STa binds GC-C more avidly than the natural hormones causing hypersecretion of Cl^-. The severe diarrhoea that this causes rapidly dehydrates infected individuals (much like cholera) and promotes dissemination of the bacterium.

Key Point

Toxins can mimic host cell events to adapt favourable environment for growth or colonization of the host or to promote dissemination of the pathogen more broadly in the human population.

SELF-CHECK 15.14

Why does STa produce an exaggerated hypersecretion?

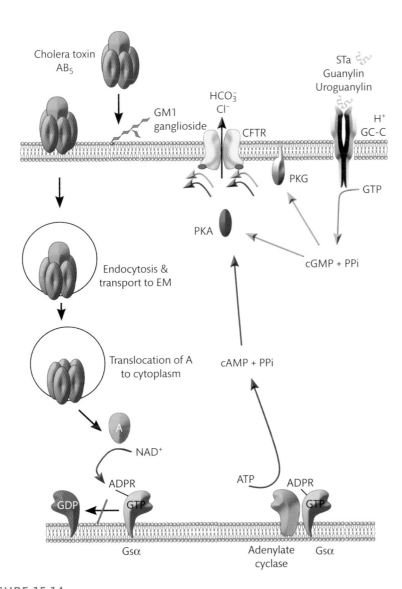

FIGURE 15.14

The B subunits of cholera toxin bind a glycolipid receptor GM1 ganglioside at the enterocyte surface. The AB_5 toxin is taken into the cell by endocytosis eventually arriving in the endoplasmic reticulum (EM). Here the B subunits are involved in translocation of the enzymatically active A-subunit to the cytoplasm. Here the A- subunit catalyses the covalent modification of a signalling GTPase $Gs\alpha$ with ADP-ribose (ADPR, for structure see Figure 15.16), maintaining it in its GTP-bound active form (consequences are indicated by blue arrows). This essentially locks adenylate cyclase on, over-stimulating the production of cAMP. Protein kinase A (PKA) is activated and it phosphorylates (red circles) the chloride ion channel CFTR leading to the hypersecretion of chloride, bicarbonate, Na^+, K^+ and water leading to diarrhoea. *E. coli* heat stable toxin STa also influences CFTR but via a different secondary messenger system (green arrows). STa mimics the peptide hormones guanylin and uroguanylin in binding the guanylate cyclase GC-C. Binding of these peptides causes production of cGMP which activates both PKA and protein kinase G which can both activate CFTR by phosphorylation. STa causes diarrhoea by being an inappropriate trigger for this system and also through its stronger binding of GC-C than the natural hormones.

15.6.2 Cytolytic toxins

Various bacteria produce toxins that compromise the integrity of host cell membranes. Although many are described as haemolysins to reflect the fact that they were discovered through their ability to lyse erythrocytes, they can disrupt the membranes of various cell types. These cytolytic toxins can be subdivided further into those toxins that degrade the fabric of the membrane and those that puncture and permeabilize it. Any toxin that compromises the barrier function of a plasma membrane will ultimately allow the leakage of cellular components, the loss of membrane potential (depolarization) and an uncontrolled influx of water leading to swelling and lysis.

15.6.3 Phospholipases

Cross reference

See Chapter 7.

An example of the first type is the α-toxin of the *Clostridium perfringens*, which is essential for its pathogenesis of gas gangrene. α-Toxin is a two-domain zinc metalloenzyme with phospholipase C activity; its C-terminal domain recognizes membrane phospholipid headgroups at the cell surface. The N-terminal domain carries the phospholipase C activity; it catalyses the hydrolysis of phospholipids including phosphatidylcholine and sphingomyelin, two of the major constituents of the outer leaflets of eukaryotic plasma membranes. Mutation of the toxin has shown that the N-terminal domain is required for all enzymatic activity and is sufficient for hydrolysis of phosphatidylcholine. An intact C-terminal domain is required for sphinogmyelinase activity and haemolysis or cytotoxicity. High concentrations of the toxin induce rapid release of phosphocholine from cell membranes and leakage of cytosolic contents such as nucleotides. Damaged cells change size and shape, lose microvilli, and membrane fistulas develop.

Cells exposed to α-toxin do not always lyse. Four factors influence the outcome of an interaction of α-toxin with a cell (1) the toxin dose, (2) the composition of the membrane including the presence of components such as proteoglycans, N-linked glycoproteins, and glycosphingolipids, (3) the capacity of the cell to activate phosphatidylcholine biosynthesis, and (4) the availability of the precursor molecules with which to make new phosphatidylcholine. However, other effects can arise from signalling processes initiated by rising concentrations of the enzyme's bioactive lipid products, ceramide and diacylglycerol (DAG), in the membrane.

Our own phospholipase C plays an important role in human physiology, it is activated in response to neurotransmitters and hormonal signals (such as acetylcholine and adrenaline) to release a secondary messenger molecule (DAG) within the cell that drives physiological responses. Figure 15.15 summarizes how DAG produced by the actions of α-toxin subverts this system. Firstly, it activates protein kinase C. This enzyme can then activate phosphoinositide phospholipase C, which generates a further second messenger inositol trisphosphate (I3P) by hydrolysing phosphatidylinositol-4,5-biphosphate (PIP2). I3P causes the endoplasmic reticulum to release Ca^{2+} and the accumulation of the metal ion in the cytoplasm triggers a range of physiological effects such as smooth muscle contraction. DAG can also activate phospholipase A2, leading to the deployment of yet another second messenger system based around arachidonic acid and its metabolites, such as thromboxane A2. These lipids are inflammatory mediators and can cause vasoconstriction which would promote the hypoxia that the obligate anaerobe *C. perfringens* requires to grow. All of the cellular effects described previously dysregulate further signal transduction pathways in endothelial cells, platelets, and neutrophils, which ultimately inhibit bacterial clearance or induce **thrombosis**, further **ischaemia** and promote the anaerobic niche that suits this bacterium.

FIGURE 15.15

Clostridium perfringens α-toxin is a phospholipase C which can lyse cells with certain membrane compositions. Its phospholipase C activity is described in the box illustrating the structure of one of its primary substrates phosphatidyl choline. It cleaves the bond between the hydroxyl group of the central glycerol unit and phosphocholine (yellow box), releasing it and its other product, diacylglycerol (DAG). α-Toxin can influence cellular physiology without causing lysis. Human phospholipase C has a key physiological role in releasing DAG a second messenger to indicate neurotransmitter or hormone binding within the cell. The production of DAG by the action of α-toxin can generate inappropriate signals. Protein kinase C (PKC) can be activated by DAG and then activate another phospholipase C that is specific for phosphoinositide, releasing inositol trisphophate (IP3), which acts as a second messenger that alters calcium management in the cell. Phospholipase A2 is also activated by DAG producing lipid intermediates that promote inflammation and vasoconstriction.

SELF-CHECK 15.15

What is the natural function of second messenger systems?

15.6.4 Cholesterol-dependent cytolysins

Pneumolysin is a well-studied member of the large cholesterol-dependent cytolysin family of pore-forming proteins. Although their amino acid sequences vary enormously, structural comparisons have revealed many similarities between the bacterial CDCs and human pore-forming immune proteins, like perforin and the membrane attack complex of the complement system.

FIGURE 15.16

Streptococcus pneumoniae produces the cholesterol-dependent cytotoxin, pneumolysin.
The protein binds cholesterol at the plasma membrane and can oligomerize to form a
circular pre-pore of about 44 monomers (top). The organization of the four domains of
pneumolysin is triggered which causes the penetration of the lipid bilayer to form a large
pore. The membrane is depolarized as ion gradient equilibrate through the large pore.
Osmosis drives the influx of water to the cell via the pore leading to cytolysis. The binding
of low doses of toxin to a cell can create smaller pores. Pneumolysin might also operate as
an invasin. It can generate actin polymerization at the cytoplasmic face of the membrane
by binding actin related protein (ARP) 2/3 complex.

As can be seen in Figure 15.16, after CDCs monomers bind cholesterol at the membrane surface they oligomerize (up to 44-monomers) to form a pre-pore. Extensive reorganization of
important α-helices forms a pair of β-hairpins; these associate with those formed in neighbouring subunits and insert into the membrane to create a pore. The normal ion fluxes across
the membrane are effectively short-circuited and it rapidly depolarizes resulting in cell death.

As we have seen with other virulence factors, pneumolysin is a very multi-faceted toxin. It
forms these characteristic membrane pores and cytolysis causes lung injury in pneumonia and
neuronal damage in meningitis. However, pneumolysin also activates the classical pathway of
complement and activates multiple signal transduction pathways; its induction of a pro-
inflammatory response through engaging TLR4 enhances tissue damage.

Furthermore, evidence is now emerging that pneumolysin also interacts with the actin cytoskeleton, both directly and indirectly. Low concentrations of pneumolysin alter the actin cytoskeleton via RhoA and Rac1 signalling; the modifications require protein kinase C and
membrane depolarization. This depolarization is brought about as membrane ion gradients

equilibrate through small pneumolysin pores that are created at low toxin concentration. Actin stress fibres, filopodia, and lamellipodia arise. The toxin itself also interacts with actin directly through the membrane. Interestingly, hepatocytes have been shown to engulf beads and bacteria coated in pneumolysin and its homologue listeriolysin from *Listeria monocytogenes*. This raises the possibility that these toxins might also function as invasins, maybe even promoting passage of these bacteria across the blood brain barrier when establishing meningitis. It has also been suggested that pneumolysin can cause damage to the cytosketal supports for the cilia of airway epitheliua, reducing the effectiveness of the mucociliary escalator and hence bacterial clearance.

15.6.5 Toxins that enter cells and disrupt cellular physiology

Thus far we have considered toxins that principally direct pathogenesis from the membrane surface either by interacting with its lipids or by engaging a surface receptor and then influencing cell biology by activating its related signalling machinery. Many toxins, however, cross membranes before exerting their toxicity and this property is reflected in a modular organization of their molecular structure. Two separable modules are recognized. One component is an active enzyme module that disrupts cellular physiology once it is in the correct cellular compartment. The second module is principally concerned with receptor binding and the translocation of the active module across membranes, directing the enzyme to the site where it exerts its effects. These modules are covalently linked but are separated to facilitate the release of the active module into the cytoplasm. This broad class of toxins is subdivided based on the molecular organization of these modules. Some toxins, like diphtheria toxin, carry all of the necessary functions on a single polypeptide and the modules are separated by proteolytic processing. Others described as binary or A-B toxins are formed from two independent polypeptides that are then covalently associated. Yet other toxins, such as cholera toxin, are constituted with an AB_5 stoichiometry.

Key Point

Despite differing molecular architectures, many toxins possess receptor binding and membrane translocation activities that support toxicity in a structural unit that is separable from a pathogenic enzymatic activity.

15.6.6 Diphtheria and cholera toxins modify key host proteins by ADP-ribosylation

Diphtheria toxin is encoded by a gene that forms part of a prophage of some strains of *Corynebacterium diphtheriae*. This is a very potent toxin that is almost entirely responsible for the pathogenesis of diphtheria, a severe pharyngitis, characterized clinically by a so-called 'bull neck' can result in the occlusion of the airways by a thick and leathery pseudomembrane.

Key Point

Some temperate or lysogenic bacteriophage can enter a 'resting' phase in which their genome is integrated into the bacterial chromosome as prophage.

The A and B modules of the toxin protein are covalently linked by a disulphide bond that is critical for the translocation of the A subunit to the cytoplasm of the host cell. The receptor binding domain of the B module uses a membrane-bound precursor of a heparin-binding epidermal growth factor-like molecule as a receptor. The peptide backbone between the two modules is then cleaved by a membrane-associated protease leaving A and B still covalently associated, but only by the disulphide bridge. The toxin is then internalized into an endosome and, as is common in endosomal trafficking, this vacuole is acidified. When the compartment reaches ~pH 5, the conformation of the translocation domain of the B module changes allowing it to enter the endosomal membrane and facilitate the passage of the A domain to the cytoplasm. Once there, the disulphide bridge that binds them is broken by reduction and the catalytic domain of the toxin is released to the cytoplasm. The enzyme activity carried on the toxin hydrolyses NAD^+ releasing nicotinamide and transferring ADP-ribose (ADPR) to a modified histidine residue (known as diphthamide) only found in elongation factor 2 (EF-2). This covalent modification of an important component of the translational machinery inhibits protein synthesis, killing the host cell.

Cross reference

See Section 15.4.2 of this chapter, and Figure 15.8.

ADP-ribosylation of a host protein is also the basis for the mode of action of the AB_5-configured cholera toxin of *Vibrio cholerae*. Figure 15.14 shows that it binds to the complex glycolipid GM1 ganglioside at the surface of enterocytes via its B subunit pentamer. After endocytosis, this toxin is directed to the endoplasmic reticulum. Here the disulphide bond between the A subunit and the B-pentamer is reduced and the active subunit is translocated to the cytoplasm. Here it modifies a subunit (Gsα) of a signalling GTPase protein by ADP-ribosylation. Its signalling is broadly analogous to what we saw with the Rho signalling GTPases, this now ADPR-modified Gsα is unable to hydrolyse bound GTP so remains permanently activated.

In turn, it activates adenylate cyclase which forms the intracellular messenger, cyclic AMP (cAMP). The rise in cAMP activates protein kinase A, which then activates the CFTR chloride ion channel. Diarrhoea then develops via the same mechanism as with STa. CFTR actively secretes Cl^- to the intestinal lumen, water, Na^+, K^+, and HCO_3^- follow. The severe diarrhoea that this causes rapidly dehydrates infected individuals and promotes dissemination of *Vibrio cholerae*.

15.7 Pan-genomes, mobile genetic elements, and the acquisition virulence factors

Like we saw with *C. diphtheriae* and diphtheria toxin, *V. cholerae* has acquired the cholera toxin gene by horizontal gene transfer, again carried on a **bacteriophage lysogen**. The acquisition of virulence factor genes from other sources via mobile genetic elements is in fact, a common theme in bacterial pathogenicity. The important Shiga-toxin of *Shigella* and *E. coli* O157:H7 is yet another prophage-encoded toxin. As you have progressed through this chapter, we have also considered the T3SS from the horizontally-acquired Spi-2 and LEE pathogenicity islands that direct the invasion of salmonellae or the development of A/E lesions in EPEC infection, the TSST-1 superantigen from the *Staphylococcus aureus* pathogenicity island SaPI-1 and the anti-phagocytic Ysc T3SS from *Yersinia* that is encoded on a virulence plasmid.

Your microbiology careers are beginning within the genomic age. The genomes of thousands of bacteria have now been sequenced. Analyses of the constantly growing databases of genomic sequence information show us that bacterial evolution is heavily influenced by

FIGURE 15.17

Diphtheria toxin B-domain binds a growth factor precursor at the cell surface as a receptor. The toxin's peptide backbone is cleaved between the enzymatically active (A) domain and the translocation domain (see scissor motif). The toxin enters the cell by endocytosis, acidification of the endosome leads rearrangements in the translocation domain (T) which allows the passage of the A domain to the cytoplasm, where it is release from the other domains by reducing the single disulphide bridge that binds them together. The A domain catalyses the hydrolysis of NAD (see structures), removing nicotinamide and transferring the ADP-ribose moiety to the unusual diphthamide (modified histidine) residue of elongation factor-2. This inhibits protein synthesis and ultimately kills the cell.

mobile genetic elements such as bacteriophage and plasmids. Collectively, a species such as *E. coli* has a core genome and an accessory genome. The core genome describes the 'essence' of the species encoding all of the basic functions that are common to each of its members. The accessory genome describes the variation within the species, the sequences that are not essential but provide advantages to bacteria in different environments. Together these core and accessory genomes are considered as the species' pan-genome. The *E. coli* pan-genome is estimated at around 13,000 genes, individual strains each carry 4,000–6,000 genes. These individual strain genomes are considered as mosaics, constructed through horizontal acquisitions as well as through conventional heredity. As *E. coli* exists in a rich and diverse niche where many opportunities arise for it to acquire genes from other organisms and increase its accessory genomic repertoire, it is considered as an open pan-genome. Consequently *E. coli* is a very diverse pathogen exhibiting considerable differences even in the six ways that its various pathotypes cause diarrhoea alone. Then we need to consider that members of this species also cause extraintestinal disease such as urinary tract infections and meningitis.

As our technical capabilities increase and sequencing costs decline, we are entering a new and exciting period of discovery in bacterial pathogenesis. We will undoubtedly learn much more about bacterial evolution and the emergence of pathogens and their genetic capabilities. As we also learn more about variation within the human genome, we should also better understand mechanisms that underpin some individuals' relative resistance to our adversaries. This fascinating subject is likely to become even more so!

 Chapter summary

Within this chapter we have seen that:

- Pathogenic bacteria can cause disease by a wide variety of mechanisms.

- Virulence is directed by defined factors that promote colonization, evade or dysregulate immunity, and disrupt tissue integrity or cellular physiology.

- Bacteria avoid mechanical clearance by firmly adhering to host surfaces using specific adhesins.

- Bacteria deploy various structural solutions to deliver adhesins to their marginal layers.

- Most pathogenic bacteria eventually invade tissues using toxins and invasins to acquire access.

- Bacteria commonly interfere with cellular signalling pathways to direct pathogenesis.

- Bacteria achieve cellular invasion by subverting the actin cytoskeleton.

- Some bacteria can directly inject effector proteins to the cytoplasm of host cells to mediate invasion or immune evasion.

- Bacteria defend against complement by producing inhibitors, recruiting host regulators of complement activation, or by hydrolysing key components.

- Bacteria coat their outer surfaces in polymers to avoid immune detection and opsonization by complement or immunoglobulins.

- Bacteria superantigens mould lymphocyte populations by stimulating large proportions of B- and T-cell repertoires.

- Bacterial toxins often interfere with second messenger systems to dysregulate cellular physiology.

- Some toxins are adapted to cross biological membranes in order to exert their toxicity.

- Virulence factors are often multifunctional and exemplify efficient use of genomic space.

- Some bacterial species have an open and extensive pan-genome that is heavily influenced by horizontal gene acquisitions.

Further reading

This chapter can best be supplemented and updated by your engagement with primary research literature. A convenient way to extend and deepen your knowledge of a particular aspect is to access these via recent review articles and database searching thereafter to catch the latest hot-off-the-press developments.

The restricted format of the chapter precludes a complete exploration of the virulence factor repertoire and its regulation in a single species or pathotypes. These are incredibly stimulating and enlightening, emphasizing the efficiencies imposed on a genome by natural selection driven by competition with other bacteria and millennia adapting to their human host and vice versa.

Here are a few that you might find useful. Explore, follow your strong personal interests, search skills and peripheral understanding should develop as you indulge yourself.

- Dubreuil JD. The whole Shebang: the gastrointestinal tract, *Escherichia coli* enterotoxins and secretion. *Current Issues in Molecular Biology* 2012; **14**(2): 71–82.

- Clements A, Young JC, Constantinou N, Frankel G. Infection strategies of enteric pathogenic *Escherichia coli. Gut Microbes*, 2012; **3**(2): 71–87.

- Marteyn B, Gazi A, Sansonetti P. Shigella: a model of virulence regulation in vivo. *Gut Microbes* 2012; **3**(2): 104–120.

  These reviews various aspects of diarrhoeal disease caused by an important group of pathogens.

  The first integrates important aspects of gut physiology well, the second describes diversity in pathotypes, and the third focuses on regulation of virulence in a related species.

- Mook-Kanamori BB, Geldhoff M, van der Poll T, van de Beek D. Pathogenesis and pathophysiology of pneumococcal meningitis. *Clinical Microbiology Reviews* 2011; **24**(3): 557–591.

  Another comprehensive review of the pathogenicity of a key bacterium.

- Kline KA, Fälker S, Dahlberg S, Normark S, Henriques-Normark B. Bacterial adhesins in host-microbe interactions. *Cell Host & Microbe*, 2009; **5**(6): 580–592.

  An accessible review article that explores structural aspects of bacterial adhesins and their interactions and ligands.

Discussion questions

15.1 What consequences might arise from a mutation in an adhesin gene of a human-specific pathogen?

15.2 What are the potential benefits of the pathogen producing both components of adhesin ligand pairing, like the EHEC/EPEC Tir/Intimin system?

15.3 *Clostridium perfringens* α-toxin can exert strong cytolytic activity and also more subtle non-lytic effects. How might the bacterium benefit from either scenario?

15.4 The *Streptococcus pneumoniae* CDC toxin pneumolysin is released from the bacterium when it lyses. How can this provide a selective advantage to the bacterium in establishing an infection?

15.5 Why have several bacteria evolved ADP-ribosylation as a pathogenic mechanism in different scenarios?

Molecular diagnostics

Jayne Harwood

Clinical microbiology laboratories have relied historically on phenotypic methods (i.e. culture and biochemical tests) or immunology-based methods (e.g. the enzyme-linked immunosorbent assay: ELISA) to detect and identify microorganisms, making this sometimes an impossible or time-consuming task with some of the more fastidious and slow growing organisms such as *Mycobacterium tuberculosis*, *Bartonella* spp., and *Mycoplasma pneumoniae*. The detection of viruses in the past was also culture based but used human/animal cell lines, as viruses do not grow under the same conditions as bacteria. Cell culture is no longer suitable for diagnosis of viral disease in particular. As a result, molecular methods have developed for the rapid detection of a range of microorganisms, but particularly for viral causes of disease.

Molecular methods are now well established as the 'gold standard' in non-clinical diagnosis of infectious disease. However, in practice, although the use of molecular methods is widespread, the number of molecular tests performed is still low compared to serological tests. The reason for this is that molecular methods are generally more complex and therefore more costly than the simple detection of an antigen or antibody.

Classical molecular techniques, such as the Southern blot, depend on the use of specific DNA/RNA probes for **hybridization**. The specificity of the reaction depends on the conditions used for hybridization.

These techniques may allow for the quantification of DNA/RNA present in the specimen. However, it is often found that the sensitivity of these techniques is comparable with other viral diagnostic methods such as serology.

More modern molecular techniques such as the polymerase chain reaction (PCR), ligase chain reaction (LCR), and nucleic acid sequence base amplification (NASBA) depend on some form of amplification of the target nucleic acid.

However, limitations in the use of molecular methods are rapidly being overcome allowing for the use of diverse technologies with expanding diagnostic capabilities. Molecular methods have been increasingly utilized to diagnose classic and fastidious pathogens since the advent of the PCR in 1983. Rapid identification methods using molecular techniques, which result in reduced turnaround times, have been introduced to deliver effective patient management and improved treatment regimes. New technologies that have been developed to detect, identify, and characterize microorganisms have significantly

Cross reference
See Chapter 13.

hybridization
Hybridization is the process of joining two complementary strands of DNA.

Cross reference
See Chapter 13.

improved the laboratory's ability to manage bacterial, fungal, and in particular, viral infections. Molecular techniques have not only enhanced the speed and sensitivity of detection but have allowed the laboratory to identify organisms that do not grow or grow only very slowly in culture. In addition to detection of the causative organism of an infection, molecular techniques also enable microbiologists to identify antibiotic resistance genes to help rationalize therapy and facilitate epidemiological studies. Many viruses do not grow in cell culture and the only way of detection is indirectly using the host's immune response by detecting IgM or IgG. However, this has changed dramatically with the advent of molecular techniques in that samples containing only a few virus particles can be examined and determined positive. This essentially means the particles themselves can be detected quickly, often days before the host's immune response in the form of IgM can be produced and in sufficient quantities to be detected. Whilst serological techniques are still widely used to diagnose viral infections, the most sensitive and specific method is the detection of the virus itself in the blood, cerebrospinal fluid (CSF), or respiratory tract.

Molecular techniques are highly sensitive and specific and have therefore revolutionized the diagnosis of disease and infections. Many large hospital laboratories and reference laboratories use techniques such as PCR, genome sequencing, molecular typing, and microarrays on a daily basis.

Learning objectives

After studying this chapter you should be able to:

- Understand and outline the principles of the PCR process.
- Recognize the different types of PCR.
- Have knowledge of the applications of molecular techniques in sample processing and routine diagnosis of infection.
- Know methods for the molecular typing of organisms in outbreak situations.

16.1 **Polymerase chain reaction (PCR)**

PCR provides an extremely sensitive method of amplifying small quantities of DNA. Despite the development of alternative amplification technologies, PCR remains the most widely used method in diagnostic laboratories for pathogen detection, since its invention in 1983 by Kary Mullis. PCR was made possible by the discovery of the enzyme *Taq* polymerase. This enzyme is a recombinant thermostable DNA polymerase from the organism *Thermus aquaticus*, and unlike normal polymerase enzymes is active at high temperatures. This enzyme joins together deoxynucleotides to form DNA.

Key Point

A polymerase is an enzyme whose function is the synthesis of polymers of nucleic acids. DNA polymerase and RNA polymerase are used to assemble DNA and RNA molecules, respectively, generally by copying a DNA or RNA template strand using base-pairing interactions.

PCR allows the *in vitro* amplification of specific target DNA sequences by a factor of 1×10^{12} after about 40 cycles and is therefore an extremely sensitive diagnostic technique. It is based on an enzymatic reaction involving the use of synthetic **oligonucleotides** flanking the target nucleic sequence of interest.

oligonucleotide
An oligonucleotide is a short fragment of single-stranded DNA that is typically 5–50 nucleotides long.

SELF-CHECK 16.1

What is unusual about the enzyme *Taq* polymerase and why was its discovery so important?

These oligonucleotides act as primers for the enzyme *Taq* polymerase. Repeated cycles of denaturation, annealing, and polymerization result in exponential production of the specific target fragment.

Key Point

Annealing means the process where complementary sequences of single-stranded DNA or RNA join by hydrogen bonds to form a double-stranded polynucleotide. The term is commonly used to describe the binding of a DNA probe, or the binding of a primer to a DNA strand during PCR.

Extraction and isolation of DNA is the key step before subsequent molecular analysis. Protocols vary and are dependent on the type of specimen, required yield, purity, and size of the nucleic acid. Most protocols are categorized as either liquid- or solid-phase extraction but they do share some common steps such as **cell lysis**, which is usually achieved through the addition of detergents, enzymes, or by physical disruption, and alcohol precipitation, which purifies and concentrates the DNA.

Key Point

The cells are lysed to allow the internal components of the cell to be exposed.

Liquid phase extraction is used when large quantities of DNA or large sample volumes are involved. Removal of cellular proteins and separation of genomic DNA through the use of an organic solvent, allows the isolation of the DNA with the removal of excess cellular proteins. This method does have disadvantages such as the unintentional loss of the DNA pellet when decanting the supernatant after centrifugation, and the use of hazardous chemicals, e.g. phenol-chloroform.

All steps of PCR are performed on the reaction mixture consisting of target DNA, primers, which need to be at least 18 nucleotides long, deoxyribonucleotide triphosphates (dNTPs: dATP, dTTP, dGTP, and dCTP), buffer and magnesium (Mg) salt, along with a DNA template, and the DNA *Taq* polymerase.

During the first stage, denaturation, the two strands of the helix of target DNA are unwound and separated by heating to 90–95°C for 15 seconds to 1 minute. Denaturation is possible because the hydrogen bonds linking the bases to one another are quite weak. The hydrogen bonds break at high temperatures, whereas the stronger covalent bonds between deoxyribose and phosphates remain intact.

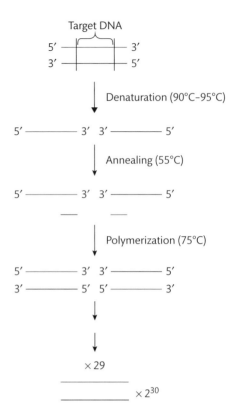

FIGURE 16.1

The basic steps of PCR showing the stages of the reaction and the temperature required for each stage.

The second stage is called annealing or hybridization. The goal of PCR is not to replicate the entire strand of DNA but to replicate a target sequence of approximately 100–600 base pairs unique to the organism being studied. Targeting the sequence is achieved using primers. Primers mark the ends of the target sequence. The primers bind (anneal) to their complementary bases on the single-stranded DNA. This step requires a much cooler temperature, 55°C for 15 seconds to 2 minutes.

Finally, during extension or polymerization (at 75°C for 15 s to 3 min), the *Taq* polymerase reads the template strand and quickly matches it with the appropriate nucleotides, resulting in two new helixes consisting of part of the original strand and the complementary strand that was just assembled (Figure 16.1). The process is repeated 25–40 times, each cycle doubling the amount of the target DNA. The more DNA there is, the easier it is to detect.

The process of transferring the tubes to different temperatures was once a labour intensive, manual process but this has been circumvented by the use of highly automated instruments called thermocyclers.

Key Point

Every cycle results in a doubling of the number of strands of DNA present.

SELF-CHECK 16.2

Why does denaturation take place at high temperatures?

Whilst the PCR process is highly automated and has been optimized over many years there are still several factors which have a significant bearing on the success of the PCR reaction. These are:

- Concentration of Mg^{2+}; since *Taq* polymerase is a magnesium-dependent enzyme, each combination of target DNA and primer requires a unique concentration of Mg^{2+}.
- Concentration and source of thermostable polymerase.
- Concentration and purity of both target DNA and primer.
- Denaturing temperature, annealing temperature, and time of reaction.
- Number of cycles.

Common problems in PCR are false negatives due to presence of PCR inhibitors, poor nucleic acid isolation, poor sample preparation, and poor amplification efficiency. False positives are due to contamination of the sample with other DNA. Common sources of error are:

- False positive reactions are caused by contamination with new or previously amplified DNA.
- Non-specific primer hybridization. Binding of primers to an area other than the desired region. This results in false positive reactions.
- Primer–dimer formation. This condition can arise if the two primers used are complementary to each other and end up hybridizing with each other rather than with the target. This may lead to little or no amplification of the target sequence.
- Background hybridization occurs as a result of non-specific binding of only one of the primers. This results in the amplification of the target DNA 30 times after 30 cycles and not exponentially.
- Primer artefact formation can occur in conditions of low **stringency**, small target amounts, too much enzyme in early cycles, high primer concentration, and excessive thermal cycling. This often occurs when the polymerase enzyme generates new primer binding sites for the same or other primer. This decreases the efficiency of PCR by consuming and competing with target for other reaction components.

Key Point

Detection of sequences with moderate or high similarity depends on how stringent the hybridization conditions were applied — high stringency, such as high hybridization temperature and low salt in hybridization buffers, permits only hybridization between nucleic acid sequences that are highly similar, whereas low stringency, such as lower temperature and high salt, allows hybridization when the sequences are less similar.

SELF-CHECK 16.3

What are the common problems with PCR?

In order to limit the spread of **amplicon** from one PCR to another, a multiple room approach is usually adopted. Preparation of primers, PCR buffers, and dNTPS is performed in one room. Preparations of PCR assay except the addition of target nucleic acid is done in another room. Processing of the specimen, preparation, and the addition of the target nucleic acid is done in yet another room. PCR cycles for amplification are performed in another room and finally the detection of the amplicon is performed in the last room. This means that at least five separated

amplicon

An amplicon is a piece of DNA or RNA that is the product of natural or artificial amplification or replication.

rooms are needed to perform PCR. The amplified products should never be carried to the preceding rooms to avoid contamination.

Key Point

Think back to how small bacteria and fungal spores are in particular and the fact they exist in large numbers environmentally. As a result one fungal spore can produce a false positive PCR if that is the species trying to be detected. Never forget the consequences of a false positive or negatives in patient management.

16.1.1 Detection of PCR products

Cross reference
See Section 16.7.1, this chapter.

Detection of DNA sequence products of the PCR assay may be performed in several ways. The least sensitive and specific method is to size fractionate the reaction product on an agarose or acylamide gel and stain the DNA with ethidium bromide (highly toxic). A more sensitive technique involves the attachment of DNA to a membrane through blot techniques followed by hybridization with a labelled homologous oligonucleotide probe. Alternatively, the PCR product may be probed directly by liquid oligomeric hybridization. However, these techniques provide no information on size of the amplified product and thus could not exclude the possibility that the product originated from a region of the human genome which exhibits homology with the target viral sequence. The most sensitive and specific detection methods result from combining the size information of gel electrophoresis with the improved sensitivity and specificity of hybridization techniques. This may be achieved by gel electrophoresis followed by Southern transfer and hybridization, or through liquid oligomeric hybridization followed by gel electrophoresis.

16.2 **Variations of PCR**

16.2.1 Reverse transcriptase PCR (RT-PCR)

Single-stranded RNA molecules cannot be amplified as described previously. In order to detect viral nucleic acid of RNA viruses (e.g. HIV) in clinical specimens, an additional step is performed before the PCR cycles are initiated. This procedure is termed reverse transcriptase PCR (RT-PCR). The RNA sequence is first converted to a double-stranded nucleic acid sequence (complementary DNA: cDNA) by using a reverse transcriptase enzyme from a retrovirus. To achieve this, a primer is annealed to the template RNA. Using this primer, reverse transcriptase synthesizes a cDNA strand by adding complementary base pairs. The template RNA is removed using an RNAse enzyme, leaving behind the newly generated single-stranded cDNA. This cDNA sequence can then be amplified using the same PCR cycles as previously described.

16.2.2 Real-time PCR

The development of 'real-time' PCR has added a huge advantage to traditional PCR. This technique allows for the real-time quantification of PCR product following each of the 40 amplification cycles. Conventional PCR methods only produce a signal of amplified product, e.g. by running an ELISA on the amplified product or by electrophoretic separation. Quantitative analysis is only possible during the early stages of the PCR assay, where reagents are in excess

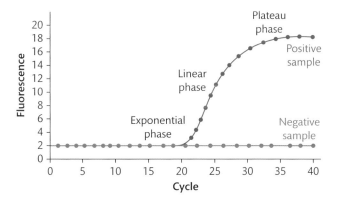

FIGURE 16.2

Real-time PCR. In this graph, the number of PCR cycles is shown on the x-axis, and the fluorescence from the amplification reaction, which is proportional to the amount of amplified product in the tube, is shown on the y-axis. This amplification graph shows two phases, an exponential phase followed by a non-exponential plateau phase. During the exponential phase, the amount of PCR product approximately doubles in each cycle. As the reaction proceeds, however, reaction components are consumed, and ultimately one or more of the components becomes limiting. At this point, the reaction slows and enters the plateau phase.

and the amount of amplified product is small. Real-time PCR allows the amplification and quantification of template DNA in a sample by establishing the number of copies present by working in the early (exponential) phase of amplification (Figure 16.2). All current methods rely on the production of a fluorescent signal.

A fluorescent dye such as SYBR Green is included in the PCR mixture and the level of fluorescence is monitored throughout the reaction. SYBR Green binds strongly to double-stranded DNA (dsDNA) and an increase in fluorescence is directly proportional to the amount of dsDNA produced. A calibration curve is produced by running a series of standards containing known amounts of dsDNA.

A computerized 'real-time' PCR instrument measures the amount of fluorescence emitted after each cycle.

As real-time PCR assays are amenable to automation, they provide a shorter turnaround time than conventional PCRs and, as such, have become a popular choice for performing molecular tests in the clinical laboratory setting. However, cost is a limiting factor in the implementation of these assays in smaller laboratories with limited resources.

SELF-CHECK 16.4

What is the difference between PCR and RT-PCR?

16.2.3 Nested PCR

Further sensitivity and specificity may be obtained by the nested PCR technique, whereby the DNA is amplified in two steps. This may be useful when the number of DNA copies is very small (i.e. a single DNA molecule from a bacterial genome) or if the sample is degraded (e.g. a sample from a forensic case).

FIGURE 16.3

Nested PCR.

In the first step, an initial pair of primers is used to generate a long sequence that contains the DNA target sequence. A small amount of this product is used in a second round of amplification, which employs primers to the final target DNA.

Nested PCR (Figure 16.3) may be performed in a single tube method or a 'two-tubes' method. In the single tube method, both the external and internal primer sets are added at the same time. There are then two different methods to accomplish nested PCR is a single tube, one method involves physical separation of the two primer sets and the other method involves differing annealing temperatures of the primers.

In the physical separation method, the tube is filled with the primary mixture consisting of target DNA, the external set of primers, and the remaining necessary components. This is overlaid with a mineral oil layer into which the internal set of primers and the necessary components have been inserted. After the first round of 25–30 cycles of PCR, the reaction mixture is spun to mix the internal primer and other components held inside the oil layer. A second round of 25–30 cycles of PCR is performed and the products are then analysed.

In the differential annealing temperature method, the reaction mixture is set up to contain both the external and internal sets of primer. These primer sets are designed so that the external primer sets hybridize with the target at a lower temperature than that required for hybridization of the internal primer sets. Switching to a higher temperature allows amplification of the internal product.

In the two-tubes method, the target is amplified using only the external primer sets after 25–30 PCR cycles. After this, the tube is opened and the mixture is transferred to a second tube containing the internal primer sets which hybridizes to the amplicon generated using the external primers. After running 25–30 CPR cycles, the products can be analysed.

16.2.4 Multiplex PCR

Multiplex PCR consists of multiple primers within a single PCR mixture to produce amplicons of varying size that are specific to different DNA sequences (Figure 16.4). By targeting multiple genes at once, additional information may be gained from a single-test run that

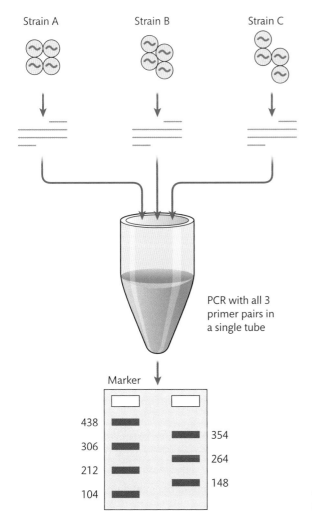

FIGURE 16.4
Multiplex PCR. This diagram shows three different strains undergoing PCR together in one tube.

would otherwise require several different PCR runs. This technique has the potential to produce savings in time and effort within the laboratory. This method is commonly used to detect multiple viruses in the same respiratory sample for example, otherwise it would require, say, six different reactions which is both time-consuming and expensive.

Advantages of multiplex PCR include:

- Potential problems in a single PCR include false negatives due to reaction failure or false positives due to contamination. False negatives are often revealed in multiplex assays because each amplicon provides an internal control for the other amplified fragments.

- The expense of reagents and preparation time is less in multiplex PCR than in PCR where several tubes of uniplex PCRs are used. A multiplex PCR is ideal for conserving costly polymerase and templates in short supply.

16.2.5 Ligase chain reaction

Ligase chain reaction (LCR) is a method of DNA amplification which differs from PCR in that it amplifies the probe molecule rather than producing amplicons through polymerization of nucleotides. Two probes are used for each DNA strand and are ligated together to form a single probe. LCR uses both a DNA polymerase enzyme and a DNA ligase enzyme, which joins together DNA fragments, to drive the reaction. Like PCR, LCR requires a thermocycler to drive the reaction and each cycle results in doubling of the target nucleic acid sequence. LCR can have a greater specificity than PCR but it is required that the exact sequence in the region being amplified is known.

SELF-CHECK 16.5

What is the difference between a DNA polymerase enzyme and a DNA ligase enzyme?

16.3 **Advantages and disadvantages of PCR**

The advantages of PCR include:

- Extremely high sensitivity – may detect down to one viral genome per sample volume.
- Easy to set up.
- Fast turnaround time.

The disadvantages of PCR include:

- Liable to contamination.
- High degree of operator skill required.
- Not easy to quantify results.
- A positive result may be difficult to interpret, especially when latent viruses such as cytomegalovirus (CMV), are detected in a previously infected individual as they will have virus present in their blood, irrespective of whether they have disease or not.
- Expensive to buy equipment and set up assays so laboratories must have sufficient samples to justify the cost and expertise required.

The first three problems have been addressed by the arrival of commercially available systems, such as the Roche Cobas Amplicor, which requires minimum sample handling. However, if using in-house PCR assays avoiding contamination is the key to successful PCR. Contamination can occur from the operator (e.g. skin cells), from previous PCR runs, airborne microbes, and positive control material used in the assay. To avoid contamination it is essential that:

- A laminar flow cabinet, which is situated in a segregated room, should be used.
- Separate supplies of PCR equipment, e.g. pipettes, reagents, microfuge tubes, should be used. There must also be separate sets for sample preparation, reagents, and product analysis to avoid cross-contamination.
- All buffers, deionized water, pipette tips, and tubes should be autoclaved to guarantee sterility.
- Disposable gloves should be worn at all times and these must be changed frequently by the operators of the assays.

The use of synthetic internal competitive targets in these commercial assays has facilitated the quantification of results. Otherwise, the same problems remain with in-house PCR methods. The sensitivity would normally be sufficient if a single PCR reaction was used followed by hybridization with a specific oligonucleotide probe. This is the approach taken by commercial assays. The fourth problem is more difficult to resolve but it is generally found that patients with active disease have a much higher viral load than those who do not. This limitation can also be overcome by using RT-PCR.

Key Point

PCR is very sensitive. One of the main problems is contamination with 'foreign' DNA. Great care is required to avoid contamination during the amplification stages.

16.4 Applications

Whilst PCR can be used for many purposes the best uses are in the detection/identification of non-culturable or slow-growing organisms such as mycobacteria and viruses. PCR is now commonly being used to identify *Mycobacterium tuberculosis* in respiratory samples. This method gives a much improved turnaround time (2–3 days compared to up to 6 weeks for culture). This quicker diagnosis allows for improved contact tracing and containment of potential outbreaks.

Cross reference
See Chapter 9.

Chlamydia trachomatis and *Neisseria gonorrhoea* are the two main agents of sexually transmitted infections. Culture of *N. gonorrhoeae* is performed using selective media and from culture, antibiotic resistance testing can be performed. *C. trachomatis* isolation requires eukaryotic cell systems because of its strict intracellular lifestyle. Serological assays for *C. trachomatis* lack specificity. PCR-based techniques are now considered reference diagnostic methods for these organisms, allowing a rapid, sensitive and specific detection of *C. trachomatis* and *N. gonorrhoeae* from urogenital samples. However, if a sample is found to be positive for *N. gonorrhoea*, a swab for culture must be taken from the patient and submitted to the laboratory to allow growth of the organism and for antibiotic resistance testing to be performed. Antibiotic resistance in *N. gonorrhoeae* is beginning to give cause for concern, with resistance to the first-line agents, ceftriaxone, and azithromycin, being reported globally.

Multiplex PCR is used commonly for the diagnosis of respiratory viruses as up to 19 viruses can be detected from one sample; these include the common causes of respiratory infections such as influenza A and B, respiratory syncytial virus and adenovirus. Multiplex PCR has proved to be a powerful tool for investigating meningitis and encephalitis caused by a variety of viruses. In neurological disease the requirement of rapid and reliable diagnosis to provide a rational basis for chemotherapy and limit unnecessary procedures and irrelevant therapy has driven development. A wide range of viruses are associated with neurological disease including herpes simplex virus (HSV), CMV, varicella-zoster virus (VZV), Epstein–Barr virus (EBV), and the enterovirus group. In view of the large number of potentially neuroinvasive viruses and because of the limited volume of the most useful diagnostic specimen – cerebrospinal fluid (CSF) – a number of multiplex PCRs have been developed.

Quantitative multiplex PCR for EBV, CMV, and adenovirus has been developed to measure the viral loads of these viruses in immunocompromised patients, such as solid organ transplant recipients and haematological-oncology patients.

16.4.1 HIV viral load monitoring

Treatment of HIV positive patients has advanced greatly by the measurement of the amount of HIV virus in the patient's bloodstream. EDTA plasma is the preferred sample for RNA-based viral load testing. A large sample volume (>1 mL of plasma) is needed for a lower limit detection level of 50 copies/mL. This lower limit level is optimal for treatment monitoring.

EDTA plasma can be stored at room temperature for 30 hours, 14 days at 4°C, or for longer periods of time at −70°C without significant decreases in viral load signal.

HIV viral load is usually reported as copies of HIV in a millilitre (mL) of blood. Changes in viral load are usually reported as a log change (in powers of 10). For example, a three log increase in viral load (3 Log10) is an increase of 10^3 or 1000 times the previously reported level, while a drop from 500,000 to 500 copies would be a three-log-drop (also 3 Log10). The HIV viral load is used to predict how long an infected person will remain healthy, or how quickly the disease will progress. A viral load greater than 100,000 copies/mL of blood within 6 months of sero-conversion, i.e. after initially getting infected, indicates that the patient has a greater likelihood of developing AIDS within 5 years. A viral load less than 10,000 copies/mL of blood in the early stages indicates a decreased risk of developing AIDS.

While receiving anti-retroviral therapy (ART) some patients with continual undetectable viral load measurements may experience a low level increase in viral load, (usually less than 500 copies/mL blood) and then on repeat testing return to an undetectable level. These transient 'blips' do not indicate that the virus is developing resistance to drug therapy. Blips appear to be more common in the winter, suggesting a connection with illness such as colds and influenza. Viral load blips are partially explained by various patient-related factors, and thought to be relatively common. High level and sustained increases in viral load are frequently related to the development of drug resistance and/or viral mutations, and often changes in ART are required.

16.5 **DNA sequencing**

DNA sequencing is the process of determining the precise order of nucleotides within a DNA molecule. It includes any method which can be used to determine the order of the four bases; adenine (A), guanine (G), cytosine (C), and thymine (T), in a strand of DNA. DNA sequencing enables us to perform a thorough analysis of DNA because it provides us with the sequence of nucleotides.

During the late 1970s, two DNA sequencing techniques were invented. These were the Sanger method, also called dideoxynucleotide sequencing or chain termination sequencing, and the Maxam–Gilbert method. The latter method is based on nucleotide-specific cleavage and is utilized mostly to sequence oligonucleotides usually smaller than 50 base-pairs in length. Because these methods use radioactive labelling and are technically complex routine use is greatly discouraged. The Sanger method is more commonly used as it is technically easier to apply and with the advent of PCR and automation, it can be applied to longer strands of DNA – including entire genes. This method is based on chain termination by dideoxynucleotides during PCR elongation reactions.

16.5.1 The Sanger method

In the Sanger method, the DNA strand to be analysed is used as a template (Figure 16.5). The region of DNA to be sequenced is amplified using PCR and then denatured to produce a single-stranded DNA. A sequencing primer is then annealed to the single-stranded DNA.

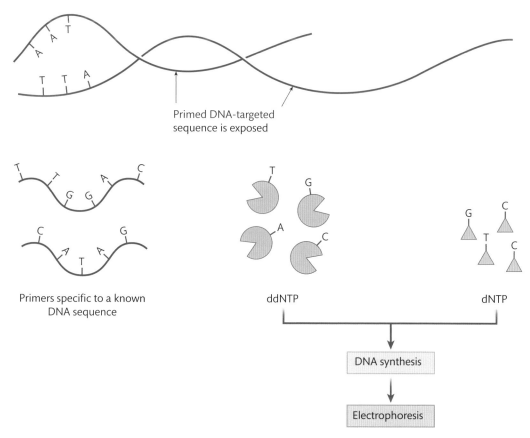

Primed DNA-targeted
sequence is exposed

Primers specific to a known
DNA sequence

ddNTP

dNTP

DNA synthesis

Electrophoresis

FIGURE 16.5
The Sanger method for DNA sequencing.

Four different PCR reaction mixtures are prepared, each containing a certain percentage of dideoxynucleotide triphosphate (ddNTP) analogues to one of the four nucleotides (ATP, CTP, GTP, or TTP). Dideoxynucleotides are essentially the same as nucleotides except they contain a hydrogen group on the 3′ carbon instead of a hydroxyl group (OH). These modified nucleotides, when integrated into a DNA sequence, prevent the addition of further nucleotides and therefore stop the elongation of the DNA chain. This occurs because a phosphodiester bond cannot form between the dideoxynucleotide and the next incoming nucleotide. Synthesis of the new DNA strand continues until one of these analogues is incorporated, at which time the strand is prematurely truncated (stopped). Each PCR reaction will end up containing a mixture of different lengths of DNA strands, all ending with the nucleotide that was dideoxy labelled for that reaction. Gel electrophoresis can then be used to separate the strands of the four reactions, in four separate lanes, and the sequence of the original template can be determined based on what lengths of strands end with which nucleotide.

Nucleic acid sequencing has emerged as an important tool for pathogen identification. Historically, DNA sequencing had been used for identification of organisms that were difficult to identify by conventional phenotypic methods and the test only offered in reference laboratory facilities. However, in recent years DNA target sequencing for rapid identification of bacterial, viral, and fungal pathogens has been increasingly utilized as a routine procedure by clinical laboratories. Guidelines have been published that provide interpretative criteria for identification of a wide range of clinically important bacteria and fungi to the species and genus levels.

In bacteria, the rRNA genes (5S, 16S, and 23S) have been commonly used for taxonomic purposes. These genes are universally present, are only minimally affected by horizontal gene transfer, and contain hypervariable regions flanked by high sequence conservation. These characteristics have made the 16S rRNA gene the most widely used region for bacterial taxonomy and identification. The sequence information retrieved from the 5' portion of the 16S rRNA gene often provides sufficient data for identification purposes. Much of the data in public databases also correlates to this region of the 16S rRNA gene.

SELF-CHECK 16.6

What are the uses of DNA sequencing and what information does it provide for patient management?

16.5.2 Applications of DNA sequencing

Amplification and sequencing of the gene encoding 16S ribosomal RNA using universal primers has become widely used in clinical laboratories for the identification of bacteria at the genus and species level, either after their isolation or increasing directly from clinical samples. The 16S RNA is the smaller subunit of the bacterial ribosome and is thought to be the most conserved sequence. It has a constant sequence that is common to most microorganisms and a variable sequence that is unique to a specific genus or species. This technique allows rapid and wide-spectrum detection of bacteria, especially in patients with culture-negative samples due to previous antimicrobial administration, as it can detect bacterial nucleic acid present in a sample through targeting conserved bacterial sequences. Nucleic acid sequencing of amplicon allows identification of the organism(s) by comparison with known sequences in public databases. It is often successful, provided that a single bacterium is present in the clinical sample. Almost all clinical samples can be tested by this technique, but those that are contaminated with commensal flora are not suitable. Examples of possible applications include detection of bacteria responsible for meningitis (CSF), endocarditis (heart valves), arthritis (joint fluid), and deep abscesses. Increasingly, this approach is also being used to identify the putative pathogen(s) in a number of inflammatory diseases, and for detection of known pathogens that are not easily diagnosed using standard methods. *Tropheryma whippelii* was identified as the cause of Whipple's disease using this method.

Substantial increases in the sensitivity of the 16S sequencing reactions can be achieved when clinical samples undergo prior culture enrichment in broth.

The universal 16S rRNA gene target and the high sensitivity of PCR can be a limitation due to false positive test results when analysing clinical samples. Even small amounts of bacterial DNA contamination either within the clinical sample, or introduced during some part of the molecular procedure may result in a false positive result, or a result that is difficult to interpret because of the amplification of one or more common commensal organism(s).

SELF-CHECK 16.7

If 16S testing is so accurate and detects both viable and non-viable bacteria in clinical samples, why are all samples not just analysed in this way?

16.6 **Molecular typing**

There are a number of scenarios where it is necessary to characterize a microbial isolate beyond the species level and determine its sub-species or strain. Molecular typing is used to:

- Relate individual cases to an outbreak of infectious disease e.g. *Salmonella* typing in an outbreak of food poisoning.

- Establish an association between an outbreak of food poisoning and a specific food vehicle.

- Study variations in pathogenicity, virulence, and antibiotic resistance of individual strains within a species.

- Trace sources of contaminants within a manufacturing process.

Pulse-field gel electrophoresis (PFGE) has been the 'gold standard' technique used by clinical laboratories to examine the molecular relatedness of bacterial and fungal isolates.

Pulse-field gel electrophoresis is a technique used for the separation of large DNA molecules by applying an electric field to a gel matrix that periodically changes direction (Figure 16.6). The procedure for this technique is relatively similar to performing a standard gel electrophoresis except that instead of constantly running the voltage in one direction, the voltage is periodically switched among three directions; one that runs through the central axis of the gel and two that run at an angle of 60° either side. The pulse times are equal for each direction resulting in a net forward migration of the DNA. For extremely large bands (up to around 2 Mb), switching-interval ramps can be used that increases the pulse time for each direction over the course of a number of hours: take, for instance, increasing the pulse linearly from 10 seconds at 0 hours to 60 seconds at 18 hours.

This procedure takes longer than normal gel electrophoresis (Figure 16.7) due to the size of the fragments being resolved and the fact that the DNA does not move in a straight line through the gel.

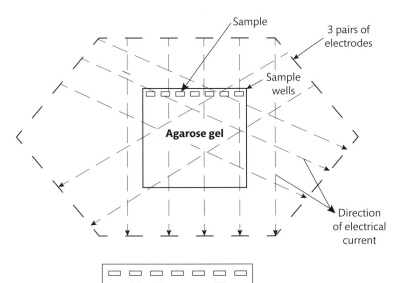

FIGURE 16.6

Pulse-field gel electrophoresis. This diagram shows the three different directions of the electrical current. The bands on the gel represent the DNA fragments.

FIGURE 16.7
Gel electrophoresis. This photograph shows the bands generated by PFGE. The bands at either end are produced from a DNA ladder. A DNA ladder is a solution of DNA molecules with known molecular weights. It is applied to an agarose gel as a reference to estimate the size of unknown DNA molecules. The test samples can be compared to this to ascertain the molecular size of the components.

Lanes 1 and 10: DNA ladder – Solution of DNA molecules of different lengths used in agarose gel electrophoresis.

Lanes 2–8: Samples.

PFGE may be used for genotyping or genetic fingerprinting. It is commonly considered a gold standard in epidemiological studies of pathogenic organisms. Subtyping has made it easier to discriminate among strains of *Listeria monocytogenes* for example and thus to link environmental or food isolates with clinical infections.

16.6.1 Multilocus sequence typing (MLST)

Multilocus sequence typing (MLST) is a technique which characterizes isolates of microbial species using the DNA sequences of internal fragments of multiple housekeeping genes. Approximately 450–500 base pair internal fragments of each gene are used. For each housekeeping gene, the different sequences present within a bacterial species are assigned as distinct alleles and, for each isolate, the alleles at each of the loci define the profile or sequence type.

The principle of MLST is simple; the technique involves PCR amplification followed by DNA sequencing. Nucleotide differences between strains can be checked at a variable number of genes depending on the degree of discrimination required.

MLST has been used in the typing of *Campylobacter* species, *Staphylococcus aureus*, *Streptococcus pyogenes* (Group A streptococcus), and *Candida albicans*.

16.6.2 Restriction fragment length polymorphism (RFLP)

RFLP is a technique which relies on the base pair changes in restriction sites, which arise due to mutations. Restriction site sequences range from 4–12 bases in length. When cleaved by the specific endonuclease enzyme, the average length of the fragment obtained is determined in part by the base pair recognized by the enzyme.

Once the desired target DNA, for example, a bacterial chromosome or plasmid, is cut using a known restriction enzyme, the resultant fragments are separated by electrophoresis on agarose or polyacrylamide gel. Upon separation on gel, the fragments can be visualized as bands after staining with ethidium bromide (which binds to dsDNA) and viewed under UV light. Depending on the numbers of fragments and their sizes either discreet or overlapping bands are seen. These bands can be transferred to nylon membranes for hybridization.

This technique is very useful as an epidemiological tool as it can be used to type isolates. The DNA of two or more isolates is subjected to digestion by the same restriction endonuclease enzyme, the fragments are separated by electrophoresis and the bands are compared. Another important application is ribotyping. The 16S RNA is the smaller subunit of the bacterial ribosome and is thought to be the most conserved sequence. It has a constant sequence that is common to most microorganisms and a variable sequence that is unique to a specific genus or species. Such sequences can be subjected to RFLP to determine relatedness with other organisms and can be confirmed by following with Southern blotting (discussed in Section 16.7.1).

Similar DNA fragment-based methods have also been developed and used for clinical analyses including: restriction endonuclease finger-printing analysis, plasmid typing, and ribotyping.

Key Point

Restriction sites are strands of DNA that are specifically recognized and cleaved by restriction endonucleases. A restriction endonuclease is an enzyme that cuts DNA at or near specific recognition nucleotide sequences known as restriction sites.

16.7 DNA microarrays

Two relatively recent advances have revolutionized research and the clinical management of infectious disease; these being the completion of the human genome project (2003) along with the sequencing of many pathogen genomes, and the development of microarray technology. These two together allow for exploring the molecular pathogenesis of infectious disease. The complex genetic processes underlying the interaction between microorganisms and their hosts have proved invaluable to the understanding of these diseases with the consequent improvements in the diagnosis, treatment, and prevention of infectious disease.

A microarray is a tool for analysing gene expression that consists of a small glass membrane or glass slide containing samples of many genes/nucleic acids arranged in a regular pattern. Microarrays have been a significant advance because they may contain a very large number of genes and because their small size is useful when trying to survey a large number of genes quickly, or when the sample to be studied is small. This technology is still considered to be in its infancy in terms of routine use but the technology is likely to be very important in the future diagnosis of infection.

DNA microarrays are small, solid supports onto which the sequences of thousands of different genes are immobilized, or attached, at fixed locations. These are created by robotic machines. The supports themselves are usually glass microscope slides, but may be silicon chips or nylon membranes. The DNA is printed, spotted, or synthesized directly onto the support. Researchers have a database of over 40,000 gene sequences they can use for this purpose.

It is important that the gene sequences in a microarray are attached to their support in an orderly or fixed way, because the operator uses the location of each spot in the array to identify a particular gene sequence. The spots can be DNA, cDNA, or oligonucleotides.

The whole process is based on hybridization probing, a technique that uses fluorescently labelled nucleic acid molecules as 'mobile probes' to identify complementary molecules; sequences that are able to base-pair with one another. Each single-stranded DNA fragment is made up of four different nucleotides; adenine, thymine, guanine, and cytosine, linked end to end. Adenine is the complement of thymine, i.e. it will always pair with thymine. Guanine is the complement of cytosine. Therefore, the complementary sequence G-T-C-T-A will be C-A-G-A-T. When the two complementary sequences find other, such as the immobilized target DNA and the mobile probe DNA, cDNA, or messenger RNA (mRNA), they will lock together (hybridize). The principle of nucleic hybridization is not new, however microarrays have allowed the parallel detection and analysis of the patterns and expression of thousands of genes in a single experiment. A DNA microarray experiment is performed as shown in Figure 16.8.

There are two main types of microarrays, these being spotted DNA and oligonucleotide arrays.

The spotted DNA method entails attaching a single-strand or dissociated double-strand DNA to the slide. This DNA may come from a cDNA library or it may be genomic products amplified by PCR. In most slides, duplicate spots are attached as controls. The DNA in each spot is usually a whole gene or expressed sequence tag and is about 300–800 nucleotides long. Two DNA samples, usually a test and a control, are fluorescently labelled with dyes. One is usually labelled with Cy5 (red) and the other with Cy3 (green). This enables differentiation of the two samples. The two samples are then incubated with the microarray slide and the fluorescently labelled probe DNA hybridizes to the immobilized target DNA with high sensitivity and specificity. The slide is then read in a scanner which consists of a laser, microscope and camera. The fluorescent labels are excited by the laser, and the microscope and camera create a digital

FIGURE 16.8
DNA microarray.

image of the array. This can be stored on a computer and the red-to-green fluorescence ratio can be calculated using computer software. The intensity of the red and green fluorescence at each spot is proportional to the amount of Cy5 and Cy3-labelled cDNA respectively that has hybridized to the DNA at that spot. If a particular gene is very active, it produces many molecules of mRNA, thus, more labelled cDNAs, which hybridize to the DNA on the slide and generate a very bright fluorescent area. Genes that are less active produce fewer mRNAs, thus, fewer labelled cDNAs, which result in dimmer fluorescent spots. If there is no fluorescence, none of the messenger RNA molecules have hybridized to the DNA, indicating that the gene is inactive.

For the oligonucleotide arrays, the oligonucleotides are either spotted as described earlier or directly synthesized *in situ* on to the solid substrate. There is no need for an attachment method using this array. Each nucleotide is usually about 50–70 nucleotides long. Over the slide there are several different oligonucleotide sequences from the same gene. The same gene can be probed independently several times in the same experiment allowing for more robust results to be generated. For every approximately 20 nucleotide sequence there is a duplicate sequence with a single base change. This is termed a mismatch, which allows comparison between hybridization to a specific sequence and background hybridization to a non-specific sequence. This generates a 'true' quantification of sample.

SELF-CHECK 16.8

What are the two types of DNA microarray? What are the differences between the two?

16.7.1 Applications of DNA microarrays

Microarrays appear to be an ideal technology for clinical microbiology laboratories because pathogens can be detected, identified, genotyped, and further profiled to determine antimicrobial resistance and virulence traits (Table 16.1). Traditionally this work was carried out on laboratory cultures. Often this was limited by slow growing organisms. Consequently, information regarding phenotypes cannot be produced in a timely manner to be clinically relevant.

Microarrays are commonly used in epidemiological investigations. Genomic variations can be characterized and differentiation between strains can be performed.

The use of DNA arrays for typing has been demonstrated in both HIV and *M. tuberculosis*. Resistance genes against rifampicin in *M. tuberculosis* have been detected using this method.

There are various analysers being developed, which employ DNA microarray technology for the identification of bacterial isolates. One such analyser is the PLEX-ID (Abbott Laboratories) whereby bacterial and fungal DNA can be detected directly from samples thus bypassing the need for culture. It is likely that such systems whilst very expensive will become more embedded in diagnostic laboratories of the future.

Key Point

Just because something is expensive for a laboratory to buy should not necessarily preclude its purchase, as there may be enormous clinical benefits in determining septicaemia rapidly, for example. Think of morbidity, mortality, more appropriate use of antibiotics, etc. when examining such systems.

TABLE 16.1 Applications of DNA microarrays.

Application	Explanation
Diagnosis – organism identification, identification of novel pathogens	The use of DNA sequences to identify organisms
Epidemiology – outbreaks	Look for differences in DNA sequences to determine the relatedness of organisms isolated in outbreak situations
Antimicrobial resistance	Look for mutations and genes that give rise to antimicrobial resistance, e.g. *UL97* and *UL54* genes in CMV giving rise to ganciclovir resistance

16.8 Nucleic acid hybridization

The two strands of a DNA molecule can be separated by exposing the DNA to high temperature, low salt concentration, or by the addition of various chemicals. The process of denaturation or melting can be reversed by lowering the temperature, lowering the salt concentration, or removing the denaturation agent. The separated strands re-associate into the double helix and the process is known as annealing.

Since the hybridization requires sequence homology, a positive hybridization reaction between two nucleic acid strands each derived from a different source indicates genetic relatedness between the two organisms. Hybridization assays require that one nucleic acid strand is from a known organism while the other is derived from the organisms to be identified.

Requirements for hybridization include target nucleic acid (DNA/RNA), restriction endonuclease enzyme, labelled probes, polyacrylamide gel/agarose, electrophoresis equipment, and stringent conditions.

Steps involved in hybridization reactions include:

1. Production and labelling of single-stranded probes.
2. Preparation of single-stranded target nucleic acid.
3. Mixture of target and probe to allow annealing.
4. Detection of reaction.

Probes are short nucleic acids with known nucleotide sequences designed to hybridize with the target nucleic acid. The probes are labelled to facilitate their detection following hybridization to the target sequence. This can be done using radioactive or non-radioactive labels. Commonly used radioactive labels are ^{32}P, ^{35}S, and ^{125}I. Common non-radioactive labels include biotin, digoxygenin, and acridinium ester.

16.8.1 Southern blot

Southern blot is a method for probing for the presence of a specific DNA sequence within a non-amplified DNA sample. DNA samples before or after restriction enzyme digestion are separated by gel electrophoresis and then transferred to a membrane by blotting via capillary action. The membrane is then exposed to a labelled DNA probe that has a complement base sequence to the sequence of the DNA of interest. The resulting fragments can be visualized on film through chemiluminescence or directly on the membrane photometrically. The method is named after its inventor, Edwin Southern. Other blotting methods, i.e. Western blot, Northern blot, and Eastern blot employ similar principles but using RNA or protein (e.g. antigens or antibodies), have been later named in reference to Edwin Southern's name.

METHOD The method for Southern blot

- Restriction endonucleases are used to cut high molecular weight DNA strands into smaller fragments.

- The DNA fragments undergo electrophoresis on agarose gel to separate them by size.

- A sheet of nitrocellulose membrane is placed on top of the gel. Pressure is applied evenly to the gel, usually by placing a stack of paper towels and a weight on top of the membrane and gel, to ensure good and even contact between the membrane and gel. Buffer transfer by capillary action from a region of high water potential (agarose gel) to a region of low water potential (filter paper) is used to move the DNA from the gel onto the membrane. Ion exchange interactions bind the DNA to the membrane due to the negative charge of the DNA and positive charge of the membrane.

- The membrane is then baked at 80°C for 2 hours to permanently attach the transferred DNA to the membrane.

- The membrane is then exposed to a hybridization probe – a single DNA fragment with a specific sequence whose presence in the target DNA is to be determined. The probe DNA is labelled so that it can be detected, usually by labelling the molecule with a fluorescent or chromogenic dye.

- After hybridization, excess probe is washed from the membrane and the pattern of hybridization is visualized on X-ray film (fluorescence) or by the development of colour on the membrane if a chromogenic detection method is used. See Figure 16.9.

Hybridization of the probe to a specific DNA fragment on the membrane indicates that this fragment contains the DNA sequence that is complementary to the probe.

16.8.2 Northern blot

This is similar to the Southern blot in all aspects except that the target nucleic acid is single-stranded RNA.

16.8.3 *In situ* hybridization

In order to obtain microbial nucleic acid for hybridization, the nucleic acid extraction technique destroys the tissue and the histopathological architecture is lost. Sometimes, it is very significant to localize the microbial nucleic acid in the tissue section. Both the DNA and RNA in routine histopathologic tissue sections remain intact and accessible for hybridization even after fixation in formalin and embedding in hot paraffin. In *in situ* hybridization the microscopy glass slides act as the solid phase.

The tissue section is deparaffinized and to expose the nucleic acid targets the sample undergoes protease digestion. The probe is applied and denaturation of the DNA at high temperature takes place. Hybridization then takes place and the signals are detected. This method allows molecular hybridization while simultaneously viewing the histopathological structure

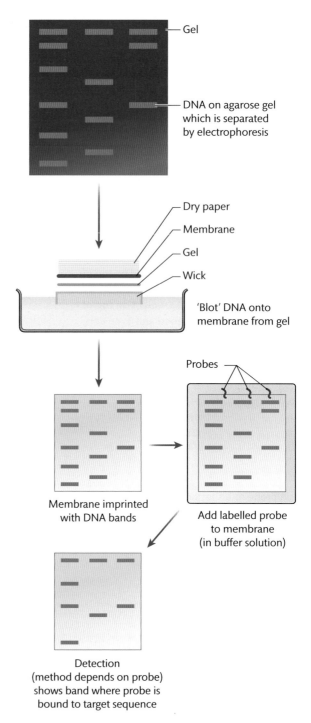

FIGURE 16.9
Southern blot method.

of the specimen. This technique allows precise detection of infected cells in the tissue. Information provided by this assay can confirm the target organism's role in the infectious process as well as giving additional information on its distribution and abundance. This technique is used when looking for Epstein–Barr virus-driven tumours in solid organ recipients for example.

CASE STUDY 16.1 *Viral resistance*

A 24-year-old is admitted to hospital for lung transplantation for end-stage lung disease associated with cystic fibrosis. On routine serological testing of the patient's blood and the donor's blood at the time of transplant, the recipient was found to be cytomegalovirus (CMV) IgG negative, which showed that he had never been infected with CMV. The donor was found to CMV IgG positive which showed that he had previously been infected with CMV. The patient was given oral valganciclovir (900 mg once daily) prophylaxis for 3 months post-transplant to protect him from CMV infection for the immediate post-operative period. The patient was discharged from hospital 6 weeks after admission following an uneventful transplant. He was given instructions to carry on taking the oral valganciclovir for the full 3 months. Two weeks after the stopping the valganciclovir, the patient was to have weekly blood tests performed for 3 months to monitor the CMV viral load by quantitative CMV PCR.

The patient was readmitted to the transplant unit, 18 weeks post-transplant with shortness of breath and spiking temperatures. On examination he had a temperature of 38°C, was markedly short of breath with an oxygen saturation of 87%. An urgent CMV viral load was performed and the results were available later that same day. The results showed his viral load had increased significantly to 3.2×10^6 copies/mL. He was changed to oral valganciclovir (900 mg twice daily) and a repeat CMV viral load was performed 7 days later. The result for this sample was 4.8×10^7 copies/mL. Due to the increase in viral load, he was changed to intravenous valganciclovir to overcome any problems he may have been having with absorption of the drug from the gut. His viral load was checked again 3 days later and was found to be 6.8×10^7 copies/mL. At this point the sample was sent for DNA sequencing to determine ganciclovir resistance. As his viral load was not decreasing, his treat-

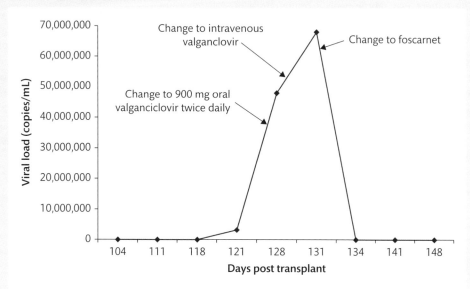

FIGURE 16.10

This graph shows the increase in CMV viral load during the course of the illness. Treatment initiation and modifications are highlighted.

ment was changed to intravenous foscarnet and his CMV viral load was repeated again 3 days later. The result for this sample was 2.4×10^3 copies/mL (Figure 16.10).

The patient was continued on foscarnet until his CMV viral load was undetectable. He made a full recovery and was discharged home.

The ganciclovir resistance test was reported as having mutations UL97 which confer ganciclovir resistance. On further questioning of the patient, it was discovered that he had been taking one valganciclovir tablet per day (450 mg) instead of two. This sub-optimal level of valganciclovir had allowed mutations within the virus to take place which would deem the virus resistance to ganciclovir. When changing anti-viral therapy his viral load decreased and he recovered.

CASE STUDY 16.2 Importance of 16S testing

A 48-year-old lady was admitted to hospital with new-onset congestive heart failure. The lady had no significant past medical history and reported that she had been feeling unwell for the past few weeks. She had a 4-day history of flu-like symptoms, including myalgia, and a 2-day history of increasing shortness of breath, chest pain, and fever. She was on no current medications. On examination, she had mild respiratory distress, blood pressure of 200/96 mmHg, heart rate of 153 beats/min, respiratory rate of 41 breaths/min, and an oxygen saturation of 89% on 15 L of oxygen. The patient was febrile, with a temperature of 38.9°C. Cardiac examination revealed a murmur consistent with mitral regurgitation.

Laboratory investigations revealed a raised white blood cell count and anaemia. Blood cultures were sent to the laboratory and antibiotic therapy with flucloxacillin and gentamicin was started. An echocardiogram was performed which showed vegetations on the mitral valve. On day 2 of admission, the patient was taken to theatre for mitral valve replacement. During surgery, extensive destruction of the mitral valve was discovered and a diagnosis of endocarditis was determined. The patient's mitral valve was sent to the microbiology laboratory for culture.

The blood cultures received from this patient grew a Gram-negative rod 3 days after collection. At this point antibiotic therapy was changed to amoxicillin and gentamicin. She was to continue this combination for 2 weeks and then stop the gentamicin but continue the amoxicillin for a further 4 weeks. The bacterium was not identified by conventional methods and was referred to a reference laboratory for identification. The mitral valve failed to yield any growth from both direct culture and enrichment culture. To determine the causative agent of the endocarditis the mitral valve was sent to the reference laboratory for 16S RNA studies to determine a diagnosis. The reference laboratory reported the organism from the blood culture to be a *Cardiobacterium hominis*. The 16S RNA profile also showed that the mitral valve was infected with *C. hominis*, showing this to be the causative organism of the endocarditis.

CASE STUDY 6.3 Controlling PCR reactions

A 32-year-old male was admitted to ITU with respiratory failure. The ITU Consultant suspected influenza A (H1N1) infection. Bronchoscopy was performed and a sample of bronchalveolar lavage fluid (BAL) was sent to the laboratory for PCR testing. The laboratory performed a standard multiplex PCR for respiratory viruses, which included influenza A (H1N1). The PCR also included an internal positive control (IPC), which was added to the

Influenza A RT-PCR: result sheet

Well	Sample	Target	Extraction method	PCR result	ct value
A1	Negative control	H1	EasyMag	Not detected	N/A
A2	Negative control	N1	EasyMag	Not detected	N/A
A3	Negative control + IPC	IPC	EasyMag	Detected	26.85
A4	Positive control	H1	EasyMag	Detected	26.19
A5	Positive control	N1	EasyMag	Detected	29.07
A6	Positive control + IPC	IPC	EasyMag	Detected	26.17
A7	BAL sample + IPC	H1	EasyMag	Not detected	N/A
A8	BAL sample + IPC	N1	EasyMag	Not detected	N/A
B1	BAL sample + IPC	IPC	EasyMag	Not detected	N/A

Extraction Run No: 432
Operator: JH
Mastermix Preparation: JH
Authorized by: MF

PCR Set up: JH
Read by: JH
Checked by: NM
Date Authorized: 24/04/2013

File Name: 2013/FLU
Reported by: JH
Date report: 24/04/13

FIGURE 16.11
Results for H1N1 PCR run.

sample prior to extraction. The results are displayed in Figure 16.11.

The H1 and N1 positive control results were as expected, as were the H1 and N1 negative controls. The internal positive controls within the negative and positive controls were also found to be as expected. However, the IPC which was added to the BAL sample was negative but should have been positive. The PCR run for this sample failed due to the internal control giving the incorrect result. The reasons for this could be either an extraction failure, therefore no DNA has been in that particular well which contained the sample and the IPC; PCR inhibition, i.e. there is something within the sample that is interfering with the PCR test; or human error.

Chapter summary

After reading this chapter you should know and understand:

■ The molecular methods available within the clinical laboratory.

■ The applications of available molecular methods.

Further reading

- **Clinical Virology Network. www.clinical-virology.org.**

  Website dedicated to virology. News, clinical tests and current viruses in circulation are all contained within the pages.

- **Mahony JB, Petrich A, Smieja M. Molecular diagnosis of respiratory virus infections.** *Critical Reviews in Clinical Laboratory Sciences* 2011; **48**(5–6): 217–249.

- **Sibley CD, Peirano G, Church DL. Molecular methods for pathogen and microbial community detection and characterisation: Current and potential application in diagnostic microbiology.** *Infection, Genetics and Evolution* 2012; **12**: 505–521.

- **Shinde SB, Fernandes CB, Patracale VB. Recent trends in** *in-vitro* **nanodiagnostics for detection of pathogens.** *Journal of Controlled Release* 2012; **159**: 164–180.

- **Wilks M ed.** *PCR Detection of Microbial Pathogens*, **2nd edition. Humana Press, 2012.**

  Authoritative and accessible, *PCR Detection of Microbial Pathogens*, Second Edition, serves microbiologists regardless of their particular interest.

 Discussion questions

16.1 'There is no longer a need for microbiology laboratories to culture samples.' Discuss this statement.

16.2 Discuss the quality assurance of molecular methods.

16.3 Discuss how you would implement a new molecular service within your laboratory.

Procedures for sample collection, transport, and processing

Malcolm Holliday

Microbiology is a little like a computer – if you put the wrong information in, you may get a bad result out. This means that great care must be taken to make sure that the quality of samples for microbiological investigations are as good as possible. You could say that collecting the sample properly is the single most important stage of the whole process of microbiological examination. If the way the sample is collected isn't correct, contaminating organisms may be introduced which will confuse the result, and it is always possible that a poorly taken sample may not have actually collected anything from the site of infection.

Learning objectives

After studying this chapter you should be able to:

- Discuss the principles of specimen collection for microbiological investigations.
- Outline the processes necessary to ensure good quality samples are received in the laboratory.
- Explain how contamination and improper transport and storage can affect the end result.
- Describe the health and safety risks of collecting, transporting, and processing microbiology samples.
- List common types of sample and the correct collection and transport methods for each.
- Discuss the principles behind the different types of transport media available.
- Outline the legislation covering the collection and transport of microbiological samples.
- Discuss basic microbiological sample processing methods.
- Outline the methods of inoculation of culture media.
- Describe the different organism hazard groups and containment levels used to process microbiological samples.

> **Key Point**
>
> A poorly collected microbiology sample will produce a poor result no matter how good the laboratory is.

This chapter will look at the important issues around sample collection, how the various sample types can be sent to the laboratory, the correct way of collecting them and transporting them to the laboratory, basic sample processing and some of the regulations and safety considerations concerned.

17.1 The importance of sample collection

When a sample is taken for microbiology, it is a snapshot of what is happening at the sample site at the moment it is taken. What we really want to find out is what organisms were in the sample at that point. Some of these organisms may be highly infectious!

Laboratory workers have to be very mindful of the health and safety risks associated with samples received and have protocols in placed to ensure laboratory staff are protected as far as possible from infection. The laboratory has to assume that the sample is infected and match appropriate protection to the risks. For example, all respiratory samples should be processed in a Class I safety cabinet due to the risk of the laboratory staff contracting TB which could be aerosolized upon opening the sample container. Staff who handle body fluids, urine, and blood samples need to protect against the risks of contracting hepatitis or even HIV. Whilst body fluids may appear visually free from blood, universal precautions such as the wearing of gloves and safety glasses is advisable when processing such samples as you must always assume the worst.

It needs to be remembered that because organisms are living things, their situation begins to change rapidly after the sample is taken. Some organisms start to die quickly, while others can multiply rapidly, depending on the conditions. This means that if the sample isn't collected properly and transported to the laboratory in the correct way and then processed appropriately, the results we get may bear little resemblance to the original organisms present at the site of infection.

Incorrectly collected specimens can also be a common reason for samples being rejected by the laboratory as unsuitable for examination.

There are a number of principles that we can apply to microbiology specimen collection.

contaminant

A contaminant is a microorganism that wasn't present in the original sample, but somehow gets into it before or while it is cultured.

Cross reference

See Chapter 5.

1. The sample must be collected from the correct infected site with a minimum of **contamination**.

   Example: Urine samples may be highly contaminated if they are not collected properly.

   Solution: Patients must be told exactly how to clean the surrounding area and collect the sample to minimize contamination.

2. The sample must be collected at the most appropriate time to recover the pathogens of interest.

   Example: In septicaemia, the maximum number of pathogens in the blood occurs when the patient's temperature rises significantly and blood cultures must be taken at this time.

Taking blood cultures when the patient's temperature has settled to normal may not detect very low numbers of the pathogen(s).

Solution: Clinical staff must be given clear instructions to take blood cultures during episodes of peaking temperature (pyrexia).

3. Enough sample must be collected to perform all the required tests.

   Example: A patient is found to have an infected abscess where **pus** is draining from a tonsil, and a swab of the discharge is sent to the laboratory. This may not allow all the different cultures required (including extended anaerobic and broth enrichment culture) to be done before all the material is wiped off the swab. A pus sample would have been better.

   Solution: Clinical staff should be given clear instructions about the best types of sample to send. It's always better to send too much rather than too little.

4. The correct collection devices and specimen containers must be used for each type of sample.

   Example: A urine sample for culture is collected in an old medication bottle. Even if washed out, this may contain traces of the original medication, which may kill some pathogens and give a misleading culture result. Even if the medication had no antibacterial effect, it is unlikely that the container would be sterile and contaminants may be introduced to the sample.

   Solution: Provide suitable containers to all users, along with appropriate instructions, and reject any samples in incorrect containers.

5. Whenever possible, samples for microbial culture must be collected before antibiotics are given.

   Example: Throat swabs taken after antibiotics have been administered to the patient may not grow the infecting pathogen.

   Solution: Where possible, samples for microbiological culture should always be taken before giving antibiotics.

6. Specimen containers must be properly labelled and sealed before being sent to the laboratory and the details must match those on the request form.

   Example: A request for *N. gonorrhoeae* culture is sent from a Genitourinary Medicine Clinic with no label and no identification on the swab. The laboratory cannot be sure that this swab is from the patient whose details are on the separate request form. If the sample was not from that patient and *N. gonorrhoeae* was isolated, reporting it would cause the wrong patient unnecessary harm, inappropriate treatment and possible family problems. If this was later shown to be a mistake, the hospital could be sued.

   Solution: Provide clear instructions to all clinical staff regarding requirements for correct labelling of samples, and enforce a policy of rejecting and not culturing any samples that do not meet these requirements.

7. Specimens should be promptly transported to the laboratory.

   Example: A swab from an anaerobic abscess is taken at 08:00 am and is sent for culture. The sample is not collected from the ward until late afternoon and does not reach the laboratory until it is closed except for urgent on-call samples. This swab will not be cultured until the next day, by which time many **anaerobes** could have died, and the pathogen may not be isolated.

   Solution: Ensure that porters, ward and clinical staff know that microbiology samples must be transported promptly to the laboratory. Contact the staff that do not comply and educate them appropriately.

pus
Pus is a discharge made up of white blood cells and fluid which is present in infected wounds.

Cross reference
See Chapter 7, Section 7.7.

anaerobe
Anaerobes are organisms that only grow in the absence of oxygen.

pathogen

A pathogen is a microorganism that has the ability to grow in the human body and cause disease.

The key to successful diagnosis depends on taking the appropriate sample correctly, at the proper time and transporting it to the laboratory without delay. This practice will help to ensure the best possible methods to ensure isolation of the target **pathogen(s)**.

SELF-CHECK 17.1

What do you consider to be the main problems associated with sample collection and ensuring that the target organism is grown from the sample?

17.2 Overview of different sample types and specimen containers

There are lots of sample containers we can use to collect samples and transport them to the laboratory; however, we must be careful that we use the correct container for the job, or the results may be affected.

17.2.1 Sterile plastic or glass 'universal' containers

These are normally sterile bottles with a screw top which are used for urine, sputum, fluids, biopsies and tissues, catheter tips, and almost any other small specimen.

Plastic containers tend to be used now, as glass containers can pose a safety hazard to staff if they break.

The 60-mL variety has a wider mouth and is sometimes preferred for sputum samples, as it's easier for patients to produce the sample directly into the container. Trying to get a sputum into a narrow-mouthed 30-mL container usually ends in a failure, with sample on the outside of the container as well as the inside.

17.2.2 Boric acid containers

These are sterile plastic universal containers with enough boric acid inside to give a concentration of 1.8% when 15 mL of urine is added and may be used when urine samples are likely to be delayed significantly before reaching the laboratory (for example overnight). The boric acid acts as a preservative and stops bacteria growing while the sample is transported. These containers are now rarely used due to improvements in sample transport.

Some bacteria may be killed if the volume of urine is insufficient.

17.2.3 Dipslides

These are sterile plastic universals with a large, flat plastic slide attached to the lid (Figure 17.1). This has bacterial culture media on each side. The slide is dipped in the urine after collection to inoculate it, the urine is then discarded, and the slide put back into the container and secured. It can then be sent to the laboratory where it can be incubated just like any other culture plate.

As no urine is received, no cell counts can be done.

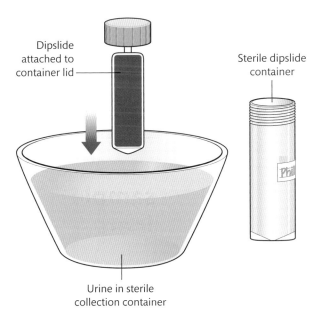

FIGURE 17.1
Dipslide urine sample.

17.2.4 Sterile plastic universals with spoons (faeces containers)

The spoon is attached to the container lid. It is used to collect a portion of faeces (stool) and transfer it to the container. It is not practical to attempt to fill a container directly while on the toilet, as the outside of the container is certain to become contaminated.

17.2.5 Swabs

Swabs are available with different tips (cotton wool, fibre, serum coated), shafts (wood, metal, plastic) and transport media (with or without charcoal, Hanks, *Chlamydia*), and may be in tubes or be broken off into bijoux bottles (Figure 17.2).

- Serum coated swabs: these are dry swabs and are only used for hardy bacteria when there will be minimal delay in delivery to the laboratory (e.g. MRSA). Moistening the swab may increase the amount of material collected.

- Transport medium swabs: these are designed to maintain microorganisms alive while being transported to the laboratory and are preferable if there is any delay in transport.

- Fine-tipped swabs on flexible wire shanks: these are useful for sampling from difficult to reach areas where a normal swab is too large, or where the shaft has to bend slightly to allow the tip to reach the sample site (e.g. ear swabs or pernasal swabs).

- Plastic shaft swabs: these may be used where a wooden shaft would adversely affect the result of the investigation (e.g. *Chlamydia* investigation). Some plastic shaft swabs have a 'nick' in the shaft which conveniently snaps off, allowing the swab to fit into a bijou bottle.

17.2.6 Blood cultures

Most blood culture bottles are designed for automated systems and consist of a bottle containing sufficient culture broth to remove the antibacterial effects of normal blood or antibiotics

Cross reference
See Chapter 5, Section 5.1.

| Pernasal swab with transport medium | Plain swab with transport medium | Ear swab with transport medium | Plain swab with no transport medium |

FIGURE 17.2
Swab types.

by dilution, or substances such as specialized resins, activated charcoal, or sodium polyethanolsulfonate (SPS) which inactivate these substances.

Systems where anticoagulated blood is lysed and centrifuged to concentrate any microorganisms before being cultured are also available.

SELF-CHECK 17.2

What are the main types of sample containers used for sample collection in microbiology?

17.3 **Methods of sample collection**

If microbiological specimens aren't collected properly, we can face all sorts of problems. These range from picking up contaminating organisms from around the site we want to sample, to missing the target altogether and sampling the wrong area. This is particularly relevant with children (who wriggle a lot and are a moving target, especially for swabbing etc.).

Whenever a sample is going to be taken, the procedure must be discussed with the patient beforehand. No one likes unpleasant surprises and having someone come up to you in hospital and start doing strange and often embarrassing things to you without any warning is not acceptable. Privacy must be ensured while the procedure is being carried out.

Samples for microbiological culture should be taken before antibiotic therapy is started if possible. This will avoid the results being distorted by the effects of the antibiotics.

All samples must be appropriately labelled before sending to the laboratory.

Hands must be washed thoroughly with bactericidal soap and water or alcohol hand gel and gloves must be worn when taking microbiological samples to avoid transferring organisms from one patient (or from your hands) to another patient. This is a key initiative to combat **health-care-acquired infections** (HCAI).

Let's look at all the different sample types and how each should be collected to get the best quality sample.

17.3.1 Urine samples

Urine grows microorganisms quite well, therefore urine samples should be sent to the laboratory as quickly as possible to avoid overgrowth of contaminants. However cleanly a sample is taken, there is always the possibility that small numbers of contaminants may enter.

Midstream urine (MSU)

These are the commonest and easiest to collect. They are the most reliable non-invasive urine samples but may not be possible in some patients.

- Male: pull back the foreskin and clean the tip of the penis with soap and water or saline to remove contaminating organisms.
- Female: clean the outer part of the vagina and labia with soap and water or saline. Clean from front to back to avoid contamination from around the anus.

Ask the patient to urinate, directing the first and last part of the stream into the toilet, but collecting the middle part into a sterile container (bedpan, kidney bowl, bottle, etc.). This can then be transferred to a labelled, sterile laboratory specimen container which is then sent to the laboratory.

It is not a good idea to ask the patient to urinate directly into the laboratory container, as these are narrow, and there is a risk that the outside of the bottle may be contaminated with urine, which is unpleasant and hazardous for anyone then handling it.

Catheter stream urine specimen (CSU)

When a patient has a catheter in place, it is not possible to collect an MSU sample. Catheter bags have a collection point provided (Figure 17.3). This should be cleaned using 70% alcohol and a sterile needle and syringe should be inserted into the collection point and sufficient urine withdrawn. This should be placed in a sterile sample container and be sent to the laboratory.

Where MSU or CSU samples can't be collected easily (e.g. from children and babies) the following techniques can be useful to ensure the most accurate diagnosis.

Bag urine

Choose the correct size of urine bag and remove the protective seal. Place the bag over the penis or vulva, working from back to front and sticking the bag to the skin. Watch the bag until urine is passed, then remove the bag, empty it into a sterile urine container and send to the laboratory.

The genital area should be washed after collection to prevent soreness.

Cross reference
See Chapter 12.

health-care-acquired infection
Health-care-acquired infection (HCAI) occurs when pathogenic microorganisms are transferred from health-care workers, other patients or the hospital environment, to a previously uninfected patient, who then develops an infection.

FIGURE 17.3
Catheter specimen of urine.
Source: Courtesy of M. Ford.

Pad urine

The baby's groin should be cleaned with warm water and the urine collection pad (UCP) placed in the nappy, towards the front. The pad should be checked every 15 minutes to see if urine has been passed. Wear gloves and remove the wet pad. Put the tip of a sterile syringe into the pad and remove as much urine as possible. Place this in a sterile container and send to the laboratory.

Suprapubic aspirate (SPA)

The abdominal skin over the bladder is cleaned thoroughly with alcohol-based disinfectant and allowed to dry, to ensure that possible contaminants are removed. A needle on a syringe is passed through the skin and directly into the bladder (which must be fairly full). A sample of the urine is withdrawn and placed into a sterile container and sent promptly to the laboratory. The needle is removed and safely disposed of.

17.3.2 Swab samples

Swabs are a convenient way to take samples for culture from superficial areas of the body. Samples may be taken from infected sites to look for the presence of pathogens, from any area to look for colonization with potential pathogens such as MRSA, or for specific organisms such as *Bordetella pertussis*, *Neisseria gonorrhoeae*, etc.

Wound swabs

aseptic technique
Aseptic technique is the use of sterile equipment and procedures to avoid possible contamination.

Select the area of wound to be sampled and gently rotate the tip of the swab in the chosen spot. Collect as much material as possible, especially if there is pus present. Ideally, old pus should be removed to allow collection of the freshest sample possible. If not, contaminants may be present and this will interfere with isolation of the target pathogen. Using an **aseptic technique** place the swab back in the sample tube and send to the laboratory.

Nasal swabs

If the swab is moistened beforehand it will help prevent discomfort to the patient. The patient should tilt their head backwards to make sample collection easier while the swab is placed into the nose, without touching the sides, and moved upwards into the tip of the nose. The swab should be gently rotated before withdrawing it and aseptically placed back in the sample tube.

Throat swabs

The patient should face the light. The patient's tongue should be depressed with a spatula to ensure that it does not rise up and contaminate the swab if the patient gags. Insert the swab into the mouth without touching the sides and quickly rub it gently over any inflamed area or any visible exudates at the back of the throat or the tonsil region before aseptically placing it back into the sample tube.

Eye swabs

The patient must be asked to try not to flinch when the sample is being taken. Moistening the swab with sterile water or saline may help. Ask the patient to look up, put on sterile disposable gloves and pull gently on the eyelid to expose the pink conjunctiva. Gently rub the swab across the lower eyelid from the inner corner outwards. Try to collect as much discharge as possible. Place the swab aseptically back in the sample tube.

Ear swabs

Use a fine-tipped swab with a flexible wire shaft. If any pus is present, sample this with the swab. Place the swab into the outer ear and gently rotate to collect any discharge. Do not push the swab too far into the ear to avoid damaging the eardrum. Place the swab aseptically back in the sample tube.

Deeper ear samples may be collected using a speculum; however, this should only be done by an experienced person to avoid causing damage.

The middle ear and inner ear cannot be sampled using a swab. Rarely, middle ear fluid can be aspirated if the eardrum is perforated, or by passing a fine needle through it.

Pernasal swabs (for Bordetella pertussis)

Use a fine-tipped swab with a flexible wire shaft and pass along the floor of the nasal cavity to the back wall of the nasal cavity (Figure 17.4). Rotate the swab gently, withdraw it carefully, and place it aseptically back in the sample tube.

17.3.3 Blood samples

Blood samples via a **venepuncture** should only be taken by suitably trained and qualified health-care workers (phlebotomists, nurses, doctors, etc.), as these are invasive samples and can pose significant risks to both the patient and the health-care worker if carried out incorrectly.

venepuncture
Taking blood via a needle placed into a vein.

Blood cultures

It is particularly important not to introduce any contaminating bacteria into blood cultures, as these can cause misdiagnosis and unnecessary antibiotic therapy.

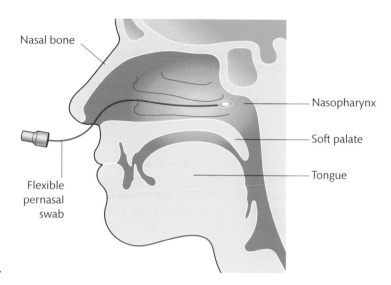

Nasal bone

Nasopharynx

Soft palate

Tongue

Flexible
pernasal
swab

FIGURE 17.4
Method of sampling using a pernasal swab.

The tops of the blood culture bottles must be removed to expose the rubber septum through which blood is injected. The septum must be cleaned with alcohol and allowed to dry immediately before the sample is taken.

The patient's skin where the blood is to be taken must be cleaned thoroughly with alcohol-based disinfectant and allowed to dry to ensure that potential contaminants are removed.

METHOD Taking blood for culture

- Blood for culture may also be taken from central venous and midline catheters in some cases.
- The line connectors must be cleaned with chlorhexidine in 70% alcohol or aqueous povidone iodine before a syringe is used to withdraw blood.
- The first 5 mL should be discarded.
- A sterile needle is attached to the syringe and the bottles inoculated as before.
- Separate syringes must be used for each culture bottle to prevent contamination.
- Forward blood cultures to the laboratory as soon as possible so the incubation process can begin.

After withdrawing the blood, the syringe is removed and a new sterile needle is placed on the syringe. This removes any possibility of introducing skin contaminants on the outside of the needle into the bottle.

Insert the needle into the bottle through the septum and allow the appropriate amount of blood to enter. The volume of blood is critical, as overfilling the bottle can lead to false-positive results with some automated blood culture systems. Too little blood reduces the chance of growing a pathogen.

Syringe needles must be safely disposed of and must never be re-sheathed. Most blood culture systems require around 5–10 mL of blood for adults, but often only 1–4 mL for neonates.

Many systems use two (or more) bottles, usually for aerobes and anaerobes, although systems for yeasts and mycobacteria are also available. Unless anaerobic infection is strongly suspected, the aerobic or general purpose bottles should be filled first. Special paediatric bottles are provided for neonates as the volume recovered is likely to be much lower than from an adult.

Blood culture bottles may have a vacuum inside, and if only a small blood sample is available, care must be taken to ensure that all the sample is not drawn into the first bottle, if more than one are required.

Inoculation of blood culture bottles should always be performed before putting blood into other containers for other laboratory tests, as these containers may not be sterile and accidental contamination may occur.

The bottles should be mixed gently by inversion and sent to the laboratory.

Key Point

Remember, a single contaminating organism going into blood culture media will grow rapidly and generate a positive signal. Rapidly growing organisms can quickly outgrow more fastidious organisms and a false result generated. Remember how misleading this could be to patient management.

Blood samples for antibiotic levels

Because the result of antibiotic levels is required before the next dose can be calculated, these are often urgent.

METHOD Blood samples for antibiotic assay

- Blood is collected by venepuncture and 10 mL placed in a clean blood tube. This may contain chemicals to aid blood clotting and serum separation, or they may not and allow blood clotting to occur naturally.
- The container is capped tightly and is sent to the laboratory as quickly as possible.
- Details of the drug, dosage, and mode of administration must be supplied to the laboratory as well as whether the sample is a 'pre' or 'post' dose sample, to aid interpretation.

Blood samples for bacterial and viral serology

These samples are taken in the same way as above. If only a small sample is available and many tests are required, it's important that the laboratory is informed which tests are the most important.

Blood samples for molecular investigations

EDTA

EDTA (ethylenediaminetetraacetic acid) is an anticoagulant to prevent blood samples from clotting.

Many of these require an **EDTA** blood sample; however, some investigations need clotted blood. Ward and clinical staff need to be aware of the specific requirements for the tests they are requesting and it is the laboratory's duty to inform them.

17.3.4 Cerebrospinal fluid (CSF)

cerebrospinal fluid

Cerebrospinal fluid is the fluid that fills the spinal column.

Cerebrospinal fluid is normally obtained by lumbar puncture, which is a specialized procedure performed by medical staff. The patient either lies or sits so that their back is arched and maximum widening of the spaces between the vertebrae is achieved.

White and red blood cells in CSF can deteriorate or lyse rapidly, especially if refrigerated, so analysis is required as soon as possible and CSF should never be put in the refrigerator prior to microbiological examination.

METHOD CSF sample collection

- The skin over the area to be punctured is cleaned with antiseptic and a spinal puncture needle is introduced between the second and third lumbar vertebrae and into the subarachnoid space (see Figure 8.2).
- The appropriate samples of CSF are obtained, after which the needle is withdrawn. Usually about 10 mL in total is required for microbiological and biochemical analysis. The usual volume is 2 mL per container.
- Samples for microbiology are placed into sterile universal bottles and transported to the laboratory promptly.

17.3.5 Sterile body fluids (e.g. joint fluid, pleural fluid, etc.)

Skin over the site must be disinfected with chlorhexidine or alcohol. The sample must be obtained using a needle and syringe and placed directly into a sterile container, then transported to the laboratory.

17.3.6 Vesicle fluids for virology

The top of the vesicle or ulcer should be lifted and a swab from a viral transport kit should be used to swab the entire base of the vesicle firmly (without causing bleeding) to collect cellular material. Place the swab in viral transport medium and send promptly to the laboratory.

17.3.7 Catheter and line tips

The skin around the catheter must be cleaned with alcohol or chlorhexidine before the catheter is removed. Around 4–5 mm of the very tip is cut off with sterile scissors and placed into a sterile container, which is then sent to the laboratory.

17.3.8 Skin, hair, and nails for dermatophyte fungi

These samples are sent for the isolation of dermatophyte fungi. For all samples, the site should be cleaned with 70% alcohol to reduce bacterial contamination, and especially if greasy ointments have been used. Samples are placed in folded black paper or universal containers for transportation to the laboratory.

Cross reference
See Chapter 14, Section 14.4.3.

Skin scrapings

Scrape outwards from the edge of the site with a blunt scalpel (or the back of the blade) or a glass slide and collect scales or flakes of skin into black paper. If there is no material being removed, a strip of Sellotape™ applied to the site and then placed on a slide can be useful. Slides must be transported inside a plastic slide holder.

Hair

Hairs should be plucked from the scalp with forceps so that the roots and follicles are attached. Ultraviolet light from a Wood's lamp may be used to detect infected hairs, which fluoresce.

Nail

Clippings should be taken from discoloured or brittle parts of the nail and cut back as far as possible from the edge. Scrapings should also be taken from beneath the nail.

SELF-CHECK 17.3

Why is it important for so many microbiological samples that the skin is cleaned first, before the sample is taken?

17.3.9 Tissue, **prostheses**, etc.

These are usually removed in theatre, and should be placed into a sterile container. A few drops of sterile saline will help stop tissues and biopsies drying out. Samples should be sent to the laboratory as quickly as possible.

prosthesis
A prosthesis is a mechanical or electronic device placed in or on the patient's body to help it function. Examples include artificial knees, hips and pacemakers.

17.3.10 Sputum

Sputum samples can easily be contaminated by passing through the mouth. Encourage the patient to cough deeply until a deep sputum specimen can be obtained (often best results are found first thing in the morning). This should be spat out into a clean (but not necessarily sterile) container such as a disposable kidney bowl.

The sample must be checked to ensure it is sputum, not saliva, and it can then be transferred to a sterile container and sent to the laboratory. Remember patients who are immunosuppressed may not produce a purulent sample.

Sputum can be induced by having the patient inhale 20–30 mL of 3–10% sterile saline using a nebulizer.

If sputum cannot be produced, a physiotherapist may be able to help the patient produce a satisfactory sample.

17.3.11 Nasopharyngeal aspirates (NPA) for virology

The patient's head should be reclined to a 70° angle. A container with a fine tube is attached to a suction pump and the tube is inserted gently into the nose. When the tube is at the very back of the nasal cavity the suction is switched on and the tube slowly withdrawn using a rotating movement. The tube should not remain in the nose more than 10 seconds. The sample should be transferred to a sterile container and transported to the laboratory.

Sputum samples are unsuitable for viral investigations.

17.3.12 Faeces

The patient should pass faeces (stool) into a clean container such as a bedpan. The spoon on the faeces container lid is used to scoop up enough faeces to fill one-quarter to one-third of the container, and the lid (with spoon still attached) is closed securely. The sample is then sent to the laboratory. If parasites are requested it is important in some cases to transport to the laboratory as soon as possible.

If the sample is diarrhoea, using the spoon to fill the container is preferable to pouring from the bedpan, where there is a significant risk of contaminating the outside of the container.

Rectal swabs

When a faeces sample cannot be collected, a rectal swab may be used. This is obtained by passing a swab carefully through the anus into the rectum, rotating gently and withdrawing it. The swab is placed back in the sample tube and sent to the laboratory.

Key Point

Rectal swabs are not as good as faeces for microbiological examination.

17.3.13 Perianal swabs and Sellotape™ preparations

These are useful in diagnosing threadworm infections. A swab may be taken from the perianal (around the anus) region, or a piece of Sellotape™ may be stuck onto the skin around the anus and then removed and stuck onto a glass slide. These are done first thing in the morning and both techniques collect *Enterobius* eggs laid by adult worms, which emerge during the night and lay eggs around the anus. Often in such cases, a diagnosis can be made clinically without the requirement to forward samples for analysis. Due to health and safety concerns from aerosolization of *Enterobius* eggs, a moist swab is preferred for laboratory examination.

17.3.14 Vaginal swabs

Cross reference

See Chapter 7, Section 7.7, *T. vaginalis* infection.

To collect a high vaginal swab, a speculum is introduced into the vagina to separate the vaginal walls and a swab is inserted and rotated gently as high as possible in the vaginal vault. The outer areas of the vagina should be avoided. The swab should be placed into transport media and sent to the laboratory. If *Trichomonas vaginalis* is suspected, Diamond's or Feinberg's transport media can be used.

Low vaginal swabs may also be sent to the laboratory. These are collected by inserting a swab into the vaginal entrance and rotating gently. This is not a suitable specimen for detecting vaginal pathogens as it will be heavily contaminated with organisms from the **perineum** area.

perineum
The perineum is the area between the anus and the vagina.

17.3.15 Cervical swabs

A speculum is introduced as above and a swab is gently inserted into the mouth of the cervix and rotated. If examination for *N. gonorrhoeae* is required, the swab should be placed into transport media containing activated charcoal to remove toxic substances and sent to the laboratory without delay. Cervical swabs are used for the diagnosis of *N. gonorrhoeae* and *Chlamydia*.

17.3.16 Penile (urethral) swabs

The prepuce (foreskin) is pulled back and a fine-tipped swab is placed 4 cm into the urethra and rotated gently. This is removed, placed in the sample tube and sent to the laboratory.

17.4 Methods of sample transport

In a hospital, most samples will be taken from wards and clinics to the laboratory by the portering services.

We need to realize that the porters will prioritize moving patients around, delivering meals, and obtaining items such as oxygen cylinders before they transport laboratory samples, so don't be surprised if samples taken in the morning don't reach the laboratory until late in the day.

Many hospitals have air-tube systems, where samples are put into a plastic 'pod' which is placed into the sending station and is forced through a system of tubes to the chosen destination. This is often the fastest method of getting samples to the laboratory.

Often, however, wards may be discouraged from sending microbiology samples by this system because samples may break and there is an infection risk. This is illogical, especially for blood samples, when samples for haematology and biochemistry laboratories are sent routinely by the air tube system, but microbiology bloods from the same patients cannot be sent.

There may be fears that if a spillage occurs inside the system, a large quantity of infected specimen may be spread around the interior of the air tubes. These are very difficult to access, and even more difficult to disinfect.

Disinfection may be accomplished by closing the system for routine use and sending 'pods' with disinfectant–soaked cloth or sponge through the tubes to every location, sometimes repeatedly – a very long and complicated procedure.

For this reason, specimens known to be a high infection risk (hepatitis B, hepatitis C, HIV, *M. tuberculosis*, etc.) and anything likely to break easily, should never be sent through an air-tube system.

Laboratory samples should always be transported in safe, leak–proof containers, so that if dropped, any breakages and spills will be contained.

Because the patient's personal and clinical details can be seen on the request form (and these may be extremely sensitive or confidential, such as HIV status), transport containers should be opaque to stop these being seen by other patients, staff, or members of the public. There are several types of carrier used, ranging from aluminium and plastic boxes to plastic bags.

Samples from GP surgeries are often collected by a regular courier service. Because these travel by road, they have to comply with the relevant road transport legislation. They must be transported in sealable, leak-proof boxes, which must carry the appropriate hazard labels, and should be securely fastened in the vehicle.

A risk assessment should have been carried out and all necessary measures put in place to minimize the dangers if there should be an accident. This includes driver training.

CASE STUDY 17.1 *Sample collection and transport*

A young child has been admitted to your Accident and Emergency Department with possible septicaemia that the clinicians think is a result of a suspected UTI.

1. What samples would you suggest are taken and how should they be transported to the laboratory?

You receive a call from one of the nursing staff on the unit saying that they have sent them down in a sealed pod in

the air tube system but it looks like they have become stuck.

2. What would you advise the nurse to do and who else would need to be contacted?

Overnight the air tube blockage was cleared but the blood culture bottle was cracked and a lot of blood was released.

3. How would you proceed and who would you contact?

SELF-CHECK 17.4

What do you think is the best method of transporting microbiology samples and why?

17.5 **Transport regulations**

pathogens

Pathogens are microorganisms that can cause disease in humans or animals.

Microbiology samples and cultures are regarded as dangerous goods because they are infectious, and could contain a variety of **pathogens**. As such, they come under several different regulations including Control of Substances Hazardous to Health (COSHH), the Health and Safety at Work Act (1974), and, more specifically, the Carriage of Dangerous Goods and Use of Transportable Pressure Equipment Regulations (2004) and its amendment in 2005 which enacts the European Directive concerning the carriage of dangerous goods by road. International Air Transport Association (IATA) regulations cover dangerous goods transported by air.

Key Point

Infectious substances are those known or reasonably expected to contain pathogens.

Wastes from laboratories can also be infectious.

Infectious substances can be divided into two categories, A or B, based on how infectious they are likely to be.

TABLE 17.1   Category A samples.

UN number and name	Microorganism
UN 2814 Infectious substances affecting humans	*Bacillus anthracis* (cultures only)
	Brucella abortus (cultures only)
	Brucella melitensis (cultures only)
	Brucella suis (cultures only)
	Burkholderia mallei – Pseudomonas mallei – glanders (cultures only)
	Burkholderia pseudomallei – Pseudomonas pseudomallei (cultures only)
	Chlamydia psittaci – avian strains (cultures only)
	Clostridium botulinum (cultures only)
	Coccidioides immitis (cultures only)
	Coxiella burnetii (cultures only)
	Crimean–Congo haemorrhagic fever virus
	Dengue virus (cultures only)
	Eastern equine encephalitis virus (cultures only)
	Escherichia coli, verotoxigenic (cultures only)
	Ebola virus
	Flexal virus
	Francisella tularensis (cultures only)
	Guanarito virus
	Hantaan virus
	Hantaviruses causing hantavirus pulmonary syndrome
	Hendra virus
	Hepatitis B virus (cultures only)
	Herpes B (cultures only)
	Human immunodeficiency virus (cultures only)
	Highly pathogenic avian influenza virus (cultures only)
	Japanese encephalitis virus (cultures only)
	Junin virus
	Kyasanur Forest disease virus
	Lassa virus
	Machupo virus
	Marburg virus

continued

TABLE 17.1 Category A samples. (*Continued*)

UN number and name	Microorganism
	Monkeypox virus
	Mycobacterium tuberculosis (cultures only)
	Nipah virus
	Poliovirus (cultures only)
	Rabies virus
	Rickettsia prowazekii (cultures only)
	Rickettsia rickettsii (cultures only)
	Rift Valley fever virus
	Russian spring–summer encephalitis virus (cultures only)
	Sabia virus
	Shigella dysenteriae type 1 (cultures only)
	Tick-borne encephalitis (cultures only)
	Variola virus
	Venezuelan equine encephalitis virus
	West Nile virus (cultures only)
	Yellow fever virus (cultures only)
	Yersinia pestis (cultures only)
UN 2900 Infectious substances affecting animals only	African horse sickness virus
	African swine fever virus
	Avian paramyxovirus Type 1 – Newcastle disease virus
	Blue tongue virus
	Classical swine fever virus
	Foot and mouth disease virus
	Lumpy skin disease virus
	Mycoplasma mycoides – contagious bovine pleuropnemonia
	Peste des petits ruminants virus
	Rinderpest virus
	Sheep-pox virus
	Goatpox virus
	Swine vesicular disease virus
	Vesticular stomatitis virus

If we are going to transport any infectious substance (samples or cultures) we have to decide which category it falls into and make sure that it is transported in a manner that complies with the regulations.

The substances that fall into Category A, which includes the higher risk infectious organisms, are shown in Table 17.1.

All samples not included in Category A come under Category B, and these must be packaged and transported according to Packaging Instruction 650 and labelled UN 3373.

This means that a leak-proof primary receptacle (normally the specimen container) must be placed inside an approved leak-proof secondary container containing absorbent material. This must be contained inside a rigid outer packaging, which is appropriately marked as in the example in Figure 17.5.

Category A samples must be packaged and transported under similar arrangements according to Packaging Instruction 620 and labelled UN 2814. Additional requirements include providing a leak-proof seal on the specimen container (e.g. heat seal, paraffin film), an itemized list of contents must be enclosed between the secondary and outer packaging and the words '*Suspected Category A infectious substance*' must be shown on this document.

FIGURE 17.5
Example of a specimen transport label.

CASE STUDY 17.2 *Sample courier incident*

Two courier vans have an accident at a crossroads in the middle of the city. Both are badly damaged and the driver of the specimen courier is unconscious. The emergency services arrive and find the contents of the van broken and all over the driver and the road. There is a lot of broken plastic/glass and lots of red and brown fluid everywhere.

1. What would you advise the emergency services to do based on sample release?

2. What would you need to investigate?

The driver of the courier has sustained wounds which samples have clearly been in contact with.

3. What would you suggest is the next stage in the process?

Twelve months later the courier driver develops an HIV infection which he is adamant was as a result of the accident.

4. What would be your response?

5. Was the advice you gave initially and your actions sufficient?

6. What do you need to ensure is in place with your courier drivers and the owners?

17.6 **Basic sample processing**

The different parts of the body can have very different physical and chemical conditions. For example, the skin under your big toe is very different from the skin inside your ear, or the skin around your genitals. Conditions inside your lungs are different from the conditions in your bladder or intestines. This means that the bacteria that might live there as normal flora, and the ones that might enter as pathogens and cause disease, can be very different in each specific part of the body.

When we grow microorganisms in the laboratory, we usually try to put them onto culture media that provide similar conditions to the part of the body the sample came from originally.

This means we try to make sure that the pH, nutrients such as sugars and proteins, gaseous conditions (aerobic, anaerobic, microaerophilic, increased CO_2, etc.) are the same as the body site we are interested in.

Cross reference
See Chapter 3.

You can look at it as though we are trying to fool the pathogens into thinking they are still at the original body site, because if they were growing and multiplying happily there, then if we provide the same conditions in culture media, the pathogens should grow happily for us. This means that we have to provide many different culture media with different ingredients. There is no single 'best' culture medium that is suitable for all specimen types and sites.

Specimens from sterile sites, such as cerebrospinal fluids (CSF), joint aspirates and blood cultures, can be cultured onto the most nutritious culture media available, because these samples have no resident normal flora that might overgrow any pathogens, and there may only be small numbers of the pathogens present.

In contrast, samples such as faeces, which come from areas with large numbers of normal flora, might require culture on media containing selective agents to help suppress some of the normal organisms and allow any pathogens to be detected.

Another way to achieve this is to use differential agents in the culture media, which will allow the pathogens to stand out from the normal flora, usually by being a specific, easily recognized colour.

Cross reference
See Chapter 3.

In practice, many specimens will be cultured onto several different culture media (either culture plates or bottles of liquid media) to ensure that the widest possible range of pathogens can be grown.

Some samples, such as urine and CSF, will have microscopy performed on them before culture. This can help indicate whether the sample is infected, and may help in deciding whether antibiotic susceptibility tests should be put up directly.

Cross reference
See Chapter 14, Section 14.4.

Skin, hair, and nail samples will have a portion of each type of sample placed into 30% potassium hydroxide (KOH) in a test tube and left for 10–120 minutes to digest the hard tissue. A drop of this will then be placed on a slide, a cover slip is applied and the specimen is examined under the microscope to look for fungal cells.

Microbiology specimens are usually processed in batches, keeping the different sample types together. All urines would be done together, in one section of the laboratory, while all blood cultures would be done in another section and all MRSA swabs in yet another. This allows maximum efficiency, as each section need stock only the culture media required for that particular type of specimen. As all the specimens will be processed using the same method, it is easier and more efficient for the person doing them.

Many microorganisms start to die as soon as they are taken away from the body, and it is necessary to process samples as soon as is reasonably possible, to get the best and most relevant result.

17.7 Inoculation of culture media

Because culture media will grow both contaminants and pathogens, it is important to use aseptic technique to avoid introducing contaminating organisms or allowing pathogens from the sample to come into contact with workers.

Culture media such as blood agar, which don't contain any inhibitors, should be inoculated first when possible. This prevents antibiotics and other selective substances killing microorganisms.

Sometimes, when only small numbers of pathogens may be present, a specific medium with inhibitors may be inoculated first (e.g. gonococcal culture plates).

If smears (wet preparations or stained slides) are needed, they should always be made after all culture media have been inoculated. This prevents contaminants that may be on the slides being transferred to the plates.

If smears must be made first (for example, if the result of the smear would guide the type of culture done) then a sterile slide must be used. These should be dipped in alcohol which is allowed to evaporate before use.

Liquid media (culture broths) should be inoculated after culture plates for swabs, but inoculated first with fluid samples.

Where possible, the following order should be followed:

- Media without inhibitors (e.g. blood agar, chocolate agar).
- Media with indicators (e.g. CLED agar, chromogenic agar).
- Media with inhibitors or selective agents (e.g. DCA agar, *B. cepacia* agar).
- Fluid media (e.g. nutrient broth, cooked meat broth).
- Smears for staining (e.g. Gram's stain, mycobacteria).

SELF-CHECK 17.5

Why is it best to inoculate non-selective media first?

17.7.1 Urine samples

Urine may be inoculated onto culture plates in several ways as follows:

- A sterile calibrated loop (1 µL, 2 µL, or 10 µL) is dipped into the urine just below the surface and removed without tilting from vertical. This is then inoculated onto a culture plate. A whole plate may be used, or two samples may be inoculated onto half a plate each. Four samples onto a quarter plate each has been used, but is not recommended.
- A sterile filter paper strip (available commercially, e.g. Bacteruritest) is dipped into the urine to the line on the strip. The strip is removed and any excess urine drained off onto the inside of the container. The strip is bent at the line and the inoculated area of the strip is then placed onto the culture plate, held for several seconds and removed. Ten to twelve urine samples may be inoculated onto a single culture plate using this method. More is not recommended.
- A number of urines (21, 36, 54, or 96) may be pipetted into sterile cups in a rack. A multipoint inoculator, which has an equivalent number of sterile pins, one of which goes into each cup, is used to pick up 1 µL of each urine. The multipoint inoculator pins are touched to the surface of an agar plate or agar in microtitre plates to inoculate spots with 1 µL each.

Some samples may also have antibiotic susceptibility tests performed directly from the sample, rather than from isolated colonies after culture. The process is similar for all samples. A sterile pipette, swab or loop is used to inoculate the sample on the centre of a plate, and the inoculum is spread all over the plate using a fresh swab, either from side to side by hand or in a circular pattern using a plate rotator, prior to placing antibiotic discs on the plate. Culture plates containing antibiotics can be inoculated directly with urine in the same way as above using a multipoint inoculator.

17.7.2 Swab samples

Swabs are inoculated onto plates by rolling the tip over a quarter or a third of each plate to form a primary **inoculum**. Fluid media is inoculated by inserting the swab into the bottle and breaking (or cutting) it off near the tip.

Simply putting the swab in the fluid medium, agitating and removing the swab again is not sufficient as many organisms remain attached to the swab fibres and will be removed when the swab is, and so maximum inoculum will not be achieved.

17.7.3 Blood cultures

Blood samples are inoculated into the blood culture bottles at the time the sample is taken. The bottles are incubated in the laboratory; often an automated system is used. When a bottle is suspected of being positive (i.e. having microorganisms present) it must be inoculated onto culture plates to grow the organism.

Most commercial systems supply a method for safely and aseptically removing a sample of the blood from inside the bottle. Often, this is a type of needle that can be pushed through the septum of the bottle and which allows a few drops of blood to escape when the bottle is inverted. These drops can be placed onto culture plates.

17.7.4 Fluids, pus, and CSF

Fluid, pus, and CSF samples may be centrifuged to concentrate small numbers of pathogens in the deposit, or may be inoculated uncentrifuged if the sample is thick or thought to contain lots of pathogens.

Either a sterile pipette or a sterile loop can be used to transfer around 10 µL of specimen to each culture plate or broth. If the sample is very thick, using a sterile swab to do this may be more convenient.

17.7.5 Tissue and biopsy samples

Tissue and biopsy samples are usually homogenized (ground up) in a little sterile saline using a sterile Griffiths tube, which is like a small enclosed pestle and mortar. This releases any organisms from inside the tissue sample.

A loopful or few drops from a sterile pipette are inoculated onto each plate or into fluid media, and generally onto both due to the precious nature of the sample.

17.7.6 Prostheses

These are usually made of metal or plastic and cannot be easily homogenized or sampled with a swab. Often the best way to culture these samples is to aseptically place them in a sterile container and add culture broth until the specimen is submerged. This can then be incubated.

17.7.7 Catheter tips

A catheter tip (or cannula) is rolled over the whole surface of the plate five times using a sterile swab, forceps or loop to move the tip, which is then removed. Any fluid or blood from the **lumen** of the catheter should be allowed to run onto the plate for culture.

---

inoculum

The inoculum is the portion of the specimen that is put onto the culture plate or into the fluid medium.

Cross reference

See Chapter 5, Section 5.1.

lumen

The lumen is the inside of any hollow, tube-like structure.

17.7.8 Skin, hair, and nails

A small flake of skin should be picked up with a sterile needle or forceps and pressed onto the surface of the culture plate or slope. This should be repeated for as many flakes as possible over the whole area of the plate.

Hair and nail samples should be picked up with sterile forceps and pushed onto the surface of the culture plates in the same way.

17.7.9 Sputum

Sputum samples are normally quite sticky and mucoid, which makes picking a suitable portion of the sample to inoculate onto culture plates difficult. There are two common methods of inoculating sputum.

METHOD *Digestion of sputum samples prior to culture*

- An equal volume of a chemical that will break down the sticky mucus (e.g. Sputasol or *N*-acetyl-L-cysteine) is added to the sample.
- Mix well.
- The mixture is incubated at 37 °C with periodic shaking until it is liquefied (around 10 min).
- Finally, the sample can then be inoculated onto culture plates with a sterile pipette or loop.

METHOD *Decontamination of sputum samples for TB culture*

- An equal volume of 4% NaOH is added to the specimen and mixed well for 20 min. Continual mixing is best, but mixing several times may be used. TB is more resistant to the alkaline NaOH than contaminating bacteria.
- 0.2 mL of the digested mixture is inoculated onto culture media in slopes using a pipette. The culture slopes are at an acid pH, and adding the alkaline sample results in a neutral pH in the end.

  OR

- An equal volume of 4% NaOH is added to the specimen and mixed well for 20 min. Continual mixing is best, but mixing several times may be used. TB is more resistant to the alkaline NaOH than contaminating bacteria.
- An equal volume of 2% HCl is added to the mixture to neutralize it
- 0.2 mL of the digested mixture is inoculated onto culture media in slopes using a pipette. The culture slopes are at a neutral pH, therefore the inoculum must be neutralized before being put on the slopes.

> **homogenized**
> Homogenized means liquefied and mixed, so that all parts of the whole sample are the same.

Some laboratories choose to dilute the **homogenized** sputum and inoculate 10 µL of the dilution onto culture plates. This helps to remove small numbers of contaminants picked up from the mouth and also to provide an estimate of the quantity of pathogens in the sample.

purulent

Purulent means containing a lot of pus.

Cross reference

See Chapter 9, Section 9.2.2.

A **purulent** fleck of the sample is selected and is removed with a sterile swab or loop. This can be quite difficult to achieve due to the stickiness of sputum, and takes a little practice. The chosen fleck is inoculated onto culture plates using the loop or swab.

Sputum samples for tuberculosis (TB) culture need to be pre-treated with a digestion/decontamination stage to remove all non-TB microorganisms before culture. TB is slow-growing and any contaminants in the sample can hide the growth of TB. These organisms are more resistant to chemicals than other bacteria. There are two methods of achieving this.

SELF-CHECK 17.6

Why are samples for TB treated with harsh chemicals before culture whereas other samples are not?

17.7.10 Faeces

Liquid faeces samples can be inoculated onto culture plates and broths using a loop, wooden stick, or swab. These do not need to be sterile. Faeces are not sterile, and the pathogens that are looked for are not found as environmental contaminants, therefore it is unlikely that any contamination will cause a problem.

Solid faeces samples should be broken up using a loop, stick, or swab and, if soft enough after this, it can be inoculated onto culture plates. If it is still solid, emulsifying it in a little saline or nutrient broth can be helpful.

Usually, several selective culture plates are inoculated for faecal pathogens.

Liquid media are also used for faeces culture, as there may only be very few pathogens present and enrichment may be necessary. These liquid media also contain selective agents to remove normal faecal organisms which may otherwise overgrow any pathogens present.

Cross reference

See Chapter 11.

Wet preparations are made when looking for faecal parasites. These can be made in saline, or with a little fresh iodine added to help differentiation.

17.7.11 Smears and wet preparations for microscopy

Smears are made by rolling the swab across a circle marked with a diamond or a wax pencil on a slide. Smears of fluid or pus samples are made using a sterile pipette, loop or swab to transfer some of the sample to a marked circle on a slide.

If the sample is thick, a smear can be made from it directly; however, if it is very thin, it may need to be centrifuged first. The supernatant is then removed and the deposit resuspended in a small amount of liquid. This is used to make the smear.

Wet preparations may be useful for detecting parasites such as *Trichomonas* spp. or clue cells (indicating bacterial vaginosis) in genital samples, or faecal parasites from stools.

Wet preparations are made by dabbing a transport medium swab onto a slide and covering the removed material with a coverslip. The same effect can be achieved with a dry swab by placing a drop of saline on the slide and dabbing the swab into it.

A drop of a fluid sample is placed on the slide with a loop and covered with a coverslip. Solid faeces samples are emulsified in a drop of saline on the slide before the coverslip is added.

CASE STUDY 17.3 *Insufficient sample*

A patient on a neurology ward has had a CSF taken for suspected meningitis. The patient was started on cefotaxime before the sample was taken. The sample arrives quickly into the department for processing. Unfortunately there is only a very small amount which is not enough for microscopy AND culture.

1. How would you proceed?

2. How would you contact and why?

3. What would be your choice of culture and why?

The doctor who is managing the patient telephones you and requests you just put it onto some culture plates to ensure the best chance of isolating the causative organism.

4. Is this the best course of action?

After 24 hours the culture plates show no growth.

5. What is your next course of action regarding the culture plates?

6. What other investigations would you suggest to the clinicians?

17.7.12 Spreading culture plates

In order to get the most out of bacterial cultures, the initial inoculum on a culture plate must be spread over the rest of the plate so that individual colonies grow. This allows mixed cultures to be easily detected and picked off for antibiotic susceptibilities or identification. This is known as 'spreading', 'plating out', or 'streak dilution'.

There are many different ways to achieve a good spread but the aim is to produce well-isolated, single colonies after incubation. There are now instruments that can plate out swabs and achieve excellent results.

The initial inoculum should cover between a quarter and a third of the total area of the plate. If half plates are used, this should be reduced accordingly.

The initial inoculum is spread over the rest of the plate in several separate streaks using a sterile loop, as shown in Figure 17.6. A fresh loop may be used for each set of streaks if desired.

When quarter plates are used, it is normal for the initial inoculum to cover the entire segment of the plate.

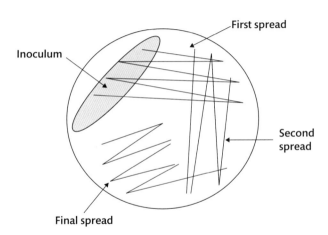

FIGURE 17.6
Method of spreading a culture plate.

17.8 **Safety considerations**

Why are samples sent to the microbiology laboratory in the first place? It is usually because the clinician thinks that the site the sample was taken from may be infected, but it is also a fact that there will always be patients or specimens that haven't been identified as infected, but which turn out to be afterwards. All microbiology samples must therefore be regarded as potentially infected from the moment they are taken, and during transport, storage, sorting, processing and disposal. The correct specimen collection techniques must be observed, and samples must be collected into the correct laboratory approved container.

The container should not be overfilled. However generous the patient has been in supplying copious amounts of specimen, it doesn't all have to be sent to the laboratory. The rim and the outside of the container should not be contaminated when the sample is placed in it. If contamination occurs, the container should be discarded and a clean one used. The caps must be tightened correctly on all specimen containers to avoid leaking and spilling while in transit to the laboratory.

Anyone taking specimens is responsible for correctly completing all details on the sample container and request form, and must label any particularly high-risk samples (such as hepatitis or HIV-positive bloods) appropriately.

Samples should only be transported to the laboratory inside a sealed plastic bag. These may be attached to the request form, or may be separate, with a pocket to hold the request form. It is important to remember that porters and couriers who may transport specimens have little knowledge of microbiology, and may not understand the dangers of leaking or contaminated specimens. However, porters and couriers must be given appropriate training in handling specimens safely and how to deal with spillages.

All staff who handle specimens should be instructed to wear the appropriate, fastened protective clothing and to cover any cuts and grazes with waterproof dressings. Hands must be washed after each spell of duty and before breaks. Porters must wash their hands on entering and leaving each ward, and when leaving the laboratory.

In the laboratory, the following points should be considered at all times:

- Whenever specimens are handled, aerosol production should be minimized. Swabs should be removed from tubes gently and caps and lids of fluid samples should be opened slowly.
- Fluid samples may be under increased pressure, especially if microorganisms in the sample have been allowed to grow and produce gas during transport. If the top is removed too quickly, the contents may discharge explosively.
- Samples should not be mixed or shaken vigorously before opening.
- Disposable gloves must be worn when handling fluid samples and any high-risk specimens.
- If there is a danger of the specimen splashing during processing, eye protection (safety glasses, goggles, or visors) must be worn.
- Leaking specimens should be assessed by a senior member of the technical staff to determine if they can be processed safely.
- Spills kits and disinfectants must be available, and staff must have appropriate training.
- All spills must be dealt with immediately and must be cleaned and disinfected using the most appropriate method.

All microorganisms in the laboratory are potentially infectious, but some pose a greater hazard than others. They are categorized into hazard groups as follows:

Hazard Group 1: A biological agent unlikely to cause disease.

Hazard Group 2: A biological agent that can cause human disease and may be a hazard to employees; it is unlikely to spread to the community and there is usually effective prophylaxis or effective treatment available.

Hazard Group 3: A biological agent that can cause severe human disease and presents a serious hazard to employees; it may present a risk of spreading to the community, but there is usually effective prophylaxis or treatment available.

Hazard Group 4: A biological agent that causes severe human disease and is a serious hazard to employees; it is likely to spread to the community and there is usually no effective prophylaxis or treatment available.

There are different containment levels that are appropriate for the different hazards of each group.

Microorganisms in Groups 1 and 2 are handled in Containment Level 1 or 2 laboratories. Level 2 is the normal standard for microbiology laboratories.

Microorganisms in Hazard Group 3 require Containment Level 3, which needs additional safety features such as a microbiological safety cabinet, **HEPA** filtration of exhaust air, a sealable laboratory for disinfection and access only to authorized people.

Hazard Group 4 microorganisms require Containment Level 4. This requires a separate laboratory with a fully sealed Class III safety cabinet, an airlock, an autoclave, and extremely rigorous safe working practices over and above those for Level 3. There are very few of these laboratories in the UK.

SELF-CHECK 17.7

What are the highest and lowest containment levels? At which level are most routine microbiology samples processed?

Chapter summary

After reading this chapter you should know and understand:

- Sample quality is the single most important stage of microbiological examination.

- A poorly collected sample will produce a poor result.

- Some microorganisms start to die as soon as the sample is taken, while others can multiply rapidly.

- Insufficient or inappropriate samples may mean that the required investigations cannot be carried out.

- Wrongly collected, transported, and labelled specimens should be rejected to ensure that incorrect results are not reported.

- Microbiology samples are potentially hazardous and must be handled and transported safely at all times.

Further reading

- **Health Services Advisory Committee.** *Safe Working and the Prevention of Infection in Clinical Laboratories*. **The Stationery Office, 1991.**

  Essential publication which covers the health and safety requirements for clinical laboratory work.

- **Hawkey P, Lewis D, eds.** *Medical Bacteriology*, **2nd edition. Oxford University Press, 2003.**

  Excellent general text covering many aspects of sample processing and other areas of microbiology.

- **Mallett J, Bailey C, eds.** *Manual of Clinical Nursing Procedures*, **6th edition. Blackwell Science, 2005.**

  Text which explains further the procedures for taking clinical samples.

- **Collins CH, Lyne PM, Grange JM, eds.** *Collins and Lyne's Microbiological Methods*, **8th edition. Arnold, 2004.**

  This is a useful text which provides further detail on many aspects of this chapter. Essential laboratory handbook.

 # Discussion questions

17.1 Why do you think there are different types of swab available?

17.2 Why is it important to take blood cultures before blood for other laboratory tests and before antibiotic therapy is started?

17.3 Why is it important to transport microbiology samples correctly?

17.4 Why are microorganisms categorized into different groups and how does this affect laboratory handling?

Hints and tips for discussion questions

Chapter 1

1.1. Size of colony, colour of colony, and shape of the colony on conventional media. Other characteristics can include smell and type of haemolyis (α, β). On nutrient agar examples would be staphylococci are typically white in appearance, enterococci are grey. *Proteus* spp. will swarm across the plate and *C. difficile* colonies smell of horse manure.

1.2 There may not be enough nutrients in the medium to grow fastidious organism such as *Neisseria* spp. The depth of the medium may be inadequate to grow anaerobic organisms. Also consider what could be in the sample that may inhibit the growth of organisms.

1.3 (a) This is probably how you would clean surfaces in your home – soap and water is generally sufficient, take into consideration how 'dirty' the surface is first.

(b) Think about the chemicals which will kill viruses – most viruses do not survive long out of the body anyway and will perish in a matter of minutes.

(c) You need to consider the features associated with *C. difficile* which are different to most other bacteria. Can these be killed with alcohol? If not what agents could you use?

1.4 Consider what functions are associated with the cell wall and how important it is. Structures of the bacterial cell are a target for potential destruction and the cell wall is no exception. What agents target the bacterial cell wall and how effective are they?

Chapter 2

2.1 Think about the number and types of organism that are isolated on a daily basis in microbiology laboratories. Are all of them pathogens – if not what are they? What is the cost of bacterial identification both in terms of staffing and reagents? Does it matter clinically if an organism is called an *E. coli* or just a 'coliform'?

2.2 Consider if automated systems perform all the different types of identification required. What do automated systems identify? Think about when an immunological test is required, and would it still be required if an automated system was used?

Chapter 3

3.1 Consider the advantages of chromogenic media in differentiating organisms in mixed culture. Think about the savings in biomedical scientists' time. Are less organisms forwarded for identification? Are there certain sample types where chromogenic media are becoming more popular based on clinical need?

3.2 In your laboratory has PCR replaced routine culture in any areas? If not why do you think this is? You need to consider workload and cost. What pathogens are isolated from clinical samples? Is it always a single pathogen? Urine samples would be a good area to consider in your answer.

3.3 Consider quality of the media – are commercially prepared media of a higher quality? You need to discuss how the media are quality assured. Are any problems associated with commercial deliveries? If so what would be the consequences of this? Consider the flexibility of having media production facilities on-site.

Chapter 4

4.1 Think about your answer in terms of ease of use, reproducibility, and standardization. What methods are used routinely – will this always be the case? Remember cost and staff required need to be considered in your answer, as well as the scientific reasons for performing susceptibility tests using both these methods.

4.2 This is quite controversial as some laboratories don't perform direct susceptibility tests – why would this be the case? Discuss the situations in which they can be performed and is there an obvious clinical benefit? Are costs and turnaround times important or are these potential benefits outweighed by the lack of standardization?

4.3 Consider how many people are on antibiotics at any one time worldwide. What antibiotics are monitored and why are they more 'important' than others? Are different patient groups of any significance?

4.4 Consider where we are now and how effective antibiotics are currently. Are there any strains of bacteria currently that cannot be treated? If not are some carrying resistance to most antibiotics? Think of these in terms of the cost of developing new antimicrobials and the regulatory approval required. What are pharma companies' priorities for new drug development? Are antibiotics higher up their R+D programme than anti-cancer agents, drugs to combat obesity, etc.? Is it profitable to make new drugs when so many countries make generics?

Chapter 5

5.1 Think about the situation if the clinician is correct and consequences if not. What can be done with a positive blood culture isolate to aid patient management?

5.2 Does the Gram stain tell you exactly what the organism is? Does it tell you its significance? What does the Gram stain *really* tell you?

5.3 Think about the organism isolated and what species is it. Are some species more important than others? What about the patient – how ill are they?

5.4 Are some organisms more important than others? Think about contaminants, the cost and time of identifying all isolates. Are suspect contaminants always so – do patients ever develop other conditions later?

5.5 You need to understand how blood cultures are taken and the techniques used. What are the consequences of using a poor technique? Will it have any clinical consequences when the results are relayed back to the wards?

Chapter 6

6.1 For both parts of the question think about the differences between the two locations and what type of patients they are likely to be. Are they likely to be simple or complicated infections? What organism would you expect to commonly isolate?

6.2 You need to consider what is meant by bacteriuria and what is significant – is it the type of organism, patient type, number of bacteria present, or other factors?

6.3 Consider the types of method available. Think about tests that are performed outside of the laboratory. Consider the advantages and disadvantages of these.

6.4 How many antibiotics can be used? Consider which are the best and for what reason. Think about the organisms being treated and what they are likely to be susceptible to. Why are some better than others, and why are some prescribed more than others?

6.5 Are all urine samples sent because the patient has a suspected UTI or can it be for other reasons? Are all causes of a UTI likely to grow on the media used? Consider factors present in the urine which may cause the organism not to grow.

6.6 Consider the different types of media used and how susceptibility tests can be performed. Does the identification have any relevance and is it better with certain media? Is cost important?

Chapter 7

7.1 Would a molecular method be better than culture – if so, why? Think about how you would perform a susceptibility test before deciding on your answer.

7.2 Where does *S. aureus* commonly reside on the human body? Would this explain why it occurs so frequently as a cause of wound infections? Are there other reasons, apart from colonization, why its incidence is so high? What properties does the organism possess to enable it to cause wound infections?

7.3 Remember the human body is covered in normal flora – think about the types of flora involved in your answer and the pathogens you would look for.

7.4 How many methods are there currently? How different are they? What are the obstacles to having only one method?

Chapter 8

8.1 Think about the age of the patient and perhaps their surroundings when they develop meningitis. Which bacteria colonize humans and at what age? Think of immunization – is it always effective? Has everyone been vaccinated?

8.2 What are the other departments in laboratory medicine (pathology)? Think about the tests they perform. Can these tests rule out meningitis?

8.3 Think about how easy it is to see small numbers of organism in a smear. If you got it wrong what consequences would this have for patient management?

Chapter 9

9.1 Does smoking damage the respiratory tract? If so, how will this promote bacterial growth? What other things can damage the respiratory tract (think seasonal)?

9.2 Think about the patient types and how quickly organisms can change from normal flora to being involved in disease. Consider environmental factors also.

9.3 Think about the cell properties of certain mycobacteria, think of how they are transmitted. What is it that gives some organisms an advantage over others?

9.4 Consider the patient types they infect. What advantage do they have over other, similar organisms? What are their characteristic properties?

Chapter 10

10.1 Consider the causes of bacterial gastroenteritis and how the disease progresses. Are cases always so severe that the patient would seek medical advice? Would it be worldwide?

10.2 What culture media are used to isolate the various pathogens? You will need to consider the problems associated with culture of faeces samples in general as well as what is likely to grow. Do other organisms 'interfere' with the isolation of target pathogens and is this important?

10.3 First of all, do you believe gastrointestinal infections will ever be eradicated – what are the barriers to this? Consider the source(s) of the pathogens involved and how they could be eliminated. Your answer must be broad enough to consider all causes of infective diarrhoea.

10.4 Consider what GI infections are most common in children of this age group, particularly viral infections. In the elderly male, consider the impact of a broad-spectrum antibiotic on the patient's normal flora and what can colonize. Patients with a history of foreign travel will need extended sample processing and the cause may not be bacterial. With a diagnosis of profuse watery diarrhoea in a patient from Somalia you need to consider any possible outbreaks which may have arisen.

Chapter 11

11.1 Consider the feasibility of reducing parasitic worldwide when many people are symptomatic and reservoirs of infection. Consider the sources of parasitic infection e.g. imported foodstuffs from endemic areas, contaminated water, foodstuffs contaminated with infected human faeces: what could be done to address this? Travel is a major risk factor – consider the general public's awareness of parasitic infections and what can be done to increase awareness of infections associated with travel. Global warming is definitely a risk factor: consider the implications of this over the next century or so and possible proactive interventions to prevent infection.

11.2 Consider those parasites which have the ability to penetrate the intestinal mucosa and migrate to distant sites including muscle and neural tissue and vital organs. Consider those parasites whose infections are kept under control by effective immune systems and what may happen if the immune system becomes suppressed or compromised. How does the immune system become suppressed or compromised?

11.3 Consider measures to target weak links in the life cycle of parasites, for example, consider screening and treating patients carrying helminths which shed eggs into the environment. Consider the environments in which the infective stages of the parasite are found; e.g. pastures, watercress, crustacens, lakes, and what measures can be put in place to prevent infection. Consider those parasites whose life cycle utilize animals consumed by humans; e.g. pigs, cattle, lamb, fish. However, beavers and numerous other wild animals can harbour infective protozoa cysts or oocysts, and these animals continue to act as reservoirs of infection. So can we really effective control human parasitic infection?

Chapter 12

12.1 Consider the factors that allow the organism to spread – are they environmental or human? What unique properties does the organism have that enable it to become established?

12.2 Consider the environment and the staff within it. How have both of these changed to enable health-care acquired infections to reduce and what have been the drivers for such change?

12.3 Evaluate why spread of the organism occurs and what patient groups are affected. What is happening to the age of the population and what effect is this having both in hospital and community patients? Does the organism have any specific pathogenic properties that make it such a problem organism? Are there any mechanisms that can be applied to reduce infection rates of any organism?

12.4 Multi-drug resistance is increasing in a wide range of microorganisms including TB, and controlling the spread is a major public health and IPC challenge. Carbapenemase-producing Gram-negative organisms are on the increase and must be managed effectively. With viruses, influenza is changing, e.g. swine flu variants. Limiting spread of infection is going to take significant resources. Also consider problems associated with norovirus. Whilst MRSA and C. *difficile* infections have declined, IPC teams must remain vigilant to ensure infections caused by these organisms are minimized.

Chapter 13

13.1 You need to consider the range of tests you would offer clinicians – what tests would they want? Would you perform all serological investigations, for example? What use can be made of reference laboratories and other referral centres? Consider financial as well as space considerations in your answer.

13.2 Your answer must include the advantages and disadvantages of cell culture in comparison with other methods. What other methods are available? Are cost, turnaround times, and staffing issues important? Which methods are considered as gold standard?

13.3 In your answer you should consider:
- Actual requirements.
- Practical considerations.
- Cost.

What sensitivity and specificity would you require? Is the assay a screening assay or a confirmatory one? You must also consider other factors important to requesting clinicians – what would these be? Also, think about how the assay will be performed, by whom and when.

13.4 Is quality control important? How is it performed and when is it performed? How do you know you have achieved the required level of quality? Consider how you record this and make reference to external methods of quality assurance.

Chapter 14

14.1 Think about how many specialized mycology staff are in routine microbiology departments and what this means to service provision. What services would be required? Also, think of other things that are required to provide the service.

14.2 How many spores does one *Aspergillus* head contain? What happens when one spore lands on a culture plate? Think of the consequences of this.

14.3 In what patients are fungal infections seen? Are these conditions likely to decrease? Think about what improvements have been seen in fungal diagnosis and therapies.

Chapter 15

15.1 Consider consequences around loss-of-function as well as gain-of-function. What consequences might there be for the eradication of this disease by vaccination?

15.2 Consider how these bacteria acquired the genes encoding these proteins.

15.3 At what stage in establishing a gas gangrene infection would a strong lytic activity have relevance?

15.4 What unit of life is the advantage relevant to? Gene, individual bacterium, or species? Might release of potentially devastating local concentrations of pneumolysin be reserved for the emergence of critical episodes in infection that are evidenced by limited lysis?

15.5 Why might NAD^+ represent a good substrate?

Chapter 16

16.1 Your answer should include the methods which can be utilized to identify microorganisms causing infection. You should comment on antibiotic resistance testing and nature of the work undertaken by the laboratory. What is the nature of the work performed? Is it cost-effective to perform by molecular methods – will it work on all samples? Are scanty organisms always important? Is PCR too sensitive – will it just detect normal flora?

16.2 Why is quality control important? How is it performed and when is it performed? How do you know you have achieved the required level of quality? Consider how you record this and make reference to external methods of quality assurance.

16.3 In your answer you should consider: what are the clinical benefits to implanting a new service? Consider the design and what is important, especially contamination issues. Would you perform all the molecular investigations within your own department or would you send certain tests away to a reference laboratory? You need to consider the financial implications as well as space and expertise of the staff within the department. Will your turnaround times per test meet clinical need?

Chapter 17

17.1 Think of the sites of the body that swabs are used to take samples from – this should indicate in what way they need to be different.

17.2 Are blood tubes for haematology and biochemistry samples sterile? If blood is taken from a patient on antibiotics what will be the concentration? What would be the consequences of a high concentration of antibiotics in the bloodstream on isolating a pathogen?

17.3 Consider how long bacteria survive outside the body. Are there any legal or health and safety issues associated with sample transport?

17.4 Look at why organisms are categorized into groups and the effect on the laboratory worker if there is a spillage, for example.

Self-check answers

Chapter 1

1.1 Fimbriae are more numerous than flagella, and its main role is adhesion. Flagella are only possessed by motile bacteria. Sex pili are involved in attachment of one bacterium to another to facilitate transfer of genetic material.

1.2 Lag, exponential, stationary, and decline phases. The main differences between them are how quickly the bacterial cell is dividing until they reach the decline phase where the cells start to die.

1.3 Viruses do not grow on agar plates, so if a viral particle passed through a filter and into the culture medium it would not grow. There would be no interference with detection of bacterial pathogens on the culture plate.

1.4 Some disinfectants are not active against spores for example and as such a range of disinfectants need to be used according to the situation. Some are toxic to human skin so careful consideration needs to be given when choosing a disinfectant.

1.5 Irregular, raised, filamentous, etc. Other colonial features include the colour of the colony and if they are causing haemolysis of the blood in the agar plate. The colour of the colony is extremely important on chromogenic agars as the colour in most cases provides a definitive identification.

Chapter 2

2.1 Firstly, there are health and safety issues if it is not performed correctly as aerosols are produced which could be very hazardous to the operator. The test should not be performed from blood agar as this can lead to a false-positive result and therefore a mis-identification.

2.2 Carbohydrates can be linked to chromogenic or fluorogenic substrates so that upon enzymic hydrolysis a coloured or fluorescent compound is released, which is easily visualized. Examples include o-nitrophenol and 4-methyl umbelliferone.

2.3 In the main, chromogenic substrates are used, as the reaction product is easily visualized and there is no need for a UV light source. However, fluorescent substrates are more sensitive and, as a result, a positive test will be determined much sooner. Substrates are therefore chosen depending upon the rapidity of the result required and the ease by which the tests are set up and results obtained.

2.4 (a) Oxidase. (b) Indole or tryptophan deaminase; also swarming on blood agar could be used. (c) Hydrogen sulphide production or fermentation of several carbohydrates. Serological tests can also be used. (d) Catalase would be the most useful differentiator.

2.5 The tube coagulase test is considered the gold standard for the detection of coagulase activity. However, it is impractical to set up one of these tests every time a *Staphylococcus* is grown. As a result, slide coagulase tests have been introduced which make detection of coagulase activity simple and rapid.

2.6 Several groups of organisms fail to ferment carbohydrates (e.g. *Pseudomonas* spp.) and as a result other tests, such as carbon source utilization tests, need to be used to differentiate between species.

2.7 Generally, biochemical tests would be better to differentiate between species. In general, there are a wide variety of tests that can be used compared to substance susceptibility tests. Even with established tests, such as optochin susceptibility, there are still problems with other closely related strains showing susceptibility to this agent.

2.8 Commercial kits have the advantages of utilizing a wide range of substrates to provide an accurate identification and differentiation from organisms which can be closely related. They are easily inoculated and results are generally easy to read. Powerful software packages are available containing databases of thousands of strains to allow for accurate identification.

Chapter 3

3.1 Like most living things bacteria require a 'balanced' diet in order to survive and multiply. The nutrients supplied are required for cell wall production, enzymes, etc.

3.2 Since pathogenic organisms require a host in order to survive and multiply, the pH for growth reflects that of the host.

3.3 Horses are large animals and as such a large amount of blood can be withdrawn. Human blood is not available in such quantities, and there are ethical issues also. Additionally, the blood would need to be screened for HIV and hepatitis before it could safely be used. Horse or sheep blood is therefore used.

3.4 For the selective isolation of Gram-positive organisms, bacitracin and aztreonam are commonly used agents. For Gram-negative strains, vancomycin is commonly used to suppress the growth of Gram-positive organisms and allow the Gram-negative strains to flourish.

3.5 The main advantages are that it eliminates the need for further confirmatory testing, compared to conventional media such as DCA or XLD. This reduces labour and lowers turnaround times for results. In the majority of cases, a coloured colony on a *Salmonella* chromogenic medium is highly likely to be a *Salmonella* spp.

3.6 The susceptibility profile of *Candida* spp. can vary widely with some species often 'intrinsically' or naturally resistant to antifungal agents. Finding these species can alter patient management. Differentiation of mixed *Candida* spp. is very difficult if not impossible on non-chromogenic media.

3.7 In general serum or blood would break down if added to media that was too hot. More importantly, antibiotic supplements for selective media would be totally inactivated by adding to media not cooled to the right temperature. If this was to happen the media would no longer be selective and important pathogens could be missed.

3.8 Media are one of the most important products used in a microbiology laboratory and as such ensuring high-quality media is essential. The consequences of poor quality or contaminated media could be disastrous in that target pathogens from clinical samples may not grow or may be covered in contaminants. The consequences for the patient could be significant.

Chapter 4

4.1 If the agar was too thin, larger zones may be encountered. With the medium too thick, the zones of inhibition would be reduced. Remember the antibiotic will diffuse downwards as well as across the plate.

4.2 If the temperature of incubation is incorrect the expected growth of the test organism will not occur. This could result in reduced or larger zone sizes depending upon the conditions. Incubation in carbon dioxide can affect the zone sizes of macrolide antibiotics such as erythromycin. Incubation of aminoglycosides anaerobically can also result in reduced zones.

4.3 Briefly, the MIC for the organism is determined at the same time as a zone size is produced. Since, from pharmokinetic studies, the serum concentration of the antibiotic is produced there is a relationship between them. From these data a zone size is produced which allows an organism to be called sensitive, resistant, or intermediate.

4.4 Potentially, the same consequences as for any incorrect result issued. For antibiotics it would mean the patient may be on inappropriate therapy. For a patient with life-threatening septicaemia, for example, this could result in serious consequences, even death.

4.5 The main problem is that the inoculum is not standardized and could be incorrect by several orders of magnitude. As a result, it can be difficult, if not impossible, on some occasions to interpret the susceptibility test result. The benefit is that for certain clinical conditions, such as septicaemia, a 'direct' result can confirm the patient is on appropriate therapy, or indicate antibiotic therapy should be changed more quickly than setting up the test after the culture result is known.

4.6 Broth tests are often performed in tubes or in microtitre plates and are often more labour intensive than conventional agar disc tests. Broth tests are considered more accurate due to the many problems that can be encountered with agar methods. Unless the process is automated, laboratories often prefer the convenience and cost benefits of agar susceptibility methods.

4.7 There are a number of species that appear to be susceptible to the antibiotic *in vitro* but are known to produce inducible enzymes which are expressed *in vivo*, for example AmpC enzymes. It is also important to recognize unusual patterns of resistance. For example, Group A streptococci are very unlikely to show resistance to penicillins and *S. aureus* strains are very rarely resistant to glycopeptides. This can be highly useful in stopping the spread of such organisms if they are identified fully.

4.8 Most antibiotics are relatively non-toxic to the host in the correct dose. Some, however, such as the aminoglycosides, can have serious side effects such as ototoxicity if the level is too high.

4.9 Generally, the automated immunoassay method is considered the best method for routine diagnostic use as it is relatively simple to perform with accurate results available in less than 30 minutes.

Chapter 5

5.1 Septicaemia is a fatal condition if not treated early and effectively. Clinicians will always treat if the indications are the patient has septicaemia.

5.2 Virtually any organism can cause septicaemia and some are highly nutritionally dependent. As a result, the blood culture systems use highly nutritious media to maximize isolation of the pathogen.

5.3 The Gram stain can provide information as to the possible identity of the infecting organism and allow appropriate antibiotic treatment to start before the culture result is obtained.

5.4 Having an indication of the susceptibility pattern of the organism growing in a blood culture bottle can aid significantly in the management of the patient.

5.5 Whilst numerous organisms cause septicaemia, the commonest are *S. aureus*, Enterobacteriaceae, *Enterococci*, *Pseudomonas*, and *Candida* spp.

5.6 If multiple organisms are involved then finding a single antibiotic to which they are all susceptible is difficult.

5.7 They may receive antibiotics which they do not need, and these may be costly, cause side effects, reduce the chance of a correct diagnosis, and increase length of hospital stay.

5.8 Yes – remember the most nutritious media are used in blood culture systems and one organism will rapidly grow into millions and a positive bottle will result. Some contaminants will grow faster than pathogens and as a result can outgrow and even inhibit their growth.

5.9 Most commonly the oropharynx in cases of native endocarditis. For prosthetic valve endocarditis it is contamination of the valve during surgery.

5.10 Symptoms can be quite vague and non-specific, such as the patient feels generally unwell and lethargic with low-grade pyrexia. Other symptoms can be heart murmurs, nodules in the eye or fingernails, as well as a raised white cell count.

Chapter 6

6.1 The commonest cause of a UTI is *E. coli*. The body has a number of mechanisms to prevent a UTI, such as urinary flow to flush the organism out. Other mechanisms include antibodies (IgA) and high osmolarity.

6.2 Whilst essential for patients with bladder problems and those post op there are disadvantages also. Colonization by bacteria and trauma, which can result in bacteraemia and septicaemia, are two major problems associate with urinary catheters.

6.3 A complicated urinary tract infection means an infection in a patient who has a structural abnormality, who is immunocompromised or who may be infected with a highly resistant organism.

6.4 In most cases upper urinary tract infection starts from infection of the lower tract. It can progress to bacteraemia in over one-third of cases. Upper urinary tract infections are considered clinically very important and essential to treat effectively.

6.5 Excretion of mycobacteria into the urine is intermittent and may not be picked up in a single sample.

6.6 The first few millilitres of a urine sample are likely to be contaminated with skin organisms. If these are present in the sample then it may be sent out as contaminated or contaminants may overgrow the causative organism of the UTI.

6.7 Microscopy, especially for the presence of WBC and RBCs, is very important alongside the culture result. The lack of WBCs in a sample may indicate asymptomatic bacteruria if significant numbers of organisms are present. The presence of RBCs (haematuria) may indicate renal infection. The presence of epithelial cells suggests the sample may be contaminated.

6.8 Automated methods are useful particularly when there is a high workload. Since most urine samples submitted are likely to be negative, these samples can be screened out without the need for culture. This can save labour, time, money, and patients being put on antibiotics they don't need.

6.9 Small numbers of organisms are likely to be insignificant or possibly represent contamination. Apart from special categories of patients, $>10^5$ organisms/mL is considered as significant.

6.10 Culture methods can vary between laboratories. Whilst CLED agar is commonly used, these plates are being superseded by chromogenic agar media, as such plates can give an accurate identification of bacterial colonies without the need for further work.

6.11 Generally, contamination is assessed by the number and types of organisms present in the sample. The majority of UTIs are caused by a single organism and the presence of three or more organisms is suggestive of contamination. Remember that low WBC counts and the presence of epithelial cells also indicate a contaminated sample.

6.12 For the patient an oral antibiotic is much preferred to an IV agent. Often IV antibiotics are administered in hospital which is more of an inconvenience than the patient being at home. Preferred choices would depend on the age of the patient and other factors such as pregnancy, and the common resistance patterns prevailing. Ideally, it would be oral agents such as amoxicillin, trimethoprim, nitrofurantoin, or a first-line cephalosporin such as cefalexin.

Chapter 7

7.1 Some organisms have more virulence mechanisms which makes them more likely to cause disease. *S. aureus* colonizes the nose, so skin infections are likely to be more common due to its occurrence on human skin.

7.2 In the tissue necrosis which occurs with gangrene there is very limited oxygen. This is an ideal environment for rapid-growing anaerobes such as *C. perfringens* to thrive.

7.3 Most throat infections are caused by a virus and antibiotics are of no use. Also, most infections get better on their own. Using antibiotics unnecessarily will only encourage resistance and limit the use of antibiotics in the future.

7.4 Both *S. aureus* and Group A streptococci produce numerous toxins which cause tissue damage, haemolysis, and evasion of phagocytosis. Serious infections caused by Group A streptococci are monitored epidemiologically so that the spread can be monitored. Think about the range of infections caused by *S. aureus* and at the same time how it is harmlessly carried in the nose of most people. What changes in the host occur to make *S. aureus* invade?

7.5 Firstly, it can be difficult to get good 'sample material' from a swab and as such it may be difficult to see any organism. Secondly, it is impossible to say with any accuracy that Gram-positive cocci seen, for example, are pathogenic strains or part of the normal flora.

7.6 Some organisms may only grow in CO_2 or under anaerobic conditions. Since organisms that grow under such conditions may be present, plates are incubated under a variety of conditions. In some cases β-haemolysis is best observed under anaerobic conditions and this can be very important in determining the identity of β-haemolytic streptococci in particular.

7.7 The biofilm will consist of organisms with a very low metabolic rate; thus antibiotics which are designed to kill rapidly growing cells will have a much lower effect on these organisms. Secondly, the organism in the biofilm will be encapsulated in a polysaccharide matrix making penetration of antibiotics difficult.

7.8 The number of organisms causing an infection in such sites may be very low. Culturing the samples direct may fail to yield the causative organism. Secondly, antibiotics may have damaged the organisms present. It is therefore essential to use broth enrichment to ensure any organisms present are isolated.

7.9 *N. gonorrhoeae* may be difficult to isolate because of the large numbers and diversity of the normal flora which may be present. In addition, the target organism may only be present in small numbers.

7.10 This is complex to answer and may be due to the fact that many infections are asymptomatic with no obvious signs – people wrongly think that protection is therefore not needed.

7.11 The organism cannot be grown by conventional culture methods, hence the need for alternative methods of detection. Screening tests for syphilis look for IgA or IgM antibodies depending upon the length of the disease.

7.12 The use of endocervical swabs is most common in females or urethral swabs in males. Culture is still used as the most common method of detection. Isolation media include antibiotics such as vancomycin, colistin, and antifungal agents such as amphotericin. Molecular methods (combined with detection of *Chlamydia*) are now proving to be useful for detection of the organism but culture still needs to be performed if susceptibility tests are required.

Chapter 8

8.1 The commonest causes of bacterial meningitis are *Neisseria meningitidis*, *S. pneumoniae*, and *S. agalactiae* (Group B).

8.2 Polymorphonuclear cells are often associated with bacterial meningitis, whereas lymphocytes are often associated with viral infections.

8.3 Bacteria will not always be seen, especially if it is an early infection where there may be few organisms infecting the CSF. Obviously the biomedical scientist won't be able to see viruses in a Gram stain!

8.4 It is important to identify any pathogen infecting a sterile site as it can have an impact upon patient management and in the case of meningitis it may be important to determine precisely what the organism is in an outbreak situation. The latter allows contacts to be traced and ensures prophylaxis is given promptly. Also, remember the problems associated with incorrect identification of *Listeria* and Group B streptococci.

8.5 Definitely not! This is one of the most serious clinical conditions which has a very high mortality rate if not treated promptly. Clinicians would always treat promptly if suspected.

8.6 In general it depends on the site. For example, respiratory organisms are likely to be encountered in pleural fluid. In peritoneal fluid it is more likely to encounter 'faecal' organisms, although any sterile site can be infected with virtually any bacteria.

8.7 Bacteria may be inside white blood cells – lysis causes them to be released allowing them to grow on culture media.

Chapter 9

9.1 Patients who are immunocompromised fail to produce as many white cells as a normal healthy individual. As a result the secretions from these patients may be mucoid.

9.2 Normal sputum samples should contain a mixture of mouth flora and the pathogen(s) in question. If diluted the mouth flora will diminish, making it easier to see the target pathogens. Other respiratory samples, for example pleural fluid, will contain no 'normal flora' organisms so there is no need to dilute the sample.

9.3 PCP is a disease only associated with patients who are immunocompromised.

9.4 Pathogens and 'normal flora' organisms will grow on basic isolation media. Selective media are used so it is easier to find the pathogen.

9.5 Bcc organisms can indicate a poor prognosis in transplant patients if they are colonizing or infecting them. As a result, it is vitally important to identify these organisms, which can be very difficult.

9.6 Decontamination agents are used to kill off the contaminating organisms in the sample so that the mycobacteria can grow unhindered. Mycobacterial cells are resistant to the decontamination procedure.

9.7 The most common species are *M. tuberculosis*, *M. bovis*, and *M. africanum*. These are Hazard Group 3 organisms.

Chapter 10

10.1 Think about the symptoms associated with most gastrointestinal infections. Do patients require hospitalization and how long do symptoms last? Do patients like submitting a stool sample to a GP?

10.2 There are many such mechanisms including the pH of the stomach. White blood cells and immunoglobulins such as IgA are abundant which also provides defence against infection. Digestive enzymes and the presence of normal colonizing bacteria are also important mechanisms.

10.3 In the Western world these infections are generally less severe, which is often due to the better health status of the individuals. Poor nutrition and sanitation contribute to the severity and length of disease in the developing world.

10.4 Think about the number of different types of gastrointestinal infection that an individual can acquire. Most have viral causes and it is very difficult to detect these routinely. Infections caused by parasites are often associated with foreign travel and it is not worth looking if there is no supporting clinical history.

10.5 For both the answer would be viral infections. If bacterial infections are considered then in developing countries it is mainly *Salmonella* and *Campylobacter* infections, although *Shigella* can be a significant cause. The same infections also occur in developing countries plus *Vibrio* and parasite infections.

10.6 The use of sodium selenite, the main ingredient of selenite broth, inhibits the growth of other interfering bacteria and allows preferential growth of *Salmonella* spp. There are no selective agents that would allow the enrichment of *Shigella* spp. at the expense of other intestinal flora.

10.7 It is highly suggestive but other organisms that are not causes of gastrointestinal disease, such as *Proteus* spp. and *Citrobacter freundii*, would produce similar colonies on XLD.

10.8 Whilst cell culture is often considered the gold standard it does not detect strains that only produce toxin A. In addition, faeces may contain chemicals and other toxin-producing bacteria, which produce a similar cytotoxic effect. The method is considered to be quite labour intensive.

10.9 Other Gram-negative organisms can have similar antigens to both *Salmonella* and *Shigella*, and cross reactions (false positives) do occur. It is generally considered that biochemical tests provide the most definitive identification in routine laboratories.

10.10 Most definitely not. This is because a patient with diarrhoea could potentially infect a whole ward or other unit before the laboratory confirmed the cause of the infection.

10.11 Think about what types of *Salmonella* cause enteric fevers and where are they causing infection in the body. What are the symptoms and length of illness of a *Salmonella* infection? Do antibiotics prolong carriage states?

10.12 Most viral illnesses are mild and self-limiting and it would be very difficult and expensive for routine laboratories to look for all potential viral causes. Generally, most laboratories would look for viruses such as adenovirus and rotavirus which cause significant disease in children. Laboratories would often look for viruses such as norovirus in outbreak situations.

10.13 Since most gastrointestinal infections are self-limiting, generally rest and fluid replacement are sufficient.

Chapter 11

11.1 Parasites are eukaryotic microorganisms which may be unicellular or multicellular. They reproduce through a variety of mechanisms (parasite dependent), for example, some undergo asexual reproduction (e.g. protozoa), whilst others are dioeciois (nematodes) or hermaphroditic (cestodes/ trematodes). Parasites require a host (or multiple hosts) to obtain nutrition and a 'parasite' may be transmitted to its host through a number of routes including: vectors (e.g. mosquitos), faecal–oral (contaminated food and water) and direct contact (sexual intercourse/skin penetration/congenital transmission).

11.2 Several risk factors are associated with the transmission and acquisition of parasitic infection, these include: travel to endemic regions, consumption of undercooked foods or contaminated food and water, immunosuppression (e.g. HIV, age), and global warming.

11.3 The 'active' stage of gastrointestinal protozoa is the feeding stage which is commonly associated with symptoms of disease, for example, gastrointestinal trophozoites. The 'infective' stage is the 'vector' of infection, for example a protozoan cyst or oocyst. The infective stage is able to withstand environmental extremes for extended periods of time, thus, this stage is readily transmitted to the host. Once consumed by the host, the infective stage is able to transform to the active stage.

11.4 *Cryptosporidium* species and *Toxoplasma gondii* both have complicated life cycles comprising sexual and asexual stages. *T. gondii* utilizes intermediate hosts including mice, birds, sheep, cattle, and pigs to undertake the asexual stage of its life cycle. As sexual reproduction cannot take place in the intermediate host, tachyzoites of *T. gondii* are released from the infective oocysts in the intestine of the intermediate host which then migrate into muscle and neural tissue where latent tissue cysts are formed.

11.5 Infections due to *Enterobius vermicularis* tend to be more common in young children for a couple of reasons. Firstly, effective hand hygiene amongst children is likely to be less than that of adults. As *E. vermicularis* promotes itching around the anus, children are more likely to scratch the anal region thus picking up numerous pinworm eggs on their hands and under their fingernails. If the hands are not washed correctly the eggs may then be transferred into the environment (door handles, surfaces) through touch, or reintroduced into the mouth of the infected host through faecal–oral/hand–mouth contact. Secondly, young children spend much time within schools and nurseries with other children and the highly infectious eggs of *E. vermicularis* are readily transmitted to many hosts through poor hygiene and contact. Whilst hygiene is the key factor, *E. vermicularis* takes advantage of the close proximity of numerous hosts for transmission.

11.6 The nematodes (roundworms) are morphologically different from the cestodes and trematodes in several ways. Unlike the trematodes and cestodes, nematodes are cylindrical, segmented parasites and have an outer cuticle. They are able to attach to their host through the use of 'lips' and 'teeth' and consume nutrients through a developed intestinal system. Both male and female sexes (dioecious) are required for reproduction within the nematode.

11.7 Human cysticercosis occurs when humans accidentally take the place of the intermediate host (*T. solium*) in the life cycle. In cysticercosis, humans ingest the eggs of *T. solium* (rather than the larval stage in contaminated undercooked pork as in taeniasis). The eggs hatch in the intestine of humans releasing aggressive first stage larvae (oncospheres) that cannot develop to adults in the intestine of humans. The oncospheres then penetrate the intestine of the human (as it would in the pig) and migrate to the muscle, eyes, central nervous system and heart. Here, cysticerci larvae develop in the human.

11.8 Following a suitable concentration technique, faecal concentrates can be examined using a number of techniques. Firstly, wet preparations, usually following staining with iodine, may be examined using light microscopy. This is probably the most common method adopted by routine clinical microbiology laboratories. In addition to this, stained smears may be examined. These include modified Ziehl–Neelson, trichrome, and iron-haematoxylin stained smears which may be examined for parasitic structures using light microscopy. Furthermore, fluorescent stains or fluorescent antibody smears such as auramine and Ig-FITC may be used to visualize parasites by fluorescent microscopy.

11.9 The optimal clinical sample for detection of active gastrointestinal trophozoites is fresh liquid faeces. Ideally, multiple samples should be obtained and transported to the laboratory as quickly as possible (within 30 min) as the trophozoites will begin to encyst over time. Active, motile trophozoites may be visualized with a light microscope using 100× or 400× magnifications.

11.10 1 EPU will equate to 6.3 μm

11.11 Several antiparasitic agents may be used to treat nematode infections, however, those commonly used include: albendazole, mebendazole, and pyrantel pamoate.

Chapter 12

12.1 Most commonly, the nose is the site of carriage of MRSA. In order to ensure that the best attempt has been made to locate MRSA, a nasal swab must be sent.

12.2 Because on mannitol salt agar the acid generated from fermentation of mannitol changes the pH throughout the medium, so the whole plate can become yellow, making the individual MRSA colonies difficult to detect in mixed culture. On chromogenic media there is no diffusion of the reaction product, making the colonies easier to detect.

12.3 The molecular methods offer significant advantages in the rapidity of results (<1 hour) and the simplicity of the methodology is now evident. However, the cost of each assay is more than 20-fold that for a chromogenic medium so its use for widespread screening is difficult to imagine financially. If large-scale screening is required the space must also be available to house multiple platforms. Several institutions advocate the use of molecular for certain situations combined with chromogenic/enrichment culture for the majority of 'routine' screens.

12.4 Screening is important for picking up MRSA carriage and such information is useful to help stop spread of infection. Most important are ward procedures such has hand washing, general cleanliness, and avoiding poor practice when inserting IV lines. These will have the most impact on MRSA bacteraemia rates.

12.5 These organisms can be highly drug resistant and vancomycin is an extremely important antibiotic for treatment of Gram-positive infections in general. If these organisms become common in a hospital environment, clinicians will be faced with difficult therapeutic decisions.

12.6 In winter months, patients often succumb to respiratory infections (especially elderly patients) and antibiotics can alter the gastrointestinal flora and allow overgrowth of *C. difficile*. In general, more antibiotics are used in the winter than in summer months.

12.7 It must be remembered that no single method is optimal for detection of *C. difficile* infection. New algorithms are being developed which initially screen for GDH as this has a high NPV. Samples positive for GDH would then be tested for the presence of toxins A + B. Some authors advocate the use of culture as part of any diagnostic algorithm. More recently, molecular methods are becoming popular due to the speed of results (<1 hour).

12.8 Gram-negative organisms are commonly susceptible to a wide range of antibiotics, including several β-lactam agents.

There are likely to be only 3-4 useable to treat MDR strains of *A. baumanii*. Think about the potential toxicity of these agents and how to determine susceptibility. Will disc testing be enough?

12.9 No. This is because *C. difficile* is likely to exist as spores in a ward environment and these gels have poor activity against spores.

12.10 If a group of infected individuals all have the same infection then it is prudent to manage them in the same environment. It would be very difficult to allocate such individuals a separate ward environment as most health-care institutions have only limited resources of this nature.

Chapter 13

13.1 Viruses have a characteristic very small size when compared to bacteria. They also have a very different genome (DNA or RNA but not both) and they are metabolically inert. In addition, they will not grow on artificial agar media.

13.2 Latency is a state of inactivity and reactivation is to become active again after a period of quiescence or as in a viral infection, latency. An example of a virus that can be latent and then reactivate is herpes simplex.

13.3 Viral transport medium should contain antibacterial and antifungal agents to prevent the overgrowth of contaminating bacteria and fungi. The presence of bacteria and fungi, particularly in cell culture, can lead to contamination of the culture and render it impossible to interpret.

13.4 Serology tests are easy, quick, and relatively cheap to perform.

13.5 These tests are rapid and results can be obtained in relatively short time spans. However, they can be tedious and labour intensive. These tests can be difficult to interpret and have a low sensitivity and specificity. The quality of the sample must be good to produce optimal results.

13.6 Molecular methods are much more sensitive and specific than other direct detection methods. They are also quick and easy to perform.

13.7 Cell culture is still used for many viral infections because it is a relatively inexpensive way to diagnose such infections. PCR is expensive to set up and so many smaller laboratories may not be financially in a position to set up a molecular laboratory.

13.8 Washing steps in an ELISA test rid the reaction well of any excess antibody or antigen that may be present. If excess antibody or antigen is present in the well, false-positive reactions will occur giving rise to inaccurate results.

13.9 HIV infection does not necessarily produce symptoms/ clinical disease for many years after the initial infection; therefore although the patient may be completely free of clinical disease, they may still be infected with HIV, and as such will produce antibodies.

13.10 Mild local infections such as HSV genitalis (genital herpes) may not produce a detectable humoral immune response as such and antibodies may not be produced.

Chapter 14

14.1 The main difference is that the bacteria are prokaryotic organisms and fungi are eukaryotic organisms.

14.2 More patients are immunosuppressed, there is better diagnosis of fungal infections and there are better treatments, which has prompted a demand for earlier diagnosis and better diagnostic aids.

14.3 Factors predisposing to fungal infections are immune state of the patient, age, use of broad-spectrum antibiotics and diabetes. These are the same factors that will predispose to many bacterial infections.

14.4 They are very unlikely to cause systemic infections as they require a lower temperature for optimal growth, hence they cause superficial infection. They are also of low virulence.

14.5 The result is available several weeks before culture. This allows therapy to be started earlier if the microscopy is positive.

14.6 The respiratory tract is the most common site of invasive *Aspergillus* infections because spores are infective and present in the air and are commonly breathed into the lung.

14.7 Allergic bronchopulmonary aspergillosis, aspergilloma, non-invasive aspergillosis, and acute invasive aspergillosis are associated with *Aspergillus*.

14.8 They are often labour intensive, require specialist media, and there is a lack of standardized protocols. They are also more costly to perform than bacterial susceptibility tests.

Chapter 15

15.1 Outside of the cell, either at the surface or at a distance from it.

15.2 Adhesins secure the bacteria to the host. Invasins promote invasion of sub-mucosal sites. Evasins help the microbe to avoid or limit damage caused by the immune system. Impedins actively disrupt the regulation of the immune system. Toxins damage cells or their physiological processes.

15.3 They are a series of molecules that are common to many tissues.

15.4 Many biological surfaces are heavily glycosylated and hence suitable for binding by lectins.

15.5 They secure a subset of proteins exported by Gram-positive organisms to the peptidoglycan to retain their activities at the cell surface.

15.6 They are unusual in expressing B1-integrins at their apical surface, i.e. the surface accessible to the gut lumen.

15.7 Integrins naturally transduce physical signals sensed via ECM molecules into cells. Physical interaction with bacteria will mimic natural events to which the integrins initiate a response.

15.8 These signalling GTPases are active in signalling when they have GTP bound to them. GAPs activate their GTPase activity, which then causes GTP hydrolysis. Thus the Rho protein enters its non-signalling GDP-bound form.

15.9 SgtP resets the actin cytoskeleton. It needs to last longer than the two other effectors SopE and SopE2 (both bacterial GEFs) to correct the balance after invasion.

15.10 To ensure that a pathogen never encountered before can be recognized and an initial response can be mounted to it. The development of an adaptive response to that pathogen might provide better handling of subsequent exposures to similar bacteria.

15.11 The three main pathways respond to different stimuli increasing the likelihood that bacteria are detected and challenged by complement. The classical pathway ensures that bacteria recognized by antibodies are targeted. The lectin pathway responds to common MAMPs. The alternative pathway is spontaneously activated to covers other scenarios and kills cells that are not specifically equipped to protect themselves from MAC.

15.12 In fact, few bacteria are sensitive to MAC. Opsonization with C3b might represent a greater threat to many.

15.13 They bind to areas of receptors that vary in structure much less than the specific antigen binding sites. Where a conventional, specific antigen can influence a single clone of B or T cells, a superantigen influences all clones in a sub-type.

15.14 STa simply binds the GC-C receptor with greater avidity than the natural hormones that regulate gut ion balances. It remains attached to it for longer.

15.15 Second messengers such as DAG, cGMP, and cAMP are generated intracellularly as a consequence of hormone or neurotransmitters binding to their cell surface receptors. They effectively transmit the 'impulse' around the cell to direct its physiological response. Toxins interfere by mimicking receptor binding or by generating the second messenger artificially.

Chapter 16

16.1 *Taq* polyermase is active at high temperatures. Its discovery allowed PCR to be developed.

16.2 Hydrogen bonds which link the bases together in DNA are weak. When subjected to high temperatures, these bonds break and allow the DNA to separate into two single strands.

16.3 The common problems with PCR are the generation of false positive reactions, little or no amplification of the target sequence, insufficient amplification of the target sequence due to background hybridization, and primer artefact formation.

16.4 Real-time PCR allows for quantification of the PCR product whereas PCR does not.

16.5 A DNA polymerase enzyme is an enzyme that synthesizes DNA molecules from their nucleotide building blocks whereas a DNA ligase enzyme is an enzyme that facilitates the joining of DNA strands together by catalysing the formation of a phosphodiester bond.

16.6 DNA sequencing is used to identify pathogens, especially ones which cannot be identified by phenotypic means, or those which cannot be cultured because they are fastidious or they are present in the sample in very low numbers. DNA sequencing has also been used to look for antimicrobial resistance genes. This has led to an improvement in patient management as antimicrobial therapy can be targeted with the appropriate treatment being administered.

16.7 16S testing will give the identification of the organism responsible for the infection but will not give antimicrobial sensitivity/resistance patterns unless a certain mutation/gene is being looked for. The organism responsible will still need to be cultured to perform antibiotic susceptibility testing, and lead to appropriate treatment.

16.8 The two different types of DNA microarray are the spotted DNA array and the oligonucleotide array. The spotted DNA array requires the attachment of a single-strand-strand or dissociated double-strand DNA to the slide, whereas the oligonucleotide arrays are directly spotted onto the slide or synthesized *in situ* onto the slide.

Chapter 17

17.1 The main problems are taking the incorrect sample, delays in transport, unlabelled samples, delays in inoculation of samples, and taking samples after the patient has received antibiotics. Selective media may need to be used to eliminate contaminating organisms.

17.2 The main types of sample containers are sterile containers (with or without spoon), swabs, blood tubes, and blood culture bottles.

17.3 The skin may contain numerous organisms which can grow on the culture media used to isolate the target pathogen. By cleaning it, their numbers are reduced significantly and this will allow pathogens to grow unhindered.

17.4 Probably the best method of sample transport is the fastest, although all methods have limitations. Air tube systems are most likely to allow samples to get to the laboratory quickly.

17.5 Since selective media contain inhibitory substances it is best to inoculate non-selective media first to allow maximum isolation of target pathogens.

17.6 Chemical treatment will not kill the mycobacteria but will kill or inhibit the growth of any contaminating organisms.

17.7 The highest is Level 4 and the lowest Level 1. Level 2 is most commonly used for processing routine microbiology samples.

Glossary

α- or β-haemolytic streptococci bacterial colonies can be described as α-haemolytic or β-haemolytic depending on their action on the red blood cells in the culture medium.

acid-fast microorganisms that resist decolorization with acid; typically applies to mycobacteria.

acyclovir an antiviral agent with activity against herpesvirus types 1 and 2 and varicella zoster virus. Acyclovir is converted by a herpesvirus enzyme into a molecule that inhibits the synthesis of deoxyribonucleic acid (DNA) molecules in the virally infected cells. This has the effect of inhibiting viral replication.

adaptive immunity an acquired immune response directed by specific antigens and featuring memory functions.

adenylate cyclase an enzyme that catalyses the conversion of adenosine triphosphate (ATP) to inorganic pyrophosphate and cyclic adenosine monophosphate (cAMP).

adhesins appear to mediate bacterial adherence to host epithelial cells thereby assisting in pathogenesis.

aglycone a molecule that is not a sugar but is linked to a natural sugar (e.g. galactose) via a glycosidic bond (e.g. nitrophenol in o-nitrophenyl-b-D-galactopyranoside).

AIDS disease of the immune system caused by HIV.

aminoglycosides a group of antibiotics, including gentamicin and tobramycin. They are considered broad-spectrum agents and are particularly active against *S. aureus* and aerobic Gram-negative bacilli. These agents can be both nephrotoxic and ototoxic.

aminopeptidase a peptidase enzyme that targets amino acids with a 'free' amino group.

amnionitis infection of the membrane sac that surrounds and protects the embryo.

AmpC β-lactamase an inducible enzyme occurring in Gram-negative species such as *Enterobacter* and *Serratia* spp. They hydrolyse broad- and extended-spectrum cephalosporins.

amphotericin B a polyene antifungal drug; it shows high patient toxicity.

amplicon an amplicon is a piece of DNA or RNA that is the product of natural or artificial amplification or replication.

anaerobes organisms that only grow when oxygen is absent.

anaphylatoxin proteolytic product of complement activation that mediate chemotaxis and inflammation.

anaphylaxis serious allergic reaction that is rapid in onset. Symptoms include itchy rash, throat swelling, and low blood pressure. May result in death.

antagonist essentially a compound which will neutralise the effect of another.

antibiotic a chemical compound that has the ability to kill or inhibit the growth of microorganisms. They are sufficiently non-toxic to be administered to the host.

arthritis the term used to describe inflammation in a joint. Septic arthritis is the name used to describe inflammation of a joint caused by infection.

arthropathy a disease or abnormality of a joint.

arthroplasty surgical procedure where an arthritic or problem joint is replaced.

asepsis the practice of trying to eliminate contaminants from entering samples; also used in surgical and other situations to ensure organisms don't enter the patient during the procedures used.

aseptic technique the use of sterile equipment and procedures to avoid possible contamination.

aspergilloma a ball of fungi found in the lungs; typically occurs with *Aspergillus* spp.

aspiration pneumonia occurs when the epiglottis fails to cover the larynx during swallowing. Food and saliva, which would normally be directed down the oesophagus, enter the trachea and can lead to pneumonia.

asymptomatic the presence of an organism but without symptoms developing.

attenuation a reduction in virulence.

atypical pneumonia organisms that cause pneumonia without characteristic symptoms, e.g. lack of sputum production.

auramine–phenol stain auramine O is a fluorescent dye and this is a common stain used to detect mycobacteria in clinical samples.

autoclave a strong, pressurized, steam-heated vessel, used to sterilize bacterial cultures or culture media.

autolysis when an organism produces enzymes that lead to the breakdown of its own cells.

avidity the combined strength of multiple intramolecular bonds.

avirulent non pathogenic.

β-lactam antibiotics a family of antibiotics which contains penicillins, cephalosporins and some other antibiotics. They are composed of a β-lactam ring and some, e.g. penicillin, are used mainly to treat Gram-positive infections. Cephalosporins are more broad-spectrum agents.

β-lactamase enzymes that break down penicillin and related antibiotics (β-lactams) such as ampicillin and destroy their antibacterial activity.

bacitracin a naturally produced antibiotic that targets bacterial cell walls.

bacteraemia the presence of bacteria in the bloodstream.

bacteriophage a bacterial virus.

bacteristatic refers to an antibiotic that inhibits the growth of an organism but doesn't necessarily kill it. Bactericidal antibiotics are those that are likely to kill the organism.

bacteriuria presence of bacteria in the urine.

balanitis inflammation of the glans penis.

barrier nursing this involves putting the patient in a side room or with other individuals with exactly the same infection in the same room. The nursing staff wear disposable aprons and gloves when dealing with these patients to minimize any spread of the infection to other patients.

Bartholin's gland two glands situated below the vagina.

biofilm a collective community of microorganisms encapsulated in a polysaccharide matrix.

β-lactam a lactam in which the amide bond is contained within a four-membered ring, which includes the amide nitrogen and the carbonyl carbon. Antibiotics which possess this feature include penicillin.

blind subculture subculture of the bottle regardless of the presence or absence of turbidity or indications of growth.

breakpoint this refers to when only certain antibiotic concentrations are tested, normally two. These concentrations would be appropriate for differentiating between susceptible, intermediate and resistant.

broad-spectrum antibiotics drugs that show activity against a wide range of organisms, typically both Gram-negative and Gram-positive species.

bronchiectasis disease that causes a localized and irreversible dilatation of the bronchi.

Burkholderia cepacia complex a group of bacteria that are most often associated with patients who have cystic fibrosis.

Buruli ulcer an infectious disease caused by *Mycobacterium ulcerans*.

butyrous resembling butter.

candidiasis infections caused by yeasts from the genus Candida.

capsule a polysaccharide coat that covers some organisms such as *C. neoformans*. Capsules help resist ingestion by white blood cells.

carbapenemase an enzyme that hydrolyses not only penicillins but also cephalosporins, monobactams, and carbapenems. Strains that produce these enzymes are highly drug resistant.

carbuncles a large abscess made up of several skin boils, filled with fluid and pus.

carrier state this is where an individual, who is not ill, can harbour an infectious organism which may cause disease if it is passed on.

casein a protein precipitated from cow's milk.

catalase an enzyme that catalyses the decomposition of hydrogen peroxide, forming water and oxygen.

catheter a hollow tube that can be inserted into a body cavity. The procedure is known as catheterization.

CD4 counts a measure of the number of helper T cells per mm^3 of blood, used to analyse the prognosis of patients infected with HIV.

cell culture the growth of cells *in vitro*.

cell line one derived from a primary culture which has been cultured for the first time.

cell lysis where cells can burst open resulting in cell death.

cellulitis a spreading infection of the skin and connective tissue.

cerebral palsy a name for a group of conditions which are non-progressive and result in physical disability.

cerebrospinal fluid a clear fluid that fills the spinal column.

chancroid an uncommon sexually transmitted infection which presents as painful sores on the genitalia.

chemiluminescence the emission of light by a substance as a result of a chemical reaction that does not involve an increase in its temperature. Chemiluminescence occurs when a highly oxidized molecule, such as a peroxide, reacts with another molecule. The bond between the two oxygen atoms in a peroxide is relatively weak, and when it breaks the atoms must reorganize themselves, releasing energy in the form of light.

chemotaxis the movement of an organism or cell along a chemical concentration gradient either toward or away from the chemical stimulus.

chromogenic media differential culture media that contain chromogenic enzyme substrates. When such substrates are metabolized (typically by hydrolysis), they release a coloured dye or 'chromogen' indicating the presence of a specific enzyme.

chromogenic substrate may be natural or synthetic and is metabolized (usually by a hydrolase) to release a coloured dye.

cilia hair-like beating structures which protrude from respiratory epithelial cells.

ciliates a class of cilia containing protozoa.

Clostridium difficile an organism involved in outbreaks of gastrointestinal disease which can be fatal, especially in the elderly. Production of two protein toxins A + B is responsible for production of disease.

coliform a loose term used for bacteria that are '*Escherichia coli*-like'. They are members of the Enterobacteriaceae family which ferment lactose to produce acid and gas at 35–37°C.

colonization an organism that is found at a particular body site but is playing no role in disease. Colonization can be transient in that individuals can be colonized with MRSA at the start of a shift and be clear at the end and vice versa.

commensal organisms organisms involved in a relationship with a host, causing no ill effects.

complement a series of proteins found in blood; when activated the proteins have an antibacterial action and help the body to fight infection.

complement fixation test an immunological test that can be used to detect the presence of either specific antibody or specific antigen in a patient's serum. However, in clinical diagnostics labs it has been largely superseded by other serological methods such as ELISA and by DNA-based methods of pathogen detection, particularly PCR.

computed tomography scan (CT scan) a medical imaging technique which generates a 3D image.

conjunctivitis an infection of the outermost layer of the eye (the conjunctiva).

containment levels describes the facilities and practices that are appropriate for the control of microorganisms.

contaminant an organism that is not deemed to be pathogenic. This can also mean an organism that was not present in the original sample.

convalescent the time where the patient is returning back to full health following an illness.

cord factor one of the mycolic acids in mycobacteria. This promotes the formation of strings of cells that give a cord-like appearance microscopically.

C-reactive protein (CRP) a protein found in blood; levels of CRP increase when there is inflammation or infection.

crepitus the medical name for sounds under the skin. Typically this is popping or cracking sounds.

crystalluria presence of crystals in the urine.

cuticle flexible, tough, outer coverings of the nematodes that provides protection. The cuticle is secreted by the epidermis.

cycloheximide a chemical that has antifungal properties. It suppresses growth of fungi such as *Aspergillus* and *Penicillium* spp. which are common in the environment and may contaminate skin and nail samples.

cysticeri larval form of *Taenia species*, consisting of a single scolex enclosed in a bladder like cyst. Hexacanths, released from eggs, develop into cysticeri in the muscle of the intermediate host over a period of 3–4 months.

cystitis acute cystitis is acute inflammation of the bladder.

cytokine a regulatory protein, released by cells of the immune system.

cytology the study of cells.

cytomegalic inclusion bodies nuclear or cytoplasmic aggregates of stainable substances, usually proteins. They typically represent sites of viral multiplication in a bacterium or a eukaryotic cell and usually consist of viral capsid proteins.

cytomegalovirus (CMV) a member of the herpesvirus family and one of the most common human viruses. The virus occurs worldwide, and most people become infected with CMV sometime during their lives.

cytopathic effect the presence of the virus often gives rise to morphological changes in the host cell. Any detectable changes in the host cell due to infection are known as a cytopathic effect. Cytopathic effects (CPE) may consist of cell rounding, disorientation, swelling or shrinking, death, or detachment from the surface.

cytotoxic agents a chemical that is toxic to host cells.

cytotoxin a toxin that kills cells.

decontamination when samples are treated with chemicals to kill or reduce the numbers of other organisms leaving the target pathogen undamaged.

definitive host the host in which a mature parasite resides and replicates/reproduces.

degranulation release of intra-cellular antimicrobial agents stored in intracellular compartments known as granules.

dermatome an area of skin that is mainly supplied by a single spinal nerve.

dermatophytes a group of three slow growing fungi which cause infections of skin, hair, and nails.

diabetic nephropathy damage to the small blood vessels within the kidney seen in patients with longstanding diabetes mellitus.

differential media culture media that include an indicator system for detection of biochemical activity, thus enabling differentiation of species or groups of microbes. A typical example would be inclusion of a sugar plus a pH indicator to demonstrate oxidation/fermentation.

dimorphic a fungus that can exist in two forms, a yeast or a filamentous hyphal form.

dioecious separate male and female organisms are required for sexual reproduction.

diphtheria an acute upper respiratory tract disease caused by *Corynebacterium diphtheriae*.

diptheroids a loose term to describe a range of Gram-positive rods that appear 'coryneform' on Gram stain.

direct susceptibility test a sensitivity test carried out directly on a sample rather than on an isolated bacterial culture.

disinfection the process of destroying harmful micro-organisms at points of transmission.

disseminated spread throughout the body.

dysentery an inflammatory disorder of the lower intestinal tract, which may be bacterial, parasitic, or protozoan. Typical symptoms include abdominal pain, fever, and severe diarrhoea. Characteristically the patient will pass blood and mucus in the stool.

dysuria pain on passing urine; patients often describe this as a burning or stinging feeling on passing urine.

echinocandin antifungal drugs which inhibit cell wall synthesis.

ectoparasite a parasite(s) which lives on the surface of the host such as head lice.

EDTA ethylenediaminetetraacetic acid is an anticoagulant to prevent blood samples from clotting.

electron microscope a type of microscope that uses a particle beam of electrons to illuminate a specimen and create a highly magnified image. An electron microscope has a much greater resolving power than a light microscope and can obtain a much higher magnification of up to 2 million times, while the best light microscopes are limited to magnifications of 2000 times.

embryonate pertaining to or resembling an embryo.

emetic toxin a toxin that causes severe, often projectile vomiting; such a symptom can be characteristic of *B. cereus* food poisoning.

empiric therapy the commencement of therapy before it is known what the infective organism is or what its susceptibility is.

empyema a collection of pus and necrotic tissue in a body cavity, e.g. the pleural cavity.

encephalitis inflammation of the brain usually caused by a viral infection.

endocarditis an infection of the heart valves.

endocytosis a process where substances are taken into the cell.

endoparasite a parasite such as tapeworms which live within the internal organs or tissues of a host.

endotoxin is a component of Gram-negative bacterial cell walls; when released into blood it causes fever.

enrichment culture a method that utilizes a nutrient liquid medium so that very small numbers of organism(s) are encouraged to multiply to large numbers. This method is used so that small numbers of potential pathogenic organisms can be detected where they may be missed on direct culture.

enrichment media culture media (typically broth based) that are designed to favour or 'enrich' the growth of specific target pathogens.

enterotoxin a toxin released by an organism in the intestine. They are protein in nature and frequently cytotoxic and kill host cells.

eosinophils a type of WBC associated with allergy. They may be detected in sputum microscopically.

epidemiology the study of the distribution of disease and its impact upon the population.

epiglottitis inflammation of the epiglottis which when inflamed can cause serious breathing difficulties.

epithelium cellular tissue which covers the external body surface, or the lining of internal surfaces.

epitopes the part of a macromolecule that is recognized by the immune system.

Epstein–Barr virus (EBV) a member of the herpesvirus family and one of the most common human viruses. The virus occurs worldwide, and most people become infected with EBV sometime during their lives.

erysipelas a diffuse infection of the upper layers of skin; often has a defined edge.

erysipeloid a cutaneous form of an infection caused by *Erysipelothrix rhusiopathiae*.

esculin a naturally occurring glucoside consisting of glucose linked via a glycosidic bond to 6,7-dihydroxycoumarin; a substrate for detecting β-glucosidase.

esterase a hydrolase enzyme that splits esters into an acid and an alcohol.

ethylene oxide a gas used as a fumigant, fungicide, and sterilizing agent. It is highly irritating to the eyes and mucous membranes and is carcinogenic.

evasin a virulence factor whose primary function is related to avoiding recognition by the immune response.

exocytosis the passage of material to the cell surface and subsequent release from the cell.

exopolysaccharide high-molecular-weight compounds composed of sugar residues. These are produced by microorganisms and released into their surrounding environment.

exotoxin a component of Gram-negative bacterial cell walls; when released into blood it causes fever.

exponential phase the period of optimal cell growth following the lag phase.

extended-spectrum β-lactamases enzymes that can be produced by bacteria making them resistant to penicillins and cephalosporins, e.g. cefuroxime, cefotaxime, and ceftazidime. These antibiotics are some of the most important antibiotics available for the treatment of infectious disease.

extracellular matrix the intercellular materials that support tissues.

faecal concentrate a method widely used in parasitology to concentrate the stool sample and allow the best chance of visualizing ova, cysts, and parasites.

faecal lactoferrin presence of leucocytes in a stool sample. Can be used as a marker for intestinal inflammation; not specific for *C. difficile*.

fastidious organisms that require additional nutrient in order to grow.

fatty acids acids found in fats and oils. They consist of long hydrocarbon chains with a carboxyl acid group at one end.

fish tank granuloma skin lesions caused by *Mycobacterium marinum*, also known as swimming pool granuloma.

flagella hair-like projections that extend from some bacteria which aid in their movement.

flagellates one of four phyla of parasitic protozoa. They can cause a range of disease in humans which depends upon the flagellate involved. Typically this involves enteritis, urethritis, and vaginitis.

fluke a parasitic flatworm that has external suckers. Flukes are sometimes called trematodes. Typical example would be *Fasciola hepatica* (liver fluke).

fluorogenic substrate may be natural or synthetic and is metabolized (usually by a hydrolase) to release a fluorescent compound.

folliculitis inflammation of a hair follicle anywhere on the skin.

free radicals an atom or chemical species that has at least one unpaired electron and is therefore highly unstable/reactive.

fumigation describes the process of sterilizing a safety cabinet with the use of formaldehyde vapour.

galactomannan a polysaccharide component of the cell wall of *Aspergillus* spp.

galactosidase a glycosidase that hydrolyses a glycosidic bond between galactose and a second sugar molecule, e.g. glucose.

gangrene a complication of cell death (necrosis) where tissues of the body start to decay.

gas gangrene the decay or necrosis of body tissues infected with a *Clostriduim* spp. where gas is formed, which results in extreme swelling of the infected area.

genetic probe a nucleic acid sequence that is complementary to the target sequence.

genome the entire genetic content of an organism.

glomerulonephritis inflammation of the glomeruli, or small blood vessels of the kidney.

glucuronidase a glycosidase that hydrolyses a glycosidic bond between glucuronic acid and a second sugar molecule.

glutamate dehydrogenase (GDH) marker for *C. difficile* strains, present in large amounts. Samples screened for the presence of GDH have a high negative predictive value (NPV); as such, the test is becoming widely used as part of a *C. difficile* detection algorithm for faeces samples.

glutaraldehyde a disinfectant used in aqueous solution for sterilization of heat-sensitive equipment and instruments. Also used as a broad-spectrum microbicide effective against all vegetative bacteria, fungi, and viruses. It is also sporicidal.

glycopeptides these antibiotics bind to cell wall peptidoglycan which affects cell wall synthesis. They are mainly used for the treatment of serious staphylococcal and enterococcal infections.

glycopeptides these are a class of antibiotics that are used for the treatment of Gram-positive infections, e.g. teicoplanin and vancomycin.

glycosaminoglycans sugar polymers consisting of repeats of alternating uronic acids and amino sugars.

glycosidase a hydrolase enzyme that hydrolyses a glycosidic bond, e.g. linking sugar units.

growth factor a nutrient or nutrients which improves the growth of microrganisms.

Guillian–Barré syndrome an autoimmune disease usually triggered by an acute infection which affects the peripheral nervous system causing paralysis.

HACEK a group of organisms, namely *Haemophilus* spp., *Aggregatibacter actinomycetemcomitans* (previously named *Actinobacillus*), *Cardiobacterium hominis*, *Eikenella corrodens*, and *Kingella* spp. whose initial letters form the acronym. They are CO_2 dependent and initial infections can lead to endocarditis.

haemadsorption when cultured cells acquire the ability to stick to mammalian red blood cells.

haemagglutinin a substance that causes red blood cells to agglutinate.

haematogenous originating in or spread by the bloodstream.

haematogenous spread an agent that spreads through the bloodstream.

haemocytometer a device for counting blood cells.

haemoptysis literally means the 'spitting of blood'.

hazard groups microorganisms belong to certain hazard groups depending upon the seriousness of the disease caused. The highest level is 4.

headspace the gas in a blood culture bottle above the liquid.

health-care-acquired infections these occur when pathogenic organisms are transferred from health-care workers, patients or the hospital environment, to a previously uninfected patient, who then develops the infection.

helminths worm parasites of the intestines, e.g. roundworm or tapeworm.

HEPA high efficiency particulate air (HEPA).

hepatocellular carcinoma (HCC) a primary carcinoma of the liver.

hermaphroditic male and female reproductive systems contained within a single organism.

heterologous antibody is an antibody derived from an individual of a different species.

heterotrophic requiring complex organic compounds (growth factors) for growth.

homogenized a process where tissue or sputum samples in particular are broken down to aid the release of microorganisms.

homologous antibody an antibody derived from an animal of the same species.

homologues are evolutionarily-related (evidenced through amino acid sequence conservation) entities. These might carry out identical (orthologues) or similar (paralogues) functions.

horizontal gene transfer the transfer of genetic materials by mechanisms not associated with conventional (vertical) heredity.

hospital-acquired infection also called a nosocomial infection, it is an infection that appears more than 48 h after a patient has been admitted to hospital or other health-care facility.

host range the range of hosts that can be infected by a pathogen.

humoral immune response an immune response mediated by secreted antibodies produced in B lymphocytes.

hybridization the process of forming a double stranded nucleic acid from two complementary DNA or RNA strands.

hydatid sand scoleces, hooks, and daughter cysts of Echinococcus tapeworms found within a primary or daughter hydatid cyst.

hydrocephalus literally means water on the brain. It is a build-up of CSF around the brain and it causes enlargement of the head in neonates.

hydrolase an enzyme that catalyses the hydrolysis of a chemical bond.

hydrophobic water hating.

hyphae long, branching filamentous cells of a fungus, hyphae are the main mode of vegetative growth, and are collectively called a mycelium.

immunocompromised or immunodeficient a state where the patient's immune function is absent or impaired so the ability to fight infection is impaired.

immunoglobulin G (IgG) an immunoglobulin, built of two γ heavy chains and two light chains. Each IgG has two antigen binding sites. It is the most abundant immunoglobulin and is approximately equally distributed in blood and in tissue liquids. IgG antibodies are predominantely involved in the secondary antibody response which occurs approximately 1 month following antigen recognition; thus the presence of specific IgG generally corresponds to maturation of the antibody response.

immunoglobulin M (IgM) an immunoglobulin built of μ heavy chains. It is the first immunoglobulin to appear on the surface of B cells and the first to be secreted. IgM is by far the physically largest antibody in the human circulatory system.

impedin a virulence factor whose primary function is related to dysregulate the immune response.

impetigo generally appears as scabs on a superficial skin infection.

in vitro in an artificial environment such as the laboratory.

in vivo inside the living organism.

incubation period the time between the receipt of infection and the onset of illness.

index patient the individual who first shows signs of the disease.

indicator antibiotics agents that are generally the least microbiologically active member of a family of antibiotics and are therefore more likely to detect low-level resistance. Examples of agents that have been used for this purpose include oxacillin for the detection of penicillin resistance in *Streptococcus pneumoniae* and methicillin-resistant *S. aureus*.

induced sputum sample that is induced in the patient by inhaling nebulized saline to promote the production of sputum.

innate immunity the generic immune response directed against pathogens that does not rely on previous exposure.

inoculum the portion of the specimen that is put onto the culture plate or into the fluid medium.

inspissation a process for heating and thus solidifying high-protein media via dehydration. The process, classically used for the coagulation of egg-based media, typically involves heating at 80–85°C and is not a process of sterilization, but most vegetative bacteria are killed.

intermediate host the host in which parasitic larval stages reside or non-sexual reproduction occurs.

interstitial fluid is the fluid that bathes and surrounds cells; produced in capillaries it is also known as tissue fluid.

intracellular organisms organisms that can be seen or multiply inside the host's cells.

intraluminal the inside space of a tubular structure (lumen).

intrathecal refers to an event that happens inside the spinal column.

intrauterine contraceptive device a device placed in the uterus for birth control.

intrinsic/inherent resistance resistance to antibiotics which occurs naturally within most or all species of a particular organism.

invasin a virulence factor whose primary function is related to entering host tissues.

ischemia the lack of oxygen supply to a particular body site.

Kauffmann–White scheme the definitive listing of all essential serological characteristics of *Salmonella*.

keratin a protein found in the outer layers of skin; it serves to protect skin.

keratitis inflammation of the cornea.

lactic acid bacilli bacteria that produce lactic acid as the main metabolic end product of carbohydrate fermentation.

lactophenol blue a good background dye to visualize fungal structures.

lag phase the period of very low physiological activity and cellular division following inoculation of a bacterial suspension into to a new culture medium.

latent virus any virus that remains in its host organism without undergoing replication. Latent viruses may be induced to replicate and cause cell lysis some time after the initial infection, for example when the host's immunity is reduced.

lecithinase a type of phospholipase enzyme that acts upon lecithin.

lectin a carbohydrate binding protein.

Lemierre's disease a disease mainly caused by *Fusobacterrium necrophorum* but other fusobacteria can be involved. It mainly affects young adults. Lemierre's syndrome follows a streptococcal throat infection which has led to a peritonsillar abscess. *Fusobacterium necrophorum* can flourish in this abscess and can penetrate into the neighbouring jugular vein. Bacteria can then disseminate into the bloodstream. It is associated with a high mortality rate.

lenticules and vitroids solid matrices designed for preserving microbes. They are typically presented as small discs containing microbial cells and spontaneously re- hydrate and dissolve on addition to culture media thus delivering a specified microbial inoculum. May be used for quality control of culture media.

leucopenia a reduction in the total number of white blood cells.

ligand a specific binding partner.

lipids fat soluble, naturally occurring compounds such as fats, oils or waxes. Cells of mycobacteria have high lipid content.

lipooligosaccharide a glycosylated complex lipid component of the outer membrane of Gram-negative bacteria featuring a small number of repeated sugar motifs.

lipopolysaccharide a heavily glycosylated complex lipid component of the outer membrane of Gram-negative bacteria featuring repeated sugar motifs.

lipophilic lipid loving; some fungi require the addition of lipids to the medium in order to grow.

lumbar puncture the procedure used to obtain a CSF sample from a patient.

lumen the inside of any hollow, tube-like structure.

lymphoma a form of cancer that originates in the lymphocytes of the immune system.

lysogen a bacterium that contains an integrated bacteriophage genome.

lysosyme a family of enzymes that damage bacterial cell walls.

M cells specialised epithelial cells which absorb matter from the intestinal contents. Associated with Peyer's patches in particular.

macrolides a group of antibiotics containing erythromycin and clindamycin. They are most often used for the treatment of staphylococcal and streptococcal infection, particularly in patients allergic to penicillins.

macrophages white blood cells (WBCs) that engulf then digest foreign bodies, including organisms.

malabsorptive state a characteristic state marked by subnormal intestinal absorption of dietary constituents, and thus excessive loss of nutrients in the stool, with chronic diarrhoea and weight loss.

mandatory reporting this is the obligatory reporting of a particular condition to local or national authorities. This often applies to communicable disease. Reporting of MRSA bacteraemia and *C. difficile* infection is mandatory in the UK.

***mec*A** this is a gene that codes for an altered penicillin binding protein (PBP2 or PBP2a). These proteins have a lower affinity for β-lactam antibiotics and confer resistance to the organism.

median lethal dose the quantitiy of a toxic substance (e.g. an antibiotic) which will kill 50% of the organisms exposed to it.

meningitis inflammation of the meninges.

metacercariae resistant, encysted final stage larval forms of some trematodes.

metachromatic describes granules (also known as volutin granules) that are cytoplasmic inclusions composed mainly of polyphosphates. They appear red-purple when stained with methylene blue.

metronidazole an antimicrobial agent with excellent activity against anaerobic bacteria and protozoa.

micro- and macroconidia names given to the spores produced by dermatophyte fungi. They differ in size; microconidia are small often spherical or tear drop shaped, 2–4 μm in diameter; macroconidia are much larger.

microaerophillic a term applied to organisms such as *Campylobacter* spp. whereby the organisms require an environment containing a reduced oxygen level for optimal growth. Many microphiles also require an elevated concentration of carbon dioxide (>5%).

microbial associated molecular pattern conserved structural elements used to detect microbes to trigger innate immunity.

microconidia and macroconidia small and large structures seen on microscopy when identifying dermatophytes.

minimum bactericidal concentration the lowest concentration of an antibiotic which is cidal to ≥99.9% of the test inoculum.

minimum inhibitory concentration the lowest concentration of an antibiotic needed to inhibit bacterial growth.

monolayer a single layer of cells growing on a surface.

monomicrobial bacteraemia bacteraemia where only one significant organism is isolated.

mucinase an enzyme that catalyses the breakdown of mucopoly-saccharides such as mucin.

mutualism a co-existence in which both partners derive benefit.

mycolic acids these are long fatty acid molecules with one long chain and one short chain. They are commonly found in the cell wall of mycobacteria.

nasogastric feed a tube, generally made of soft rubber or plastic, that is inserted through a nostril and into the stomach.

nebulized antimicrobials antibiotics are inhaled using a device which creates a cloud of small particles. High drug concentration in the lung is achieved and minimal systemic absorption reduces toxicity.

necrotizing fasciitis a rare infection often known as 'flesh eating disease' affecting the deeper layers of skin and subcutaneous tissue.

necrotizing pneumonia when multiple abscesses can be found in the lungs.

needlestick injury when a needle used to take a blood sample from a patient accidentally pierces the skin of a health-care worker.

Negri bodies eosinophilic inclusion bodies found in the cytoplasm of certain nerve cells containing the rabies virus.

nematodes a collective term for parasitic roundworms, such as hookworm and pinworm.

neuraminidase frequently found as an antigenic determinant on the surface of influenza virus. It is also a drug target for the prevention of influenza infection.

neutropenia a reduction in the number of phagocytic white blood cells.

non-dermatophyte fungi other filamentous fungi that can cause infections. There are several species that can cause infections of nails.

non-selective agar media that support the growth of a wide range of organisms; they do not contain inhibitory substances.

normal flora (human microbiotica) the collective term for the organisms colonizing a given body site.

nosocomial infections infection associated with health care which develops more than 48 h after the patient is admitted. For example, a urinary tract infection occurring as a complication of a procedure such as urinary catheter insertion.

novobiocin a naturally produced antibiotic and an inhibitor of DNA gyrase enzyme.

number needed to treat a statistical term that assesses the effectiveness of a health-care intervention, for example seven pregnant women with asymptomatic bacteriuria would have to be treated to prevent one case of pyelonephritis.

'O' antigen an antigen that is part of the lipopolysaccharide layer of the wall of Gram-negative bacteria.

oligonucleotide a short nucleic acid polymer, typically with 20 or fewer bases.

onychomycosis term given to a fungal infection of the toe or finger nails.

oocyst the resistant stage in the life cycle of coccidial parasites. The cyst may remain infective for long periods in dry conditions.

operculum a 'lid' at the top of many trematode eggs which allows release of larval trematodes. A useful distinguishing feature when attempting to identify the egg.

ophthalmia neonatorum also known as neonatal conjunctivitis. An eye infection of newborn infants contracted during delivery.

opportunistic pathogen an infection caused by a pathogen(s) that doesn't normally cause disease in healthy individuals.

opsonins an antibody in the blood stream which enhances phagacytosis of the infecting bacterium by attaching to it.

optochin a shorthand term for ethylhydrocupreine hydrochloride, a chemical that inhibits the growth of most strains of *Streptococcus pneumoniae* but not other α-haemolytic streptococci.

orbital cellulitis infection of orbital tissue

otitis externa infection of the outer ear; often called 'swimmer's ear'.

otitis media inflammation of the inner ear.

ovaritis inflammation of the ovaries.

oxidase shorthand for cytochrome oxidase which oxidizes compounds and therefore utilizes oxygen with an electron transfer chain.

pandemic an epidemic that occurs over a wide geographical area such as a region or even worldwide.

pan-genome the combined genomic content possessed by members of a species.

parasite an organism which lives on or in an organism of another species from which it derives nutrients which aids its survival.

parasitology the study of parasites,

paratope the part of the antibody which attaches to the antigen.

passage the subculture of cells from one culture vessel to another.

pathogen an organism that has the ability to grow in the human and animal body and initiate disease.

pathogenicity the ability to cause disease.

pathogenicity island a DNA region acquired in the pan-genome by horizontal gene transfer that is particularly related to pathogenesis and virulence.

pathotype a subset of a species that produces pathology via a distinct mechanism.

pattern recognition receptors triggers of innate immunity that recognise MAMPs.

pelvic inflammatory disease describes any infection in the lower female reproductive tract that spreads to the upper female reproductive tract.

peptidase a hydrolase enzyme that hydrolyses a peptide bond, e.g. linking amino acids.

peptidoglycan a polymer found in bacterial cell walls. It is composed of polysaccharide and peptide chains to make a strong structure. Target for antibiotics, especially of the β-lactam type.

peptones a protein derivative which is produced upon partial hydrolysis of a protein.

pericarditis inflammation of the pericardium (the fibrous sac surrounding the heart).

perineum the area between the anus and the vagina.

peristalsis the rhythmic, wavelike motion of the walls of the alimentary canal. These motions move the contents of the alimentary canal onwards.

pernasal swab a thin flexible swab that passes through the nose to the back of the throat, often used to diagnose whooping cough.

personal protective equipment equipment that creates a physical barrier between a worker and potential hazards; in its simplest form this could be a laboratory coat.

Peyer's patches oval elevated patches of closely packed lymph follicles on the mucosa of the small intestines.

phagocytosis the cellular process of engulfing solid particles such as bacteria.

pharmacodynamics the study of the biochemical and physiological effects of drugs and the mechanisms of their actions.

pharyngitis inflammation of the throat or pharynx.

phenol formerly carbolic acid. Acts like a detergent; it reduces the hydrophobic effect of lipids, enabling the dye to penetrate the cell wall.

phenotype a typical characteristic of an organism. This could be seen as its colonial appearance or biochemical properties. Atypical *E. coli*, for example, may show different biochemical properties but it is still an *E. coli*.

phosphatase an enzyme that removes a phosphate group from its substrate.

photophobia a dislike of bright lights.

pigbel a fatal type of food poisoning caused by a specific type of *C. perfringens* toxin (β-toxin).

pleural effusion fluid that accumulates in the pleural cavity.

pleural fluid the fluid between the two layers of pleura.

point of care testing (POCT) these are tests that can be done at the point of care, for example the GP surgery, the outpatient clinic, on the ward or even in the patient's own home. It is often used as a rapid assay to help immediate management and to decide which patients need further laboratory work up.

polymerase chain reaction (PCR) a technique involving amplification of specific DNA sequences which can be used to rapidly identify pathogens.

polymicrobial bacteraemia bacteraemia where two or more significant organisms are isolated.

pouch of Douglas the extension of the peritoneal cavity situated between the uterus and rectum.

primary culture any culture derived from cells, tissues or organs taken directly from an organism.

primary culture plates those plates onto which the clinical samples are directly inoculated. Organisms from primary plates can be inoculated onto further plates; these secondary plates are called subcultures.

productive cough this results in the expectoration of sputum.

prokaryotic an organism (bacteria and cyanobacteria) characterized by the lack of a distinct, membrane-bound nucleus or membrane-bound organelles. Also characterized by the fact that the DNA is not organized into chromosomes.

prophage the integrated bacteriophage genome of a lysogen.

prophylaxis the administration of a treatment to prevent disease developing.

prosthesis a mechanical or electronic device placed in or on the patient's body to help it function, e.g. artificial knees and hips, and pacemakers.

proteoglycan a heavily glycosylated protein often featuring glycosaminoglycans.

proteolytic describes the action of protein digestion by microbial enzymes such as proteases.

prothrombin glycoprotein precursor of thrombin that is produced in the liver and is necessary for the coagulation of blood.

protozoa small single cell or acellular organisms (generally parasites) that are usually found in soil or water.

prozone the phenomenon exhibited by some sera, in which agglutination or precipitation occurs at higher dilution ranges but is not visible at lower dilutions or when undiluted.

pruritis ani irritation of the skin of the anus causing patients to scratch.

pseudomembranous colitis an infection of the colon, the symptoms of which are severe diarrhoea, abdominal pain and fever. The disease can often be fatal, particularly in elderly patients.

puerperal sepsis also known as childbed fever. Infection of the female reproductive system following childbirth or abortion.

PUO pyrexia of unknown origin – increase in a patients temperature but no obvious cause can be found.

purpuric rash the appearance of red or purple discolorations on the skin, caused by bleeding underneath the skin.

purulent containing a lot of pus.

pus a discharge made up of white cells and fluid which is present in infected wounds.

pyelonephritis an infection of the kidney, which is a complication of urine infection.

pyrexial spike a transient increase in the patient's body temperature.

quinolones a group of antibiotics containing nalidixic acid. The newer agents such as ciprofloxacin are known as fluoroquinolones because of a fluorine atom added to the quinolone nucleus. They are generally well tolerated by the patient and display a broad spectrum of activity.

radiolabelled the tagging of a compound with a radioisotope.

rapid-growing mycobacteria mycobacteria that produce colonies within 7 days.

redox potential this is measured in volts under standardized conditions and expresses the propensity of a chemical to acquire electrons and thereby be reduced or release electrons and undergo oxidation. A lower redox potential will favour reduction and vice versa.

resident organisms (also known as normal flora or commensals) organisms deeply seated within the epidermis in skin crevices, hair follicles, sebaceous glands, and beneath fingernails. Their purpose is protecting the skin against colonization by transient organisms. They are not readily removed by hand washing.

ribosomes round particles composed of RNA and protein found in the cytoplasm of living cells. These structures serve as the site of assembly for polypeptides.

ribotyping the process of 'fingerprinting' an organism by detection of specific genomic DNA.

ringworm the common name for fungal infections of the skin and hair.

salpingitis inflammation of the fallopian tubes; can be acute or chronic.

saponin compounds found generally in plants which have a detergent-like action.

satellitism growth of *H. influenzae* on blood agar around colonies of other organisms producing V factor, e.g. *S. aureus*.

search and destroy a programme of screening all individuals on admission and discharge from hospital for the presence of MRSA.

selective media culture media that contain growth inhibitors (often antibiotics) to preclude the growth of unwanted commensal bacteria and facilitate the isolation of target pathogens.

senescence cells which are metabolicaly still active but no longer capable of cell division.

sensitivity that proportion of true positives which the test correctly identifies, calculated as the number of true-positive results divided by the number of true-positive and false-negative results.

septicaemia an infection of the bloodstream caused by toxic microorganisms.

seroconversion the development of detectable specific antibodies to viruses in a patient's serum as a result of infection or vaccination.

serogroup a grouping of microorganisms based on cell surface antigens.

skin antisepsis preparing the skin with disinfectant to remove bacteria before a blood sample is taken.

slow-growing mycobacteria colonies of mycobacteria that take longer than 7 days to appear.

Southern blot a method used to check for the presence of a DNA sequence in a sample. Southern blotting combines agarose gel electrophoresis for size separation of DNA with methods to transfer the size-separated DNA to a filter membrane for probe hybridization.

specificity the probability that an individual who does not have the particular disease being tested for will be correctly identified as negative, expressed as the proportion of true-negative results to the total of true-negative and false-positive results.

splenectomy removal of the spleen.

sporicidal a substance or preparation which will kill bacterial and fungal spores.

staphylocoagulase a protein secreted by some staphylococci. It activates prothrombin to cause the conversion of flbrinogen to fibrin, thus stimulating coagulation or clotting.

stationary phase the period after the end of the exponential growth phase where the number of bacteria in culture remains relatively constant for a period of time.

sterile pyuria pus or lots of white blood cells in the urine but no infectious cause detected.

sterilization the process which destroys all forms of microbial life.

stringency the molecular reaction conditions which are required for the annealing of single stranded DNA for example.

subarachnoid haemorrhage bleeding into the area between the pia mater and the arachnoid membrane around the brain.

subculture the transplantation of cells from one culture vessel to another.

superantigens a bacterial or viral antigen that have a powerful effcect in the body by activating T-cells resulting in cytokine release and system wide inflammation.

superficial fascia the soft tissue part of the connective tissue.

superoxide a compound containing the highly reactive superoxide ion O_{2-}, an important killing mechanism generated in the lysosomes of phagocytes.

synergy testing tests to determine if antibiotic combinations would have an additive, indifferent or antagonistic effect.

synthetic substrate designed for detection of enzymes and not usually occurring in nature, synthetic substrates link sugars, fatty acids or amino acids to indicator molecules such as coloured or fluorescent dyes that are released to indicate enzyme activity.

syphilis a sexually transmitted disease caused by the bacterium *Treponema pallidum*.

systemic relating to the entire body e.g. systemic infection.

tachyzoite a rapidly multiplying stage in development of the tissue phase of *T. gondii* infection.

tegument protective outer body covering of the flatworms that has both secretive and absorptive functions.

therapeutic index the ratio between the toxic dose and the therapeutic dose of a drug, used as a measure of the relative safety of the drug for a particular treatment. A drug with little difference between toxic and therapeutic doses is referred to as having a narrow therapeutic index.

thermocycler a piece of laboratory apparatus most commonly used to amplify segments of DNA in PCR. The device has a *thermal block* with holes where tubes holding the reaction mixtures can be inserted. The cycler then raises and lowers the temperature of the block in discrete, pre-programmed steps.

thermonuclease a nuclease is an enzyme capable of cleaving the phosphodiester bonds between the nucleotide subunits of nucleic acids. Staphylococci, and some other species, produce a thermonuclease capable of withstanding heat (e.g. 100°C).

thrombosis the formation of a clot or clots in a blood vessel which can be very serious e.g deep vein thrombosis DVT.

time to positivity the time taken from when a blood culture bottle is inoculated to when it is identified as being positive.

tinea the name given to a fungal infection of the body; it is usually followed by a term to describe the body site, e.g. tinea capitis.

tissue tropism a preference or selectivity of colonization displayed by a pathogen for a particular tissue.

toxic shock syndrome a serious, often life-threatening syndrome caused by bacterial toxins, commonly from *S. aureus* or *S. pyogenes*.

toxin a virulence factor whose primary function is related to disrupting cellular physiology or damaging cellular integrity.

transient colonization colonization by a microorganism that occurs for a short time only.

transmissible plasmids small, circular molecules of DNA that are separate from the bacterial chromosome. These can be transferred between bacteria and may carry resistance genes.

traumatic tap where a capillary or blood vessel is 'nicked' when a CSF sample is taken. Samples become blood stained. Serial samples can help identify whether the blood is due to a traumatic tap.

trematodes a collective term for some parasitic worms such as *Paragonimus*. These worms commonly exist in contaminated water supplies and cause human infection.

Triton X a non-ionic detergent used to lyse cells.

trophozoite the active feeding stage of a protozoal parasite, as distinct from its encysted stage typically seen in *G. lamblia*.

tuberculin skin test involves the subcutaneous inoculation of a purified protein derivative of MTB.

undulate bacterial colonies which have a wavy outline or appearance.

urea produced by the liver and excreted in the kidney, it is the means by which the body removes potentially toxic ammonia, a breakdown product of proteins.

urease a hydrolase that decomposes urea to form water and ammonia.

urethral syndrome patient experiences symptoms of a UTI but significant bacteriuria is not detected.

uropathogens organisms that can infect the urinary tract.

urticaria skin rash characterized pale red, raised, itchy bumps; often associated with an allergic response.

vaccination the administration of material (an antigen) to produce immunity to a disease, usually by production of antibodies.

venepuncture taking blood via a needle placed into a vein.

vesicle a small, clear blister-like eruption on the skin that eventually ruptures, ulcerates, crusts over, and heals without scarring unless it becomes infected with a bacterial pathogen.

vesicoureteric reflux failure of the one-way valve mechanism that usually prevents bladder urine flowing back in to the ureter.

Vincent's angina a polymicrobial infection of the gums which leads to their necrosis.

viraemia presence of viruses in the bloodstream.

virucidal a substance capable of killing or neutralizing a virus.

virulence the ability of an organism to produce disease; highly virulent organisms are able to produce disease easily.

Wood's light a long-wave ultraviolet light used as a diagnostic tool by dermatologists to distinguish dermatophyte infections from other causes of scalp irritation and hair loss.

xanthochromia the yellow coloration of CSF samples caused by lysed blood.

Ziehl-Neelsen (ZN) used to stain mycobacteria using fuchsin combined with phenol. Malachite green is used as a counter stain. In modified form can be used to stain some intestinal parasites.

zoonosis a disease that normally exists in animals but can be transmitted to humans.

References

Chapter 2

Barrow GI, Feltham RKA, eds. *Cowan and Steel's Manual for the Identification of Medical Bacteria*, 3rd edition. Cambridge University Press, 2004.

Bascomb S. Enzyme tests in bacterial identification. In: Colwell RR, Grigorova R, eds. *Methods in Microbiology*, Vol. 19, pp. 105–160. Academic Press, 1987.

Collier L, Balows A, Sussman M, eds. *Topley and Wilson's Microbiology and Microbial Infections*, 9th edition. Arnold, 1998.

Collins CH, Lyne PM, Grange JM, Falkinham JO, eds. *Collins and Lyne's Microbiological Methods*, 8th edition. Arnold, 2004.

Isenberg HD, ed. *Clinical Microbiology Procedures Handbook*, 3rd edition. American Society for Microbiology, 2010.

Manafi M, Kneifel W, Bascomb S. Fluorogenic and chromogenic substrates used in bacterial diagnostics. *Microbiology and Molecular Biology Reviews* 1991; **55**: 335–348.

Perry JD, Ford M, Hjersing N, Gould FK. Rapid conventional scheme for biochemical identification of antibiotic resistant *Enterobacteriaceae* isolates from urine. *Journal of Clinical Pathology* 1988; **41**: 1010–1012.

Chapter 3

Barrow GI, Feltham RKA, eds. *Cowan and Steel's Manual for the Identification of Medical Bacteria*, 3rd edition. Cambridge University Press, 2004.

Collier L, Balows A, Sussman M, eds. *Topley and Wilson's Microbiology and Microbial Infections*, 9th edition. Arnold, 1998.

Difco Laboratories. *Difco Manual: Dehydrated Culture Media and Reagents for Microbiology*. 1953.

Madigan M, Martinko J, eds. *Brock Biology of Microorganisms*, 13th edition. Prentice Hall, 2011.

Snell JJS, Brown DFJ, Roberts C, eds. *Quality Assurance: Principles and Practice in the Microbiology Laboratory*. Public Health Laboratory Service, 1999.

Chapter 4

Andrews J, Brenwald N, Brown DFJ, Perry J, King A, Gemmell C. Evaluation of a 10 µg cefoxitin disc for the detection of methicillin resistance in *Staphylococcus aureus* by BSAC methodology. *Journal of Antimicrobial Chemotherapy* 2005; **56**: 599–600.

Andrews JM, Brown DFJ, Wise R. A survey of antimicrobial susceptibility testing in the United Kingdom. *Journal of Antimicrobial Chemotherapy* 1996; **37**: 187–204.

Andrews JM. Determination of minimum inhibitory concentrations. *Journal of Antimicrobial Chemotherapy* 2001; **48** (Suppl. 1): 5–16.

Andrews JM. The development of the BSAC standardized method of disc diffusion testing. *Journal of Antimicrobial Chemotherapy* 2001; **48** (Suppl.1): 29–42.

Andrews JM. BSAC standardized disc susceptibility testing method (version 6). *Journal of Antimicrobial Chemotherapy* 2007; **60**: 20–41.

Berenbaum MC. A method for testing for synergy with any number of agents. *Journal of Infectious Diseases* 1978; **137**: 122–130.

Berenbaum MC. Correlation between methods for measurement of synergy. *Journal of Infectious Diseases* 1980; **142**: 476–480.

Ericsson H, Sherris JC. Antibiotic sensitivity testing. Report of an International Collaborative study. *Acta Pathologica et Microbiologica Scandinavica Section B* 1971; **217** (Suppl.): 1–90.

Hakanen AJ, Linggren M, Huovinen P, Jala J, Kotilainen P. New quinolone resistance phenomenon in *Salmonella enterica* nalidixic acid-susceptible isolates with reduced fluoroquinolone susceptibility. *Journal of Clinical Microbiology* 2005; **43**: 5775–5778.

Hoffner SE, Svenson SB, Kallenius G. Synergistic effects of antimycobacterial drug combinations of *Mycobacterium avium* complex determined radiometrically in liquid medium. *European Journal of Clinical Microbiology* 1987; **6**: 530–555.

Lang BJ, Aaron SD, Ferris W, Herbert PC, MacDonald NE. Multiple combination bactericidal antibiotic testing for patients with cystic fibrosis infected with multiresistant strains of *Pseudomonas aeruginosa*. *American Journal of Respiratory and Critical Care Medicine* 2000; **162**: 2241–2245.

Louie L, Matsumura SO, Choi E, *et al. Performance Standards for Antimicrobial Susceptibility Testing*; Fifteenth Informational Supplement, M100-S15, Vol. 25. Clinical and Laboratory Standards Institute, 2005.

MacGowan AP, Wise R. Establishing MIC breakpoints and the interpretation of in vitro susceptibility tests. *Journal of Antimicrobial Chemotherapy* 2001; **48** (Suppl. 1): 17–28.

MacGowan AR, Bowker K, Bedford KA, Holt HA, Reeves DS. Synergy testing of macrolide combinations using the chequerboard technique. *Journal of Antimicrobial Chemotherapy* 1993; **32**: 913–915.

Metzler CM, DeHaan RM. Susceptibility tests of anaerobic bacteria: statistical and clinical considerations. *Journal of Infectious Diseases* 1974; **130**: 588–594.

Muller-Serieys C, Andrews J, Vacheron F, Cantalloube C. Tissue kinetics of Telithromycin, the first ketolide antibacterial. *Journal of Antimicrobial Chemotherapy* 2004; **53**: 149–157.

Olsson-Liljequist B, Larsson P, Walder M, Miörner H. Antimicrobial susceptibility testing in Sweden. *Scandinavian Journal of Infectious Diseases* 1997; **105** (Suppl.): 3.

Ragunathan PL, Ison C, Livermore DM. Nalidixic acid-susceptible, ciprofloxacin-resistant *Neisseria gonorrhoeae* strain in the UK. *Journal of Antimicrobial Chemotherapy* 2005; **56**: 437.

Nightingale CH, Murakawa T, Ambrose PG, Drusano GL, eds. *Antimicrobial Pharmacodymanics in Theory and Clinical Practice*, 2nd edition. Marcel Dekker, 2007.

Ragunathan PL, Ison C, Livermore DM. *Methods for Antimicrobial Susceptibility Testing of Anaerobic Bacteria; Approved Standard*, 4th edition, M11-A4, Vol. 17, No. 22. Clinical and Laboratory Standards Institute, 1997.

Comité de l'Antibiogramme de la Société Français de Microbiologie. Technical Recommendations for in vitro susceptibility testing. *Clinical Microbiology and Infectious Diseases* 1996; **2** (Suppl. 1): S11–S25.

Snell JJS, Brown DFJ, Perry SF, George R. Antimicrobial susceptibility testing of enterococci: results of a survey conducted by the United Kingdom National External Quality Assessment Scheme for Microbiology. *Journal of Antimicrobial Chemotherapy* 1993; **32**: 401–412.

Working Party on Antibiotic Sensitivity Testing of the British Society for Antimicrobial Chemotherapy. A guide to sensitivity testing. *Journal of Antimicrobial Chemotherapy* 1991; **27** (Suppl. D): 1–50.

Yeo SF, Livermore DM. Effect of inoculum size on the in-vitro susceptibility to beta-lactam antibiotics of *M. catarrhalis* isolates of different beta-lactamase types. *Journal of Medical Microbiology* 1994; **40**: 252–255.

Chapter 5

Elliott TSJ, Foweraker J, Gould FK, Perry JD, Sandoe JAT. Guidelines for the antibiotic treatment of endocarditis in adults: report of the Working Party of the British Society for Antimicrobial Chemotherapy. *Journal of Antimicrobial Chemotherapy* 2004; **54**: 971–981.

Finch RG, Greenwood D, Norrby SR, *et al.* eds. *Antibiotic and Chemotherapy: Anti-Infective Agents and Their Use in Therapy*, 8th edition. Churchill Livingstone, 2003.

Freeman R, Gould FK. *Infection in Cardiothoracic Intensive Care*. Hodder Arnold, 1987.

Shanson DC. *Sepicaemia and Endocarditis: Clinical and Microbiological Aspects*. Oxford University Press, 1990.

Standards Unit, Evaluations and Standards Laboratory, Centre for Infections. *Investigation of Blood Cultures (for Organisms other than Mycobacterium Species)*, BSOP 37, 2005.

Chapter 6

Fallon D, Ackland G, Andrews N, Frodsham D, Howe S, Howells K, Nye KJ, Warren RE. A comparison of the performance of commercially available chromogenic agars for the isolation and presumptive identification of organism from the urine. *Journal of Clinical Pathology* 2003; **56**: 608–612.

Graham JC, Galloway A. The laboratory diagnosis of urinary tract infection. *Journal of Clinical Pathology* 2001; **54**: 911–919.

Leigh DA, Williams JD. Method for detection of significant bacteriuria in large groups of patients. *Journal of Clinical Pathology* 1964; **17**: 498–503.

National Institute for Health and Care Excellence. *UTI in Children: Urinary Tract Infection in Children: Diagnosis, Treatment and Long-term Management*, 2007. Available at www.nice.org.uk/nicemedia/pdf/CG54NICEguideline.pdf (accessed 14 August, 2013).

Smyth M, Moore JE, McClurg RB, Goldsmith CE. Quantitative colorimetric measurement of residual antimicrobials in the urine of patients with suspected urinary tract infection. *British Journal of Biomedical Science* 2005; **62**: 114–119.

Chapter 7

Beers MH, Robert Berkow R. *The Merck Manual of Diagnosis and Therapy*, 19th edition. John Wiley & Sons, Inc., 2011.

Hay PE, Morgan DJ, Ison CA, *et al.* A longitudinal study of bacterial vaginosis during pregnancy. *British Journal of Obstetrics and Gynaecology* 1994; **101**: 1048–1053.

Health Protection Agency/Public Health England. *Investigation of Genital Tract and Associated Specimens*. BSOP 28. National Standard Method. www.hpa.org.uk/ProductsServices/MicrobiologyPathology/UKStandardsForMicrobiology Investigations/TermsOfUseForSMIs/AccessToUKSMIs/SMIBacteriology/smiB28InvestigationofGenitalTractand Associated/ (accessed 14 August, 2013) Currently under review.

Health Protection Agency. *Investigation of Skin, Superficial, and Non-surgical Wound Swabs*. BSOP 11. National Standard Method. www.hpa.org.uk/ProductsServices/Microbiology Pathology/UKStandardsForMicrobiologyInvestigations/TermsOfUseForSMIs/AccessToUKSMIs/SMIBacteriology/smiB11InvestigationofSkinSuperficialandNonSurgic/ (accessed 14 August, 2013).

Holmes KK, Sparling PF, Stamm WE, *et al. Sexually Transmitted Diseases*, 4th edition. McGraw-Hill Medical, 2008.

Nugent RP, Krohn MA, Hillier SL. Reliability of diagnosing bacterial vaginosis is improved by a standardised method of Gram stain interpretation. *Journal of Clinical Microbiology* 1991; **29**: 297–301.

Rogstad K ed. *ABC of Sexually Transmitted Infections*, 6th edition. Wiley-Blackwell, 2011.

Chapter 8

Bain BJ. *Blood Cells – A Practical Guide*, 4th edition. Blackwell Publishing, 2006.

Finch RG, Greenwood D, Norrby SR, *et al. Antibiotic and Chemotherapy: Anti-Infective Agents and their Use in Therapy*, 8th edition. Springer, 2004.

Merck online manual. www.merck.com/mmhe/index.html (accessed 14 August, 2013).

Standards Unit, Evaluations and Standards Laboratory, Centre for Infections. *Investigation of Fluids from Normally Sterile Sites*. National Standard Method BSOP 26.

Standards Unit, Evaluations and Standards Laboratory, Centre for Infections. *Investigation of Continuous Peritoneal Dialysis Fluids*. National Standard Method BSOP 25.

Standards Unit, Evaluations and Standards Laboratory. Centre for Infections. *Investigation of Cerebrospinal Fluid*. National Standard Method BSOP 27.

Tunkel A. *Bacterial Meningitis*. Lippincott Williams and Wilkins, 2001.

Chapter 9

BTS Pneumonia Guideline Committee. *BTS Guidelines for the Management of Community Acquired Pneumonia in Adults – 2004 update*. www.brit-thoracic.org.uk/Portals/0/Guidelines/Pneumonia/MACAP2001gline.pdf (accessed 14 August, 2013).

Cystic Fibrosis Trust. *Antibiotic Treatment for Cystic Fibrosis*, 3rd edition 2009. www.cysticfibrosis.org.uk/media/82010/CD_Antibiotic_treatment_for_CF_May_09.pdf (accessed 14 August, 2013).

Drake R, Vogl W, Mitchell A. *Gray's Anatomy for Students*, 2nd edition. Churchill Livingstone, 2009.

Goering R, Dockrell H, Zuckerman M, Roitt I. *Mims' Medical Microbiology*, 5th edition. Mosby, 2012.

Ratledge C, Dale JW. *Mycobacteria*. Wiley Blackwell, 1999.

Versalovic J, Carroll KC, Jorgensen JH, *et al. Manual of Clinical Microbiology*, 10th edition. American Society for Microbiology, 2011.

Chapter 10

Ash LR, Orihel TC. *Atlas of Human Parasitology*, 5th edition. ASM Press, 2007.

Collier L, Balows A, Sussman M, eds. *Topley and Wilson's Microbiology and Microbial Infections*, 9th edition. Arnold Publication, 1998.

Garcia LS. *Diagnostic Medical Parasitology*, 5th edition. ASM Press, 2007.

Mims C, Nash A, Stephen J. *Mims' Pathogenesis of Infectious Disease*, 5th edition. Academic Press, 2000.

Standards Unit, Evaluations and Standards Laboratory, Centre for Infections. *Investigation of Faecal Specimens for Bacterial Pathogens*. National Standard Method BSOP 30. www.hemltd.ru/publications/sections/Normativ/foreign/samples/medicine/NHS001/article.pdf (accessed 14 August, 2013).

Standards Unit, Evaluations and Standards Laboratory, Centre for Infections. *Investigation of Specimens other than Blood for Parasites*. National Standard Method BSOP 31. www.hpa.org.uk/webc/hpawebfile/hpaweb_c/1317132857407 (accessed 14 August, 2013).

Chapter 11

Audicana MT, Kennedy MW. *Anisakis simplex*: from obscure infectious worm to inducer of immune hypersensitivity. *Clinical Microbiology Reviews* 2008; **21**(2): 360–379.

Doyle E. *Foodborne Parasites: A Review of the Scientific Literature*. FRI Briefings 2003. http://fri.wisc.edu/docs/pdf/parasites.pdf (accessed 14 August, 2013).

Murray PR, Rosenthal KS, Pfaller MA. *Medical Microbiology*, 6th edition. Mosby, 2009.

Winn W, Allen S, Janda W, Koneman E, Procop G, Schreckeberger P, Woods G. *Koneman's Colour Atlas and Textbook of Diagnostic Microbiology*, 6th edition. Lippincott Williams and Wilkins, 2006.

Chapter 12

Care Quality Commission. Several publications from the Commission and previous bodies on health-care-acquired infection. www.cqc.org.uk.

Casewell M, Philpott-Howard J. *Hospital Infection Control. Policies and Practical Procedures*. W.B. Saunders, 1994.

Centre for Evidence Based Purchasing, NHS. *Evaluation Report: Clostridium difficile Toxin Detection Assays*. CEP08054, 2009.

Conterno LO, *et al.* Real-time polymerase chain reaction detection of methicillin-resistant *Staphylococcus aureus*: impact on nosocomial transmission and costs. *Infection Control and Hospital Epidemiology* 2007; **28**: 1134–1141.

Department of Health, Chief Medical Officer. *Winning Ways: Working Together to Reduce Health Care Infection*, 2003. http://webarchive.nationalarchives.gov.uk/20130107105354/http://www.dh.gov.uk/prod_consum_dh/groups/dh_digitalassets/@dh/@en/documents/digitalasset/dh_4064689.pdf (accessed 14 August, 2013).

Department of Health. HTM 07-01. *Safe Management of Healthcare Waste*, 2006. www.gov.uk/government/publications/guidance-on-the-safe-management-of-healthcare-waste (accessed 14 August, 2013).

Kuijper EJ, Coignard B, Tüll P, *et al.* Emergence of *Clostridium difficile*-associated disease in North America and Europe. *Clinical Microbiology and Infection* 2006; **12** (Suppl. 6): 2–18.

National Audit Office. Health-care-acquired infection audits. www.nao.org.uk.

Planche T, Aghaizu A, Holliman R, Riley P, Poloniecki J, Breathnach A, Krishna S. Diagnosis of *Clostridium difficile* infection by toxin detection kits: a systematic review. *Lancet Infectious Diseases* 2008; **8**: 777–784.

Standards Unit, Evaluations and Standards Laboratory, Centre for Infections. *Investigation of Specimens for Screening for MRSA.* National Standard Method B29. www.hpa.org.uk/ ProductsServices/MicrobiologyPathology/UKStandards ForMicrobiologyInvestigations/TermsOfUseForSMIs/ AccessToUKSMIs/SMIBacteriology/smiB29Investigation ofSpecimensforScreeningforMRSA/ (accessed 14 August, 2013), Currently under review.

Standards Unit, Evaluations and Standards Laboratory, Centre for Infections. *MRSA Select Culture Medium.* National Standard Method MSOP 30. www.hpa.org.uk/webc/ HPAwebFile/HPAweb_C/1194947389820 (accessed 14 August, 2013).

Standards Unit, Evaluations and Standards Laboratory, Centre for Infections. *Processing of Faeces for Clostridium difficile.* National Standard Method BSOP10. www.hpa.org.uk/webc/ hpawebfile/hpaweb_c/1317132856426 (accessed 14 August, 2013).

Chapter 13

Desselberger U. *Medical Virology – A Practical Approach.* IRL Press, 1995.

Jerome KR. *Lennette's Laboratory Diagnosis of Viral Infections,* 4th edition. Informa Healthcare, 2010.

Mahy BWJ, Collier L, eds. *Topley and Wilson's Microbiology and Microbial Infections,* Vol. 1 Virology, 9th edition. Arnold, 1998.

Schachter J, Stamm WE. *Chlamydia.* In: Murray PR ed. *Manual of Clinical Microbiology,* 7th edition, pp. 795–806. ASM Press, 1999.

White DO, Fenner FJ. *Medical Virology,* 4th edition. Academic Press, 1994.

Zuckerman AJ *et al. Principles and Practice of Clinical Virology,* 6th edition. Wiley, 2009.

Chapter 14

Anaissie EJ, McGinnis MR, Pfaller MA. *Clinical Mycology,* 2nd edition. Churchill Livingstone, 2009.

Bancroft D, Gamble M. *Theory and Practice of Histological Techniques,* 6th edition. Churchill Livingstone, 2007.

Dr Fungus. Website available at: www.doctorfungus.org (accessed 14 August, 2013).

Kibbler CC, Mackenzie DWR, Odds FC, eds. *Principles and Practice of Clinical Mycology.* Wiley Blackwell, 1996.

Stevens DA. Diagnosis of fungal infections: current status. *Journal of Antimicrobial Chemotherapy* 2002; **49** (Suppl S1): 11–19.

Chapter 15

Bowden MG, Heuck AP, Ponnuraj K, *et al.* Evidence for the 'dock, lock, and latch' ligand binding mechanism of the staphylococcal microbial surface component recognizing adhesive matrix molecules (MSCRAMM) SdrG. *Journal of Biological Chemistry* 2008; **283**(1): 638–647.

Brady MJ, Campellone KG, Ghildiyal M, Leong JM. Enterohaemorrhagic and enteropathogenic *Escherichia coli* Tir proteins trigger a common Nck-independent actin assembly pathway. *Cell Microbiology* 2007; **9**(9): 2242–2253.

Fliegauf M, Sonnen AF, Kremer B, Henneke P. Mucociliary clearance defects in a murine in vitro model of pneumococcal airway infection. *PLoS One* 2013; **8**(3): e59925. doi: 10.1371/ journal.pone.0059925.

Hupp S, Förtsch C, Wippel C, Ma J, Mitchell TJ, Iliev AI. Direct transmembrane interaction between actin and the pore-competent, cholesterol-dependent cytolysin pneumolysin. *Journal of Molecular biology* 2013; **425**(3): 636–646.

Koretke KK, Szczesny P, Gruber M, Lupas AN. Model structure of the prototypical non-fimbrial adhesin YadA of *Yersinia enterocolitica. Journal of Structural Biology* 2006; **155**(2): 154–161.

Pentecost M, Otto G, Theriot JA, Amieva MR. *Listeria monocytogenes* invades the epithelial junctions at sites of cell extrusion. *PLoS Pathogens* 2006; **2**(1): e3. doi:10.1371/ journal.ppat.0020003.

Wong AR, Raymond B, Collins JW, Crepin VF, Frankel G. The enteropathogenic *E. coli* effector EspH promotes actin pedestal formation and elongation via WASP-interacting protein (WIP). *Cell Microbiology* 2012; **14**(7): 1051–1070.

Chapter 16

Desselberger U. *Medical Virology – A Practical Approach.* IRL Press, 1995.

Lennette EH, Smith TF. *Laboratory Diagnosis of Viral Infections,* 3rd edition. Marcel Dekker, 1999.

Mahy BWJ, Collier L, eds. *Topley and Wilson's Microbiology and Microbial Infections,* Vol. 1 Virology, 9th edition. Arnold, 1998.

Maurin M. Real-time PCR as a diagnostic tool for bacterial diseases. *Expert Review of Molecular Diagnostics.* 2012; **12**(7): 731–54.

Rampini SK, Bloemberg G, Keller P, *et al.* Broad-range 16S rRNA gene polymerase chain reaction for diagnosis of culture-negative bacterial infections. *Clinical Infectious Diseases.* 2011; **53**(12): 1245–51.

White DO, Fenner FJ. *Medical Virology,* 4th edition. Academic Press, 1994.

Zuckerman AJ *et al. Principles and Practice of Clinical Virology,* 4th edition. Wiley, 1999.

Chapter 17

Advisory Committee on Dangerous Pathogens. *Biological Agents: Managing the Risks in Laboratories and Healthcare Premises*. Health and Safety Executive, 2005.

Advisory Committee on Dangerous Pathogens. *Categorisation of Biological Agents According to Hazard and Categories of Containment*, 4th edition. HSE Books, 1995.

Carriage of Dangerous Goods (Classification, Packaging and Labelling) and Use of Transportable Pressure Receptacles Regulations 2004, SI No 568. The Stationery Office, 2004.

Church D. The seven principles of accurate microbiology specimen collection. *Microbiology Newsletter*, Calgary Laboratory Services. Vol. 6, 2005.

Clinical Practice Committee, Great Ormond Street Hospital for Children. *Microbiological Specimen Collection*, version 2.0, 2006.

Control of Substances Hazardous to Health Regulations 2002. The Stationery Office, 2002.

Evans EGV, Richardson MD, eds. *Medical Mycology. A Practical Approach*. Oxford University Press, 1989.

Gilchrist B. Wound infection – sampling bacterial flora: a review of the literature. *Journal of Wound Care* 1996; **5**: 386–388.

Health and Safety Executive. *Biological Agents: Managing the Risks in Laboratories and Healthcare Premises*. The Stationery Office, 2005.

Higgins C. An introduction to the examination of specimens. *Nursing Times* 1994; **90**: 29–32.

Isenberg HD, ed. *Clinical Microbiology Procedures Handbook*, Vol 1. American Society for Microbiology, 1992.

Garcia LS. *Diagnostic Medical Parasitology*, 5th edition. ASM Press, 2007.

Miller MJ. *A Guide to Specimen Management in Clinical Microbiology*. American Society for Microbiology, 1999.

Richardson MD, Warnock DW. *Fungal Infections. Diagnosis and Management* 4th edition. Blackwell Scientific Publications, 2012.

Standards Unit, Evaluations and Standards Laboratory, Centre for Infections. *Inoculation of Culture Media*. QSOP 52. Issue date 2007.

Standards Unit, Evaluations and Standards Laboratory, Centre for Infections. *Investigation of Blood Cultures (for Organisms other than Mycobacterium Species)*, BSOP 37, 2005.

Weinbaum FI. Doing it right first time: quality improvement and the contaminant blood culture. *Journal of Clinical Microbiology* 1997; **35**: 563–565.

Index